The Malalignment Syndrome
Implications for Medicine and Sport

To Alison, 'My Fair Lady', always
                                        WS

For Churchill Livingstone:

Editorial Director, Health Professions: Mary Law
Project Manager: Derek Robertson
Design Direction: Judith Wright

The Malalignment Syndrome

Implications for Medicine and Sport

Wolf Schamberger

Clinical Associate Professor, Department of Medicine, Division of Physical Medicine and Rehabilitation, and The Allan McGavin Sports Medicine Centre, University of British Columbia, Vancouver, Canada

With contributions by

Fredric T. Samorodin RPT BSR MCPA
(Chapter 8: Treatment: The Manual Therapy Modes)

Cynthia Webster BSR PhD(C) RPT
(Chapter 6: Horses, Saddles and Riders)

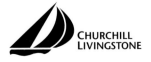
CHURCHILL
LIVINGSTONE

CHURCHILL LIVINGSTONE
An imprint of Elsevier Science Limited

First published 2002

ISBN 0 443 06471 7

British Library Cataloguing in Publication Data
A catalogue record for this book is available from the British Library

Library of Congress Cataloging in Publication Data
A catalog record for this book is available from the Library of
Congress

Note
Medical knowledge is constantly changing. As new information
becomes available, changes in treatment, procedures, equipment and
the use of drugs become necessary. The author, contributors and the
publishers have taken care to ensure that the information given in this
text is accurate and up to date. However, readers are strongly advised
to confirm that the information, especially with regard to drug usage,
complies with the latest legislation and standards of practice.

The
publisher's
policy is to use
**paper manufactured
from sustainable forests**

Printed in China by RDC Group Limited

Contents

v

Preface

Malalignment of the pelvis, spine and extremities remains one of the frontiers in medicine, unrecognized as a cause of over 50% of back and limb pain. The associated biomechanical changes – especially the shift in weight-bearing and the asymmetries of muscle tension, strength and joint ranges of motion – affect soft tissues, joints and organ systems throughout the body and, therefore, have implications for general practice and most medical subspecialty areas. Because of the accentuation of these biomechanical changes with athletic activity, their impact is particularly significant to those practising orthopaedic or sports medicine. Athletes who are out of alignment may have difficulty progressing in their sport and as a result sometimes have to abandon their efforts altogether. Malalignment also puts athletes at increased risk of injury, and once injured, they are likely to take longer to recover, or may even fail to do so at all.

The author describes the more common presentations of malalignment, the signs and symptoms that comprise the 'malalignment syndrome', and a treatment approach that is simple yet effective and proven in clinical practice. Success depends largely on involving the patient or athlete in regular self-assessment to allow for the early recognition of recurrence of malalignment in order to initiate appropriate self-treatment or seek help as quickly as possible. The intent is to create a degree of independence for patients or athletes by opening their eyes and those of the attending doctors, coaches and trainers to the hitherto unrecognized problems relating to malalignment.

Acknowledgements

The author is deeply indebted to the following: The American Association of Orthopaedic Medicine, which, at the inaugural meeting in 1984, planted the kernel of recognition that malalignment is a medical entity in its own right, and for having provided the opportunity to develop that thought through the many workshops at subsequent meetings, both of the AAOM and of its 'offspring', the Canadian Association of Orthopaedic Medicine; Miss Diane Lee, PT, and Drs Vincent Pratt, Duncan Murray, and Ian Murray, who provided the support over the following years to continue working in this area, at a time when the recognition of malalignment-related problems continued to prove a challenge; Miss Cynthia Webster and Mr Fred Samorodin, for having contributed a chapter to the book and for having provided the many opportunities to discuss the contents; Mr Jeff MacDonald-Bain, for steadfastly providing the skills needed to transform ideas into clear-cut, easy to understand yet aesthetic illustrations; members of the Division of Physical Medicine and Rehabilitation, Department of Medicine, Faculty of Medicine, University of British Columbia, for encouragement and the financial support provided for research and other costs; Drs Patrick Foran, Donald Grant, Wolfgang Kliem, Else Larsen, and Dorthea McCallum, for the insight they have given from the chiropractic field; Drs Doug Clement, Donald McKenzie, Rob Lloyd-Smith, Navin Prasad, and Jack Taunton of the Allan McGavin Sports Medicine Clinic at the University of British Columbia, for having provided access to the many athletes presenting with problems relating to malalignment, and for reviewing the manuscript, along with Drs Vincent Pratt and Gulraj Thauli and the staff of the Burnaby Physiotherapy Clinic; Karen Moskal, whose secretarial skills, computer knowledge, and dedication to her work were invaluable; Carol Atkinson, Iona Schamberger, Paul Truelove, Marty Wanless, and in particular Ms Dena Gaertner, for modelling; Roman Sabo, for his help with photography; Sharon Spinder and Neil Bendle, for having assisted with the scientific studies and analysis of the data; Steven and Paul Paris (Paris Orthotics), and Mark McColman and Deborah Mitchell (Kintec Orthotics), for gait analysis on the Amfit TM and Footmaxx TM, respectively; for having reviewed specific sections, contributed information, or helped in other ways – Caitlin Adamson, Margaret Byrne, Sharon Card, Magdy Conyd, Shandra Darby, Graham and Susan Arthur, Laura Harmse, Deirdre and Gary Hetherington, Leigh Holyoak, David Southard and Keith Nichol (Rackets and Runners TM), Sheila Moore, J. J. Rogers, Jodi Russell, Gloria Schellenberg, Hugh Smythe, B. J. Thomas.

My heartfelt thanks go to my family: Alison, Anton, Iona, Adrian and Jodi, without whose encouragement, tolerance, help and understanding this book would never have come about.

Introduction

At one time, I was a national caliber, 2 hours 20 minutes marathon runner. My running career from high school in the 1960s through 39 marathons in the 1970s had been relatively injury free. It was in 1980, following a run on narrow, winding trails, that I first became aware of the right heel pain. There had been no obvious injury, no twisting or unexpected jarring. The pain fluctuated in intensity and could be present both on weight-bearing and at rest. Sometimes there was no pain at all; the pain was most likely to recur with running. There was not even a temporary improvement with standard physiotherapy, anti-inflammatory medication, acupuncture and a lift for a right leg supposedly shorter than the left.

The tendency to pronation was so pronounced on the right side that the heel cup of a racing flat or lighter running shoe would start to collapse noticeably inwards on the right within 3 or 4 weeks (Fig. I.1).

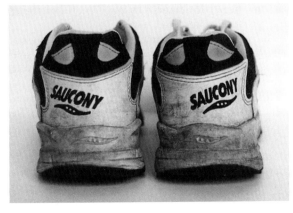

Figure I.1 Heel cup collapse, inwards on the right and outwards on the left running shoe, reflecting a malalignment-related tendency to right pronation and left supination respectively.

Orthotics with a 4 degree medial raise on the right failed to control this marked pronation. An injection of local anaesthetic around the heel did not provide even short-term relief. The pain impaired heel strike and push-off, and with time resulted in noticeable wasting of the entire right leg. With runs of 10 miles or more, the right thigh muscles – particularly the quadriceps – would ache as with overuse, similar to how the leg muscles usually felt just after having completed a marathon.

In 1987, 7 years after the onset of the pain, I attended the annual meeting of the American Association of Orthopedic Medicine in Montreal. One speaker projected a drawing of patterns of pain and/or paraesthesias referred from the sacrotuberous and sacrospinous ligaments, as delineated by Hackett (1958) with hypertonic saline injections (Fig. I.2). It was the circle around the heel that caught my eye – I wondered whether my pain could be on the basis of referral from these more proximal structures. That would explain why the injection around the right heel had failed to affect the pain.

My suspicions were confirmed at a workshop that afternoon. One of the instructors, an osteopath, noted that I was out of alignment: my right innominate bone was rotated anteriorly relative to the sacrum. He proceeded with correction using a gentle muscle energy technique (MET), described in detail in Chapter 7 (Figs 7.8, 7.9). Basically, I lay supine and he offered resistance to my attempts to extend my flexed right thigh. This MET in effect reversed the origin and insertion of the right gluteus maximus, resulting in posterior traction and rotation of the right innominate.

The manoeuvre, simple as it may seem, was successful; better still, my heel pain disappeared immediately on realignment. However, on stepping back into my shoes I felt awkward: the right side of my pelvis now seemed higher than the left. Then I remembered

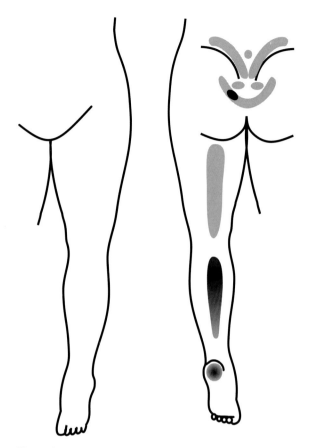

Figure I.2 Referred pain – sacrospinus and sacrotuberous ligaments (sacroiliac joint instability). (After Hackett 1958, with permission.)

the lift incorporated into the right orthotic for the 'shorter' right leg. After removing the orthotics, the pelvis felt level again. The best part was yet to come, when I went for a 12 mile run later that day and, for the first time in years, came back without the ache in my right thigh muscles. Within 3 months, the muscle bulk on the right leg had increased to match that on the left. I continued to do the MET daily.

Over the next 4 years, I occasionally went out of alignment, usually as a result of some asymmetrical activity such as hiking or climbing. Eventually, I came to recognize these recurrences just from the fact that my gait pattern felt different, with my right foot not only pronating excessively, but also pointing outward from midline more than the left. If I delayed correction, the right heel pain would come back within 24 hours. Much less often, I would switch sides: the left innominate rotating forward and the right backward, with associated pain from the left posterior pelvic ligaments.

In addition, although frequency of this rotational malalignment decreased gradually over the years, and correction was usually fairly immediate, my shoes continued to collapse in the same pattern: right inward, left outward. It was not until more recently that I realized this problem was attributable to a recurrent left outflare and right inflare (see Figs 2.10 and 2.14), causing the pelvis and the legs to rotate to the left. Barring the occasional recurrence, which I can usually correct easily on my own, I am now staying in alignment more or less continuously.

The months following the meeting in Montreal stand out as the most exciting of my years in sports medicine as I gradually became aware of other changes that occurred with malalignment. I began to piece together the biomechanics, symptoms and signs that constitute what I now call the 'malalignment syndrome'. Probably foremost was the awareness that my right leg was no longer rotated outward, and that I was no longer pronating with my right foot; in fact, I have turned out to be a supinator.

Athletes and other patients presenting with malalignment were noted to show consistent patterns of asymmetry involving muscle function, weight-bearing and ranges of motion in particular. Eventually, knowledge of a certain presentation of malalignment allowed for the prediction of the associated pattern of asymmetry or vice versa. In addition, the specific changes could be related to specific problems with which the athlete or patient presented. Even more important was the recognition that simply correcting the malalignment was often adequate treatment for problems that had evaded cure for months, sometimes years, using standard therapy approaches. This aspect has now been corroborated by my clinical experience and the studies presented here.

The concept of malalignment often evokes feelings of anxiety in those not familiar with the terminology and the examining techniques. The reader has to realize that, like anything else practised by any one group to the exclusion of all else, the subject can appear more difficult than it really need be to someone looking from the outside. I myself had arrived on the scene by accident and from the feet up, so to speak, rather than through one of the traditional approaches (e.g. chiropractic or osteopathy) that teaches a detailed examination of the alignment of the various parts of the pelvis and spine. In the intervening period, I have learned some of these more detailed assessments and have obtained more training in manual therapy techniques. This additional knowledge has repeatedly emphasized the fact that the initial assessment should always establish whether or not malalignment is one of the problems one may be dealing with, and that, as I will try to show in this book, it is usually not a complicated matter.

I recognize that the majority of the readers are, like myself, primarily interested in being able to establish whether malalignment is present, and whether it might be the cause of the athlete's or patient's complaints, in which case they can then refer him or her to someone who has the skill to correct it. I have tried to provide an easy method for determining the presence of malalignment. To this end, I have limited discussion to the four most common, and usually treatable, presentations: vertebral malrotation, rotational malalignment, sacroiliac joint upslip, and outflare/inflare.

I am also a strong believer that the more athletes/patients can do for themselves, the better their chances of recovery. I look at the therapist as doing the 'fine-tuning', whereas the athletes and patients need to get involved in their day-to-day treatment to help to maintain alignment between visits. It is important that they learn to recognize any recurrence of malalignment; the sooner they do, the sooner they can get on with self-correction manoeuvres and/or seek help. A spouse or friend can easily be taught how to help with the assessment, although most athletes/patients will quickly learn how to do this on their own – they themselves can usually carry out some of the techniques that may correct the malalignment or, failing that, at least achieve partial correction and decrease their discomfort until they can reach their therapist for further treatment. By these means, they can often speed up their recovery and, at the same time, decrease their dependence on the therapist.

Most of them will eventually come to recognize the changes that occur at the time of recurrence, such as a shift in gait pattern. An earlier recognition of recurrence allows for an earlier initiation of treatment, usually easier correction and often an avoidance of the pain and other problems that are likely to bother the athlete the longer malalignment persists.

My intent here is to create an awareness of the malalignment syndrome and the problems it can create in anyone afflicted with it, particularly athletes, who may be more at risk of becoming symptomatic because of the very nature of their sport. If I can get others to start looking at those presenting for help in what may at first seem a completely different way, and hopefully stimulate some research along new lines, then I will have succeeded.

1

The malalignment syndrome: a synopsis

Medicine has, to date, been relatively unaware of malalignment and its related problems. Sports medicine, in particular, has failed to recognize the malalignment syndrome as one of the major causes of back pain and other musculoskeletal problems, also capable of mimicking disturbances, or actually causing disturbances, in every organ system (see Chapter 4). The concern in sports medicine relates primarily to the problems caused by the biomechanical changes inherent to malalignment: specific sports injuries, impaired recovery from injury and a failure of athletes to realize their full potential (see Chapters 5 and 6).

In addition, much of the research dealing with matters relating to weight-bearing, ground reaction forces and muscle strength has failed to take into account the biomechanical effects of malalignment. Side-to-side differences in upper and lower extremity ranges of motion or muscle strength, for example, lack meaning when we do not know whether the athletes enrolled in a particular study were in alignment or not. This chapter will serve to outline:

- the various presentations of malalignment with which the malalignment syndrome has been associated
- the basic implications of the malalignment syndrome in terms of altered biomechanics, diagnostic features and appropriate treatment.

MALALIGNMENT AND TRADITIONAL THINKING

Malalignment has traditionally been thought of in terms of involvement of the pelvis and spine. Three presentations of pelvic malalignment, and their specific planes of movement (see Fig. 2.6), are particularly prevalent (Box 1.1).

Box 1.1   Common presentations of pelvic malalignment

- **Rotational malalignment.** 'Anterior' or 'posterior' rotation of an innominate (pelvic bone) relative to the sacrum, referring to the direction of movement of the upper part of the innominate (e.g. iliac crest, anterior superior iliac spine or posterior superior iliac spine) in the sagittal plane (see Fig. 2.29)
- **Upslip of the sacroiliac joint.** Direct upwards translation of an innominate relative to the sacrum in the vertical plane (see Fig. 2.39)
- **Inflare/outflare.** Inward or outward movement of an innominate, respectively, in the transverse (horizontal) plane (see Fig. 2.10)

Box 1.2

- Distortion of the pelvic ring
- Associated changes in the alignment of the axial and appendicular skeleton, so that there appears to be a reorientation of the body from head to foot
- Compensatory changes in the soft tissue structures
- Occasionally also visceral involvement, affecting the genitourinary, gastrointestinal and reproductive systems

All three cause some form of asymmetry. In addition, both rotational malalignment and sacroiliac joint upslip result in:

- distortion of the pelvic ring and the joints that are part of that ring: the symphysis pubis and the two sacroiliac joints (see Fig. 2.29)
- pelvic obliquity (see Fig. 2.43)
- compensatory curvatures of the spine (see Figs 3.6 and 3.7)

In addition, there may be excessive rotation, or 'malrotation', of one or more vertebrae, which can either have resulted from the pelvic malalignment or may actually be responsible for the occurrence of the pelvic malalignment in the first place.

Rotational malalignment and upslips form but one component of a clinical entity here designated as the 'malalignment syndrome'.

MALALIGNMENT SYNDROME

The malalignment syndrome is characterized by the features listed in Box 1.2.

Diagnosis rests on the findings of:

- asymmetrical alignment of the bones of the pelvis, trunk and extremities
- compensatory curvatures of the spine, with or without associated malrotation of one or more vertebrae
- asymmetrical ranges of motion of the head and neck, trunk, pelvis and joints of the upper and lower extremities
- asymmetrical tension in the muscles, tendons and ligaments
- asymmetrical muscle bulk and strength
- an apparent (functional) leg length difference
- an asymmetrical weight-bearing pattern.

Findings associated with inflare/outflare relate primarily to pelvic ring distortion, asymmetrical tension on the soft tissues and an asymmetry of weight-bearing and of some ranges of motion.

Associated with these findings there may be:

- tenderness to palpation in joints and soft tissues that are put under increased tension, compressed or otherwise subjected to increased stress as a result of these asymmetries
- pain localizing to these joints and soft tissues, as well as typical patterns of referred pain and/or paraesthesias originating from these structures, and possibly visceral symptoms.

Investigations may be required to rule out pathological conditions that can present with symptoms overlapping with those related to malalignment (e.g. disc degeneration, nerve root compression, sciatica and sacroiliitis) or predispose to the recurrence of malalignment following correction (e.g. ovarian cyst, uterine fibroids or central disc protrusions).

Treatment consists primarily of a correction of the malalignment using manual therapy techniques. The chance of recovery is improved by teaching the athlete:

- self-assessment techniques to determine whether or not there is malalignment and of what type
- some self-treatment methods, such as muscle energy techniques, which can often be helpful in achieving realignment
- 'core' muscle strengthening to increase the stability of the pelvis and trunk.

The addition of foot orthotics, a sacroiliac belt or compression shorts may help to increase the stability of the pelvis. Prolotherapy injections are worth trying, particularly when there is evidence of laxity that allows malalignment to recur; these injections can strengthen connective tissue (e.g., the ligaments of the pelvis and spine), by inducing an inflammatory response that then stimulates new collagen formation. Cortisone injections, and other injection techniques such as neural therapy, may be helpful when ligament or joint pain fails to settle even though realignment is being maintained. As long as malalignment keeps recurring, the emphasis is on symmetrical exercises, unless the therapist specifically recommends an asymmetrical stretching or strengthening routine. The response to this treatment approach has been excellent in athletes who have often failed to respond to standard therapeutic approaches.

MALALIGNMENT AND SPORTS

One of the more common complaints of athletes/patients presenting with malalignment is that of back pain and dysesthesias referred to the lower extremities. A failure to recognize this and other manifestations of the malalignment syndrome sets the stage for misdiagnosis and mistreatment. Minor changes seen with imaging techniques receive more attention than is their due. Neurological and/or orthopaedic lesions are considered and may be extensively investigated, all to no avail. Further confusion arises from a tendency to attribute differences in the style and recurrence of injuries, especially unilateral injuries, to preferences acquired over a lifetime, the repetition of certain patterns of movement and right or left handedness and footedness, yet these factors may have little or nothing to do with style or the injury in question. Consider the following examples:

- a downhill skier who finds it easier to execute a turn to the right than to the left
- an ice hockey player who easily makes a quick stop turning to the left but feels awkward on attempting the same stop turning to the right
- a horseback rider whose horse keeps veering off to the left is chagrined to find that switching to another horse does not solve the problem.

Side-to-side differences of this type can all occur on the basis of the biomechanical changes that occur with malalignment, as will become apparent throughout the following chapters.

So where does the problem of malalignment start? Perhaps we can take some comfort from the fact that most of us go out of alignment somewhere between the ages of 8 and 12 years (see Ch. 2). The initiating factor may be as basic as a fall or a collision while playing in the school yard or at home. More likely, however, it is a developmental problem related to a subtle asymmetry of muscle tension determined at the spinal tract or cranial level, possibly by something as simple as the fact that most of us are either right or left motor dominant (see Ch. 2), although the picture is probably more complicated, involving something such as a disturbance of craniosacral rhythm, a facilitation of the reticular activating system or pressure on central nervous system structures as they exit from the cranial foramina (see Ch. 8).

One might think of malalignment as being one of the prices that we have to pay for walking upright, were it not for the fact that quadrupeds such as horses can also be afflicted by this condition (see Ch. 6). In addition, we now know that pelvic malalignment may result from a problem elsewhere, such as a disc protrusion, vertebral malrotation, temporomandibular joint dysfunction or antalgic weight-bearing pattern. The malalignment of a specific bone or joint is known to result in an increase (facilitation) or decrease (inhibition) of tension in specific pairs of muscles.

The important thing is to keep an open mind, to be aware that malalignment can be triggered by various mechanisms and to search for these if the athlete/patient fails to respond to initial attempts at realignment. The correction of malalignment, and maintenance of realignment, can be achieved in the majority and may well be what finally puts them back on the road to recovery, allowing the athlete to return to and/or finally progress in his or her chosen sport.

References henceforth will be primarily to 'athletes' with the understanding that most of the material discussed applies also to the 'non-athletic' and 'patient' populations.

2

Common presentations and diagnostic techniques

An understanding of the malalignment syndrome requires a knowledge of the common presentations of malalignment and the techniques used to diagnose these presentations. Key to this is an understanding of the sacroiliac (SI) joint and the role it plays in the normal and abnormal functioning of the unit formed by the lumbosacral spine, the pelvic girdle and the hip joints. Interestingly, in the early 20th century, the SI joint was thought to be the main source of low back pain and was the focus of many scientific investigations. The publication in 1934 of a paper by Mixter and Barr on rupture of the intervertebral disc quickly changed the direction of these investigations: over the next four decades, the SI was more or less ignored in favour of the disc as a primary cause of back pain.

The resurgence of interest in the SI joint since the 1970s can be traced to the following:

● a failure of disc resection, and subsequent desperation-measure fusions, to relieve low back pain in a considerable percentage of patients
● the recognition of the short- and long-term complications of chymopapaine 'discectomy'
● the evolution of the computed tomography scan and subsequently magnetic resonance imaging, with a recognition of the fact that disc protrusions were common but did not necessarily cause back pain (Magora & Schwarz 1976).

From the late 1930s into the 1980s, research focused largely on SI joint anatomy and biomechanics (Bernard & Kirkaldy-Willis 1987, Bowen & Cassidy 1981, DonTigny 1985, Vleeming et al 1989a, 1989b, 1990a, 1990b, 1992a, 1992b). More recent interest in rehabilitation involving the SI joint may be attributed in large part to two factors. First was a recognition of the fact that approximately 20–30% of low back and referred pain comes from the SI joint itself and/or the surrounding ligaments, muscles and other soft tissues involved in the functioning of the joint (Maigne et al 1996,

Schwarzer et al 1995). Second was the international forum for ongoing research on the SI joint and the lumbo-pelvic-hip unit, provided first by the Interdisciplinary World Congress on Low Back Pain and its Relationship to the Sacroiliac Joint in San Diego in 1992 and 1995, in Vienna in 1998, and in Montreal in 2001.

This chapter will initially examine some old and new concepts regarding the SI joint and the lumbo-pelvic-hip unit. It will then look at common presentations of malalignment – rotational malalignment, SI joint upslip/downslip, sacral torsion, outflare/inflare and vertebral malrotation – before discussing the tests frequently used to examine the pelvis and spine in order to diagnose malalignment.

THE SACROILIAC JOINT

The SI joints are planar joints that function to transfer the weight of the trunk and upper body to the ilia and on to the ischial tuberosities in sitting or to the lower extremities in standing. They also act as a shock absorber, particularly at heel strike. Stresses are absorbed in large part by the complex of pelvic ligaments and by the muscles that cross each SI joint; these same ligaments and muscles help to stabilize the joint for load transfer. Some SI joint motion does occur and seemingly helps to decrease the energy cost of ambulation (DonTigny 1985, 1990). The rather flat joint surfaces also allow movement in a way that makes it possible for women to deliver what are, in evolutionary respects, rather large babies.

A basic understanding of SI joint development, configuration and biomechanics is crucial to the understanding and diagnosis of asymmetries of the pelvis and spine. At the same time, it must be emphasized that the SI joints are but two of the three joints inherent to the pelvic ring and comprise but one facet of the lumbo-pelvic-hip unit and the entity designated here as the 'malalignment syndrome'. It is unfortunate that discussion so often centers on the SI joints to the exclusion of all the other structures that are part and parcel of this syndrome. The discussion that follows in this and subsequent chapters will hopefully put the role of the SI joints into proper perspective.

The reader is referred to Vleeming et al (1997a) and Lee (1999) for a more detailed discussion of the most recent thinking and scientific studies on pelvic and SI joint embryology, development and ageing, and on the kinetic interaction of the pelvis with the spine and the hip joints.

ANATOMY, DEVELOPMENT AND AGEING

The exquisite work by Bowen and Cassidy (1981), Bernard and Cassidy (1991) and others has demonstrated the following.

First, at birth, one finds the well-defined cartilaginous surfaces, synovial fluid and capsular enclosure typical of a synovial joint (Bernard & Cassidy 1991, Bowen & Cassidy 1981, Cassidy 1992, Dihlmann 1967, Sashin 1930, Solonen 1957, Williams & Warwick 1980). A thin fibrocartilagenous cover develops over the iliac surface, in contrast to the thick layer of hyaline cartilage noted on the sacral surface.

Second, the articular surfaces of the SI joint eventually assume an L-shape, with a shorter, almost vertical, upper arm and a longer, lower arm directed posteriorly and inferiorly (Fig. 2.1C). These arms can be oriented in a different plane relative to the vertical axis, creating a propeller-like appearance (Fig. 2.1B). In addition, the sacrum widens anteriorly, creating an anterior-to-posterior wedging effect (Fig. 2.2B; see also Figs 2.6 and 2.31).

Third, the joint capsule thickens anteriorly to form the anterior or ventral sacroiliac ligament; this is a weak ligament that has been shown to be continuous with the anterior fibres of the iliolumbar ligament (Fig. 2.2A). The interosseous ligament forms the posterior border of the joint (Fig. 2.2B, 2.10a-iii); it constitutes the strongest ligament supporting the SI joint and makes up for what is usually a rudimentary or even absent posterior joint capsule. Additional support comes from the posterior sacroiliac ligaments, the long posterior (or 'dorsal') sacroiliac ligament, and the iliolumbar, sacrotuberous and sacrospinous ligaments (Fig. 2.3).

Fourth, Bellamy et al (1983) have observed that the SI joint is surrounded by the largest and most powerful muscle groups in the body but that none of these directly influences the movement of this joint. As Lee pointed out in 1992, however, very few articulations in the body are actually capable of independent motion, and although the muscles crossing the SI joint are not typically described as prime movers of that joint, motion can occur at the SI joint as a result of their contraction. Lee goes on to list 22 muscles that influence SI joint movement, ranging from latissimus dorsi proximally to sartorius distally. Richard (1986) notes that 36 muscles have their insertion on each ilium, but that only 8 of these are also attached to the sacrum; some of the others just cross the joint but provide a key function in establishing and maintaining the axes of movement (e.g. right gluteus maximus posteriorly; see Fig. 7.8) or stabilizing the joint (e.g. iliacus anteriorly; see Fig. 2.31).

The work of Vleeming et al (1989a) is of particular interest in this respect. From their initial dissections on

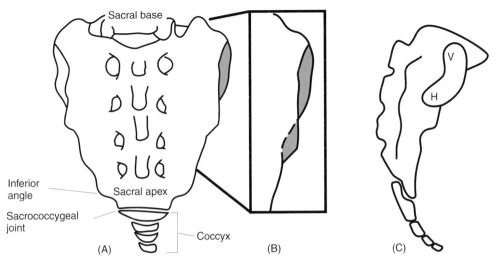

Figure 2.1 Posterior aspect of the sacrum and coccyx, and configuration of the adult sacroiliac joint. (A) Anteroposterior view: major bony landmarks. (B) Angulated inset showing orientation of the two main arms of the sacral articular surface along different planes relative to the vertical axis, which creates a propeller-like shape (see also Figs 2.12 and 2.13). (C) Lateral view: L-shape of the sacroiliac joint (H = horizontal arm; V = vertical arm). (After Vleeming et al 1997, with permission.)

12 cadavers, these authors reported that gluteus maximus was attached to the sacrotuberous ligament in all cases. In 50% of dissections, there was also a unilateral or bilateral 'fusion' of the sacrotuberous ligament with the tendon of the long head of biceps femoris at the origin (Fig. 2.4; see also Figs 2.26 and 2.37). In some specimens, 'fusion' to the ligament was complete so that there was actually no connection of this muscle to the ischial tuberosity itself.

Vleeming et al (1989b) showed how load application to the sacrotuberous ligament, either directly to the ligament or by way of its continuations with the long head of biceps femoris (see Figs 2.4 and 2.37) or the attachments of gluteus maximus, significantly diminished the ventral (forward) rotation of the base of the sacrum. They hypothesized, later finding support for this hypothesis, that these forces resulted in a compression of the sacral and iliac surface, increasing the coefficient of friction and thereby decreasing movement at the SI joint (Vleeming et al 1990a, 1990b).

These findings are but one illustration of how specific muscles may indirectly affect the sacrum, the innominate bones and hence the function of the joints of the pelvic girdle by producing joint motion, compression or both. Recent work by these and other authors has more clearly defined the role of these so-called inner and outer pelvic 'core' muscles as dynamic stabilizers of the SI joints in particular and of the lumbo-pelvic-hip girdle and trunk in general (see 'Kinetic function and stability' p. 21, and Figs 2.18–2.28).

Fifth, the prepubertal SI joint surface is described as planar – flat opposing sacral and iliac surfaces that allow for small gliding movements in all directions (Fig. 2.5A). After puberty, most individuals develop 'a crescent-shaped ridge running the entire length of the iliac surface with a corresponding depression on the sacral side' (Fig. 2.5B), and 'with increasing age the surfaces become more irregular and prominent' (Cassidy 1992, p. 41). This apparent 'roughening' of these surfaces may be an adaptation to adolescent weight gain; certainly, work by Vleeming et al (1990a, 1990b) supports the conjecture that these macroscopic changes represent functional, rather than pathological, adaptations. These authors present evidence that articular surfaces with both a coarse texture and ridges and depressions have high friction coefficients, consistent with their view that the roughening represents a 'non-pathological adaptation to the forces exerted at the SI joints, leading to increased stability' (Vleeming et al 1990a). The same authors raise two points of particular interest:

• These physiologically normal intra-articular ridges and depressions could easily be misinterpreted as osteophytes on radiological studies. They point out that:

it might well be that a textbook statement like 'The sacroiliac synovial joint rather regularly shows pathologic changes in adults, and in many males more than 30 years of age, and in most males after the age of 50, the joint becomes ankylosed ...' (Hollinshead 1962) is based on an incorrect interpretation of anatomical data

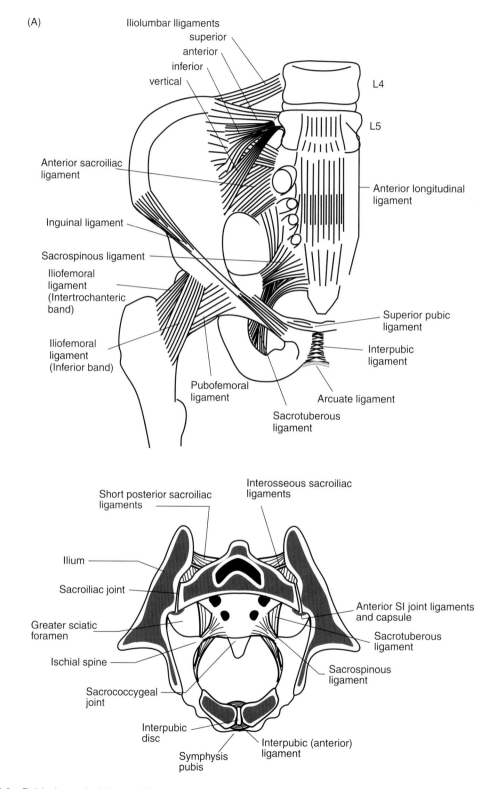

Figure 2.2   Pelvic ring: articulations and ligaments. (A) Anterior view. (B) Superior view (note the anterior widening of the sacrum).

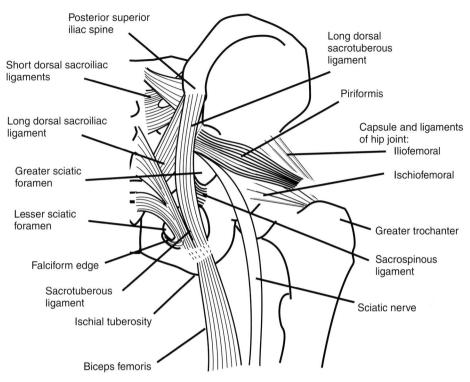

Figure 2.3   Posterior pelvic ligaments and muscles that act on the sacroiliac joint.

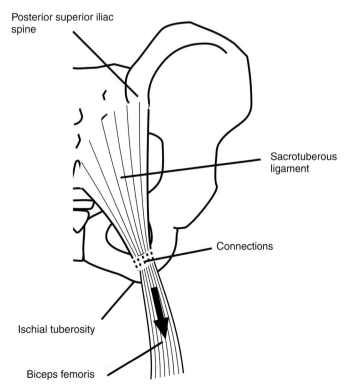

Figure 2.4   Tension in the sacrotuberous ligament can be increased by increasing tension in the biceps femoris, and vice versa, when there are fibrous connections between the ligament and the muscle (see also Fig. 2.37). (After Vleeming et al 1997, with permission.)

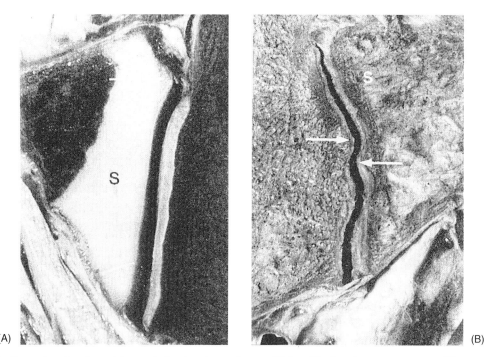

Figure 2.5   Coronal section through two embalmed male specimens. (A) Age 12 – the planar appearance of the sacroiliac joint (S denotes the sacrum). (B) Over age 60 – the presence of ridges and grooves is denoted by arrows. (From Vleeming et al 1990a, with permission.)

and that 'with standard radiological techniques, the [cartilage-covered] ridges and depressions easily can be misinterpreted as pathologic, because of the well known overprojection in SI joints' (Vleeming et al 1990a).

- SI joints with intact cartilage showed the friction coefficient to be particularly high 'in preparations with complementary ridges and depressions'. This led them to conjecture that:

Under abnormal loading conditions … it is theoretically possible that an SI joint is forced into a new position where ridge and depression are no longer complementary. Such an abnormal joint position could be regarded as a blocked joint (Vleeming et al 1990b, p. 135).

This may refer to the frequent finding of a decrease or even absence of movement, also referred to as 'locking', in one or other SI joint on clinical examination of those presenting with malalignment (discussed in detail under 'Functional or dynamic tests' below, and in Ch. 3). Note that this decrease or loss of mobility occurs 'under abnormal loading conditions'. Normal interlocking of the surfaces contributes to joint stability and limitation of range of motion of the SI joint (Snijders et al 1992a).

Sixth, the joint may retain its synovial features well into the patient's 40s or 50s. The fibrocartilage cover-

ing the iliac side consistently starts to degenerate early in life, usually by the third decade in males and the fourth or fifth decade in females. Iliac osteoarthrosis is indicated by an initial fibrillation of the cartilage, plaque formation and eventual peripheral erosions and subchondral sclerotic changes.

In contrast, osteoarthritic changes are rarely noted on the sacral side by the fifth decade. With advancing age, the typical changes of worsening osteoarthritis (deep erosions, areas of exposed subchondral bone, enlarging osteophytes and increasing fibrous connections) result in both articular surfaces becoming totally irregular. In some individuals, this change may progress to a complete replacement of the joint space with fibrous tissue, eventual calcification and a complete loss of movement. However, 'in most cases, the joint remains patent throughout life. Fusion can occur by synostosis or by fibrosis' (Cassidy 1992, p. 41).

Fibrous adhesions, although more common in older specimens, have been noted in younger male specimens, but 'to a lesser degree'. Whereas bony ankylosis is rare, para-articular synostosis has been reported by Valojerdy et al (1989) as a common finding in both males and females over the age of 50. Most will continue to show some SI joint movement well into their

70s and 80s (Bowen & Cassidy 1981, Cassidy 1992, Colachis et al 1963). Some studies have actually refuted the existence of absolute intra-articular ankylosis in the elderly (Resnick et al 1975).

Finally, the clinical significance of the premature osteoarthrosis on the iliac side is not known. However, similarly to other sites in the body, osteoarthrosis does not necessarily cause symptoms. As Magora & Schwartz reported in 1976, and others have since confirmed, osteoarthrosis of the spine correlates more with increasing age than with back pain. The same is probably true for the SI joint.

MOBILITY

There has been much debate over whether movement can occur at the SI joint, despite a wealth of studies dating from the early 1900s proving that small amounts of movement are indeed possible (Ashmore 1915, Beal 1982, Bowen & Cassidy 1981, Colachis et al 1963, Dihlman 1967, Egund et al 1978, Frigerio et al 1974, Miller et al 1987, Pitkin & Pheasant 1936, Sashin 1930, Solonen 1957, Strachan 1939, Weisl 1955). The question was settled definitively in vivo in the study by Sturesson et al (1989) using roentgen stereophotogrammetric analysis (a computerized dual-radiographic technique for assessing the relative movement of implanted titanium balls serving as reference points on the ilium and sacrum), and by Jacob & Kissling (1995) and Kissling & Jacob (1997) using Kirschner rods implanted in both ilia and the sacrum in healthy volunteers.

Figure 2.6 depicts the basic axes and planes. Movement of the SI joint is best described as triplanar and amounts to approximately 2–4 degrees of rotation in the sagittal, frontal and transverse (horizontal) planes (Egund et al 1978, Sturreson et al 1989) in addition to a similar degree of translation in a lateral, craniocaudal and anterior–posterior direction (Egund et al

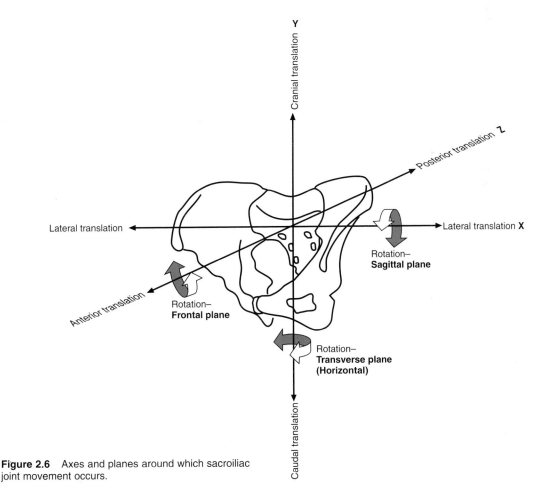

Figure 2.6   Axes and planes around which sacroiliac joint movement occurs.

1978). Stevens and Vyncke reported 3.3 degrees mean axial rotation of the sacrum in the transverse plane on side-bending in 1986. Asymmetry, both of the configuration and the amount of mobility possible on one side compared with the other, appears to be the rule (Bowen & Cassidy 1981, Vleeming et al 1992a, 1992b).

Most studies to date have, however, used a static approach to investigating a dynamic phenomenon. In addition, none of the authors cited have indicated whether malalignment of the pelvis was present. Malalignment results in asymmetrical opposition of the SI joint surfaces and can also cause unilateral SI joint hypermobility, hypomobility or even locking (see Chs 3 and 4), all factors that could result in an asymmetry of configuration and/or mobility. Few would argue with the observation by Cassidy (1992, p. 42) that 'a valid and reliable method for measuring this motion in patients has not yet been developed'.

AXES OF MOTION

Motion at the SI joint is complex, probably not occurring around one fixed axis but instead being a movement combining rotation and translation (Beal 1982, Bernard & Cassidy 1991, Egund et al 1978, Frigerio et al 1974, Kissling & Jacob 1997, Walker 1992). A good description of the directions and degrees of freedom of movement at the SI joints can be found in *Gray's Anatomy* (Williams & Warwick 1980). With the risk of oversimplification, the primary motions that can occur are outlined in Box 2.1.

Rotation of the sacrum or an innominate results in a relative displacement of the joint surfaces (Figs 2.12 and 2.13). Excessive rotation and/or translation in any direction can have a shearing effect. These surfaces may also become pathologically 'stuck' in any one position, Panjabi's so-called 'compressed' joint (see 'Kinetic function and stability' below and Figs 2.18 and 2.19). Nutation makes for stability, and counternutation for instability; the amount of nutation, or counternutation, can be of a normal or a pathological degree.

Muscles that can effect nutation (see Fig. 2.8A), and increase stability, include those that can:

- rotate the sacral base anteriorly (e.g. semispinalis or erector spinae muscles; see Fig. 2.26)
- rotate the ilia posteriorly (e.g. rectus abdominis – see Fig. 2.24A; biceps femoris – see Fig. 2.37).

Box 2.1   Axes of motion of the sacroiliac joint

1. **Rotational movement**, anterior or posterior, in the sagittal plane
   - of one or both ilia relative to the sacrum; if both rotate, this may be:
     – in the same direction (e.g. as occurs usually with flexion or extension of the trunk; see Fig. 2.83)
     – in opposite directions (e.g. as occurs in the course of normal gait; Fig. 2.7 and see Figures 2.9, 2.17 and 2.28)
   - of the sacrum relative to both ilia; forward movement of the base has been designated as *nutation* and backward movement is *counternutation* (Fig. 2.8)

2. **Upward or downward translation** along the vertical or Y-axis; this may involve one or both ilia relative to the sacrum, or the sacrum relative to the ilia (see Fig. 2.6)

3. **Axial rotation** of sacrum and ilia in the transverse plane
   - sacrum and ilia as one unit.
     – this normally occurs with clockwise or counterclockwise rotation of the pelvis when standing or walking (Fig. 2.9)
   - an ilium relative to the sacrum:
     – the anterior part of the ilium moving either outwards or inwards from the midline in the transverse plane; this is also known as *outflare* and *inflare* respectively (Fig. 2.10; see also Fig. 2.14B)
     – some outflare occurs in association with anterior, and inflare with posterior, innominate rotation during normal gait (Fig. 2.10A) and flexion/extension manoeuvres (see Fig. 2.14B)
   - the sacrum relative to the innominates in the transverse plane or around the vertical axis (see Fig. 2.58):
     – this normally occurs with trunk rotation in sitting (when the innominates are fixed by bearing weight on the ischial tuberosities) and during gait (Fig. 2.28)

4. **Torsion** of the sacrum around an oblique axis
   - torsion with rotation around the right or left oblique axis usually happens in conjunction with some rotation around the vertical axis (see point 3 above)
   - the oblique axes run from the sacral base on one side to the apex on the opposite side (Figs 2.7B, 2.11, 2.17)
   - these axes are named according to the side of origin, the right oblique axis, for example, starting at the right sacral base

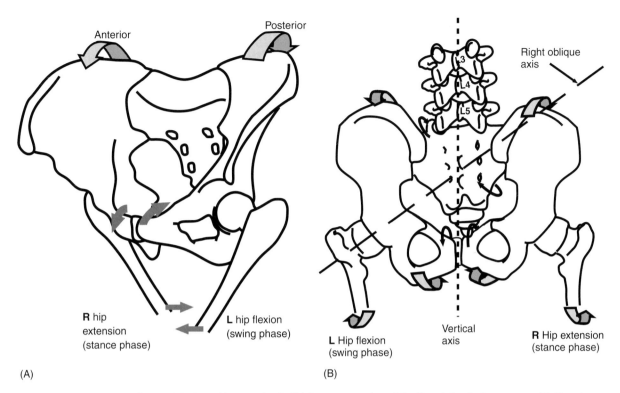

Figure 2.7 Movement of the pelvic ring with normal gait. (A) Contrary rotation of the ilia relative to the sacrum. (B) Sacral torsion around the right oblique axis associated with right anterior, left posterior innominate rotation (posterior view).

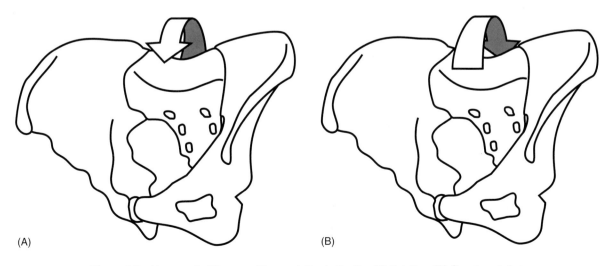

Figure 2.8 Movement of the sacral base relative to the ilia. (A) Nutation. (B) Counternutation.

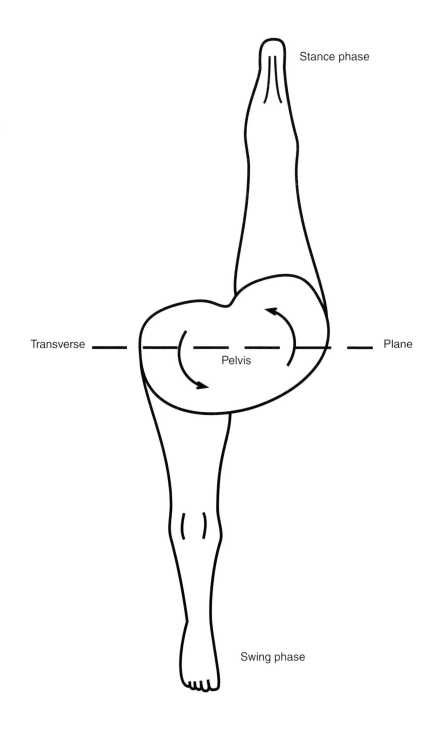

Figure 2.9 Pelvic rotation in the transverse plane with normal gait: counterclockwise during the right swing, left stance phase; clockwise with left swing, right stance.

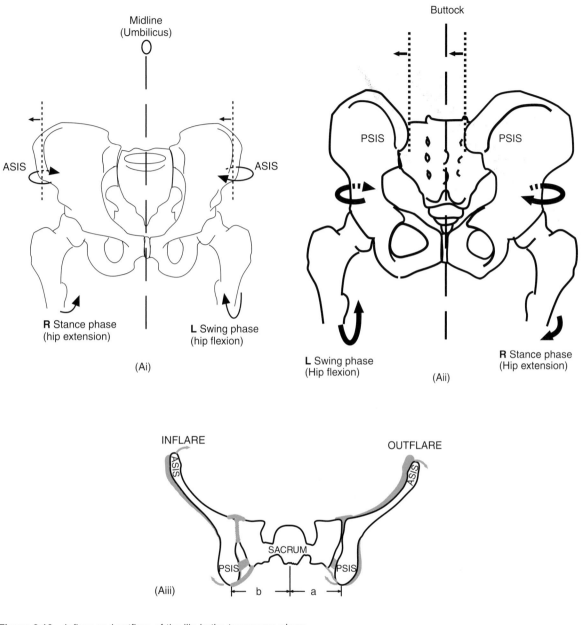

Figure 2.10   Inflare and outflare of the ilia in the transverse plane.

(A) With normal gait (right stance, left swing phase):
(i) anterior view; (ii) posterior view; (iii) superior view. ASIS = anterior superior iliac spine; PSIS = posterior superior iliac spine.

(B) Relative to umbilicus (assuming that it is central), thumbs against inside of the ASIS show:
(i) initial asymmetry with right outflare (away from the midline) and left inflare (closer to the midline); (ii) symmetry following correction (equidistant from the midline).

(C) Relative to the crease, thumbs against the inner aspect of the PSIS show:
(i) initial asymmetry with right outflare (closer to the midline) and left inflare (away from the midline); (ii) right and left equal after correction of the outflare/inflare.

Figure 2.10 B & C, see overleaf

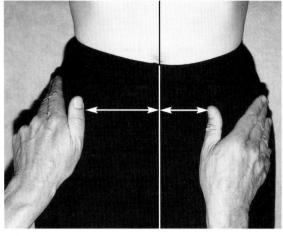

(Bi)

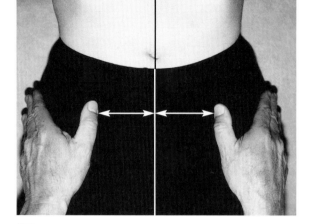

(Bii)

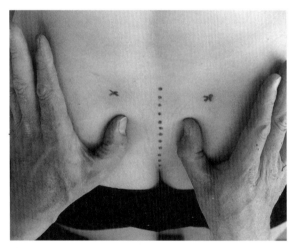

(Ci)

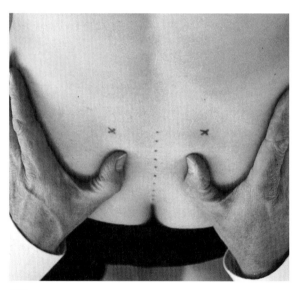

(Cii)

Figure 2.10 *Continued*

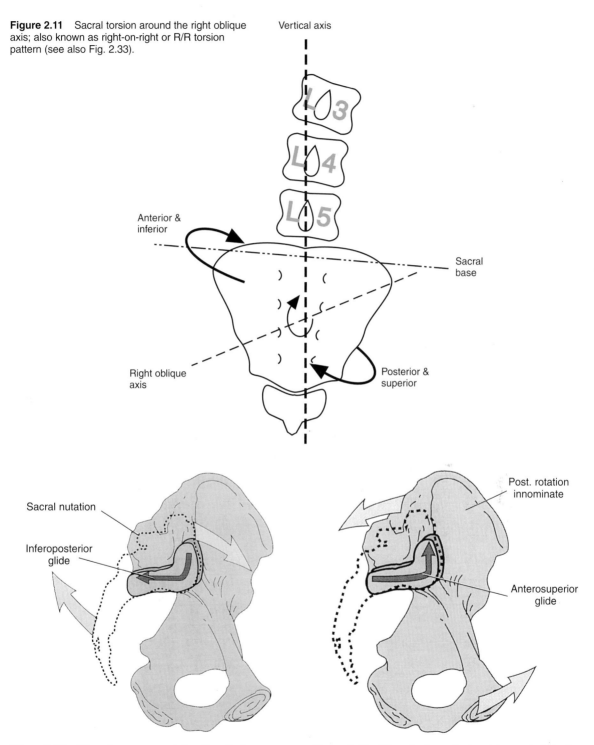

Figure 2.11 Sacral torsion around the right oblique axis; also known as right-on-right or R/R torsion pattern (see also Fig. 2.33).

Vertical axis

L3

L4

L5

Anterior & inferior

Sacral base

Right oblique axis

Posterior & superior

Sacral nutation

Inferoposterior glide

Post. rotation innominate

Anterosuperior glide

Figure 2.12 When the sacrum nutates, its articular surface glides inferoposteriorly relative to the innominate (anterosuperiorly on counternutation). (From Lee 1999, with permission.)

Figure 2.13 When the innominate rotates posteriorly, its articular surface glides anterosuperiorly relative to the sacrum (inferoposteriorly on anterior rotation). (From Lee 1999, with permission.)

Muscles that effect counternutation (see Fig. 2.8B), and decrease stability, include those that can:

- rotate the sacral base posteriorly (e.g. pubococcygeus, a levator ani muscle originating from the pubic rami and inserting into the coccyx; see Fig. 2.36)
- rotate the ilia forward relative to the base of the sacrum (e.g. iliacus, rectus femoris and tensor fascia lata/iliotibial band complex; see Fig. 2.37).

BIOMECHANICS

Movement around the various axes of the SI joints occurs as part of normal movement patterns involving the spine, pelvis and lower extremities throughout our day-to-day activities (DonTigny 1985, Greenman 1992, 1997). The sacrum influences the relative movement of the ilia, and vice versa, as tension is increased in the connecting soft tissues – primarily ligaments and muscles – that act on the SI joint(s). This is a normal phenomenon, as described, but will be influenced by the presence of tight structures, for example, a hamstring acting on an SI joint by way of a tight biceps femoris that has connections to the sacrotuberous ligament (see Fig. 2.4). In addition, the movement is likely to be asymmetrical when such tightness is worse on one side compared with the other. When sitting, the ilia are relatively 'fixed' and less mobile than when standing.

Trunk flexion (Fig. 2.14A)

In standing. Flexion initially results in a simultaneous forward rotation of the sacrum and ilia in the sagittal plane, and this may continue through full flexion (Kapandji 1974; Fig. 2.14B). Flexion somewhere past 50–60 degrees sees the ilia continuing to rotate forward symmetrically in most people; in some, however, the sacrum now counternutates, the base moving posteriorly and the apex (coccyx) anteriorly, decreasing the lumbosacral angle and therefore the lumbar lordosis (Fig. 2.15A). The counternutation from this point on may occur as a result of:

- a posteriorly-directed force applied to the sacral base by the flexing lumbar spine
- a maximal tightening of the ligaments (interosseous, sacrotuberous and sacrospinous) effected by the initial nutation (Fig. 2.16A)
- the presence of any other factor capable of opposing the progressive nutation of the sacrum, for example, tightness of hamstrings or pubococcygeus.

In sitting. The initial movement on trunk flexion is one of sacral counternutation as the ilia rotate anteriorly. Counternutation increases the tension in the long dorsal sacroiliac ligament in particular, eventually resulting in posterior rotation of the ilia on further trunk flexion (Figs 2.16B, 7.37).

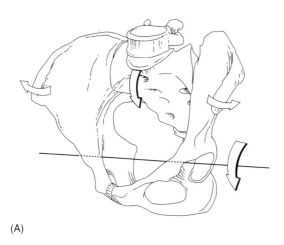

(A)

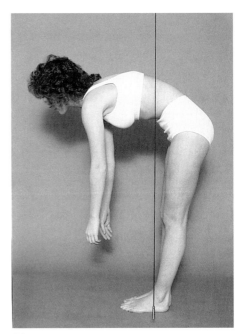

(B)

Figure 2.14 Forward flexion of the trunk from the erect standing position normally results in initial sacral nutation, anterior rotation of the innominates and a concomitant outflare of both innominates. (From Lee 1999, with permission.)

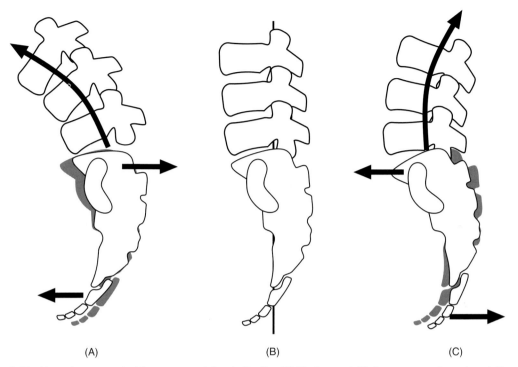

Figure 2.15 Normal movement of the sacrum relative to the ilia. (A) Flexion past 45 degrees: sacral counternutation. (B) Neutral (standing). (C) Extension: sacral nutation.

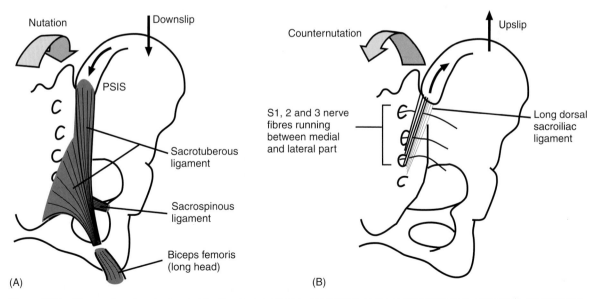

Figure 2.16 Ligaments put under tension by the movement of an innominate or the sacrum relative to each other. (A) Posterior rotation or downslip of an innominate; sacral nutation: sacrotuberous, sacrospinous and interosseous ligaments (not shown – see Figs 2.2B and 2.10C). (B) Anterior rotation or upslip of an innominate; sacral counternutation: long dorsal sacroiliac ligament.

Trunk extension

In standing. On extension, the ilia rotate posteriorly and the sacrum nutates, increasing the lumbosacral angle and hence the lumbar lordosis (see Fig. 2.15C).

In sitting. Initially, the ilia do not move as the spine extends and the sacrum nutates. Once nutation has taken up all the slack in the interosseous, sacrospinous and sacrotuberous ligaments (Fig. 2.16A), and in the pelvic floor muscles and ligaments attaching to the coccyx, further extension will result in anterior rotation of the ilia.

Standing or landing on one leg

There is ipsilateral SI joint movement consisting primarily of an upward translation of the ilium, with or without an element of anterior or posterior rotation, relative to the sacrum.

Vertical forces on the sacrum

As proposed by Strachan in 1939, a force transmitted vertically downwards from the lumbar region causes the sacrum to glide downward and flex (counternu-tate); traction applied from above causes the sacrum to move upward and extend (nutate).

Ambulation

During ambulation, there is:

- rotation of each ilium in the sagittal plane – anteriorly on the side of hip extension, posteriorly on the side of hip flexion (see Fig. 2.7)
- rotation of the pelvis as a whole in the transverse plane – forwards on the side of the advancing lower extremity (see Fig. 2.9)
- rotation of the pelvis as a whole in the frontal plane – up on the weight-bearing side, down on the other
- concomitant with displacement of the pelvis in these planes, the sacrum itself torquing alternately to the right and left around the vertical and oblique axes with each gait cycle. The left rotation of the sacrum that accompanies the posterior rotation of the right innominate as the right leg swings forward, for example, helps to ensure the tightening of the right sacrotuberous, sacrospinous and interosseous ligaments – and hence stabilization of the right SI joint – in preparation for heel strike and weight-bearing on that side (Fig. 2.17; see also Fig. 2.28).

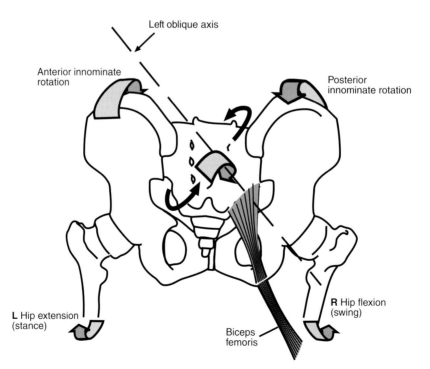

Figure 2.17 Gait: right swing, left stance phase with right posterior, left anterior innominate rotation, and sacral torsion around the left oblique axis results in a tightening of the right sacrotuberous, sacrospinous and interosseous ligaments.

KINETIC FUNCTION AND STABILITY

The ability of the SI joints to transfer weight and to absorb shock is closely linked to the proper functioning of the hip joints and the spine, in particular the lumbar segment. Normal kinetic function involves all three regions simultaneously and depends on the availability of normal ranges of motion, appropriate muscle function and the ability to stabilize the various components adequately and in a co-ordinated manner. The following concepts are helpful in understanding the interaction between the pelvis, spine and lower extremities, in particular with regard to stability.

Panjabi: active, passive and neural control systems

Panjabi's conceptual model (1992), originally intended to explain the stabilizing system of the spine, finds application 'to the entire musculoskeletal system' (Lee 1999) and is particularly helpful when trying to understand the factors that have a bearing on SI joint stability. Panjabi proposed the following interacting systems (Fig. 2.18):

1. the *'passive system'*: the 'osteoarticular ligamentous' structures; that is, the support derived from the actual shape of the joint and its ligaments and capsule

2. the *'active system'*: the 'myofascial' or contractile tissues acting on the joint

3. the *'control system'*: the central and peripheral nervous systems that co-ordinate the interaction between the passive and active systems.

The normal interplay of these systems results in a small amount of displacement of the joint surfaces with minimal resistance, the so-called *neutral zone*, and makes for stability (Fig. 2.19A). Injury to or degeneration of articulations and/or supporting ligaments (passive system), muscle weakness (active system) and the incoordination or failure of muscle function (control system) can all result in instability, with abnormal displacement of the joint surfaces around an enlarged neutral zone (Fig. 2.19B).

Contracture of the capsule and ligaments results in a loss of the neutral zone, with restriction of movement and stiffness of the joint (Fig. 2.19C). A restriction of movement within the neutral zone can also occur with active forces bringing the joint surfaces too close together, the so-called 'compressed' joint (Fig. 2.19D). A joint can also end up 'compressed', with the joint surfaces in an abnormal position because of excessive movement relative to each other, for example excessive forward rotation of the ilium relative to the sacrum in the sagittal plane, to the point of creating a so-called 'locked' SI joint. When the latter joint is 'decompressed' by moving the surfaces back into proper alignment, the neutral zone may now, however, turn out to be enlarged because the capsule and ligaments have been stretched, initially when the excessive forward rotation occurred (e.g. a shear-force injury) and/or as a result of the joint having been in this abnormal position for some time.

Failure of the control system can result in an aberrant movement of the surfaces relative to each other. Passive movement remains normal (within the neutral zone). However, active stabilization of the joint varies so that joint mobility is at times excessive, at other times normal, as the appropriate distance between the joint surfaces is repeatedly lost and regained (Fig. 2.19E). In addition to the dynamic instability, chronic failure of the control system can eventually also result in passive instability as the joint surfaces deteriorate and the supporting capsule and ligaments are repeatedly stretched. The instability that results for whatever reason may present as a sudden 'giving way' of what is often mistakenly localized to the 'hip joint', but actually is a manifestation of the 'slipping clutch' phenomenon which is discussed further below (Dorman 1994, Dorman et al 1998, Vleeming et al 1995a).

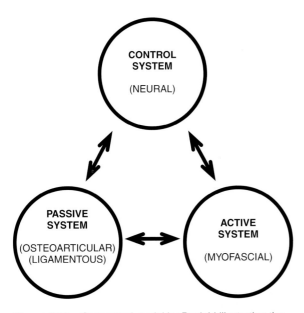

Figure 2.18   Conceptual model by Panjabi illustrating the systems that interact to provide stability. (After Panjabi 1992, with permission.)

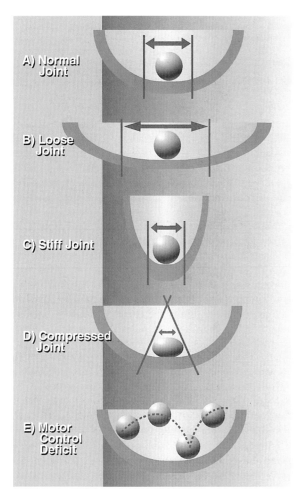

Figure 2.19   The 'ball in a bowl' concept of the joint neutral zone.
(A) Motion in a normal neutral zone.
(B) Loss of form closure results in increased motion within the neutral zone.
(C) Joint fibrosis decreases motion in the neutral zone
(D) Excessive compressive forces acting across the joint completely block motion within the neutral zone.
(E) With a motor control deficit, passive motion within the neutral zone remains normal since the dysfunction is dynamic; functionally, as the ball moves in the bowl, approximation is intermittently lost and then regained. (From Lee 1999, as redrawn from Panjabi 1992, with permission.)

'Self-locking' mechanism and 'form and force closure'

The strong ligamentous support system that allows for proper SI joint function is nevertheless felt to be inadequate to prevent dislocation of the joints under postural load unless supplemented by other forces. This has led to the concept of a 'self-bracing' or 'self-locking' mechanism based on the fact that 'In combination with load transfer through fascia, muscle forces that cross the SI-joints can produce joint compression. This counteracts mobility by friction and interlocking ridges and grooves' (Snijders et al 1993, 1995). The terms *form* and *force* closure delineate the passive and active components of this self-locking mechanism respectively (Snijders et al 1993, Vleeming et al 1990a, 1990b, 1997):

> Shear in the SI-joints is prevented by the combination of specific anatomical features (form closure) and the compression generated by muscles and ligaments that can be accommodated to the specific loading situation (force closure) … If the sacrum would fit the pelvis with perfect form closure, no lateral forces would be needed. However, such a construction would make mobility practically impossible. (Vleeming et al 1995)

Therefore, SI joint stability depends on a combination of form and force closure (Fig. 2.20).

Sacroiliac joint form closure

In the case of the SI joint, form closure is derived from the following:

● The triangular shape of the sacrum makes it fit between the ilia like a keystone in a Roman arch (Fig. 2.21); the two ends of the arch are firmly connected by the action of the sacrotuberous and sacrospinalis ligaments and the coccygeus and piriformis muscles, so that the relatively flat SI joint surfaces are loaded only with compression and shear is minimized.
● The interlocking of the variably oriented sacral and iliac articular surfaces helps to counter vertical and anterior–posterior translation (see Fig. 2.1B).
● The anteriorly widening sacrum restricts movement between the innominates by causing wedging in an anterior-to-posterior direction (see Figs 2.2B and 2.31).
● The increasing joint friction coefficient noted with advancing age as a result of:
– the formation of the interlocking ridges and grooves (see Fig. 2.5B)
– roughening of the joint surfaces, which usually starts with the deterioration of the fibrocartilagenous cover of the iliac surface.
● The ligaments that influence the SI joint: the anterior, interosseus and posterior SI joint and pelvic floor ligaments (see Figs 2.2, 2.3, 2.10, 2.16, 2.35, 2.36, 2.37, 3.59, 3.60, 3.61 and 3.63).

Sacroiliac joint force closure

SI joint force closure is derived from two sources, the first of which is any active force that results in nutation

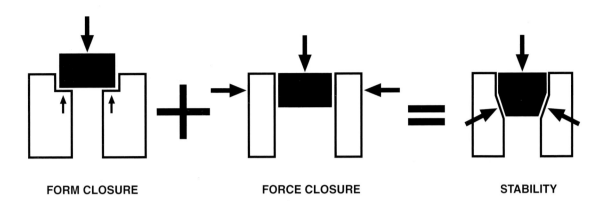

FORM CLOSURE   **FORCE CLOSURE**   **STABILITY**

Figure 2.20   Model of the self-locking mechanism: the combination of form and force closure establishes stability in the sacroiliac joint. (After Vleeming et al 1997, with permission.)

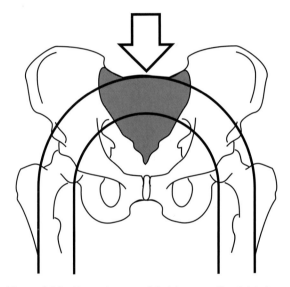

Figure 2.21   Form closure: minimizing sacroiliac joint shear through the 'keystone in a Roman arch' effect, with the sacrum being 'trapped' vertically. (After Dorman & Ravin 1991, with permission.)

of the sacrum (see Figs 2.8, 2.14, 2.15 and 2.37). Nutation comes about either by anterior rotation of the sacral base (e.g. contraction of multifidi, extensor spinae or sacrospinalis) or posterior rotation of the ilia (e.g. contraction of hamstrings or rectus abdominis). Nutation results in a tightening of the interosseous, sacrotuberous and sacrospinous ligaments (see Fig. 2.16A). The tightening appears to facilitate the force closure mechanism, thereby increasing the compression of the SI joint articular surfaces, which in turn increases the stability of the joint for load transfer

(Vleeming et al 1997). Conversely, counternutation decreases tension in these same ligaments and results in decreased stability (see Fig. 2.16B).

Second, force closure arises from the contraction of the 'inner' and 'outer' myofascial units. These units help to stabilize not only the pelvis, but also the lumbar spine and hip joints.

The 'inner' unit. The inner unit (Fig. 2.22) consists of the multifidi, thoracic diaphragm, transversus abdominis and pelvic floor muscles. Work by Sanford et al (1997), using fine-wire electromyography, suggests that the contraction of specific abdominal muscles is coupled with the contraction of specific pelvic floor muscles (e.g.

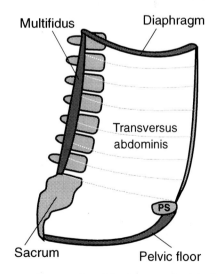

Figure 2.22   The muscles of the 'inner core' unit include the multifidus, transversus abdominis, thoracic diaphragm and pelvic floor. (From Lee 1999, with permission.)

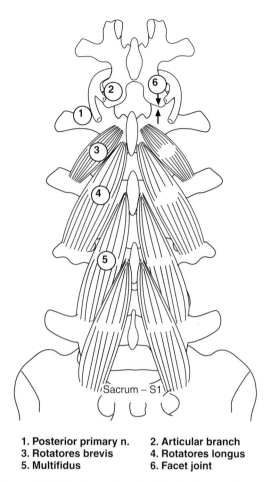

1. Posterior primary n.   **2. Articular branch**
3. Rotatores brevis   **4. Rotatores longus**
5. Multifidus   **6. Facet joint**

Figure 2.23   Posterior elements of the lumbosacral spine.

the co-contraction of transversus abdominis and pubococcygeus, the oblique abdominals and ilio/ischiococcygeus, and rectus abdominis and puborectalis).

The simultaneous contraction of some of the muscles that constitute this 'inner core' may be able to set up a force couple capable of affecting the stability of the SI joint and lumbosacral junction. For example, the multifidi, originating from the lower lumbar vertebrae, insert into the upper sacrum (Fig. 2.23), and ilio- and ischiococcygeus insert into the coccyx (see Fig. 2.36). Contraction of the multifidi causes sacral nutation; contraction of ilio/ischiococcygeus causes counternutation. The balance of these forces could move the sacrum into a stable or unstable position respectively. Transversus abdominis contraction (Fig. 2.24A) appears to occur in preparation for carrying out an action (Richardson et al 1999) and results in:

- the co-activation of pubococcygeus

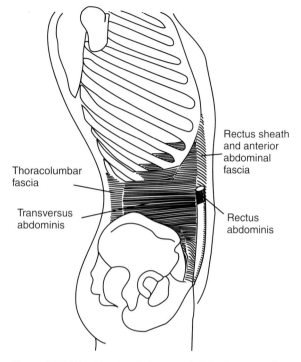

Figure 2.24 (A)   Muscles that are part of the 'outer core' unit. Transversus abdominis (also shown: rectus abdominis).

- the force closure of the anterior aspect of the SI joints; simultaneous compression of that part of the joint caused by inward movement of the ilia is resisted by the strong ligaments running across the back of the SI joint on that side (Snijders et al 1995b)
- lateral traction forces by way of insertions into the thoracolumbar fascia (Figs 2.24A, C), which in turn:
  - increases the intra-abdominal pressure, believed to contribute to lumbar spine stability (Aspden 1987)
  - increases tension within the thoracolumbar fascia, stabilizing the fascia and thereby making it more effective in its role as part of the 'outer unit', in particular as part of the posterior oblique (Fig. 2.25A) and deep longitudinal (see Fig. 2.26) systems.

The 'outer' unit. The outer unit is made up of the following systems. The *oblique* systems comprise:

- the posterior oblique system (Fig. 2.25A): the continuum of latissimus dorsi connected, by way of the thoracolumbar fascia, to the contralateral gluteus maximus will, on contraction:
  - compress the SI joint on the side of the gluteus maximus

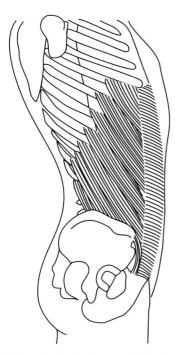

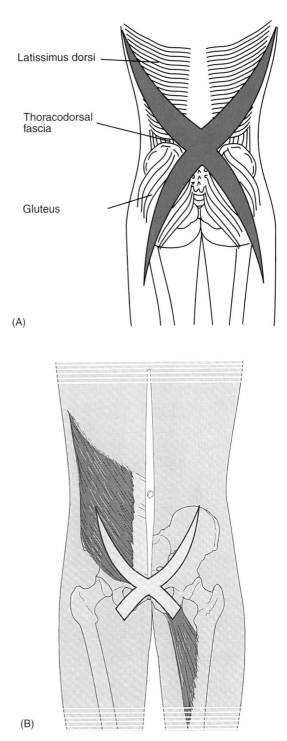

Latissimus dorsi

Thoracodorsal fascia

Gluteus

(A)

Figure 2.24 (B) Muscles that are part of the 'outer core' unit. External oblique.

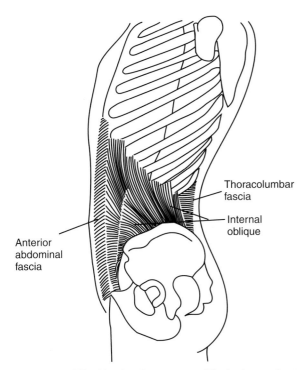

Thoracolumbar fascia

Internal oblique

Anterior abdominal fascia

(B)

Figure 2.24 (C) Muscles that are part of the 'outer core' unit. Internal oblique.

Figure 2.25 The oblique systems of the 'outer unit'.
(A) Posterior oblique system. (After Lee 1999, as redrawn from Snijders et al 1995, with permission.)
(B) Anterior oblique system (From Lee 1999, with permission.)

– contribute to load transfer through the pelvic region with rotational activities (Mooney et al 1997) and during gait (Gracovetsky 1997; Greenman 1997)

● the anterior oblique system (Fig. 2.25B): the external and internal abdominal obliques on one side are connected, by way of the anterior abdominal fascia, to the contralateral adductors of the thigh (see Figs 2.24A, B, C). Contraction of the obliques may help to initiate movement (Richardson & Jull 1995), provided that the trunk has been stabilized by prior contraction of transversus abdominis (Hodges & Richardson 1996). The lower horizontal fibres of the internal abdominal oblique may augment transversus abdominis in its role of supporting the SI joint (Richardson et al 1999).

Second is the *deep longitudinal* system (Fig. 2.26). The continuum of the erector spinae muscle connected, by way of the deep lamina of the thoracodorsal fascia, to the contralateral sacrotuberous ligament and biceps femoris (Gracovetsky 1997, Vleeming et al 1997) will, on contraction:

● compress the SI joint because of biceps femoris connections and the increase in tension on the sacrotuberous ligament (Wingerden et al 1993)

● increase tension in the thoracodorsal fascia and thereby enhance the ability of the fascia to contribute to any SI joint force closure mechanisms acting across it.

Last is the *lateral* system (Fig. 2.27). The gluteus medius and minimus, and the contralateral adductors of the thigh, are more involved with the proper function of the pelvic girdle in standing and walking rather than with SI joint force closure. SI joint instability is, however, said to result in a reflex inhibition of these muscles (Lee 1999) and may account for the feeling of the hip 'giving away', or 'slipping clutch syndrome' (Dorman 1994, 1995, Dorman et al 1998, Vleeming 1995).

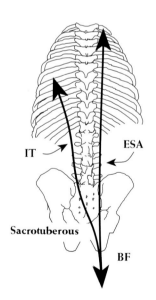

Figure 2.26 Deep longitudinal system of the 'outer unit': the biceps femoris (BF) is directly connected to the upper trunk via the sacrotuberous ligament, the erectores spinae aponeurosis (ESA) and iliocostalis thoracis (IT). (From Gracovetsky 1997, with permission).

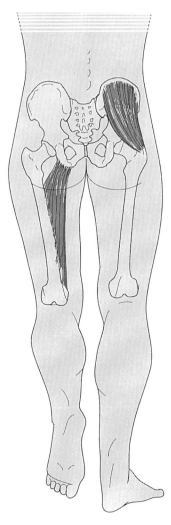

Figure 2.27 The lateral system of the outer unit includes the gluteus medius and minimus, and the contralateral adductors of the thigh. (From Lee 1999, with permission.)

Force closure of the SI joints suffers as a result of problems with the active system (e.g. muscle weakness) or the control system (e.g. the inadequate recruitment and/or improper timing of contraction of the inner/outer units). The movement patterns that a patient starts to use in order to compensate for these insufficiencies may lead to eventual decompensation of the low back, pelvis, hip and knee joints (Lee 1997a).

Functional evaluation of form and force closure

There are a number of functional tests for the evaluation of form and force closure that are coming into common usage in clinical practice, both to help to arrive at a proper diagnosis and to determine the appropriate treatment. These are discussed under 'Functional or dynamic tests' below.

Sacroiliac joint function during the gait cycle

During the right swing phase, the right SI joint becomes progressively more stable in preparation for weight-bearing, as a result of:

1. rotation of the sacrum around the left oblique axis, so that the right sacral base drops forward and down into nutation, while the apex rotates backward and to the left (see Fig. 2.17); the rotation is initiated by the contraction of the left piriformis and gluteus maximus, the key stabilizers of the oblique axes, during the left stance phase
2. rotation of the right innominate posteriorly relative to the sacrum.

Both of these actions result in increasing nutation of the right SI joint, with a passive increase in tension in the sacrotuberous, sacrospinous and interosseous ligaments (form closure). At the same time, tension in the 'posterior oblique' sling is increased both actively, with contraction of the right gluteus maximus, and passively, with the simultaneously forward swinging of the left arm and clockwise rotation of the trunk, stretching left latissimus dorsi. The right iliopsoas is already contracting to help to swing the leg forwards, at the same time acting across the right SI and hip joint (force closure). The onset of right hamstring contraction just before heel strike further increases the tension in the sacrotuberous ligament, augmenting form closure. The combined effect is a compression of the right SI joint, increasing its stability and hence ability to deal with load transfer at heel strike.

Gradual destabilization of the right SI joint, in preparation for the swing phase, is accomplished by:

- the onset of counternutation of the right sacral base, as the sacrum begins to rotate around the right oblique axis with the left leg swinging forwards (Fig. 2.7B)
- the anterior rotation of the right innominate bone relative to the sacrum, passively with hip extension and actively with contraction of the ipsilateral iliacus and rectus femoris (see Fig. 2.37)
- the contraction of piriformis (one of the prime hip extensors).

Tension in the right sacrotuberous ligament decreases even further as the hamstrings gradually start to relax. Form closure of the right SI joint is therefore gradually lost during stance so that stability during this phase is provided primarily by force closure. Active contraction of the left latissimus dorsi and right gluteus increases tension in the connecting thoracolumbar fascia and compresses the right SI joint; this contraction also starts to reverse the forward swing of the left arm and clockwise rotation of the trunk that had occurred during the right swing phase. Iliacus and rectus femoris act across the joint while helping the anterior rotation of the innominate. Once hip extension has been completed at the end of stance, gluteus maximus and piriformis begin to relax, at which point sacral torsion around the right oblique axis can proceed unhindered to its maximum range in preparation for left heel strike.

As the right leg begins to swing forwards following toe-off, the sacrum again begins to rotate around the left oblique axis, and the cycle repeats itself. During a complete cycle, therefore, the SI joints move reciprocally in a figure-of-eight pattern, combining motion in all three planes. The interaction between the spine, pelvic unit and hips is further delineated in Figure 2.28.

It is encouraging to think that we are presently encountering a groundswell of recognition for problems relating to the SI joint. Scientific studies and models of the type cited above have helped to clarify the forces normally acting on the joint. The role that the joint plays as part of the pathological presentations of malalignment will be discussed throughout the following sections.

COMMON PRESENTATIONS OF PELVIC MALALIGNMENT

The complete 'malalignment syndrome' is seen in association with two presentations of pelvic malalignment, namely *rotational malalignment* and *upslip*. Rotational malalignment is by far the most common, occurring in isolation in 80–85% of those with pelvic

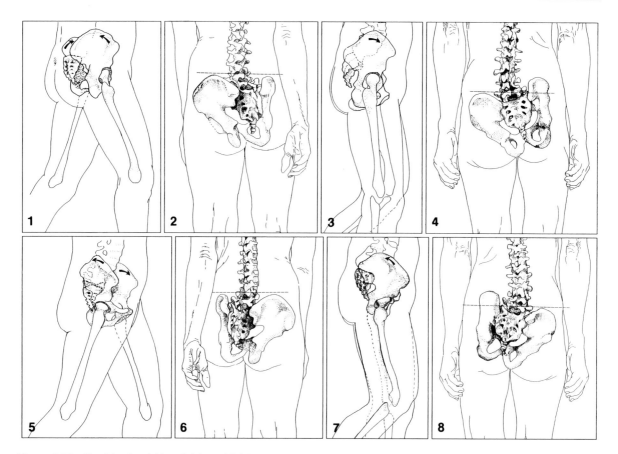

Figure 2.28 Combined activities of right and left innominates, sacrum and spine during walking. At right heel strike: 1. the right innominate has rotated in a posterior and the left innominate in an anterior direction; 2. the anterior surface of sacrum is rotated to left and superior surface is level, while the spine is straight but rotated to the left. At right midstance: 3. the right leg is straight and the innominate is rotating anteriorly; 4. the sacrum has rotated to the right and side-bent left, whereas the lumbar spine has side-bent right and rotated left. At left heel strike: 5. the left innominate begins rotation anteriorly; after toe-off, the right innominate begins rotation posteriorly; 6. the sacrum is level but with the anterior surface rotated to right. The spine, although straight, is also rotated to right, as is the lower trunk. At left leg stance: 7. the left innominate is high and the left leg straight; 8. the sacrum has rotated to the left and side-bent right, while the lumbar spine has side-bent left and rotated right. (From Greenman 1997, with permission.)

malalignment. An upslip occurs in isolation in about 5–10%, and the combination of an upslip with a rotational malalignment in another 5–10%.

Much less common is *downslip*. Some aspects of the malalignment syndrome are seen in association with an *outflare* and *inflare* when these are present in isolation; however, when these conditions are noted in combination with one of the other presentations, the complete syndrome will be evident.

ROTATIONAL MALALIGNMENT

'Rotational malalignment' refers to excessive anterior or posterior rotation of an innominate bone relative to the

sacrum in the sagittal plane. Such rotation can affect an innominate in isolation, but one is more likely to see it in association with:

- rotation of the contralateral innominate in the opposite direction, similar to that which occurs in normal walking (see Figs 2.7 and 2.17)
- a dysfunction of movement of one or both SI joints
- torsion of the sacrum, most often around one of the oblique axes
- displacement of the pubic bones relative to each other.

The overall effect is an asymmetrical distortion of the pelvic ring (Fig. 2.29). The movement dysfunction may

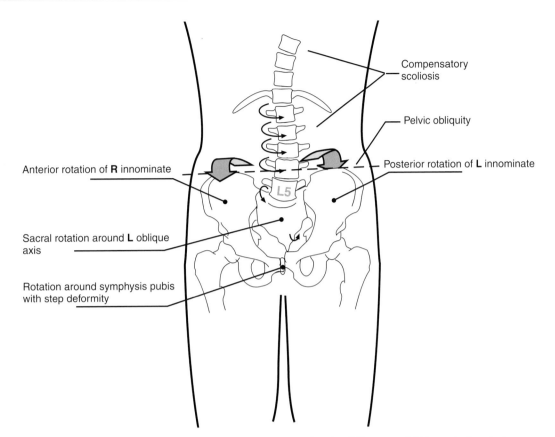

Compensatory scoliosis

Pelvic obliquity

Posterior rotation of **L** innominate

Anterior rotation of **R** innominate

Sacral rotation around **L** oblique axis

Rotation around symphysis pubis with step deformity

Figure 2.29   Typical distortion of the pelvic ring associated with rotational malalignment: right innominate anterior, compensatory left posterior, and sacrum in torsion around the left oblique axis.

occur in the form of hypomobility, or actual 'locking', of one of the SI joints; there may be compensatory hypermobility of the opposite SI joint, or a true laxity of one or both joints.

> The most common presentation of rotational malalignment is that of right anterior and left posterior innominate rotation with 'locking' of the right SI joint.

Examination findings typical of the most common presentation are detailed in Appendix 1.

Aetiology of rotational malalignment

Athletes are sometimes able to recall a specific incident that seemed to have triggered their problem. They may date symptoms to a fall, a collision or a lifting–twisting motion. Female athletes may have noticed onset around the time of the delivery of a baby. There is, however, the question of whether rotational malalignment usually occurs on a developmental or a traumatic

basis. The following are some of the mechanisms that may result in rotational malalignment.

Developmental

Several studies have found a high percentage of children already presenting with asymmetries before reaching their teens. Pearson (1951, 1954), undertaking progressive standing radiological studies on 830 children from 8 to 13 years of age, found some degree of pelvic obliquity in 93%. Longitudinal studies by Klein and Buckley (1968) and Klein (1973) showed an increasing prevalence of asymmetry on going from elementary (75%) to junior (86%) to senior high school (92%). One might think that the anterior and posterior innominate rotations are the result of an accumulation of minor traumas and insults. However, as Fowler had already indicated in 1986, the rotation is now thought to be 'primarily the result of muscular imbalances which secondarily restrict sacroiliac joint motion' (p. 810), a clearly identified traumatic or mechanical stress being a less frequent cause. Perhaps the 'muscular imbalance' relates to a C_1–C_2 instability or the fact that 70% of us are left and 15% right motor dominant, but this has not been established.

Combinations of bending, lifting and twisting

A particular traumatic incident or mechanical stress later in life is more likely to have made a pre-existing rotational malalignment symptomatic rather than actually having caused the malalignment. A common mechanism involves bending forward while twisting the trunk to either the right or the left side (Fig. 2.30A). The intent may be simply to pick up a piece of paper from the floor, but this often actually constitutes a combined action of forward flexion with side-bending and axial rotation of both the sacrum and the vertebrae. The onset of pain is usually acute, often felt on trying to get back to the upright position. The pain sometimes comes on more gradually over the next few

hours or even days, which may be more suggestive of injury to the ligaments and the prolonged time required for inflammation to develop because of the relatively poor blood supply to the ligaments.

Stevens (1992) postulates how a strong activation of gluteus maximus and biceps femoris on the side opposite to the lateral bending, in conjunction with the asymmetrical loading of the spine and pelvis inherent to side-bending while standing, may result in a side-to-side difference in the amount of anterior rotation possible in the SI joints. For example, with right lateral bending, anterior rotation in the SI joints is:

- restricted on the contralateral side through increased tension in the sacrotuberous ligament, in part due to contraction of muscles attaching to this ligament (e.g. gluteus medius, piriformis and the hamstrings)
- normal or possibly even increased on the ipsilateral side.

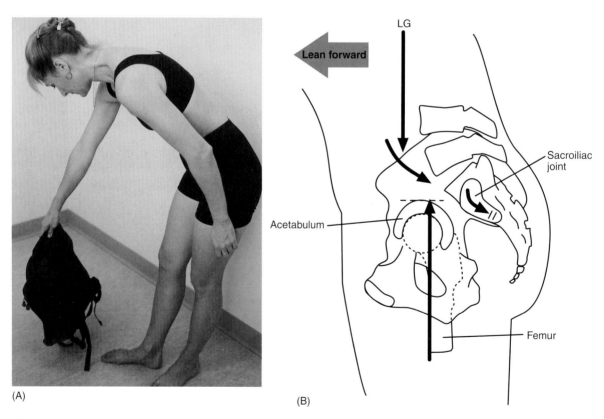

(A)   (B)

Figure 2.30 A common way of making a pre-existing rotational malalignment symptomatic. (A) Simultaneously bending forwards and twisting to the right or left (or returning back to neutral from that position), especially while hanging on to a weight. (B) When the trunk leans forwards, the line of gravity (LG) moves anteriorly, causing an anterior rotation of the pelvis around the acetabula; caudal gliding of the sacroiliac joint is impaired, relaxing the posterior pelvic ligaments and making the joint vulnerable. (After DonTigny 1990, with permission.)

DonTigny (1990) describes how, on bending forward in standing, the weight of the trunk shifts the line of gravity anterior to the acetabula and 'the innominates tend to rotate anterior and downward around the acetabula and appear to limit caudal gliding [of the sacrum]' (p. 483; Fig. 2.30B). In this position, the SI joints become vulnerable: the posterior SI joint ligaments are now in a relaxed position, and the anterior ligaments never do offer much support at the best of times (see Fig. 2.2):

Because the sacrum is placed within the innominates and is wider anteriorly, when the innominates move anteriorly and downward on the sacrum the innominates tend to spread on the sacrum. On reaching their limit of motion, they may wedge and become fixed in the anterior position. There is no problem when the spine and the innominates flex anteriorly at the same rate, or if the spine flexes prior to the innominates. Dysfunction occurs when the innominate bones rotate anteriorly prior to flexion of the spine, or if the innominates lag and the spine extends prior to posterior rotation of the innominates. (DonTigny 1990, p. 485)

The spasm of specific muscles could also result in wedging of the bones of the pelvis in an abnormal position. For example, iliacus and piriformis, which normally contract to stabilize the SI joint on the weight-bearing side, could go into spasm so that the innominate on that side becomes stuck in an anteriorly rotated position relative to the sacrum (Fig. 2.31). Iliacus would have the effect of rotating the innominate anteriorly and wedging it against the widening sacrum. Piriformis could rotate the sacrum posteriorly, in effect wedging it against the innominate as the latter is attempting to rotate forward. However, as Grieve (1988) has pointed out, and as noted in the discussion in Chapter 3:

sacroiliac sprain and pelvic torsion are so often associated with spasm or tightness of the piriformis that it is difficult to decide whether sacroiliac dysfunction is primary or secondary to piriformis overactivity. (p. 177)

Rotatory forces acting on an innominate

Forces can act directly on the innominates to cause excessive anterior or posterior rotation relative to the sacrum. This may result in a partial-to-complete impairment of movement between the sacrum and ilium. Such unilateral rotational forces can result in three ways.

Leverage effect of a lower extremity (Fig. 2.32). Excessive leverage can result on one or other innominate with passive movements of the femur, either deliberate or such as may occur in sports and during surgical, obstetric and gynaecological procedures (Grieve 1976). There comes a point on passive right hip extension, for example, at which movement of the femur independent of the ipsilateral innominate reaches its physiological limit (Fig. 2.32B). From there on, further passive hip extension will result in movement of the right femur and innominate together. The femur is now acting as a lever to rotate the innominate anteriorly. Similarly, pulling the thigh onto the chest to flex the hip will eventually engage the hip socket and cause the innominate to rotate posteriorly (Fig. 2.32A).

It is for this reason that stretches involving unilateral hip flexion are best avoided on the side of a previously corrected posterior innominate rotation during the initial period of treatment of a rotational malalignment disorder, for fear of precipitating a recurrence of the posterior rotation. Conversely, the same manoeuvre may be useful to effect the correction of an anterior rotation (see Figs 7.16, 7.17 and 7.18).

Direct rotatory force applied to an innominate. The application of specific forces, either as part of a treatment regimen or with a fall or collision, can result in innominate rotation. The axis of rotation of the sacrum is around the mean transverse axis, passing through the point at which the two parts of the L-shaped sacral articulating surfaces meet, at about the level of S2, whereas the axis of rotation of the wings of the ilia is around the inferior transverse axis, passing though the inferior pole of the sacral articulating surfaces (Richard 1986; Fig. 2.33).

Anterior rotational forces on the innominate result when:

- an anterior force is applied to its posterior aspect above the level of the inferior transverse axis (e.g. posterior iliac crest)
- a posterior force is applied to its anterior aspect below the level of the inferior transverse axis (e.g. the anterior or superior aspect of the pubic bone).

Posterior rotational forces on the innominate result when:

- a posterior force is applied to its anterior aspect above the level of the inferior transverse axis (e.g. anterior iliac crest)
- an anterior force is exerted on its posterior aspect below the level of the inferior transverse axis (e.g. ischial tuberosity).

Forces acting on a lower extremity. An impact to a lower extremity can affect the innominate if the force is transmitted upwards through the hip joint. A rotational force results if the femur is at an angle relative to the innominate at the time of impact: anterior rotation if the hip joint is in a flexed position, posterior if the joint is in extension. Typical examples include:

- falling forward and landing on one knee
- coming down hard on one extremity while the trunk is lurched either forwards or backwards, such as on

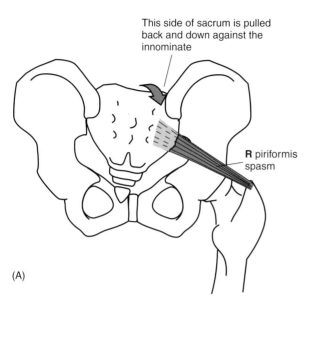

This side of sacrum is pulled back and down against the innominate

R piriformis spasm

(A)

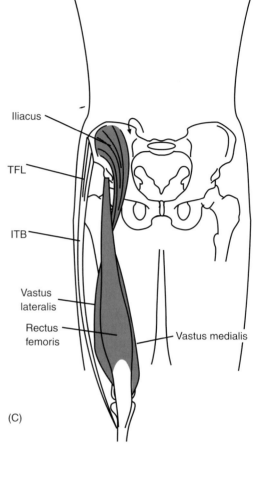

Iliacus

TFL

ITB

Vastus lateralis

Rectus femoris

Vastus medialis

(C)

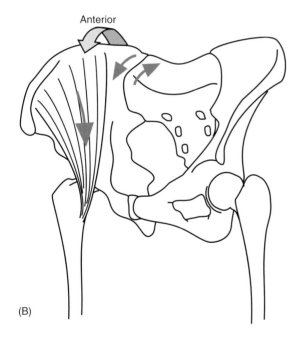

Anterior

(B)

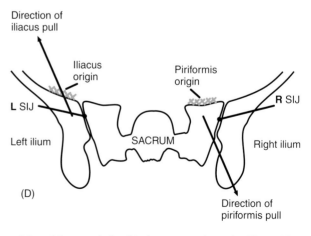

Direction of iliacus pull

Iliacus origin

Piriformis origin

L SIJ

R SIJ

Left ilium

SACRUM

Right ilium

(D)

Direction of piriformis pull

Figure 2.31 Stabilization of the sacroiliac joint (SIJ) through wedging of the anteriorly widening sacrum (see also Figs 2.2B and 2.10C). (A) Piriformis pulling the sacrum backwards against the innominate. (B) Iliacus pulling the innominate forwards against the sacrum. (C) Anterior innominate rotation through the action of iliacus, rectus femoris and the tensor fascia lata/iliotibial band complex. (D) Wedging effect viewed from the top of the joint.

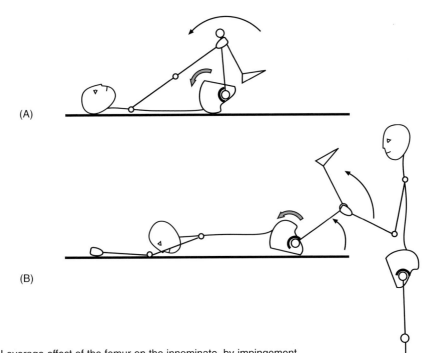

Figure 2.32 Leverage effect of the femur on the innominate, by impingement against the acetabular rim (see also Figs 7.16–7.18). (A) Against anterior rim: results in posterior rotation. (B) Against posterior rim: results in anterior rotation.

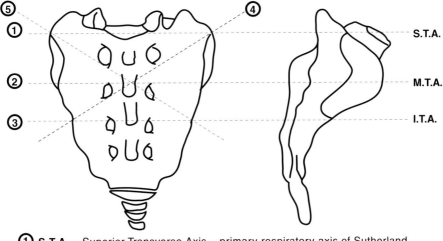

① **S.T.A.** = Superior Transverse Axis – primary respiratory axis of Sutherland

② **M.T.A.** = Mean Transverse Axis – axis of rotation of the sacrum in respect to the ilia

③ **I.T.A.** = Inferior Transverse Axis – axis of rotation of the ilia in respect to the sacrum, at the inferior aspect of the SI joint

④ Right Oblique Axis

⑤ Left Oblique Axis

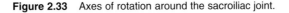

Figure 2.33   Axes of rotation around the sacroiliac joint.

an uneven dismount in gymnastics, an asymmetrical landing following a jump, or simply missing a step when going down a staircase
- the impact transmitted through an extended lower extremity on hitting against the wall in the luge, or while jammed against the floorboards of a crashing bobsled or toboggan
- the impact of a collision absorbed by the foot pushing on the clutch or brake of a vehicle (Fig. 2.34) or by the knee hitting the dashboard.

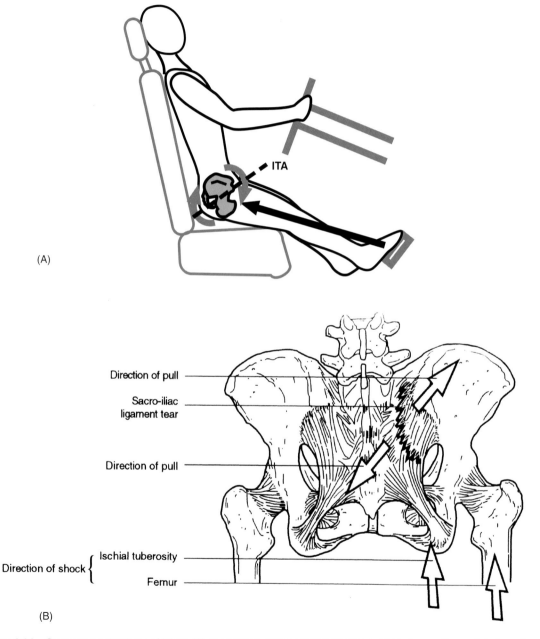

(A)

(B)

Direction of pull

Sacro-iliac ligament tear

Direction of pull

Direction of shock { Ischial tuberosity

Femur

Figure 2.34 Common mechanisms of injury. (A) In an automobile accident: the force, impacting on the acetabulum at an angle below the inferior transverse axis (ITA) (see Fig. 2.33), results in anterior rotation of the right innominate. (B) In a fall: forcing the leg upwards or landing on the ischial tuberosity can shear the ligaments between the sacrum and ilium.

The author is reminded of an athlete who initially presented with 'right anterior, left posterior' innominate rotation, and the right anterior superior iliac spine (ASIS) prominent because of counterclockwise rotation of the pelvis in the transverse plane. Two weeks later she was found to be in perfect alignment without having had any form of treatment in the interval. She recalled having recently tripped, landing initially on both knees, her trunk then being flung forward. In the process, she had seemingly effected a correction, either by exerting a left anterior or a right posterior rotational force through a femur on hitting the ground, or perhaps by way of reflex muscle contractions. Trauma can obviously work both ways!

Asymmetrical forces exerted by the spine, pelvis or legs

Torsion of the sacrum and rotation of the innominates can result from abnormal forces being transmitted to these bones from the spine, pelvic floor or lower extremities.

Spine. Excessive rotation of vertebrae from C1 down to L5 can result in forces capable of causing malalignment of the pelvis. These forces include a reactive asymmetrical increase in muscle tension and/or direct torsion and traction forces. A rotation of L4 or L5, for example, is a well-recognized cause of recurrent torsion of the sacrum and secondary malalignment of the innominates (Beal 1982, Kirkaldy-Willis & Cassidy 1985, Richard 1986).

A right (clockwise) rotation of the body of L4 or L5 results in a posterior movement of the right transverse processes, and with it the origins of the attaching iliolumbar ligaments (see Fig. 2.2A). This movement increases the tension in these ligaments, and creates a posterior rotational force on the right ilium by way of their insertions into the posterior iliac crest (Fig. 2.35A). The simultaneous anterior movement of the left transverse processes increases tension in the left iliolumbar ligaments and creates an anterior rotational force on the left ilium.

A rotation of L5 to the right also brings the surfaces of the left L5–S1 facet joint increasingly closer together. Once these surfaces have been maximally compressed, the facet joint on this side starts to act as a fulcrum so that any further rotation of L5 will now cause torsion of the sacrum around the right oblique axis (Fig. 2.35B). A rotation of L4 can have a similar effect, with compression of the left L4–5 facet surfaces eventually working as a fulcrum to rotate first L5 and then the sacrum in succession.

In these cases, treatment that corrects the malaligned lumbar vertebra(e) may automatically allow the pelvic bones to rotate back into alignment.

Pelvic floor. The components of the levator ani muscle constitute a major part of the pelvic floor (Fig. 2.36):

- *puborectalis* and *pubococcygeus*, originating from the pubic bone and anterior obturator fascia
  - puborectalis, running posteriorly to form a muscular sling by uniting at the anorectal flexure with its partner from the opposite side
  - pubococcygeus, attaching posteriorly to the midline raphe or anococcygeal body, running from the rectum to the coccyx
- *ilio-* and *ischiococcygeus*, arising from the ischial spine, posterior obturator fascia and sacrospinous ligament, and inserting posteriorly into the lowest part of the sacrum.

These various attachments of the levator ani muscles directly to parts of the pelvis, or indirectly by way of their ligamentous or fascial connections, puts them in a strategic position to influence alignment. For example, any asymmetry of tension in these muscles caused by irritation of the pelvic floor from a unilateral ovarian cyst, uterine fibroid or other mass can result in recurrent malalignment of the sacrococcygeal joint, the innominates relative to each other, the sacrum and secondarily the spine.

Lower extremities. Any condition that results in a lower extremity exerting an asymmetrical torquing force on a hip joint can in turn cause a rotational malalignment as the force is transmitted, in succession, to the innominate, the SI joint, the sacrum and finally the lumbosacral junction. Torquing forces of this kind can result from:

- asymmetrical weight-bearing with a leg length discrepancy or from a painful condition involving a lower extremity
- unilateral or asymmetrical muscle tightness or contracture, for example:
  - a rotational force exerted on the innominate bone by a tight rectus femoris by way of its origin from the anterior inferior iliac spine (AIIS), or a tight tensor fascia lata by way of its origin from the ASIS
  - a tight biceps femoris, either directly, by way of its attachments to the ischial tuberosity, or indirectly, through continuations with the sacrotuberous ligament (Fig. 2.37; see also Fig. 2.4)
- asymmetrical forces created by contracture or scarring of the fascia that envelops the muscles of the hip girdle and thigh, with its extensive connections to the hip joint capsule and ligaments, the pelvis itself and proximally to the thoracolumbar and anterior abdominal fascia.

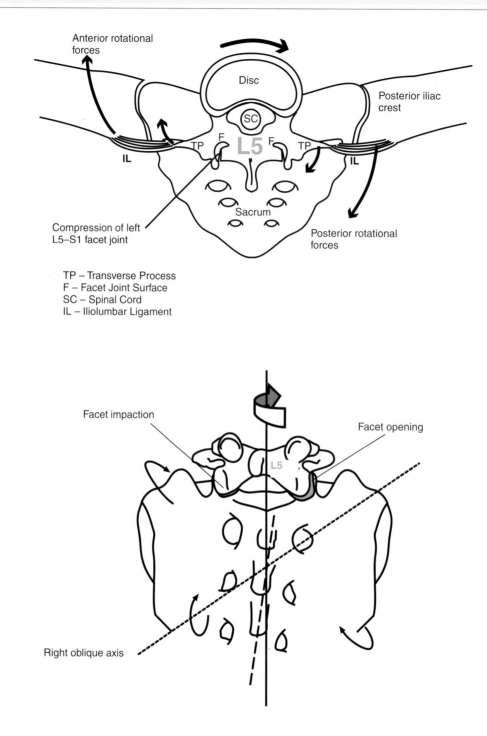

Anterior rotational forces

Disc

Posterior iliac crest

SC

TP F **L5** F TP

IL IL

Compression of left L5–S1 facet joint

Sacrum

Posterior rotational forces

TP – Transverse Process
F – Facet Joint Surface
SC – Spinal Cord
IL – Iliolumbar Ligament

(A)

Facet impaction

Facet opening

L5

Right oblique axis

(B)

Figure 2.35 Rotational effect on the innominates caused by right axial (clockwise) rotation of the L5 vertebral complex. (A) Right posterior and left anterior innominate rotation as a result of increased tension in the iliolumbar ligaments as these are being pulled backwards on the right and forwards on the left. (B) Rotation of the sacrum around the right oblique axis as a result of compression (impaction) of the left L5–S1 facet joint. IL, iliolumbar ligament; TP, transverse process; F, facet joint surface; SC, spinal cord.

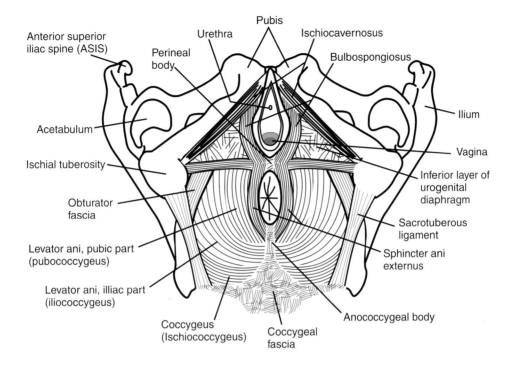

Figure 2.36 The female pelvic floor muscles and ligaments. (After Travell & Simons 1992, with permission.)

Myofascial contracture

Contracture or lengthening of the fascia, muscles, ligaments and capsules is one of the major long-term complications of any type of malalignment and a frequent cause of the recurrence, and possibly also the initial occurrence, of that malalignment. It is the nature of soft tissues to contract when placed in a shortened position and to lengthen when put under increased tension for prolonged periods of time.

Contracture can occur actively (e.g. as a result of the shortening induced by a chronic increase in muscle tension) or passively (e.g. wherever the origin and insertion are moved closer together). Alternatively, these tissues can undergo lengthening when subjected actively or passively to a chronic increase in tension, such as can occur when an origin and insertion are moved further apart. The myofascial tissue on the relatively shortened concave side of a lumbar curve will, for example, contract, whereas that on the lengthened convex side will elongate with time (Fig. 2.38).

Myofascial tissue that is constantly in some state of contraction will eventually undergo some reorganization. The end stage is a gradual replacement of the muscle element with an increasing amount of connective tissues.

Failure to treat myofascial contractures has been identified as one of the main factors responsible for the recurrence of malalignment following a realignment of the bony elements of the pelvis and spine (Shaw 1992). Recurrence may, however, also be attributable to connective tissue lengthening that has resulted in joint instability.

Contractures are often to blame for some of the new aches and pains that athletes frequently report during the first 2–4 weeks following realignment, as the tight tissues are put under tension until they finally regain their normal length.

SACROILIAC JOINT UPSLIP AND DOWNSLIP

The degrees of freedom of the SI joint normally allow for approximately 2 degrees of upward and downward (craniocaudal) translation of an innominate relative to the sacrum (Grant's Atlas 1980). Excessive upward or downward movement can result in the fixation of an innominate relative to the sacrum in what are referred to as an SI joint 'upslip' and 'downslip' respectively.

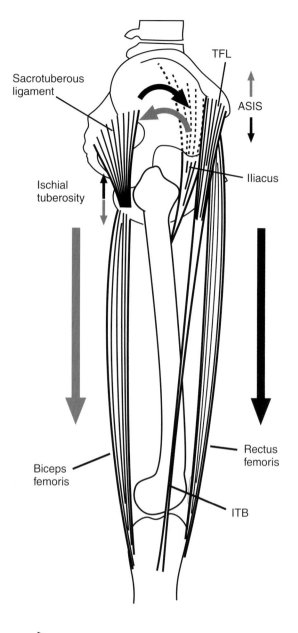

Sacrotuberous ligament

TFL

ASIS

Iliacus

Ischial tuberosity

Biceps femoris

Rectus femoris

ITB

➡ = anterior force or counternutation from rectus femoris, iliacus and TFL/ITB complex

➡ = posterior force or nutation from hamstrings (especially biceps femoris) and connections to a tight sacrotuberous ligament.

Figure 2.37 Torquing forces on the innominate caused by tightness in the attaching muscles or ligaments (see Figs 2.31B and C for an anterior view). ASIS, anterior superior iliac spine.

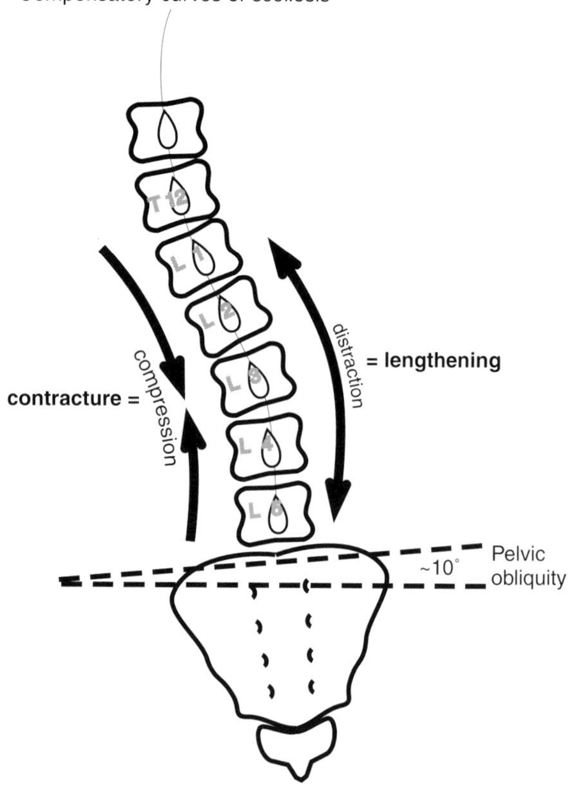

Compensatory curves or scoliosis

T12

L

L

L

L

L

contracture = | compression

distraction | = lengthening

~10° | Pelvic obliquity

Figure 2.38 Myofascial contracture and lengthening related to spinal concavity and convexity respectively.

Sacroiliac joint upslip

> Upslip:
> - occurs considerably less often than rotational malalignment (about 10–20% versus 80%)
> - may coexist with a rotational malalignment (5–10%) or an outflare/inflare

The more obvious causes of upslip include traumatic upward forces transmitted:

- through the leg to the acetabulum, with the knee straight and the hip joint in a relatively neutral position (Fig. 2.39) so that the leg does not exert a rotational force on the innominate, a situation that might occur, for example, when:
  - the foot is jammed against the floorboards of a crashing car, bobsled or other vehicle (see Fig. 2.34A)
  - landing hard on an extended extremity in a fall, on a dismount or on missing a step (see Fig. 2.34B)

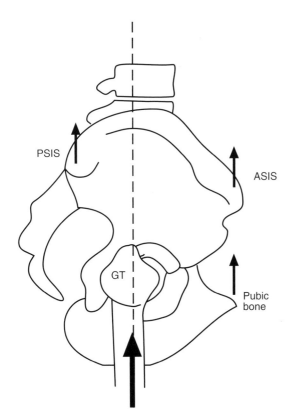

Figure 2.39 Upslip caused by a unilateral upward force transmitted to the innominate through the acetabulum. ASIS, anterior superior iliac spine; GT, greater trochanter; PSIS, posterior superior iliac spine.

- straight upwards through the innominate itself, such as on falling and landing directly on the ischial tuberosity on one side to cause a shear injury (see Fig. 2.34B).

However, more subtle forces relating primarily to an imbalance of the hip girdle muscles can also cause an upslip to occur initially and are probably the main cause for its recurrence. Typical of these is a unilateral increase in tension involving quadratus lumborum, latissimus dorsi, psoas major/minor (Fig. 2.40), the external and internal abdominal obliques (see Figs 2.24B, C) or a combination of these muscles.

As with rotational malalignment, an upslip causes a specific pattern of pelvic ring distortion. Appendix 2 gives the examination findings typically seen with the less common right SI joint upslip; these findings are detailed below in the discussion of 'Establishing the diagnosis of malalignment'.

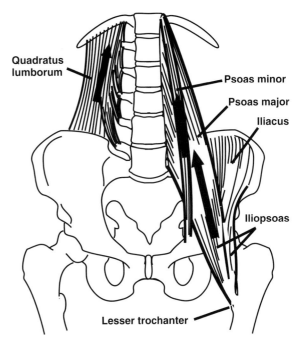

Figure 2.40 Muscles capable of generating forces (arrows) that can result in an upslip.

Sacroiliac joint downslip

Downslip occurs rarely and is frequently missed. Typically, there is a history of excessive traction on an extremity. Examples of this mechanism include:

- incidents where the athlete is hurled forward while one leg remains tethered, such as occurs with the failure of one ski binding to release, or the entrapment of one foot in the toe straps of a crashing bicycle or the stirrups while horse-riding
- trying rapidly to extract an extremity that has sunk into a hole, for example a foot suddenly stuck deep in mud on a boggy running trail.

Downslip is usually misdiagnosed initially as an upslip of the opposite SI joint. It is often only when measures aimed at the correction of the 'upslip' repeatedly fail that the therapist begins to suspect that the problem is actually a downslip on the opposite side, and appropriate treatment is instituted.

PELVIC OUTFLARE AND INFLARE

'Outflare' and 'inflare' refer to movement of the innominates outwards and inwards respectively in the transverse plane (see Figs 2.10 and 2.14). Normal outflare and inflare have invariably been linked to simultaneous movements of the innominates in the sagittal plane, but there are different descriptions offered of how and why this should happen:

1. *Outflare linked to anterior rotation*: as previously described (DonTigny 1990), the anterior widening of the sacrum causes the innominates to 'spread on the sacrum' or flare out whenever the innominates rotate anteriorly and downward relative to the sacrum; the same will occur with counternutation of the sacrum. Inflare will occur with a posterior rotation of the innominates relative to the sacrum, and with sacral nutation.

2. *Outflare linked to posterior rotation*: the posteriorly rotating innominates are described as gliding medially because of the posterior narrowing of the sacrum, causing the pelvis to open anteriorly; the same occurs with sacral nutation (see Fig. 2.14B). Inflare will occur with anterior rotation and with sacral counternutation (JS Gerhardt, personal communication, 1999).

Other facts to appreciate when considering pathological outflare and inflare include the following. First, outflare and inflare can actually exist in isolation. Movement in the transverse plane can occur in these directions, without coexisting rotation or upslip, and excessive movement can result in fixation in an outflare or an inflare position. For example, reversal of the convex-concave relationship, with a concave ilial and convex sacral surface, allows for innominate rotation medially or laterally around a vertical axis which could result in inflare or outflare dysfunction, respectively (Greenman 1990).

Second, when rotational malalignment is present, an outflare can be seen on the side of the anterior innominate rotation, and a seemingly compensatory inflare on the side of the posterior rotation. However, the reverse findings of an inflare associated with anterior, and an outflare with posterior, rotation also occur.

Finally, tightness or adhesions in the surrounding tissues may determine whether an outflare or inflare occurs with rotation. For example:

- Adhesions and/or scar tissue formation in the lower posterior pelvic ligaments (around the S3 level) or the long (dorsal) sacroiliac ligament, or involving the posterior hip joint capsule or ligaments, would tend to hold the posterior aspect of the innominate medially and predispose to outflaring on posterior innominate rotation while preventing inflaring on anterior rotation.
- Increased tension in iliacus or sartorius predisposes to inflaring on anterior rotation.

The umbilicus and the gluteal cleft conveniently demarcate the anterior and posterior midline respectively. If a right outflare and left inflare are present, the right ASIS will have moved outwards and the left inwards relative to the umbilicus (see Figs 2.10 Ai & ii; Bi); whereas the right posterior superior iliac spine (PSIS) will have moved inwards and the left outwards relative to the gluteal cleft (see Figs 2.10Aii & iii; Ci).

Correlation of the PSIS to the gluteal cleft is, however, more likely to be accurate, given that the umbilicus is frequently 'off centre' pre- and post-partum and as a result of previous surgery and visceral adhesions. In addition, the umbilicus frequently appears in the centre when an outflare/inflare is actually present, probably as a result of having been pulled towards the side of the outflare by the transversus abdominis muscle being put under increased tension (whereas those on the side of the inflare relax). An even easier, and probably more accurate, way of determining outflare and inflare is shown in Box 2.2.

The recognition of outflare and inflare is important from a treatment perspective in that:

1. they can result in specific clinical problems relating to altered biomechanics, stress being placed particularly on the SI joints, hip joints and surrounding soft tissues (see Ch. 3)
2. rotational malalignment and upslip may resist treatment efforts using the muscle energy technique until a coexisting outflare or inflare has been corrected (see Ch. 7)
3. correction attempts aimed at the outflare and inflare first are successful in simultaneously correcting a coexisting upslip and/or rotational malalignment in over 90% of cases.

Box 2.2   Determining inflare and outflare

Look for a change in the relative height of:

- the anterior superior iliac spine in the supine position, down and out with outflare and up and in with inflare; remember, however, that the height will also be affected by rotational malalignment, the anterior superior iliac spine rotating forwards and down with anterior, and backwards and up with posterior rotation
- the **posterior superior iliac spine** in the prone position, up and inwards with outflare and down and outwards with inflare; this is a more accurate way of determining outflare/inflare even if rotational malalignment is present.

ESTABLISHING THE DIAGNOSIS OF MALALIGNMENT

The initial step in the diagnosis of malalignment is to establish whether asymmetry is present and, if so, whether it is caused by an anatomical leg length difference, a form of pelvic malalignment, vertebral malrotation or a combination of these.

Examination is preferably carried out on a firm, even surface. Sitting or lying on a soft or sagging support, or across a break in the surface, may affect the assessment and lead to incorrect conclusions. If the reader is interested in carrying out manipulations or mobilization procedures other than the simple techniques presented in this text, a more detailed determination of the type of pelvic and spine malalignment present is of the utmost importance. Such a detailed determination is, however, not usually necessary in order to apply the material presented here to the clinical setting. Advanced assessment and treatment techniques are best learned in a formal teaching setting, hands-on workshops and from selected papers, books and videos (e.g. Aitken 1986, Bernard & Cassidy 1991; DonTigny 1990, Fowler 1986, Lee 1998, 1999, Lee & Walsh 1996, Richard 1986, Vleeming et al 1997, Wells 1986b).

Box 2.3 outlines the basic questions to be answered by the examination.

Box 2.3   Examination for pelvic malalignment

1. Is the pelvis level or oblique?
2. Are the bony landmarks of the pelvis symmetrical or asymmetrical?
3. What happens on the sitting–lying test (described in detail below)?
4. Is there any sacral torsion or excessive nutation or counternutation of the sacrum?
5. Is there an obvious curvature of the spine (e.g., a scoliosis) and/or any excessive rotation of isolated vertebrae?
6. Is there any gapping and/or displacement of the symphysis pubis?
7. Is there any increase in tension and/or tenderness localizing to specific muscles and ligaments?
8. What are the findings on sacroiliac joint and pelvic girdle testing for:
   – function, motion/mobility and stability
   – form and force closure?
9. Is the basic neurological and vascular examination normal?

PELVIC OBLIQUITY

The presence or absence of pelvic obliquity may become obvious from what are sometimes very easily apparent dimples of Venus on the buttocks, about 1 cm above the PSIS (Fig. 2.41A). A more accurate examination relies on a comparison of the relative height of the index and/or middle fingers lying on the lateral iliac crests (Fig. 2.41B), or the thumbs or index fingers resting on the pubic bones (Fig. 2.41C), or hugging against the lower part of the ASIS (Fig. 2.41D), PSIS (Fig. 2.41B) or of the ischial tuberosities (Fig. 2.41F). Aspects of the sacrum, such as the inferior lateral angle (Fig. 2.41G) and sacral sulci (see Fig. 2.56), and a comparison of the highest point of the ASIS and PSIS in the supine and prone positions (see Fig. 2.10A) may also prove helpful.

In *standing*:

- If the pelvis is level, this suggests (but does not confirm) equal leg length (Fig. 2.41B and 2.42A).
- If the pelvis is oblique, there may be an anatomical (true) or functional lengthening of the leg on the elevated side (Figs 2.42B and 2.43).

In *sitting and lying* supine or prone, if the pelvis is now level, this suggests an anatomical leg length difference (LLD) as the cause of any obliquity noted in standing; if that were so, the LLD would still be evident in prone and supine lying, but all the pelvic landmarks would be symmetrical (see Fig. 2.42B). If the pelvic obliquity persists while sitting, with the iliac crest elevated on the same side as in standing, pelvic malalignment is probably present (Fig. 2.43A–D; see also Fig. 2.46B); a less likely cause is an actual difference in the height of the innominates (see Fig. 3.80). If the pelvic obliquity persists, but with the iliac crest now higher on the side opposite to that noted in standing, malalignment is even more likely to be present to account for such a change. The pelvis remains level in the presence of an outflare and inflare alone.

BONY LANDMARKS OF THE PELVIS

In practice, assessment using the pelvic landmarks may not be entirely accurate because of muscle imbalance, congenital or acquired side-to-side differences of bony contours, or a unilateral tendency to pronation or supination when weight-bearing.

Attempts to establish the presence or absence of malalignment must never be limited to the assessment of landmarks alone but should be supplemented by the findings on assessment of pelvic obliquity and leg length in various positions.

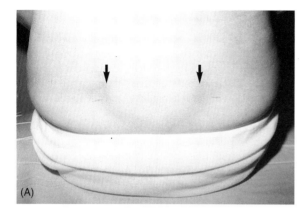

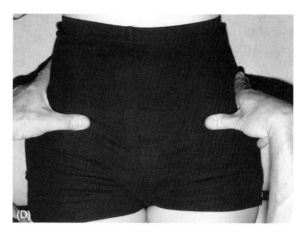

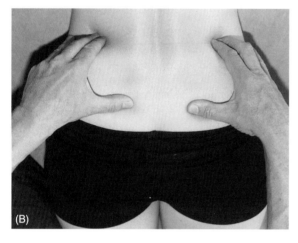

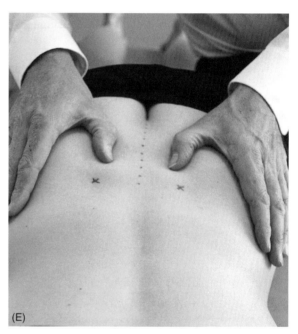

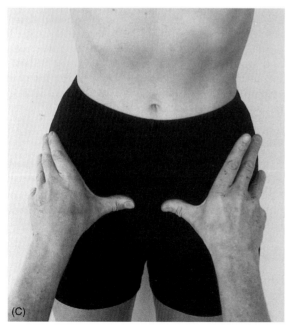

Figure 2.41 Landmarks when the pelvis is aligned and the leg length equal. (A) Dimples of Venus, about 1 cm above the inner margin of the posterior superior iliac spine (PSIS). (B) Fingers on the iliac crests, thumbs against the inferior aspect of the PSIS. (C) Superior pubic bones (thumbs resting on the superior aspect). (D) Anterior superior iliac spine (thumbs resting against the inferior aspect). (E) PSIS (thumbs resting against the inner aspect, equidistant from the midline). (F) Ischial tuberosities. (G) Inferior lateral angle at the S5 level. (Figs 2.41F and G: from Lee & Walsh 1996, with permission.)

Fig. 2.41 (F) & (G), see opposite

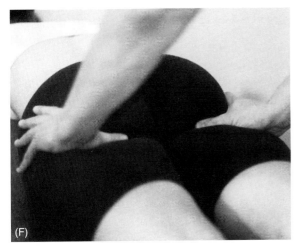
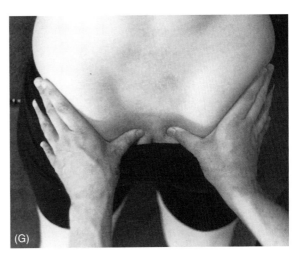

Figure 2.41 *Continued.*

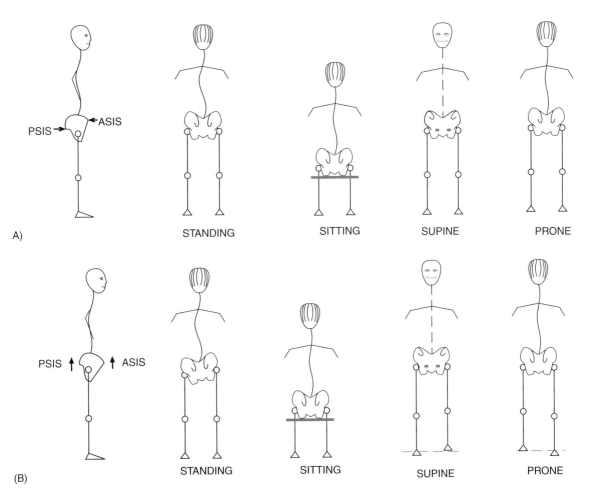

Figure 2.42 Effect of leg length on the aligned pelvis. (A) Aligned: leg length equal. (B) Aligned: an anatomically long right leg (the pelvis level sitting and lying). ASIS, anterior superior iliac spine.

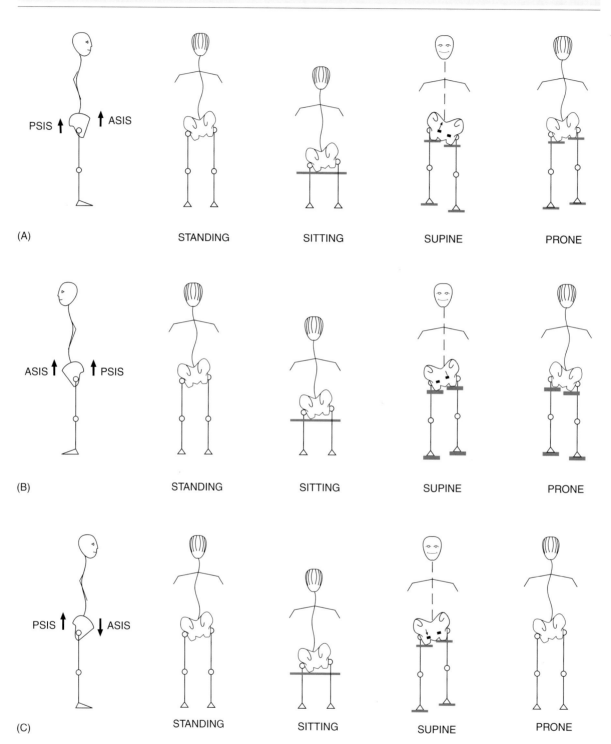

Figure 2.43 Pelvic obliquity related to malalignment (some typical presentations). (A) Right upslip (all right pelvic landmarks up in all positions). (B) Left upslip (right pelvis usually up standing and sitting, left up lying). (C) Right anterior rotation (one common presentation). (D) Left anterior rotation (one common presentation). ASIS, anterior superior iliac spine.

Fig. 2.43(D), see opposite

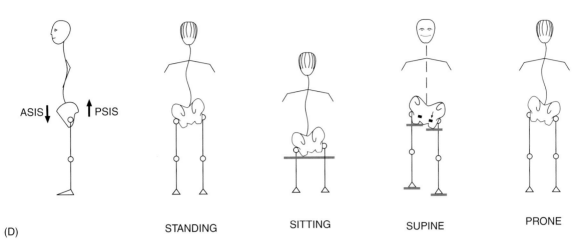

(D)   STANDING   SITTING   SUPINE   PRONE

Figure 2.43 *Continued.*

In alignment and with leg length equal (see Figs 2.41 and 2.42A)

The iliac crests will be level when standing, sitting, and lying prone or supine.

The right and left ASIS and PSIS will be level during standing, sitting and lying. On a lateral view, the ASIS is positioned upwards relative to the PSIS approximately the same amount on both sides.

The right and left superior and inferior pubic rami are level when lying supine or standing (see Fig. 2.41C), the ischial tuberosities level in lying prone or standing (see Fig. 2.41F).

The right and left ASIS will be level in the transverse plane when standing, sitting or lying supine. That is, there is no rotation of the pelvis clockwise or counterclockwise that would bring one ASIS forwards and the other backwards.

In alignment, with an anatomically long leg

Only in standing are all landmarks elevated on the side of the long leg, with a uniform obliquity of the pelvic crests and superior pubic rami on clinical examination (see Fig. 2.42B). A standing anteroposterior X-ray of the pelvis shows:

- a uniform obliquity of the sacrum and superior pubic bones, with no displacement of the right and left pubic bones relative to each other
- a difference in the height of the femoral heads, which is the true LLD (Fig. 2.44A).

Sacroiliac joint upslip

There is a simultaneous elevation of all the pelvic landmarks on the side of the upslip. One is not, however, dealing with a simple upward tilt of the pelvis as occurs with an anatomically long leg, but with an actual upward translation of all the landmarks relative to the other side.

Right upslip. There is an upward displacement of the right ASIS, AIIS, pubic rami and PSIS (see Fig. 2.43A). The right superior pubic ramus is raised by 3–5 mm relative to the left one; this can be appreciated as a step deformity at the symphysis pubis on palpation and on X-ray. The right leg is pulled upwards with the right innominate, so that it appears to be shorter than the left leg when the athlete is lying prone or supine (see Fig. 2.43A). The shortening usually amounts to some 5–10 mm. In standing, however, the iliac crest is elevated on the side of the upslip so that the right leg appears to be the longer one in that position. In fact, the elevation of the right iliac crest persists during sitting and lying, and is in part due to the associated rotation of the pelvis in the frontal plane.

Left upslip. This is most easily appreciated on examination in the supine and prone positions, in which case the left leg is noted to be shortened and the left ASIS, PSIS, pubic bone and iliac crest elevated relative to the right (see Fig. 2.43B). The pelvis, however, usually appears higher on the right in standing and sitting, possibly because of a shortened left leg (in standing) and an element of pelvic rotation in the frontal plane.

Rotational malalignment

Anterior superior and posterior superior iliac spines. With anterior rotation of the innominate bone in the sagittal plane, the PSIS moves upward (cephalad) and the ASIS and pubic bone move downwards (caudad).

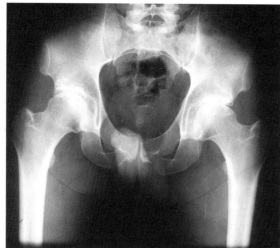

(A)

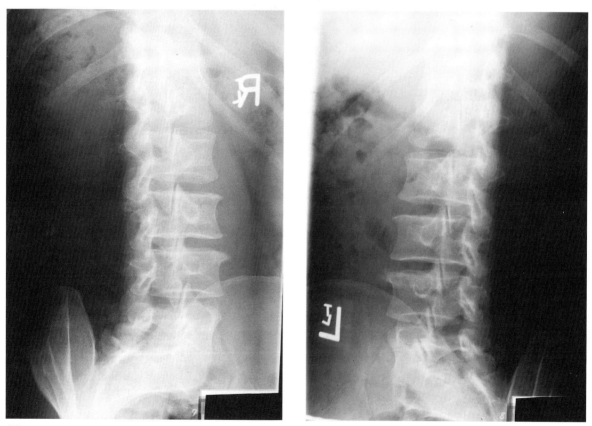

(Bi)

(Bii)

Figure 2.44 X-ray of a standing athlete with anatomical (true) leg length difference – right leg long. (A) Posteroanterior view: right femoral head higher than left; note the uniform obliquity of the superior pubic rami and the almost symmetrical appearance of the sacroiliac joints and lesser trochanters. (B) (i) Right and (ii) left oblique views: the facet joints appear to be of uniform width except for right L4–L5, narrowed by what appear to be osteoarthritic changes.

With posterior rotation, the PSIS moves downwards and the ASIS and pubic bone upwards. The anterior or posterior rotation of one innominate is usually compensated for by the contrary rotation of the opposite innominate, which has the effect of amplifying the asymmetry. One can usually make the diagnosis of rotational malalignment on the basis of this complete asymmetry of the ASIS and PSIS (see Figs 2.29, 2.43C, D and 2.46).

Pubic bones. With right anterior, left posterior innominate rotation, there will be rotation around the symphysis pubis, with the right pubic bone rotating downwards and backwards (posteriorly), and the left upwards and forwards (anteriorly). This creates a displacement at the symphysis pubis that is usually easily apparent both on clinical examination (see Fig. 2.46C) and on anteroposterior X-rays of the pelvis (Fig. 2.45).

> In other words, as a result of either anterior or posterior rotation of one innominate, all the bony landmarks of the pelvis end up completely asymmetrical in all positions of examination, both on anterior–posterior and side-to-side comparisons.

Outflare and inflare

Outflare and inflare are unlikely when the right and left ASIS are level when viewed in supine-lying and

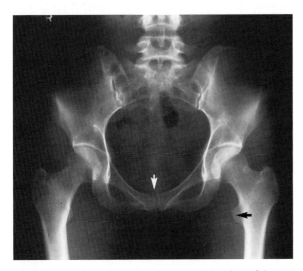

Figure 2.45 X-ray: standing anteroposterior view of the pelvis in an athlete with equal leg length and right anterior, left posterior rotational malalignment. Note the equal height of the femoral heads but the obliquity of the pelvic crests, the approximately 3 mm downward displacement of the right superior pubic ramus relative to the left at the symphysis pubis, and the apparent asymmetry of the sacroiliac joints and lesser trochanters (the left appearing larger, the right smaller – compare with Fig. 2.44).

the PSIS in prone-lying. A right ASIS lower and away from centre in the supine position, and higher and towards the centre when prone, relative to the left ASIS will, however, reflect rotation in the transverse plane, in keeping with a right outflare and left inflare (see Fig. 2.10).

The ASIS and PSIS and the pubic bones remain level on viewing the pelvis from front or back when the athlete is standing, sitting and lying prone or supine (see Fig. 2.10) and leg length also remains unchanged.

SITTING–LYING TEST

This test affords those caring for athletes, and indeed the athletes themselves, a quick way of establishing whether malalignment is actually present and, if so, whether it is a rotation, upslip or possible downslip, in order that appropriate treatment can be initiated.

Leg length is compared by noting the level of the medial malleoli in the 'long-sitting' (legs in front) and 'supine-lying' positions (Figs 2.47 and 2.48). Trying to compare the high points of the malleoli is sometimes difficult, especially if the malleoli are uneven in contour developmentally or as a result of injury, not very prominent or quite a distance apart (as occurs, for example, in the athlete with knock-knees or genu valgum). It is much easier, and more accurate, to compare the level of the thumbs placed in the hollow immediately below the medial malleolus on each side. Point the thumbs straight downwards to make the comparison more accurate. In addition, take care not to forcefully hold on to the ankles with your hands, or else the free upwards and downwards movement of the legs may be impaired.

At home, the test is best performed on a firm bed, carpeted floor or even a table: a soft bed could alter the movement of the legs by allowing the pelvis to sink into the surface unevenly. The heels must be able to slide without hindrance. If one or other heel gets caught up on the surface, it will in turn shift the pelvis on that side and make the test invalid. A sheet covering the plinth, or at least a towel placed under the heels, will prevent them getting caught up on a vinyl or leather surface; alternately, the athletes can just keep their socks on for this test. If a smooth surface is not available at home or on the field, try placing a jacket under the feet, the smooth lining facing upwards.

The athlete initially lies supine and is then asked to sit up. A shift of the pelvis or other error is less likely if one gives assistance by pulling up on the athlete's outstretched hands; when carrying this manoeuvre out

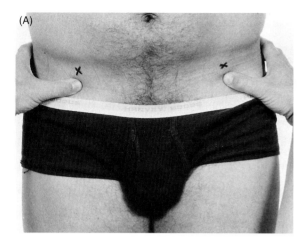

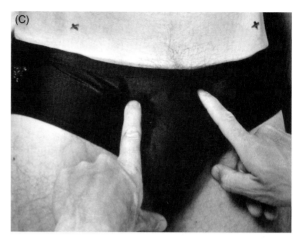

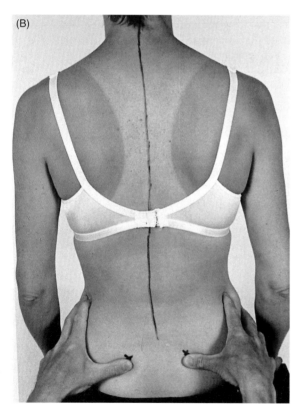

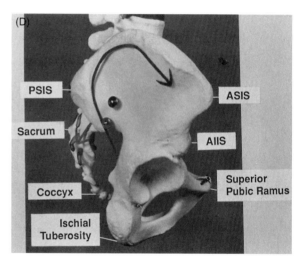

Figure 2.46 Rotational malalignment: right anterior, left posterior innominate rotation in both athletes. (A) Asymmetry of anterior superior iliac spine (ASIS) (right down, left up). (B) Asymmetry of posterior superior iliac spine (PSIS) and iliac crests (right up, left down) in standing (also in sitting – see Fig. 3.79B). (C) Right superior pubic ramus displaced downwards relative to the left. (D) Shift of the right pelvic landmarks relative to their left counterparts: right iliac crest, PSIS and ischial tuberosity move up; right ASIS, anterior inferior iliac spine and pubic ramus move down.

alone, the athlete can use a belt or rope for the same purpose (Fig. 2.49). Once the examiner has established the relative leg length, the athlete is asked to lie down, again taking care not to shift the pelvis in the process, and the comparison is repeated. The examiner also observes the direction of movement of the feet on sitting up and lying down.

Clinical correlation

Barring excessive tension or contracture in the pelvic and hip girdle structures (e.g. unilateral contracture of quadratus lumborum, or psoas major/minor pulling up on the ipsilateral innominate; see Fig. 2.40), the more common presentations on the sitting–lying test are those described below.

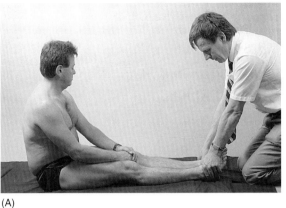
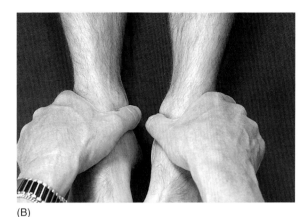

(A) (B)

Figure 2.47 Sitting part of the sitting–lying test. (A) Long-sitting. (B) Left leg longer than the right.

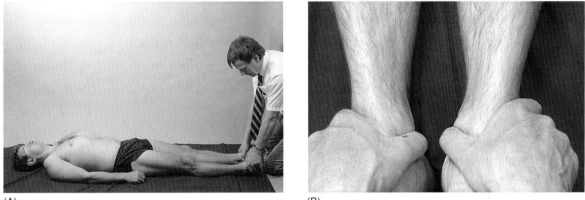

(A) (B)

Figure 2.48 Lying part of the sitting–lying test. (A) Supine-lying. (B) The right leg has lengthened relative to the left leg.

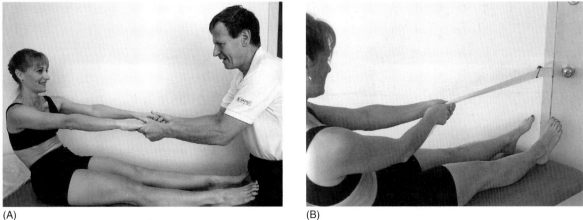

(A) (B)

Figure 2.49 Sitting–lying test: assisting sitting up to decrease error. (A) Assisted by a second person. (B) Using a strap or rope to pull up on while looking for relative leg length difference and any shift of the right versus left foot.

Aligned, leg length equal (Figs 2.50 and 2.51)

In supine-lying, the acetabula lie anteriorly and raised (craniad) relative to the ischial tuberosities (Fig. 2.50A). On moving into the long-sitting position, flexion occurs initially in the thoracic and then the lumbar spine, at which point the pelvis starts to rotate forwards and eventually pivots over the tuberosities as one unit. The acetabula are therefore moved even further anteriorly and also downwards (caudad) so that the legs appear to lengthen to an equal extent (Fig. 2.50B). On returning to

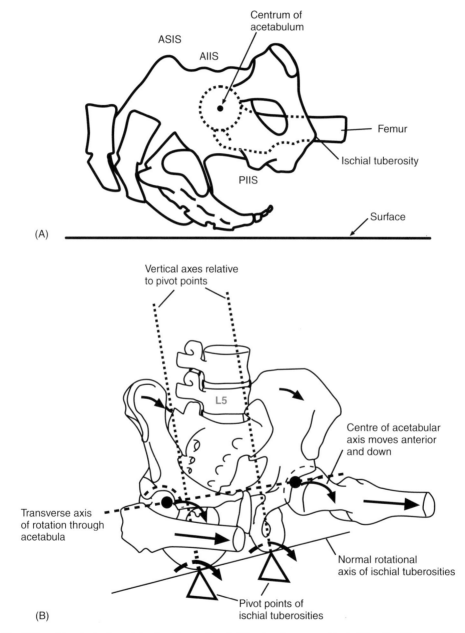

Figure 2.50 Sitting–lying test: aligned, leg length equal and all landmarks symmetrical. (After DonTigny 1997, with permission.) (A) Supine-lying: the acetabula lie anterior and craniad relative to the ischial tuberosities. (B) Moving into long-sitting: the innominates pivot over the ischial tuberosities and the acetabula move forwards and caudad, causing the legs to lengthen equally. ASIS, anterior superior inferior spine; AIIS, anterior inferior iliac spine; PIIS, posterior inferior iliac spines.

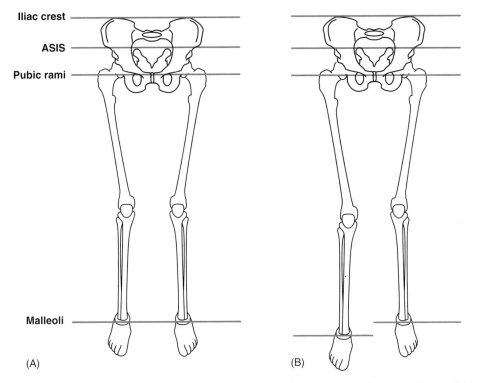

Iliac crest

ASIS

Pubic rami

Malleoli

(A)

(B)

Figure 2.51 Sitting–lying test: in alignment, the pelvic landmarks on the right match all those on the left. (A) Leg length equal: the malleoli match in sitting and lying. (B) Anatomical leg length difference: right leg longer to an equal extent in both sitting and lying. ASIS, anterior superior inferior spine.

supine-lying, the pelvis rotates backward as one unit, the acetabula are moved upwards and posteriorly, and the legs appear to shorten again to an equal extent.

The feet therefore move together: downwards as the athlete assumes the long-sitting position, upwards on supine-lying. The examiner's thumbs in the hollows just below the malleoli will match exactly in both positions (Fig. 2.51A). The pelvic landmarks are also all symmetrical when both prone and supine (see Figs 2.41 and 2.42A).

Outflare and inflare (see Fig. 2.10)

Leg movement and lengthening/shortening are as above, provided there is no LLD and/or associated upslip or rotational malalignment. In other words, the legs are of equal length and move downwards and upwards together.

Aligned, anatomical leg length difference present (Fig. 2.51B)

One leg is longer than the other (see Fig. 2.42B). The pelvis, however, still rotates forwards and backwards as

one unit on long-sitting and supine-lying respectively. Therefore, leg movement and lengthening/shortening are as in the first case above. No change occurs in the actual length of either leg, so the difference between the malleoli corresponds to the true LLD and remains the same in both positions (Fig. 2.51B). The feet move downwards and upwards together. All the pelvic landmarks are higher on the side of the long leg in standing but level when sitting and lying.

Sacroiliac joint upslip (Fig. 2.52)

With a right upslip, the right innominate is shifted upwards but not rotated relative to the sacrum (see Fig. 2.43A). The pelvis continues to move as one unit so that the legs still lengthen and shorten to an equal extent on long-sitting and supine-lying respectively. The right leg will therefore appear to be shorter in both positions by the amount of upward shift that has occurred (Fig. 2.52). Similar to the situation with an anatomical LLD, the malleoli do not match, the difference remains the same in sitting and lying, and the feet move downwards and upwards together. The anterior and posterior pelvic

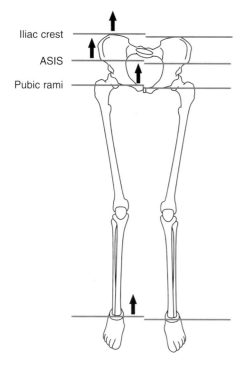

Iliac crest

ASIS

Pubic rami

Figure 2.52 Sitting–lying test: right sacroiliac joint upslip. The right leg remains short to an equal extent in sitting and lying; the anterior and posterior pelvic landmarks are all displaced upwards on the right side relative to the left. ASIS, anterior superior iliac spine.

landmarks have, however, all moved up (craniad) on the right side (see Fig. 2.43A). The findings are the reverse for a left upslip.

Sacroiliac joint downslip

In the case of a right downslip, the innominate will have moved downwards relative to the sacrum, the right leg will be consistently longer in both long-sitting and supine-lying, and all the right-side landmarks will be displaced downwards (caudad) relative to the left in both the supine and the prone position. The findings are the reverse for a left downslip.

Rotational malalignment (Fig. 2.53)

With rotational malalignment, the pelvis no longer moves as a unit because the innominate bones have rotated relative to the sacrum. When in alignment, or with an upslip present, the right and left innominates remain relatively symmetrical to the sacrum; there is no rotation around the SI joint. On sitting up and leaning forwards the pelvis continues to move as one

unit while rotating over an axis running just below the ischial tuberosities (see Fig. 2.50B). The acetabula move forwards and the two legs lengthen to an equal extent.

With right anterior, left posterior rotation, however, there is contrary rotation around the SI joints, the right acetabulum being displaced down and backwards, the left one up and forwards. The ischial tuberosities end up displaced relative to the axis running underneath them – left forward and down with posterior, right backward and up with anterior, rotation:

• When sitting up, pressure is eventually exerted on the anterior aspect of the right tuberosity, accentuating the anterior rotation and forcing all of the pelvis (and hence acetabula) to rotate in the transverse plane – backwards on the right and forwards on the left side – causing the right leg to shorten and the left leg to lengthen relative to each other.
• On lying supine, the reverse occurs so that the right leg now lengthens and the left shortens.

In other words, there is a difference in leg length that changes with a change in position. In the example above, there will be a relative lengthening of the right and shortening of the left leg on long-sitting, and a reversal of these changes on supine-lying (Fig. 2.54; see also Figs 2.47 and 2.48).

Barring any complicating factors, the leg that lengthens on moving from the long-sitting to the supine-lying position indicates the side on which the innominate has rotated anteriorly. This may be remembered by 'the rule of the 3 Ls':

Leg Lengthens on lying = side of the anterior rotation

Alternately, the rule could be:

Shortens sitting, lengthens lying *or* pulled up sitting up, pushed down lying down

The emphasis is on a 'relative' shortening and lengthening of the legs. For example, the right leg may be:

• shorter than the left in sitting but longer in lying (Fig. 2.54A)
• shorter than the left when sitting, becoming less so on lying (Fig. 2.54B)
• longer in sitting and even more so in lying (Fig. 2.54C).

In all three cases, there has been a relative lengthening of the right leg. This is consistent with a right anterior rotation, provided that there is also asymmetry of all the landmarks on both anterior-to-posterior and side-to-side comparison (see Fig. 2.46). Leg length changes and

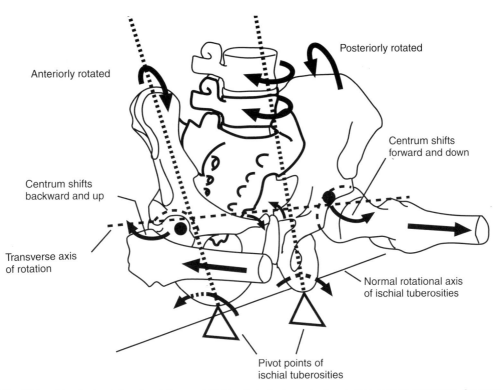

Anteriorly rotated

Posteriorly rotated

Centrum shifts
forward and down

Centrum shifts
backward and up

Transverse axis
of rotation

Normal rotational axis
of ischial tuberosities

Pivot points of
ischial tuberosities

Figure 2.53 Sitting–lying test: rotational malalignment (right anterior) – innominates pivot in contrary directions. Centrum of each acetabulum moves in an opposite direction relative to the vertical and transverse axes, causing the right leg to shorten and the left to lengthen on long-sitting; the reverse occurs on supine-lying. (After DonTigny 1997, with permission.) (See also Fig. 2.50.)

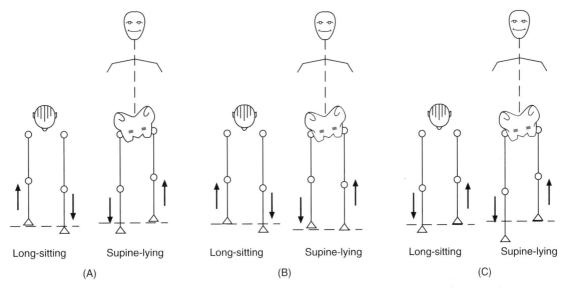

Long-sitting   Supine-lying   Long-sitting   Supine-lying   Long-sitting   Supine-lying

(A)   (B)   (C)

Figure 2.54 Sitting–lying test: rotational malalignment. Probable right anterior, left posterior innominate rotation, given the lengthening of the right leg relative to the left on moving from long-sitting to supine-lying. Note the asymmetry of the pelvic landmarks. Fig. 2.54A depicts the most common presentation. (A) The right leg is shorter sitting, longer lying. (B) The right leg is shorter sitting and still short but less so lying. (C) The right leg is longer sitting and even more so lying.

asymmetries are the reverse for a left anterior rotation (Fig. 2.55).

The true leg length will influence which leg actually ends up appearing longer or shorter in the sitting or lying position. However, the asymmetry of all the landmarks makes it impossible to discern the true length other than by a comparison of the femoral heads on a standing anterior–posterior X-ray view of the pelvis (see Figs 2.44 and 2.45). This problem is discussed in more detail under 'Functional leg length difference' in Chapter 3.

The difference in leg length noted on moving from one position to the other may be less than 5 mm or as much as 25–40 mm, most showing a change of 10–20 mm. It must again be emphasized that when carrying out the sitting–lying test, the actual length of either leg, or which leg is longer or shorter, is not what matters in the presence of a rotational malalignment. What *does matter* is that:

1. there is a relative change in leg length
2. the right foot moves in a direction opposite to that of the left

3. the side on which there is a relative lengthening of the leg on lying supine is likely to be the side of an anterior rotation, but this should always be verified by examining the landmarks
4. the pelvic landmarks all remain asymmetrical in every position of examination in the presence of an anterior or posterior rotation.

These four findings are pathognomonic of rotational malalignment. False-positive tests can occur with the sitting–lying test for a number of reasons in an athlete who is in alignment. For example, tightness of left hamstrings or gluteus maximus may impair anterior rotation of the left innominate on long-sitting. If the right innominate can still rotate anteriorly unhindered, it will cause the right leg to shorten on sitting and lengthen on lying relative to the left. This may give the false impression that there is rotational malalignment with right anterior, left posterior innominate rotation.

It is for this reason that one must always check the position of the major landmarks (ASIS and pubic rami anteriorly, PSIS posteriorly) to confirm the impression

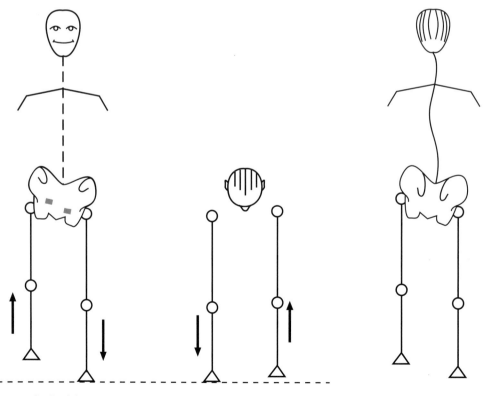

Supine-lying   Long-sitting   Prone-lying

Figure 2.55 Sitting–lying test: rotational malalignment. Probable left anterior, right posterior innominate rotation.

gained on the sitting–lying test. When one leg is short by an equal amount in both sitting and lying, a check of the landmarks is one way of differentiating a true LLD (in which all the landmarks are aligned; see Fig. 2.51B) from an upslip (in which all the landmarks are raised on the side of the upslip; see Fig. 2.52).

In order to reduce error, try to carry out the assessment of the landmarks in the same way each time, following the procedure outlined in Box 2.4.

Which eye is dominant can usually be established quite easily:

1. Hold an index finger up in front of you so that it overlies a mark, sign or other object some 6–10 m away.
2. Close your left eye, leaving the right one open:
   - if your index finger continues to overlie the object, you are probably right-eye dominant
   - if your index finger moves away from the object, see what happens when you now close your right eye and leave the left open: if the finger continues to overlie the object, you are probably left-eye dominant.
3. If your finger shifts away from the object on closing either eye, consider your 'more dominant' eye to be the one that leads to the lesser amount of shift when open.

Therefore, if you are right-eye dominant:

- approach the athlete with your right – from his or her right when lying supine, left when prone

---

Box 2.4 Assessing the anatomical landmarks

1. Whenever possible, face the athlete's front or back directly (see, for example, Figs 2.46A, B, C, 2.62 and 2.64)
2. If this is not possible, try to approach the athlete so that you can place your dominant eye as close to the midline as possible (e.g. your right, if you are right-eye dominant; see Fig. 2.10B, C)
3. Avoid looking at landmarks from an angle
4. Orientate right and left markers in the same way in order to make side-to-side comparisons easier and more accurate. For example, the thumbs should both be:
   - pointing downward while resting against the malleoli (see Figs 2.47 and 2.48)
   - pointing upwards (craniad) resting against the ASIS or PSIS to detect outflare or inflare (see Fig. 2.10B, C)
   - aligned horizontally when resting against the ASIS, PSIS or top of the superior pubic rami in order to detect upslip or rotation (see Figs 2.41, 2.46, 2.83, 2.84, 2.87 and 2.88)

- bring the right eye as close to midline as possible for making valid side-to-side comparisons of landmarks.

The reverse applies if you are left eye dominant.

It is useful to get into the habit of standing or sitting by the athlete on the correct side, both to facilitate the assessment and to make it more accurate. This approach also proves valuable at the time of carrying out alignment corrections using muscle energy and other treatment techniques as it allows for quick feedback on whether or not realignment has been achieved (see Figs 7.9, 7.11 and 7.13–7.16).

TORSION OF THE SACRUM

Torsion of the sacrum occurs naturally as part of daily activities such as reaching, throwing, walking and running. Torsion can occur around various axes and is governed by the motion of the trunk, pelvic bones and lower extremities. Normal sacral torsion into nutation on trunk flexion, and counternutation on extension, has been described above (see Figs 2.8, 2.14 and 2.15), as has movement around the oblique axes during the gait cycle (see Figs 2.7, 2.11 and 2.17) and on unilateral facet joint impaction (see Fig. 2.35).

The sacrum may actually become pathologically fixed so that there results a loss of motion in certain directions. The following are three of the more common reasons for this occurring:

- a movement that inadvertently exceeds the physiological limit available in that direction
- excessive tension or spasm in one of the muscles that attaches to the sacrum or coccyx
- contracture of ligaments, capsules, fascia or other connective tissue that can influence the position of the sacrum or coccyx.

The muscles primarily involved are the piriformis and iliacus.

Piriformis originates from the anterior aspect of the sacral base, the diagonal direction of its pull rotating the sacral base posteriorly relative to the ilium (see Fig. 2.31A). Iliacus rotates the ilium anteriorly relative to the sacrum (Fig. 2.31B). Either movement causes a wedging of the ilium against the anteriorly widening sacrum and would normally help to stabilize the SI joint; if excessive, however, it can result in a loss of mobility between the ilium and sacrum.

The diagnosis of torsion can usually be made simply by observing 'the lie of the sacrum': comparing the position of distinguishing landmarks when the athlete lies prone.

Position of the sacral base as judged by the sacral sulci. The sacral sulci are formed by the junction of the sacral ala with the ilium on either side. Locate the depression at the junction of L5 and S1 with the tip of one index finger and then run both index fingers outwards at this level until they abut the medial edge of the posterior iliac rim (approximately 1.5–2.5 cm lateral to the midline). Now push the tip of each index finger into the depression, or 'sulcus', formed at this junction of the sacrum with the pelvis (Fig. 2.56A). The depth of the sulcus is approximately 1.0–1.5 cm. The depth of the right sulcus should equal that of the left.

The position of the sacral apex. The sacral apex is the terminal part of the sacrum to which the coccyx attaches (see Fig. 2.1A). Press the pulp of the index fingers or thumbs firmly down, through the soft tissues, onto the right and left lateral edges of this caudal part of the sacrum. The fingers will normally lie at an equal depth.

The inferior lateral angle. This is the corner formed at the point where the inferior part of the sacrum rapidly starts to taper toward its junction with the coccyx (see Fig. 2.1A). It is usually easily palpable through the overlying soft tissues, 1.0–1.5 cm up and out from the sacrococcygeal junction (see Fig. 2.41G). The right inferior lateral angle usually lies at a depth equal to that of the left in the transverse plane. In addition, the inferior lateral angle will be level in the frontal plane; that is, there is no displacement either upwards (cephalad) or downwards (caudad) of one relative to the other.

The following are among the more commonly noted patterns of excessive or fixed sacral torsion. The reader is referred to Richard (1986) and Fowler (1986) for further descriptions of the various forms of sacral torsion and the effects of such torsion on the lumbar spine.

'Left/left' or 'left-on-left' sacral torsion. The sacrum is fixed in rotation around the left oblique axis (see Figs 2.17 and 2.33). Therefore, the right sacral sulcus (the right finger in Fig. 2.56B) is depressed, having rotated anteriorly and downwards; whereas the left sacral apex (left finger) is elevated, having rotated posteriorly and upwards. The right inferior lateral angle lies anteriorly and caudad, the left posteriorly and cephalad.

'Right/right' or 'right-on-right' sacral torsion. The sacrum is fixed in rotation around the right oblique axis (see Figs 2.11, 2.33 and 2.35B). The findings are the reverse of those noted for 'left-on-left' torsion (Fig. 2.56B).

Rotation posteriorly around the right or left oblique axis. Rotation occurs in the direction opposite to that described in the previous sections. The base rotates backwards instead of forwards to right and left, resulting in a 'right-on-left' and 'left-on-right' pattern respectively (Fig. 2.57). Whereas the forward rotation described above accentuates the lumbosacral angle, increasing the lumbar lordosis and making the lumbar segment more supple, the backwards rotation is associated with a reduction of the angle, and hence the lordosis, with a stiffening of this segment. Even worse,

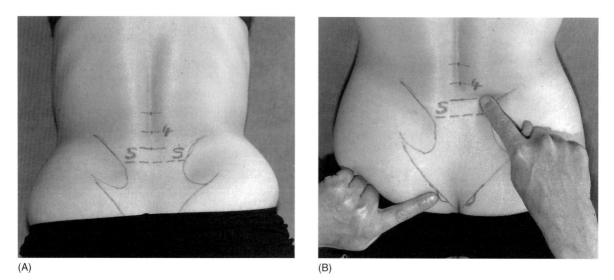

(A) (B)

Figure 2.56 Assessment of sacral landmarks in the prone-lying athlete. Note: the clinician with right eye dominance should carry out examination from the athlete's left in order to bring that eye closer to the midline. (A) In alignment; the right and left sacral sulci (S) are of equal depth and level (as is the sacral base, demarcated by the dotted line); the solid line at '4' indicates the location of the L4 spinous process. (B) 'Left-on-left' rotation: the right index finger lies in the depressed right sacral sulcus, the left index finger on the ILA denotes an elevated left sacral margin.

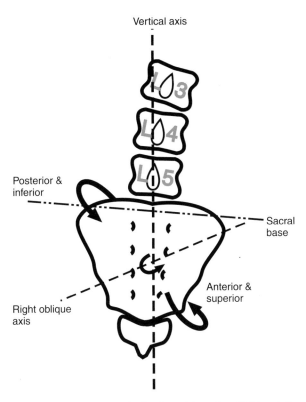

Figure 2.57 Example of a 'backwards' rotation: 'right-on-left' rotation around the right oblique axis.

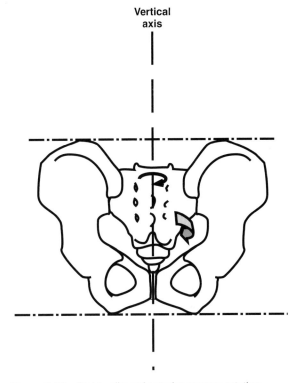

Figure 2.58 Right unilateral anterior sacrum: rotation counterclockwise around the vertical axis.

there may actually be formation of a lumbar kyphosis. These 'backward' presentations have been linked to distressing and seemingly unrelated problems (Richard 1986), including headaches and disturbed function of the gastrointestinal system (e.g. diarrhoea alternating with constipation) and the genitourinary system (e.g. frequency, nocturia and a disturbance of menstrual function).

Right or left unilateral anterior sacrum. The entire sacrum has rotated excessively to the right or left around the vertical axis in the transverse plane (Fig. 2.58). For example, a right unilateral anterior sacrum:

- brings all the sacral landmarks anteriorly on the right and posteriorly on the left side
- puts the left posterior sacroiliac (including the long dorsal), sacrospinous and interosseous ligaments, and the right anterior SI joint ligaments and capsule, under increased tension
- jams the sacrum against the innominate on the left side.

Excessive rotation in the sagittal plane (Figs 2.8, 2.12 and 2.14–2.16). This presents as either:

- excessive nutation, with the base fixed in an anterior position, and accentuation of the lumbar lordosis
- excessive counternutation, with the base fixed in a posterior position, and flattening of the lumbar lordosis or even the production of a lumbar kyphosis.

Clinical correlation

Sacroiliac joint upslip and anatomical leg length difference. There is usually no associated sacral torsion. The sacrum may be rotated around the vertical axis, but this is usually in conjunction with some rotation of the pelvis as a whole in the transverse plane (see Fig. 2.9).

Rotational malalignment. There is usually an associated torsion of the sacrum, right-on-right and left-on-left being most common forms (as discussed further in Ch. 3).

CURVES OF THE SPINE AND VERTEBRAL MALROTATION

To ascertain what is present, first examine the standing athlete from the back, looking for unlevelling of the pelvis, shoulders and inferior angles of the scapulae

(Fig. 2.59). Note any curvature(s) formed by the spinous processes. Is the spine straight or does there appear to be one uniform curve or the more probable double (or scoliotic) curve with a lumbar component convex to one side, reversing at the thoracolumbar junction to give way to a thoracic curve convex in the opposite direction (see Figs 2.42, 2.43 and 2.46B). Where does the thoracic curve reverse proximally to give way to the cervical curve? This reversal usually occurs at the cervicothoracic junction but may be seen as far down as the T4 or T5 level (Fig. 2.60).

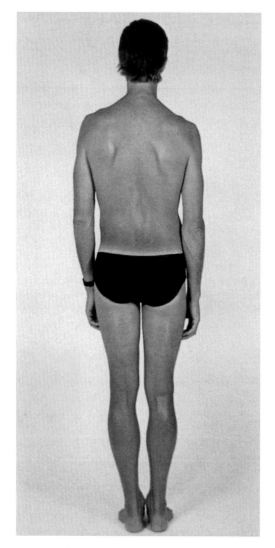

Figure 2.59 Standing photo showing pelvic obliquity (right side high), scoliotic curves (thoracic convex left, lumbar right) and scapular depression (right side down). The right knee is flexed, as if the athlete were attempting to lower the pelvis on the high side.

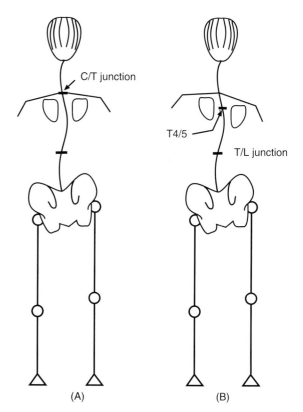

Figure 2.60 Site of curve reversal at the proximal end of the thoracic spine. (A) More common: at the cervicothoracic (C/T) junction. (B) Less common: at the T4 or T5 vertebral level. T/L, thoracolumbar.

Having the athlete bend forwards brings the spinous processes into better relief and may make these curves more obvious. On side flexion, a completely flexible scoliotic curve will usually become one uniform curve, whereas an interruption of this curve may still be evident on this manoeuvre in the presence of pelvic malalignment and/or vertebral malrotation. There may be a failure of an area, or even an entire segment, to bend along with the rest of the spine; the lumbar segment, for example, may appear stiff as a rod on bending to the right and/or left, whereas the thoracic segment flexes easily to both sides (Fig. 2.61).

Next, examine the spine with the athlete sitting. Again, note the level of the pelvis, shoulders and scapulae. If the pelvis is now level, and any curves of the spine noted on standing have decreased or disappeared, these curves were probably helping to compensate for the pelvic obliquity caused by a true LLD (see Fig. 2.42B). Any residual curves represent the 'intrinsic' curves with which most of us are blessed.

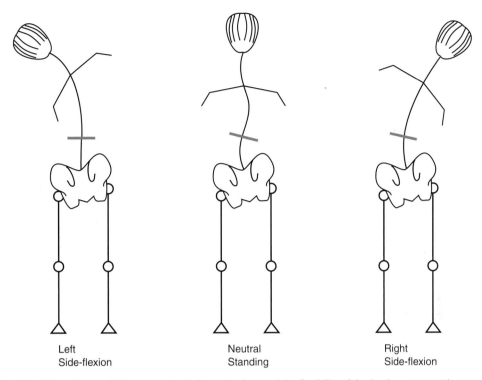

| Left
Side-flexion | Neutral
Standing | Right
Side-flexion |

Figure 2.61   Flexibility of the scoliotic curve noted when standing upright: flexibility of the lumbar segment is normal on right side flexion but restricted on left side flexion.

Then have the athlete lie supine to determine the direction of any persistent pelvic obliquity (see Figs 2.43A–D). A comparison of the right to the left clavicle and ribs will provide some indication of the effect of any thoracic convexity or rotation of the individual vertebrae. Tenderness over one or both sternoclavicular joints, and/or an anterior protrusion or recession of this end of either clavicle, suggests a torsional effect on the clavicles, which can, with time, result in ligament laxity and the subluxation of that joint (Figs 2.62A and 2.63B).

A displacement of specific ribs on one side relative to the matching ribs on the opposite side (Fig. 2.62B), tenderness over one or more of the sternochondral or costochondral junctions, and protrusion or recession of the anterior end of a rib or ribs should raise suspicions of the rotation of specific thoracic vertebrae (Fig. 2.63A, B), although these findings can also occur as a result of ribs adjusting to a pronounced thoracic convexity.

Finally, look at the back with the athlete lying prone, his or her head resting in a face-hole or chin over the edge, to protect the upper spine from being twisted by a rotation of the head and neck. Check the level of the pelvis and scapulae. If any curves are present, are they convex in the same direction as in standing and sitting (Fig. 2.64A)? Again, does the upper thoracic curve start to reverse at the cervicothoracic junction, or below that point (see Fig. 2.60)?

To help to define these curves better, stand at the head and lay the pulp of each index finger lightly on either side of the protuberant spinous process of C7. Then run these fingers down alongside the thoracic and lumbar spinous processes and onto the sacrum. Note the direction in which the tips of the fingers point as they sweep downward and the sites at which their direction changes – usually at the apex of the thoracic and lumbar convexities, and at the thoracolumbar and lumbosacral junctions (Fig. 2.64B–E).

Also note whether the smooth, contrasting curves formed by the spinous processes of the thoracic and lumbar segments are at any point acutely interrupted by an excessive rotation of one or more of the vertebrae, henceforth designated as a *vertebral malrotation*. The rotation of a vertebral body results in the rotation of its spinous process in the opposite direction. At the level of a vertebral malrotation to the right, for example, the spinous process will be displaced to the left relative to the spinous process of the vertebra above and below. The finger running down alongside the spinous

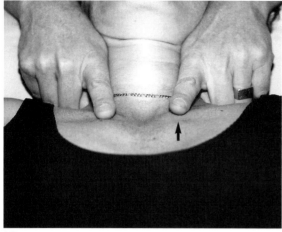

(A)

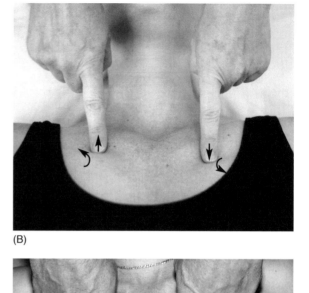

(B)

Figure 2.62 Involvement of the ribs and clavicles with malalignment. (A) Posterior rotation of the left clavicle, resulting in anterior protrusion (and possibly eventual subluxation) at the left sternoclavicular junction, with the reverse findings on the right. (B) 1st to 4th, 5th or 6th rib level inclusive: showing the more commonly seen displacement of these left ribs downwards and forwards (anterior rotation) relative to the right ones, which are displaced upwards and back by the posterior rotation of the ribs at these upper levels (thoracic convexity is to the left – see Figs 2.64 and 3.13B). (C) 5th or 6th rib level: the right and left ribs now match in both planes (near the apex of the thoracic convexity); the ribs below these levels will show the right ones displaced downwards and forwards relative to the left ones.

(C)

processes on the left side will abut the spinous process of this malrotated vertebra and be forced to move outwards to get around it, whereas the finger on the right side will dip into the hollow created by the rotation of that spinous process to the left.

For example, Fig. 2.65A shows an oblique pelvis with a uniform curve of the lumbar spine convex to right; the L1–4 vertebrae inclusive are rotated clockwise into the convexity. Superimposing an L4 vertebral malrotation to the left, that is, an excessive rotation of the body to the left and the spinous process to the right (as shown in Fig. 2.65B) would result in:

- the L4 spinous process interrupting the lumbar curve by jutting out to the right
- a matching hollow on the left at this level.

As the finger glides past the malrotated level, there is often also a reaction on the part of the athlete, most frequently a spontaneous withdrawal reaction and a reflex contraction of the immediately adjacent paravertebral muscles, sometimes radiating to involve the more distant erector spinae muscles. Sometimes the athlete complains of outright pain.

One can usually palpate, or even see, an increase in tension in the immediately adjacent paravertebral muscles, and elicit tenderness from these muscles, the supraspinous and interspinous ligaments, and other attaching soft tissues. A force applied to the spinous processes in a posterior-to-anterior and right/left translatory direction may elicit pain from the malrotated, and sometimes also adjacent, vertebrae by stressing these soft tissues, intervertebral ligaments and facet joints,

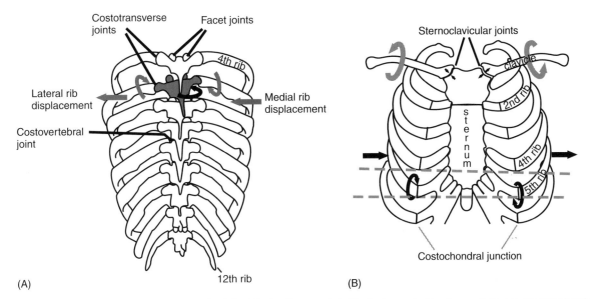

(A)

(B)

Figure 2.63   T5 vertebral malrotation to the left, with simultaneous left side flexion and either forwards flexion or extension; i.e. a left 'FRS' or 'ERS' pattern respectively (see also Figs 3.5 and 3.13). (A) Posterior view: deviation of the T5 spinous process to the right, with contrary rib displacement and rotation; note the right facet joint compression, left 'distraction' or opening, and increase in stress on the costotransverse and costovertebral joints at this level. (B) Anterior view: stress on the bilateral 5th costochondral junctions through the ribs; also illustrated are the typical opening and closing of the sternoclavicular joints caused by contrary rotation of the clavicles that can result with the compensatory scoliosis associated with pelvic malalignment.

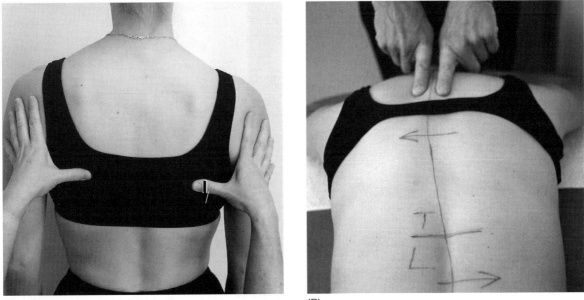

(A)

(B)

Figure 2.64   Determining the direction of a thoracic and lumbar convexity. (A) In standing, downward displacement of the right scapular apex and the depressed right shoulder suggest (but do not confirm) a thoracic curve primarily convex to left (see also Fig. 2.60). (B) Left thoracic, right lumbar convexity (the apex of each curve is marked by a horizontal arrow); fingers alongside the spinous processes above thoracic apex – pointing to left. (C) Fingers below the thoracic apex – now pointing to right. (D) Fingers above lumbar apex – still pointing to right. (E) Fingers below lumbar apex – again pointing to left.

Figure 2.64 (C)–(E), see overleaf

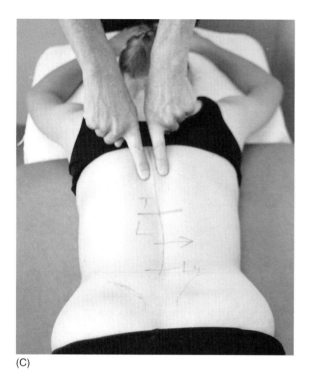

(C)

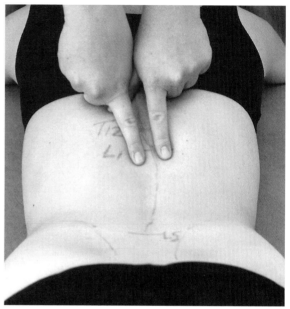

(D)

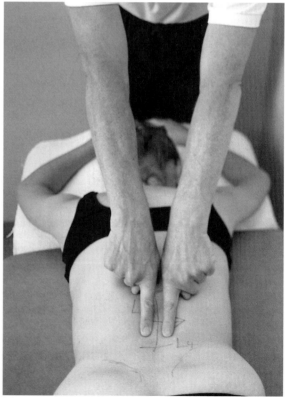

Figure 2.64 *Continued*

(E)

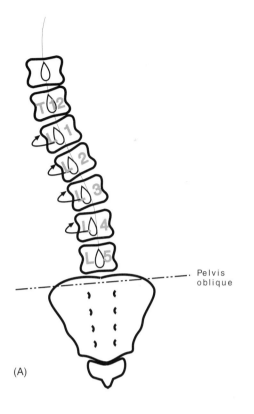

(A)

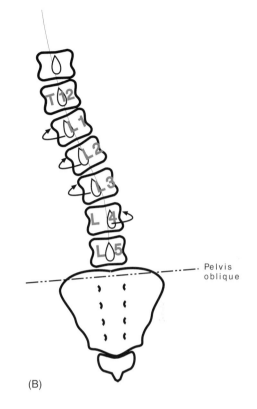

(B)

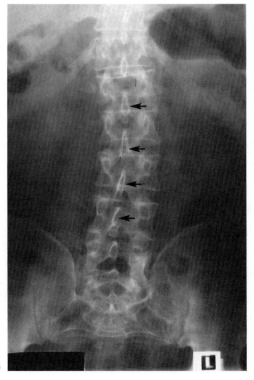

(C)

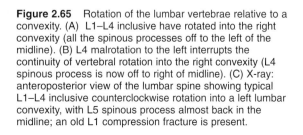

Figure 2.65 Rotation of the lumbar vertebrae relative to a convexity. (A) L1–L4 inclusive have rotated into the right convexity (all the spinous processes off to the left of the midline). (B) L4 malrotation to the left interrupts the continuity of vertebral rotation into the right convexity (L4 spinous process is now off to right of midline). (C) X-ray: anteroposterior view of the lumbar spine showing typical L1–L4 inclusive counterclockwise rotation into a left lumbar convexity, with L5 spinous process almost back in the midline; an old L1 compression fracture is present.

capsules and ligaments. It should, however, be noted that not all vertebrae that appear malrotated are necessarily tender or have an associated reactive increase in muscle tension.

Clinical correlation

Anatomical leg length difference. Triple curves – lumbar, thoracic and cervical – that compensate for the pelvic obliquity are evident on standing. They are decreased, or sometimes even abolished, as the pelvis becomes level in sitting and lying (see Fig. 2.42B).

Sacroiliac joint upslip. A right or left upslip also results in obliquity of the pelvis, and there is usually a compensatory triple curve.

In *right upslip* (see Fig. 2.43A), the pelvis is raised on the right side. The lumbar segment will be convex into either the high or the low side of the pelvis. The obliquity and the direction of the curves remain constant in standing, sitting and lying.

With *left upslip* (see Fig. 2.43B), the obliquity is again high on the right side in both standing and sitting but reverses with both prone- and supine-lying, so the left side ends up high in these situations. The direction of the curves remains constant in all positions, the lumbar curve usually convex to left and thoracic to right.

Rotational malalignment. There is typically the triple curve with reversal at the thoracolumbar and cervicothoracic junctions. The curves usually persist in standing, sitting and lying prone but may reverse direction on moving from one position to another (see Fig. 2.43C, D).

The pelvic obliquity is in part caused by:

- rotation of the innominate(s) in the sagittal plane, with elevation of the iliac crest on the side of the anterior rotation
- an associated rotation of the pelvis in the frontal plane
- the functional LLD.

Which pelvic crest is higher or lower is, however, also influenced by other factors, including whether there is an underlying anatomical (true) LLD or a coexisting sacral torsion or SI joint upslip. It may therefore vary with the position of examination. Most prevalent is a consistent elevation of the right pelvic crest.

Outflare/inflare. Innominate rotation occurs in the transverse plane so that, provided the leg length is equal, there is no pelvic obliquity.

EXAMINATION OF THE SYMPHYSIS PUBIS

The examiner should note whether any of the following occur.

Pain on palpating or stressing the joint

The symphysis may be painful on direct palpation. Pain caused by joint distraction may indicate primarily a ligament or a capsular problem as these are put under increased tension (Fig. 2.66). Pain caused by joint compression is more likely to indicate joint pathology (Figs 2.67 and 2.68). Degenerative changes on X-ray and a positive bone scan may also be helpful in this respect but are by no means pathognomonic for symptoms arising from the joint itself. Superoinferior translation gives information on joint stability; pain provoked in this way probably is less specific because the manoeuvre stresses both the joint and the soft tissue structures (Fig. 2.69).

Disturbance of the symmetry of the joint

Anterior or posterior rotation of an innominate bone cannot occur without causing the rotation of one pubic bone relative to the other. Similarly, an upslip or downslip causes a simultaneous upwards or downwards translation respectively at both the SI joint and the symphysis pubis. The displacement at the symphysis is usually 3–5 mm and readily discernible:

- on comparison of the level of a finger placed on the upper edge of the superior pubic ramus, 1.5–2.0 cm to either side of the midline (see Fig. 2.46C)
- by appreciating a sudden drop or rise in the contour as one sweeps a finger along the upper edge from one side to the other

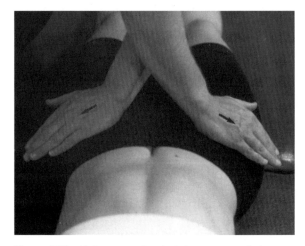

Figure 2.66 Pain provocation test: transverse anterior distraction (symphysis pubis and anterior sacroiliac joint capsule and ligaments) with simultaneous posterior sacroiliac joint compression. (From Lee & Walsh 1996, with permission.)

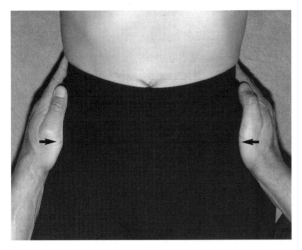

Figure 2.67 Pain provocation test: medial compression of the innominates results in anterior compression and posterior distraction.

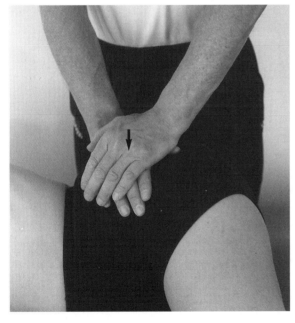

Figure 2.68 Pain provocation test: anterior compression and posterior gapping achieved with a downward force on the upper innominate in side-lying. (From Lee & Walsh 1996, with permission.)

- on the anterior–posterior X-ray view of the pelvis (see Fig. 2.45).

As previously indicated, this displacement is associated with an obliquity of the pubic bones that remains evident on standing, sitting and lying.

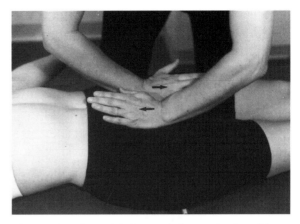

Figure 2.69 Superoinferior translation test for the pubic symphysis. (From Lee & Walsh 1996, with permission.)

Instability of the joint

This may become apparent as:

- excessive gapping (greater than 5 mm) noticeable on joint palpation
- excessive movement of the joint with the application of anteroposterior and superoinferior translatory forces
- excessive separation of the pubic bones on X-ray.

It should, however, be pointed out that even marked instability may not become readily apparent on clinical examination, or even routine anterior–posterior views of the pelvis, especially when these are taken with the athlete supine. If instability is suspected, X-rays should be taken while stressing the joint, which can be achieved by:

- carrying out an active straight leg raising test (see under 'Functional tests' below); this test has an advantage in that it can be carried out with the athlete lying supine (Fig. 2.70A)
- maintaining a 'flamingo' or 'figure-4' position, standing alternately on the right and left legs, with the hip and knee of the opposite leg flexed and the foot resting against the inside of the weight-bearing leg (Fig. 2.70B)
- alternately letting one leg hang down while bearing full weight on the other one standing on a stool (Fig. 2.70C).

Clinical correlation

Aligned, anatomical leg length difference. With an anatomical long right leg, the right pubic bone lies higher than the left in standing. There is no actual

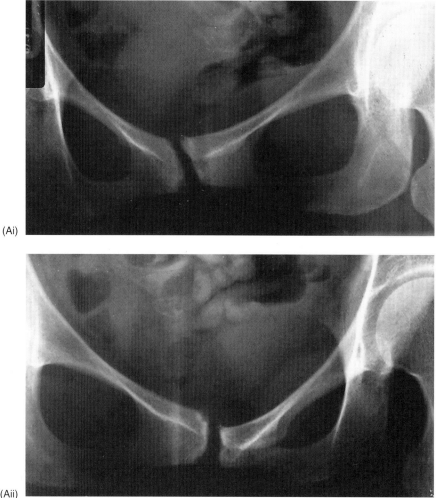

(Ai)

(Aii)

Figure 2.70 X-ray diagnosis of symphysis pubis instability. (A) X-rays during 'active SLR' (ASLR) of a patient with a large displacement: (i) During ASLR of the right leg (reference side); (ii) During ASLR of the left (symptomatic) side. No malalignment of the pubic bones is seen during ASLR on the reference side. A step of about 5 mm is seen at the upper margins on the symptomatic side. The projection of the left pubic bone is smaller than that of the right, indicating an anterior rotation of the left pubic bone about an axis in the vicinity of the sacroiliac joint. (From Mens et al, 1997 with permission.) (B) 'Flamingo' or 'Figure-4' position likely to detect displacement of the left pubic bone relative to the right one when left SI joint inadequately stabilized on left weight-bearing. (C) Left pubic bone is stressed by freely suspending the right leg to shift weight-bearing to the left.

Fig. 2.70 (B) & (C), see overleaf

displacement of the pubic bones relative to each other, just a uniform obliquity that slopes from right down to left and is abolished on sitting or lying supine (see Fig. 2.42B).

Sacroiliac joint upslip. On the side of the upslip, there will usually be a 3–5 mm upwards displacement of the pubic bone relative to that on the other side, with an obliquity slanting up towards the side of the upslip (see Fig. 2.43A, B).

Rotational malalignment. With right anterior and left posterior innominate rotation, the right pubic bone is shifted posteriorly and downwards, the left anteriorly and up. There is an actual downwards displacement of the right pubic bone shifted to the left (see Figs 2.29, 2.45 and 2.46C). Left anterior and right posterior innominate rotation results in the reverse findings.

Outflare/inflare. The pubic bones will be level.

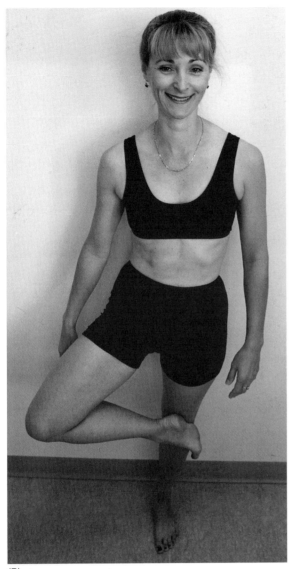

(B)

(C)

Figure 2.70 *Continued.*

HIP JOINT RANGES OF MOTION

The hip ranges of motion are symmetrical in the athlete presenting in alignment or with an anatomical LLD. These ranges of motion will be asymmetrical in the presence of rotational malalignment, SI joint upslip or downslip and outflare/inflare, as discussed in detail in Chapter 3. Asymmetry of hip range of motion in the absence of pelvic malalignment, or in a pattern inconsistent with that typically associated with malalignment (see Appendix 3), should trigger a search for tightness of the surrounding soft tissues or other hip

joint pathology. Tightness of the anterior or Y ligaments, for example, will limit ipsilateral hip extension; a capsular pattern, indicating generalized tightness, may be indicative of underlying hip osteoarthritis or of previous severe trauma with scarring.

ASSESSMENT OF LIGAMENTS AND MUSCLES

The examination for asymmetry and malalignment must include an assessment of tension and tenderness in the ligaments of the pelvic region and along the

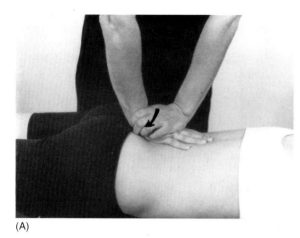
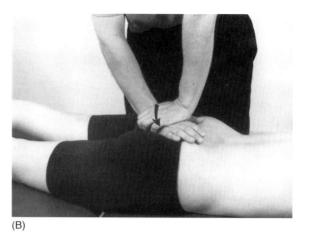

(A)   (B)

Figure 2.71 Pain provocation tests for posterior pelvic ligaments, the hands applying an anterior force for 20 seconds. (A) Hands overlying the sacral base to enforce nutation and thereby increase tension in the sacrotuberous, sacrospinous and interosseous ligaments (see Figs 2.3 and 2.16A). (B) Hands overlying the sacral apex to enforce counternutation and thereby increase tension in the long dorsal sacroiliac ligament (see Fig 2.16B). (From Lee & Walsh 1996, with permission.)

spine (see Figs 2.2 and 2.3). The sacrotuberous and sacrospinous ligaments, which are subjected to increased tension by sacral nutation for example, often prove tender to palpation but may be otherwise completely asymptomatic (see Figs 2.3 and 2.16A). A spring test to temporarily augment the nutation, and hence the tension, may provoke pain from these ligaments (Fig. 2.71A). Similarly, augmenting counternutation with anterior pressure on the apex of the sacrum may provoke pain from the already tense and often tender long dorsal sacroiliac ligament (Fig. 2.71B; see also Figs 2.3 and 2.16B). Some muscles are typically affected in terms of being tense and tender or showing a functional weakness. The importance of these structures as a source of localized and referred pain, and as a cause of recurrence of malalignment, is discussed in Chapter 3.

TESTS USED FOR THE EXAMINATION OF THE PELVIC GIRDLE

The assessment for malalignment requires an in-depth examination of the individual components – spine, pelvis and hip joints – and of the pelvic girdle as a unit. This section will concentrate on:

- tests for mobility and stability
- tests of the ability of the unit to transfer load, remain stable and maintain balance when subjected to functional or dynamic stresses.

Because some of these tests also exert forces on the lumbosacral spine, tests selective for this segment (e.g. motion palpation, springing the vertebrae and facet stress tests) must always be part of the examination. As Lee (1992, p. 475) has pointed out so succinctly:

primary pathology of the lumbar spine can lead to secondary symptoms from the pelvic girdle. Alternately, primary pathology of the sacroiliac joint can lead to secondary symptoms from the lumbar spine

The examination of gait, posture and the neurological, muscular and vascular systems is mentioned as appropriate throughout the text. The reader is referred to Lee & Walsh (1996), Lee (1999), Vleeming et al (1997) and texts specifically concentrating on neurovascular problems for a more extensive coverage of these aspects.

TESTS FOR MOBILITY AND STABILITY

The following are tests commonly used to localize pain and to determine dysfunction of SI joint movement (e.g. hyper- or hypomobility, or excessive rotation).

A caution is in order, however. First, some of these tests are not specific for the SI joint itself because they also stress the hip joint, lumbosacral region or all three sites simultaneously. In order to better localize the pain, the examination should include tests that are more specific for stressing these individual sites.

Second, tests do not differentiate between pain arising from the joint itself, the supporting soft tissues or both. Compression tests are, however, more likely to precipitate pain from the joint, distraction tests pain from the ligaments and capsule. The selective injection of local anaesthetic into the joint space or the ligaments may also be helpful in making the distinction.

Leverage tests

The following manoeuvres all depend on stressing the SI joint by using the femur like a lever to effect movement of the innominate bone. The femur can be used to rotate the innominate in the sagittal plane, to move it in an anterior or posterior direction, or to adduct or abduct it relative to the sacrum. With the exception of Yeoman's test, all are carried out with the athlete lying supine.

First, with the hip flexed between 80 and 120 degrees to put the thigh at different angles relative to the innominate, push downwards on the knee in order to move the femur, and hence the hip joint and innominate, in an anterior– posterior direction (Fig. 2.72). There will be a simultaneous anterior rotational stress of varying degree applied to the innominate, given that the acetabulum lies below the inferior transverse axis, around which the wings of the ilia turn relative to the sacrum (see Fig. 2.33).

Next, with the hip joint flexed to 90 degrees, the femur is passively adducted to stress the SI joint by forcing the anterior joint margins together and, at the same time, separating or 'gapping' the posterior joint margins to stress the posterior capsule and ligaments. The adduction force is applied with one hand on the outside of the knee while the other hand palpates the SI joint posteriorly to determine the amount of gapping (Fig. 2.73).

Whereas gapping may be quite obviously increased or decreased from normal, always make a side-to-side comparison in order to determine actual differences in contrast to a generalized bilateral joint laxity or tightness that may be normal for that athlete. This test may not be tolerated when there is tenderness or spasm in muscles such as iliopsoas that are literally 'compressed' by the manoeuvre. Alternately, posterior 'gapping' or distraction can be achieved by using a medial force applied to both innominates in supine lying (see Fig. 2.67), or to the upper innominate in side-lying (see Fig. 2.68).

Passive abduction of the flexed hip will gap the anterior part of the joint and stress the anterior capsule and ligaments, whereas the posterior aspect of the joint will be compressed.

Shear stress tests can then be carried out. *Anterior shear* can be achieved with FABER test (simultaneous hip Flexion, Abduction and External Rotation), also known as Patrick's or the Figure-4 test. It has been commonly used to test for hip joint pathology and for

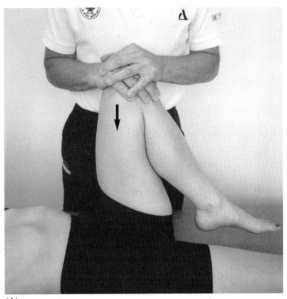

(A)

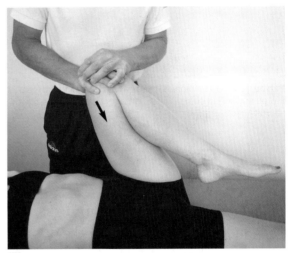

(B)

Figure 2.72 Passive displacement of the innominate relative to the sacrum by a force applied through the femur. (A) With the left hip flexed to 90 degrees: a more direct anterior–posterior force. (B) Right hip flexed to 110 degrees: relatively more anterior rotational force.

restriction of range of motion, in particular external rotation (Fig. 2.74; see also Fig. 3.73). However, given that the hip joint lies caudad to the SI joint, this manoeuvre also turns the femur into a lever capable of:

- rotating the innominate posteriorly and externally relative to the sacrum, and stretching the soft tissues (e.g. iliopsoas) in the groin

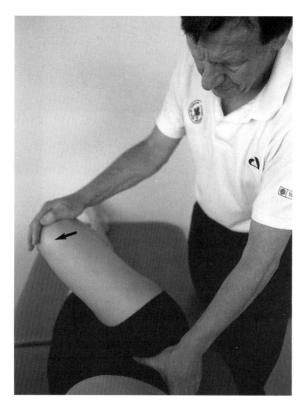

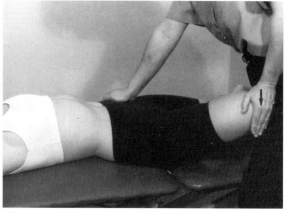

(A)

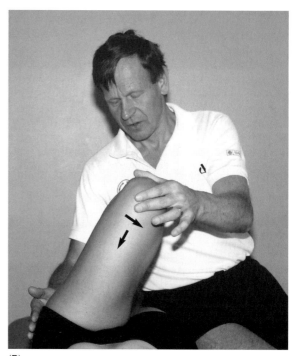

(B)

Figure 2.73 Passive adduction of the right femur to 'gap' the posterior and compress the anterior aspect of the right sacroiliac joint.

- effecting nutation and thereby stressing the sacrotuberous, sacrospinous and interosseous ligaments
- opening the SI joint anteriorly and compressing it posteriorly, thus stretching the anterior SI joint capsule and ligaments
- moving the ilium anteriorly relative to the sacrum while the pelvis is stabilized, which results in an anterior shear stress.

Posterior shear can be effected with the FADE (simultaneous Flexion, Adduction, Extension) or POSH (POsterior SHear) tests (Fig. 2.74B).

Hip extension tests are commonly used to stress the hip joint, but progressive movement of the femur will eventually also stress the SI joint by rotating the innominate anteriorly in the sagittal plane.

1. *Yeoman's test*: passive hip extension, with the athlete prone (Fig. 2.75A)
2. *Gaenslen's test*: passive hip extension, with the athlete supine and the leg hanging over the side of the plinth (Fig. 2.75B).

Figure 2.74 Shear tests for the sacroiliac joint. (A) FABER manoeuvre (Flexion, ABduction and External Rotation). After finding the physiological limit of simultaneous movement in these directions, the femur is gently moved into further abduction and external rotation; at the same time, the contralateral innominate is fixed so that the flexed right femur becomes a lever capable of rotating the innominate externally and posteriorly through the hip joint (see also Fig. 3.73). (From Lee & Walsh 1996, with permission.) (B) FADE (simultaneous Flexion, ADduction and External force) or POSH (POsterior SHear) test: the hip is flexed, the femur adducted and an axial force then exerted through the femur to push the ilium posteriorly relative to the sacrum.

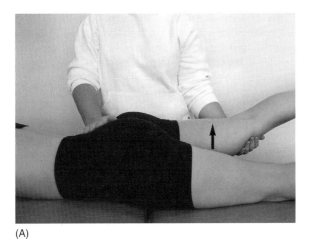

(A)

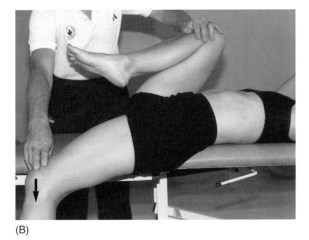

(B)

Figure 2.75 Hip extension to effect anterior innominate rotation and stress the sacroiliac joint. (A) Right Yeoman's test (passive hip extension, prone-lying). (B) Left Gaenslen's test (passive hip extension, supine-lying).

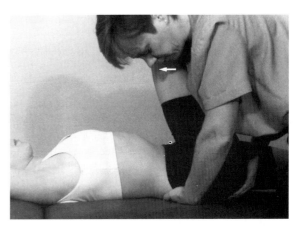

Figure 2.76 Passive hip flexion, using the right femur to effect posterior rotation of the right innominate relative to the sacrum. (From Lee & Walsh 1996, with permission.)

Passive straight leg raising, and hip flexion with the knee bent (Fig. 2.76), can both turn the femur into a lever capable of putting a torsional stress on the SI joint by rotating the innominate posteriorly in the sagittal plane. The pain thus provoked, by stressing the SI joint itself and/or putting tender posterior pelvic ligaments under increased tension, may be confused with pain elicited by putting the sciatic nerve and nerve roots under stretch or by mechanically stressing the lumbar spine as it is forced into increasing flexion.

Wells (1986) suggests that some differentiation between a lumbar as opposed to an SI joint problem should be possible. An SI joint problem is more likely if the pain produced by a unilateral test does not occur on carrying out the test on both sides simultaneously because the latter does not produce the torsional stress on the SI joint that results with a unilateral test. Pain persisting on the bilateral test argues for a lumbar cause because the stresses on the nerves and lumbar spine are the same in both tests.

Spring tests

Pain originating from the hip joint proper may interfere with the interpretation of leverage-type tests and may even make it impossible to use them. This problem can be bypassed by passive mobility tests that attempt to shift either the innominate or the sacrum relative to the other, the aims being to assess the quantity of motion and to see whether the test provokes any symptoms.

Once the end of the passive range has been reached, the application of a gentle springing force provides further information regarding end-feel and symptom provocation. As Hesch et al (1992, p. 445) have stressed, 'the spring test is ... applied as a gentle force within the physiological range'. Findings run from excessive movement to varying degrees of impaired movement or absolutely no joint play or spring detectable. On all these tests, side-to-side comparison is imperative in order to detect a relative increase or decrease in mobility. The reader is referred to Lee & Walsh (1996) and Lee (1999) for a more extensive description of these tests.

Spring tests carried out with the athlete prone

Springing of the innominate in a posterior–anterior direction creates a shear stress on the SI joint and allows for the localization of pain and the assessment of the amount of movement possible in the anterior direction.

The heel of one hand is placed on the innominate, directly on or alongside the PSIS; the heel of the other hand rests along the opposite border of the sacrum in order to stabilize the sacrum relative to the innominate (Fig. 2.77). After locking the elbow, bend forward with the trunk and apply a gradually increasing downwards pressure on the innominate until all the slack in the soft tissues surrounding the SI joint has been taken up and the initial movement of the innominate stops. At this point, apply a quick, low-amplitude force directly through the outstretched arm to the hand and the underlying innominate.

The above manoeuvre can be modified by placing the heel of the hand that rests on the innominate either above or below the PSIS in order to produce an anterior or posterior torsional stress respectively on the innominate relative to the sacrum. The sacrum is stabilized by placing the heel of the other hand on the apex.

The SI joint and specific ligaments can be stressed selectively using a quick springing action to force the sacrum into increased nutation or counternutation, similar to the pain provocative tests using a prolonged force (see above and Fig. 2.71).

Pain may be provoked by stressing the SI joint in a longitudinal direction. The heel of one hand pushes on the apex of the sacrum in a cephalad (upwards) direction as the heel of the other hand pushes caudad (downwards) on the posterior iliac crest (Fig. 2.78A). Conversely, the heel of one hand exerts pressure in a caudad direction on the base of the sacrum as the heel of the other hand applies pressure against the ischial tuberosity to move the innominate cephalad (Fig. 2.78B). If the coccyx is tender, it may be impossible to do these tests.

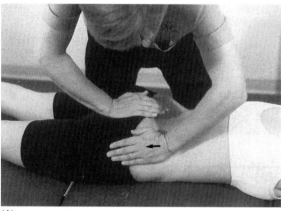

(A)

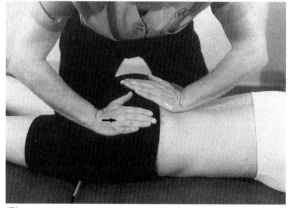

(B)

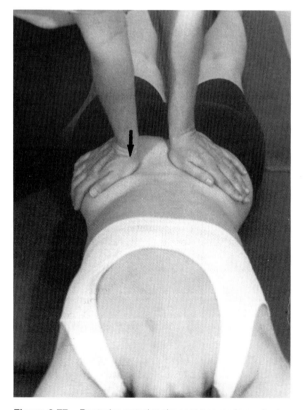

Figure 2.77 Posterior-anterior shear stress on innominate relative to the sacrum: with the left hand on the far side of the sacrum for counterbalance, the right hand applies a quick downward force on the right innominate. (From Lee & Walsh 1996, with permission.)

Figure 2.78 Translation of the right innominate relative to the sacrum. (A) Inferosuperior: sacrum cephalad, innominate caudad. (B) Superoinferior: sacrum caudad, innominate cephalad. (From Lee & Walsh 1996, with permission.)

In another test, the fingers of one hand fix the ASIS and iliac crest while the heel of the other hand forces down on the ipsilateral side of the sacrum until end-feel is perceived (Fig. 2.79). A small amount of pain-free joint play in the anteroposterior plane can normally be detected. Alternatively, with the left hand steadying the sacrum, the right hand can apply a quick upwards (anteroposterior) force on the innominate.

Spring tests carried out with the athlete supine

Compression and distraction forces. These are modifications of the pain provocative tests discussed above, with the addition of a quick, low-amplitude stress once end-feel has been perceived on stretching the surrounding soft tissues (see Figs 2.66, 2.67 and 2.68).

Glide of the innominate relative to the sacrum. The long and ring fingers are hooked around the medial edge of the posterior pelvic ring and come to lie in the sacral sulcus, where they can sense movement between the

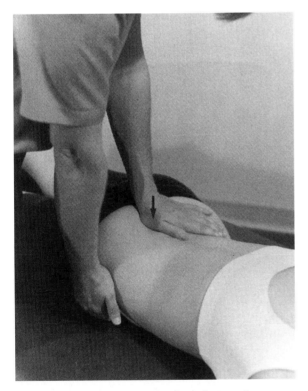

Figure 2.79 Posterior translation (innominate on the sacrum) – prone. Here the right hand applied to the right anterior superior iliac spine and iliac crest fixes the innominate while a posteroanterior force is applied with the heel of the left hand to the ipsilateral side of the sacrum. Quantity and end feel of motion and the reproduction of symptoms are observed. (From Lee & Walsh 1996, with permission.)

innominate and the sacrum. The index finger lies on the spinous process of L5 in order to sense the end of motion between the sacrum and the innominate when the pelvic girdle as a unit starts to bend laterally relative to L5 (Fig. 2.80). A note is made of the amount of movement and the actual end-feel itself (well-defined, sloppy, etc.), whether the manoeuvre elicits any symptoms and how all this compares with the opposite side.

Craniocaudal or superoinferior plane. The knee is about 20–30 degrees flexed, resting across the examiner's knee. The other hand holds the distal end of the femur or patellofemoral region in order to apply a force alternately in a superior (cephalad, Fig. 2.80) and an inferior (caudad) direction (Fig. 2.81); the latter can be augmented with pressure exerted by the examiner's knee against the proximal tibia.

Anterior–posterior and rotary planes. The heel of the free hand applies pressure on the ipsilateral ASIS to create a translatory force in an anterior–posterior direction until an end-feel is perceived (Fig. 2.82A). The manoeuvre is then repeated by applying the force just above and below the ASIS in an attempt to effect rotation of the innominate relative to the sacrum, and to assess the glide between the innominate and sacrum:

- anterior rotation to assess inferoposterior glide by applying the force just above the ASIS (Fig. 2.82B)
- posterior rotation for superoanterior glide, by applying the force just below the ASIS (Fig. 2.82C).

The failure of a leverage or spring test to provoke pain does not mean that the joint is functioning normally. The joint may, for example, be hypomobile yet asymptomatic; it is often the joint that is still mobile that proves to be painful, possibly because of the increased stress to which it is now subjected as a result of the hypomobility in the other joint:

mobility restrictions of the lumbar spine, pelvic girdle and/or hip joint will influence the function and motion of the adjacent regions. Often, all three areas require treatment and it is not rare for the most hypomobile area to be the least symptomatic. (Lee 1992, p. 475)

FUNCTIONAL OR DYNAMIC TESTS

The leverage and spring test are passive tests for SI joint mobility and stability. The following tests try to assess, in particular, the ability to transfer load through the SI joints, such as occurs during day-to-day activities. These tests need to evaluate specifically:

- the passive or form closure system – articular and ligamentous
- the active or force closure system – myofascial
- the control system – neural coordination.

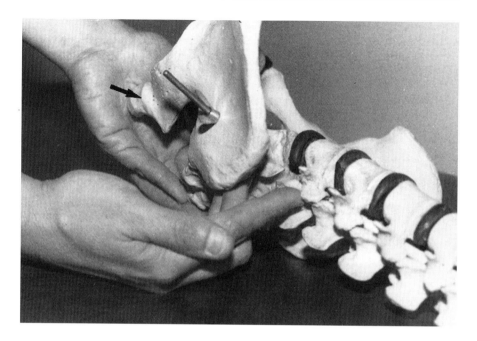

Figure 2.80 Placement of the long and ring fingers in the sacral sulcus, and the index finger on L5 for sensing innominate movement relative to the sacrum. (From Lee & Walsh 1996, with permission.)

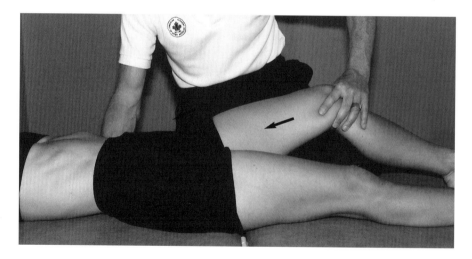

Figure 2.81 Innominate movement relative to the sacrum: craniocaudal or superoinferior plane.

Examples of the functional or dynamic tests commonly used are shown in Box 2.5.

Flexion and extension tests: pelvic, sacroiliac and lumbosacral

These tests for movement of the pelvic girdle and lumbosacral junction can be carried out with the athlete standing or sitting. If the athlete is seated, support the feet on a chair to improve stability and allow for maximum forward flexion of the trunk. When both SI

Box 2.5 Functional or dynamic testing of the pelvic girdle

- Gait analysis (see 'Joint function during the gait cycle' above)
- Lumbosacral tests in standing – bending forwards and backwards
- Tests carried out while weight-bearing on one leg, e.g. the Gillet test
- Active straight leg raising tests augmented by form and force closure

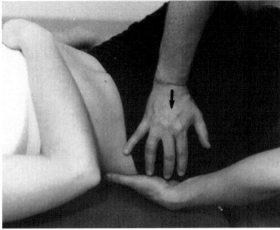

(A)

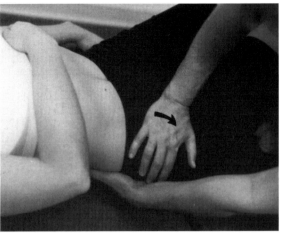

(B)

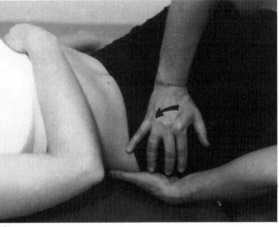

(C)

Figure 2.82   Innominate movement relative to the sacrum. (A) Anteroposterior translation or glide: a posterior translation force is applied to the innominate and the motion is noted posteriorly. (B) Anterior rotation of the innominate requires an inferoposterior glide of the sacroiliac (SI) joint (a caudad force applied above the anterior superior iliac spine). (C) Posterior rotation of the innominate requires a superoanterior glide at the SI joint (a cephalad force applied below the anterior superior iliac spine).

joints function normally, and barring other influencing factors (e.g. a functional LLD or asymmetry of muscle tension), the movement of the L5 vertebral complex, and of the ilia and the sacrum relative to each other, is symmetrical on trunk flexion and extension. The tests are carried out as described in Box 2.6.

One can encounter an abnormal sacral flexion test for reasons other than dysfunction of movement at one or other SI joint. As Lee & Walsh (1996) have emphasized, these tests examine lower quadrant function in forward flexion and extension rather than being specific for SI joint mobility. For example, a positive forward-bending test can result from unilateral restriction of flexion of the

hip joint, piriformis muscle spasm and tightness or hypertonicity of the hamstrings (Lee 1992). The presence or absence of such conditions will dictate the appropriate treatment. Carrying the test out in a sitting position will decrease, or even eliminate, some of the factors that can influence lower quadrant function.

Clinical correlation

Sacroiliac joint upslip and anatomical leg length difference. Neither an upslip in isolation nor an anatomical LLD is associated with evidence of movement dysfunction on this test. With a right upslip, for example,

---

Box 2.6 Flexion and extension tests

1. A thumb is placed on identical points on the ilium on each side (e.g. the inferior aspect of the posterior superior iliac spine). The thumbs will move in unison once the sacrum and the innominates start to move together: upwards on trunk flexion (Fig. 2.83A), downwards on trunk extension (Fig. 2.83B)
2. One thumb is then placed on the ilium, against the inferior aspect of the posterior superior iliac spine, and the other on the adjoining part of the sacral base (Fig. 2.84A)
   - On forward flexion, the sacral base will normally move forwards into nutation for approximately the first 45 degrees (see Fig. 2.15). This sacral nutation may eventually stop and the innominates start to rotate anteriorly to the sacrum (counternutation). The stability of the sacroiliac

joints is directly related to the range through which nutation can occur (Lee 1999)
   - On backward bending, the sacrum normally stays in nutation relative to the innominates (see Fig. 2.15), also causing the thumbs on the sacrum and ilium to separate
   - The amount of sacral movement that occurs relative to the ilium is equal on the right and left sides in both flexion and extension
3. L5 will also move symmetrically on these tests (Fig. 2.85). Fingers placed on the transverse processes will show these to move together. There is no evidence of vertebral:
   - rotation (moving forwards on one side and backwards on the other)
   - side flexion (moving up on one side and down on the other)

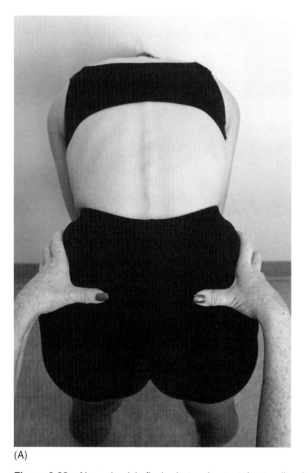

(A)

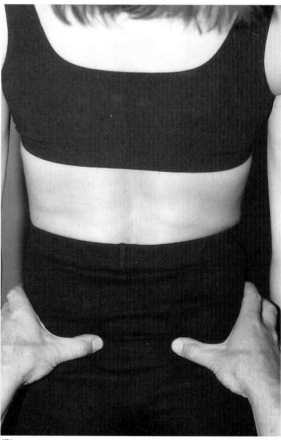

(B)

Figure 2.83 Normal pelvic flexion/extension test. In standing (neutral position), the thumbs are on matching points – the inferior aspect of the posterior superior iliac spine (PSIS) (see Fig. 2.41B). (A) On trunk flexion: the thumbs (= PSIS) move up by an equal amount. (B) On trunk extension: the thumbs (= PSIS) move down by an equal amount.

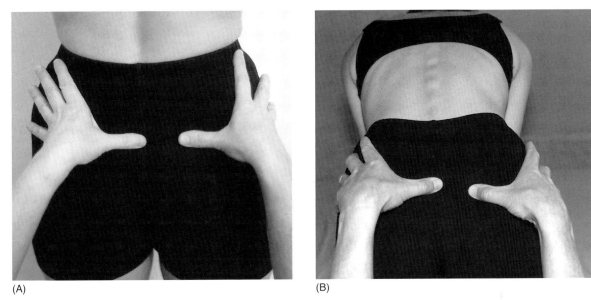

(A)   (B)

Figure 2.84   Normal sacroiliac flexion/extension test. (A) Right thumb on the posterior superior iliac spine, left on the adjoining sacral base. (B) On the initial 45 degrees of flexion, the thumb on the sacrum has moved upwards relative to that on the ilium with movement of the sacral base into nutation; a similar separation occurs as nutation is increased with extension (see Figs 2.14 and 2.15).

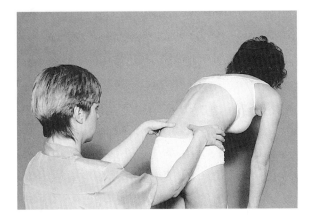

Figure 2.85   Normal lumbosacral flexion/extension test. Thumbs on the transverse processes of the L5 vertebra travel an equal distance, upwards on flexion and downwards on extension. (From Lee 1999, with permission.)

the right PSIS remains higher than the left to an equal extent in all positions. This is similar to someone with an anatomical LLD, with the right leg long, when tested standing (Fig. 2.86B).

Rotational malalignment. Assuming an otherwise normal lower quadrant function, these tests will be abnormal when the excessive anterior or posterior rotation of an innominate bone has resulted in a

decrease of movement possible at one SI joint relative to the other, or even a complete loss of movement, also referred to as 'locking' of that SI joint.

With locking of the right SI joint, for example, the sacrum and the right innominate now move as one unit on trunk flexion and extension. Therefore, the right thumb will move relatively further than the left, upwards on flexion and downwards on extension (Figs 2.86A and 2.87). Remember that, with rotational malalignment, the right and left PSIS are usually no longer level in the neutral position – standing or sitting – to start with: the right may be noticeably higher or lower than the left. Therefore, with locking of the right SI joint:

- on forward flexion:
  - a right PSIS that was lower than the left in the neutral standing position could end up level with or higher than the left
  - if the right PSIS was already higher than the left, the difference between them would increase (Figs 2.86A and 2.87B)
- on trunk extension:
  - a right PSIS that was higher in the neutral position might become level with or end up lower than the left (Figs 2.86A and 2.87C)
  - if it was lower than the left to start with, the difference between them would increase.

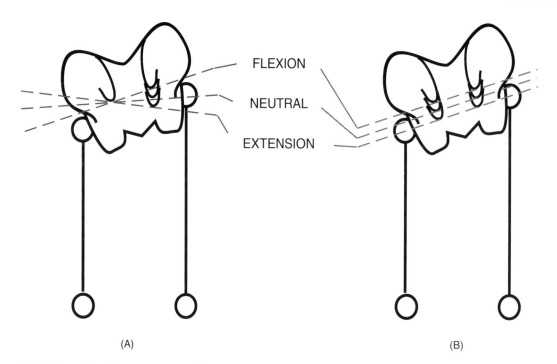

Figure 2.86 Normal and abnormal changes in the position of the right relative to the left posterior superior iliac spine (PSIS) with trunk flexion and extension in standing. (A) With locking of the right sacroiliac (SI) joint: excessive movement of the right PSIS upwards with flexion, downwards with extension. (B) With true leg length difference (right leg long) or right upslip: the right and left PSIS still move in unison and to an equal extent.

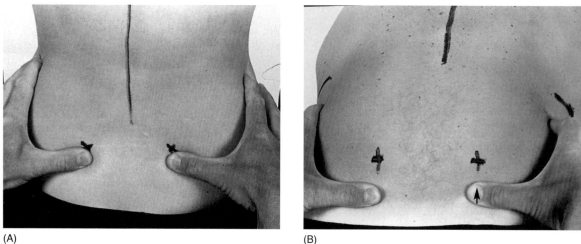

Figure 2.87 Abnormal sacroiliac flexion/extension tests with rotational malalignment: right anterior and 'locked', left posterior. (A) In standing upright, the level of right posterior superior iliac spine (PSIS) is just above that of the left. (B) On trunk flexion: the right PSIS has moved even further upwards. (C) On trunk extension: the right PSIS has moved below the left.

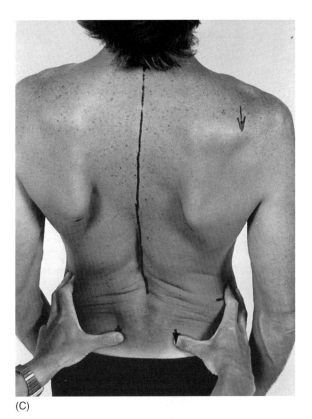

(C)

Figure 2.87 *Continued.*

Similar changes would occur on movement of the PSIS relative to the sacral base on flexion/ extension tests. In the athlete presenting with left anterior innominate rotation, the changes in PSIS level would be the reverse of those discussed above. As with the sitting–lying test, it is the relative change in position on these flexion/ extension tests that is of prime importance to help to diagnose the presence of an upslip versus a 'locking' of a joint and rotational malalignment.

Ipsilateral kinetic rotational test (Gillet test)

The Gillet test is a test for:

- the ability to balance while weight-bearing on one leg
- the ability for parts of the pelvic girdle on the non-weight-bearing side to continue to undergo some rotation while those on the weight-bearing side become 'fixed' or stabilized as load is transferred through the pelvic girdle onto that leg

For a left kinetic rotational test, the examiner places the left thumb against the inferior aspect of the left PSIS and the right thumb on the sacrum directly in line with the left thumb (Fig. 2.88A). The athlete is first asked to: flex the left hip and knee to 90 degrees (posterior rotational test):

- Left hip flexion will normally cause the left innominate to rotate posteriorly relative to the sacrum. Therefore, the thumb on the left innominate will move downwards relative to the right thumb resting on the relatively 'fixed' sacrum (Fig. 2.88C). Flexion of the left hip past 90 degrees should result in further posterior rotation of the left innominate and a downwards displacement of that thumb.
- With this test, there will also be a simultaneous left rotation of the sacrum, as well as a left rotation coupled with side flexion of the L5 vertebral complex. Standing on the right leg alone triggers contraction in the muscles that stabilize or 'fix' the right SI joint (e.g. the right piriformis and iliopsoas), so that the right innominate and sacrum can now be considered to act as one stable unit. Therefore, flexion of the left hip will not normally result in any movement between the right thumb placed below the right PSIS and the left thumb on the adjoining sacrum.
- The right kinetic posterior rotational test should show the above findings in reverse: when the right hip is flexed, posterior rotation of the right innominate with downwards displacement of the right thumb relative to the left thumb resting on the stable sacrum (Fig. 2.88E).

The athlete then extends the right hip joint (anterior rotational test). This results in findings opposite to those seen with right hip flexion: anterior rotation of the right innominate relative to the sacrum, with sacral left rotation and L5 left rotation and side flexion. The right thumb will move upwards relative to the left one on the sacrum (Fig. 2.89). There will be no detectable movement between the thumbs similarly placed on the left side. Left hip extension should result in the same findings in reverse.

A normal test will show the amount of movement of the thumb on the right innominate to be equal to that noted when doing the test on the left side (see Figs 2.88C, E). A positive (abnormal) kinetic rotational test can occur with movement dysfunction of the SI joint and may be partial or complete. There are therefore two possible findings when the dysfunction involves the right SI joint.

- *a completely abnormal test:* 'locking' of the right SI joint is present and does not allow for any rotation

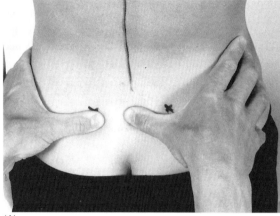

(A)

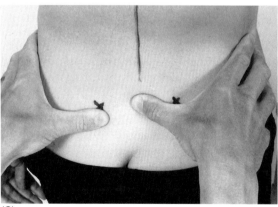

(B)

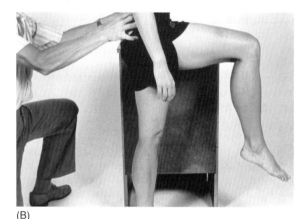

(C)

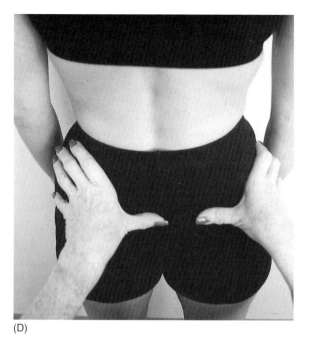

(D)

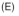

(E)

Figure 2.88 Normal posterior kinetic rotational (Gillet) tests: hip flexion. (A) Starting position for the test on the left: the left thumb placed against the inferior aspect of the left posterior superior iliac spine (PSIS), the right thumb on the sacral base just lateral to the median sacral crest and level with the left thumb. (B) Set-up for testing, with a side table to provide support should balance become a problem. (C) Left hip flexion: posterior rotation of left innominate displaces the left thumb downwards relative to that on the sacrum. (D) Starting position for the test on the right (the reverse of that seen in A). (E) Right hip flexion: posterior rotation of the right innominate displaces the right thumb downwards relative to that on the sacrum by an amount equal to that noted on the left side (see Fig. 2.88C).

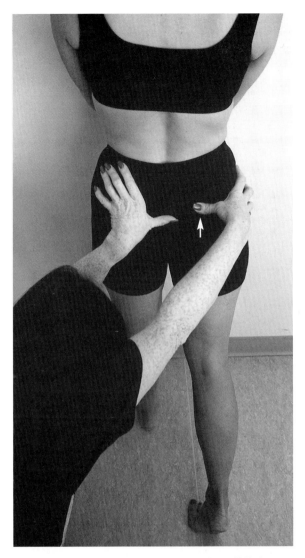

Figure 2.89 Normal anterior kinetic rotational (Gillet) test: hip extension. Starting position for the test on the right side as in Fig. 2.88D (for the left, as in Fig. 2.88A). On right hip extension: anterior rotation of the right innominate displaces the right thumb upwards relative to that on the sacrum.

between the sacrum and the right innominate. The right thumb fails to separate from the left one as the right hip is flexed or extended (Fig. 2.90A). On attempting to flex the right hip to more than 90 degrees, the right thumb will actually begin to move upwards (Fig. 2.90B). This reflects the fact that further right hip flexion is actually accomplished by having the 'locked' sacrum and right innominate rotate as one unit counterclockwise in the frontal plane. The test will be normal on the left side.

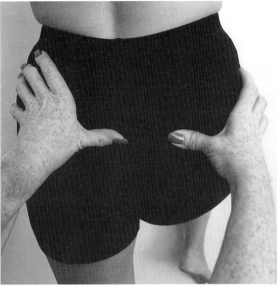

(A)

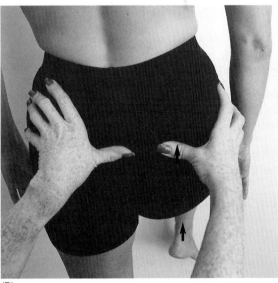

(B)

Figure 2.90 Abnormal right kinetic rotational test (right sacroiliac joint 'locked'). (A) Right hip flexion: the right posterior superior iliac spine (PSIS) fails to drop down relative to the sacral base (relatively unchanged from Fig. 2.88D starting view). (B) Increasing right hip flexion: the right PSIS actually moves upwards – the sacrum and right innominate rotate counterclockwise in the frontal plane as one 'locked' unit.

- *a partially abnormal test:* limited movement between the right sacrum and innominate is possible, allowing some separation of the two thumbs, but is perceptibly less on the right side compared with what occurs when the test is carried out on the 'unlocked' left side.

A positive kinetic rotational test may also be possible with intrinsic hip joint abnormality, lumbar spine scoliosis or leg length inequality (Bernard & Cassidy 1991) as well as with various lesions of the ipsilateral 'iliosacral' joint or the lumbar spine (Fowler 1986). Therefore, one should never rely on one test in isolation when attempting to establish the diagnosis of malalignment and SI joint malfunction.

Clinical correlation

- Anatomical LLD, SI joint upslip and outflare/inflare: the test is negative.
- Rotational malalignment: the test may be positive, with evidence of a partial or complete loss of movement on one side. This dysfunction is often reduced or abolished very quickly with early treatment even though there may be ongoing evidence of the rotational malalignment.

Evaluation of load transfer ability: active straight leg raising

Active straight leg raising, with or without reinforcement to engage the form and force closure mechanisms, can be used to evaluate the athlete's ability to transfer load from the lumbosacral junction through the pelvic girdle and hip joint to the lower extremity. Active right straight leg raising in supine-lying normally results in:

- posterior rotation of the right innominate and relative anterior rotation of the sacral base on the right, with nutation of the right SI joint (DonTigny 1985)
- a tendency of the whole pelvis to rotate around the vertical axis towards the raised right leg (Jull et al 1993)
- a simultaneous rotation at the lumbosacral junction in the opposite direction, which results in tightening of the right iliolumbar ligaments and a further decrease in movement of the right SI joint.

The overall effect is a stabilization of both the lumbosacral junction and the right SI joint, which in turn allows for a more effective load transfer from the spine to the leg on that side (Snijders et al 1993). Mens et al (1997) have described how a decreased ability to actively straight leg raise while lying supine seems to correlate with an abnormally increased mobility of the pelvic girdle, as evaluated by movement at the sym-

physis pubis on X-ray. If a dysfunction of load transfer is suspected, supplemental tests to define whether there is a problem with the passive or active system are indicated.

The active straight leg raising is carried out both supine and prone-lying. The athlete is initially observed performing a functional test, namely straight leg raising unassisted, one leg at a time (Figs 2.91A and 2.92A).

Note is made of the following:

- the degree of active straight leg raising possible on each side
- the ease with which the straight leg raising is carried out (both as observed and as reported by the athlete)
- any compensatory movements of the pelvis or trunk; these usually involve rotation of the pelvis toward the side on which the leg is being raised

---

The effect of the following supplemental tests on the ability to carry out the active straight leg raising may help to localize a problem to the passive or the active system. Any improvement would be suggested by an increase in the range of active straight leg raising accomplished and/or an increase in the ease with which this manoeuvre is carried out.

Form closure (passive)

An augmentation of form closure can be achieved by compression of the SI joints with a medially directed compression force applied to the lateral aspect of the innominates while the athlete attempts active straight leg raising (Figs 2.91B and 2.92B). Any improvement noted suggests that the problem is in part or completely caused by a loss of the passive supporting system (e.g. ligament lengthening or tear, or joint laxity resulting from osteoarthritic degeneration).

Force closure (active)

Improvement achieved by an augmentation of force closure suggests that the problem is primarily the result of a loss of strength in the supporting muscles, incoordination of muscle support or a combination of these.

Inner core (see Fig. 2.22). Active straight leg raising is attempted while contracting the transverses abdomini, multifidus, thoracic diaphragm and pelvic floor muscles.

Anterior oblique system (see Fig. 2.25B). After first carrying out right active straight leg raising in supine-lying (hip flexion), the athlete is asked to repeat the manoeuvre immediately after having activated the anterior

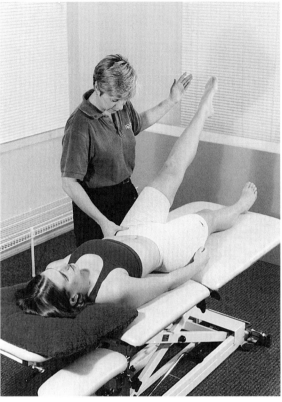

(A)

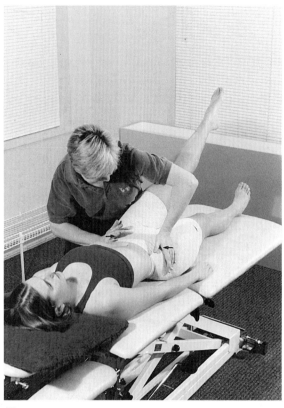

(B)

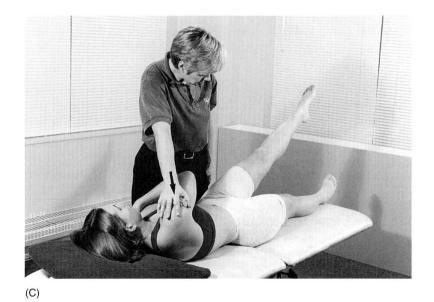

(C)

Figure 2.91 Functional test for sacroiliac joint load transfer ability in supine-lying. (A) Functional test of supine active straight leg raise. (B) With form closure augmented. (C) With force closure augmented. (From Lee 1999, with permission.)

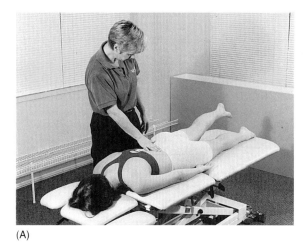

(A)

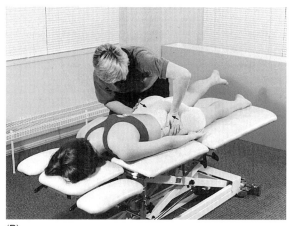

(B)

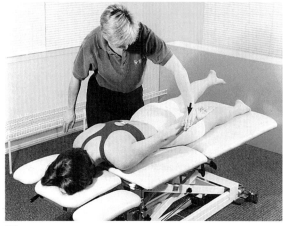

(C)

Figure 2.92 Functional test for sacroiliac joint load transfer ability in prone-lying. (A) Functional test of prone active straight leg raise. (B) With form closure augmented. (C) With force closure augmented. (From Lee 1999, with permission.)

oblique system. Activation is accomplished by having the athlete reach with the left hand over towards the right knee, effectively flexing and rotating the trunk towards the right. Activation can be augmented by resisting the trunk rotation with pressure against the left anterior shoulder (see Fig. 2.91C). The same manoeuvre is then carried out on the left side for comparison.

Posterior oblique system (see Fig. 2.25A). After first carrying out right active straight leg raising in prone-lying (hip extension), the athlete is asked to repeat this manoeuvre immediately after extending and medially rotating the left arm against a steady resistance offered by the examiner (see Fig. 2.91C). The resistance to this movement activates the left latissimus dorsi, increases tension in the thoracodorsal fascia and primes the posterior oblique system prior to actively extending the right leg. During this test, note is also made of the sequence of muscle activation on leg extension; in the

example given, this would be right hamstrings initially, followed by right gluteus maximus and finally the left erector spinae muscles (Janda 1978).

SIMULTANEOUS BILATERAL SACROILIAC JOINT MALALIGNMENT

Our discussion has been restricted primarily to the two major presentations associated with the malalignment syndrome, namely SI joint upslip and rotational malalignment. Both result in an asymmetrical distortion of the pelvis. Outflare and inflare have been mentioned, specifically for the distortion they cause to the pelvis and their interaction particularly with rotational malalignment. For the sake of completeness, a brief mention must be made of some

Case history

An athlete suffered a shear injury of her right sacroiliac joint when her right leg shot out in front of her on a wet floor and she landed on her right buttock. The right sacroiliac joint was unstable in both the anteroposterior and craniocaudal planes, making it impossible to maintain any correction of the malalignment even for short periods of time. The results of active straight leg raising tests were as follows:

1. Right active straight leg raising was 40 degrees supine, 10 prone and painful in both positions; the values for the left were 70 and 30 degrees respectively, both pain free. Lateral compression (augmented form closure) improved the values for the right side to 70 degrees supine and 30 prone, with a report of a decrease in the associated pain; the left-side values remained unchanged.

2. Activation of inner core and the anterior and posterior oblique systems (augmented force closure) failed to improve the values on either side.

The diagnostic impression was that of a shear injury of the right sacroiliac joint and a loss of form closure, the instability probably being attributable to loss of the ligamentous support. Force closure, derived from core muscle strength and coordination, appeared to be intact. The initial treatment consisted of using a sacroiliac belt and undergoing a course of prolotherapy injections to strengthen and tighten up the ligaments surrounding the right sacroiliac joint. Once ligamental support had been regained, attempts at realignment and strengthening of the back, pelvic and hip girdle muscles were successfully resumed (see Ch. 7).

problems that relate to alignment but present with pelvic symmetry and lack the features typical of the malalignment syndrome. The diagnosis is often delayed or missed altogether because of a paucity of physical findings or difficulty in interpreting the signs and symptoms.

SYMMETRICAL MOVEMENT OF THE INNOMINATES RELATIVE TO THE SACRUM

Excessive anterior or posterior rotation of both innominates and simultaneous bilateral upslips or downslips can occur (DonTigny 1985, Richard 1986). These present primarily with signs of movement restriction, along with a displacement of the landmarks that is symmetrical and may therefore be difficult to diagnose. For example, with bilateral anterior innominate rotation there is:

- bilateral restriction of hip flexion and straight leg raising as a result of the mechanical limitation caused

by anterior rotation of the acetabular rim, and the increased tension in the hamstrings, whose origins have been separated from their insertions
- a symmetrical upward movement of the PSIS, making these landmarks more prominent
- symmetrical depression of the ASIS.

SACRAL TORSION AROUND A TRANSVERSE AXIS

These conditions involve excessive torsion of the sacrum in the sagittal plane around a transverse axis. For example, falling and landing on the apex can rotate the base backwards into excessive counternutation, whereas a blow to the base can rotate it forwards into excessive nutation. Although landmarks are altered, their symmetry is preserved and that may be misleading. Richard (1986, p. 26) describes the following conditions.

'Bilateral sacrum anterior'

This lesion can result with hyperextension of the pelvis and spine. The sacrum becomes fixed, with the base actually backwards and the apex forwards (counternutation), the sacrospinous ligaments, which come to play the role of a pivot, being under increased tension and at risk of injury. The sacral sulci diminish or disappear, and the apex becomes less prominent. The lumbar lordosis is decreased or abolished, and the lumbar segment feels 'stiff' on applying pressure to the spinous processes. The athlete may complain of back pain and difficulty in stooping forward.

The lumbar plexus bilaterally is put under increased tension. A separation of their origins and insertions also increases tension bilaterally in iliacus and rectus femoris; this in turn limits hip extension and decreases the space available for the existing femoral and obturator nerves. There may be symptoms of bilateral groin discomfort and paraesthesias, suggesting femoral and/or obturator nerve irritation, and the femoral stretch test may be positive. The ASIS will have moved downwards and the PSIS upwards bilaterally and symmetrically.

'Bilateral sacrum posterior'

Excessive forward rotation of the sacral base (nutation) is sometimes seen following excessive forward flexion of the trunk and pelvis. It results in a uniform deepening of the sacral sulci and a uniform increase in the prominence of the inferolateral sacral angles and the sacral apex. The lumbar lordosis is increased; the lumbar segment feels supple and elastic when pressure is applied to the spinous processes. Pressure on the facet joints is increased. Nerve roots may be compromised by a narrowing of the intervertebral foramina.

Tension in the sacrotuberous ligaments and hamstrings is increased by a separation of their origins and insertions; hip flexion is reduced, and these structures, which may be tender to palpation, are now at increased risk of injury. The athlete may complain of recurrent cramps in the hamstrings, and of pain from the lower sacral region and ischial attachments of the sacrotuberous ligaments.

These conditions are mentioned mainly to point out that there are other presentations involving the rotation of pelvic structures that can be a major cause of debility. Unlike an upslip or rotational malalignment, however:

- the symmetry of the landmarks is preserved
- there is no associated malalignment syndrome.

STANDARD BACK EXAMINATION CAN BE MISLEADING!

It cannot be emphasized strongly enough that parts of the standard back examination are often completely normal in the athlete presenting with malalignment. In particular, this includes looking at trunk flexion, extension, side-bending and simultaneous extension and rotation to right and left. These manoeuvres may fail to stress the structures in the pelvic region or spine in such a way as to provoke pain from the sites that are typically put under stress by malalignment. Unfortunately, the fact that the limited standard examination has failed to elicit pain is sometimes interpreted as meaning that the athlete does not have a problem, when the real problem is that the clinician's examination skills are limited and, in fact, inadequate for establishing the diagnosis of malalignment.

At the same time, it must be remembered that even if the examiner is familiar with the tests for malalignment, the diagnosis of malalignment should be based on a conglomeration of findings and never on the results of just one or two tests alone. The examination should include an assessment for:

- leg length in more than one position
- asymmetry of landmarks, muscle strength, hip joint ranges of motion and other aspects of the malalignment syndrome (see Ch. 3).

> Once the presence of malalignment has been established, one must avoid falling into the trap of automatically assuming that all the athlete's complaints are related to the malalignment.

There is no excuse for not carrying out a complete orthopaedic, neurological and vascular examination in order to rule out other pathology. Only this will allow one to determine, with some degree of certainty, whether some or all of the symptoms are attributable to the malalignment, and to proceed with appropriate investigations in addition to realignment and other treatment measures. This chapter has hopefully provided a sound basis for the examination techniques that will be of help in making these distinctions in athletes presenting with malalignment.

3

The malalignment syndrome

Sacroiliac (SI) upslips and rotational malalignment never exist in isolation: there are always associated changes involving both the axial and appendicular skeleton as well as the attaching soft tissue – muscles, tendons, fascia, ligaments and capsules. In addition to various asymmetries of the skeletal and soft tissue structures, there is also a reorientation of the body segments from head to foot. The combined effect is the malalignment syndrome.

CLINICAL FINDINGS COMMONLY NOTED WITH MALALIGNMENT

Malalignment syndrome will be discussed here in terms of several findings on the physical examination that are commonly associated with malalignment (Box 3.1).

Box 3.1 Physical findings associated with the malalignment syndrome

- Asymmetry of pelvic orientation in the frontal plane
- Asymmetry of pelvic orientation and movement in the transverse plane
- Asymmetry of sacroiliac joint mobility
- Curvature of the lumbar, thoracic and cervical spine
- Asymmetry of the thoracic and shoulder girdle ranges of motion
- Asymmetry of lower extremity orientation
- Asymmetry of foot alignment, weight-bearing and shoe wear
- Asymmetry of muscle tension
- Asymmetry of upper and lower extremity muscle strength
- Asymmetry of muscle bulk
- Asymmetry of ligament tension
- Asymmetry of upper and lower extremity ranges of motion
- Apparent leg length difference
- Problems with balance and recovery

There are some significant differences in the manifestation of the malalignment syndrome seen in association with:

- rotational malalignment
- SI joint upslip.

The prevalence of malalignment, and of the three main types of presentation, has been detailed in Chapter 2. Basically:

1. approximately 80–90% of adults present with malalignment
2. rotational malalignment is far more common than upslip, presenting in isolation in approximately 80–85%, compared to upslip alone in only 10%, of those presenting with malalignment
3. upslips coexist with rotational malalignment in another 5–10% of cases
4. outflare/inflare is present in approximately 5–15%, either in isolation or combined with one or both of the other types.

The discussion will focus first on the malalignment syndrome seen in association with rotational malalignment, with reference to SI joint upslip where appropriate. A separate section emphasizes the major similarities and differences seen when the syndrome is associated with an SI joint upslip compared with rotational malalignment, this being followed by features of the syndrome associated with outflare/inflare. Significant clinical correlations are indicated at the end of most of the subheadings. Reference is also made to Chapters 5 and 6 and Appendixes 1–13 for a more detailed analysis of the sports-specific implications of this syndrome.

MALALIGNMENT SYNDROME SEEN WITH ROTATIONAL MALALIGNMENT

Rotational malalignment refers to the excessive anterior or posterior rotation of one innominate in the sagittal plane; the contralateral innominate may compensate by rotating in the opposite direction. Torsion of the sacrum around the right or left oblique axis (see Fig. 2.33) usually completes the distortion of the pelvic ring. In most cases, there is evidence of dysfunction of movement of one or other SI joint. This can range from hypermobility to various degrees of decreased mobility or complete 'locking'.

DESCRIPTION OF ROTATIONAL MALALIGNMENT

In order to prevent needless repetition, the following abbreviations will be used:

- right (or left) anterior (or posterior) rotation (see Figs 2.29 and 2.46), referring to anterior or posterior rotation of the right or left innominate relative to the sacrum in the sagittal plane
- right (or left) locked on the kinetic rotational test (see Figs 2.86, 2.87 and 2.90), referring to locking of the right or left SI joint; more common on the right side than the left.

'Right anterior, left locked' would, for example, refer to an athlete presenting with anterior rotation of the right innominate and locking of the left SI joint. For illustrative purposes, reference is frequently made to 'right anterior and locked', which refers to the combination of 'right anterior rotation and locking of the right SI joint' because this is the most common of all these presentations (see Appendix 1).

Clinical correlation

Localized pain may arise from one or both SI joints. Athletes with hypomobility or locking of one SI joint not infrequently complain of pain from the region of the other, supposedly normal, SI joint. This suggests that the pain may result from the increased stress on this 'normal' joint and its ligaments as it tries to compensate for the lack of mobility in the impaired SI joint (see Figs 2.2 and 2.3).

The pain may result from a chronic increase in tension or even spasm in muscles that may reflect:

- contraction to effect rotation of an innominate (e.g. iliacus; see Fig. 2.31B, C) or sacral torsion (e.g. piriformis; see Fig. 2.31A) as these muscles attempt to stabilize the SI joint(s) by decreasing the mobility or causing actual locking
- facilitation of these muscles as a result of the malalignment (see 'Asymmetry of muscle tension' below).

Pain may also result from an increase in pressure on the malaligned, and hence incongruent, SI joint surfaces. Bone scans frequently show increased and/or asymmetrical activity in the SI joints (see Fig. 4.31). In the absence of any indications of an inflammatory condition, such as a seronegative spondyloarthropathy or ankylosing spondylitis, these abnormalities on the bone scan may simply reflect an increase in bone turnover triggered by such an increase in pressure. The abnormalities on the bone scans usually disappear once the pressure has been relieved by maintaining realignment of the joint surfaces for several months.

Following a successful correction of the malalignment, examination may now reveal hypermobility of a previously locked joint, which predisposes to a recurrence of the malalignment and locking. Hypermobility may be indicative of ligament laxity, osteoarthritic joint degeneration, poor muscle support or control, or a combination of these. Ligament laxity may be a reflection of:

• a previous severe sprain or strain of the ligaments, such as occurs with a shear injury to the SI joint sustained by falling and landing on one buttock or leg (see Fig. 2.34B)

• ligament lengthening that has occurred with time as the ligaments are:
– put under constant stretch by the distortion of the pelvic ring seen with malalignment
– repeatedly stretched with recurrence of malalignment after correction (see Fig. 3.60)

• a generalized problem of hypermobile joints, possibly as the result of a genetically determined defect in the amount or quality of elastic tissue produced. This problem can vary in degree of severity and, at its worst, presents in the form of conditions such as the Ehler–Danlos syndrome.

The presence of generalized hypermobility is important to establish because these athletes generally do not respond as well to realignment attempts, tend to lose correction more easily and are more likely to benefit from additional measures to maintain correc-tion (e.g. foot orthotics, SI belts and ligament injections). Generalized hypermobility is more common in the group that tends to 'switch sides', for example, presenting with right or left anterior rotation on different occasions.

A quick test to assess the degree of mobility is to have the athlete flex the wrist and then passively bring the thumb towards the volar aspect of the forearm. In most tests, the thumb will end up parallel to the forearm (Fig. 3.1A). If the thumb is further away from the forearm (e.g. the athlete on the left in Fig. 3.1A), or closer to or even touching the forearm (Fig. 3.1B), the athlete may well have generalized joint hypo- or hypermobility respectively. This should be confirmed by assessing the amount of joint play possible on the passive movement of some other joints (Fig. 3.1B); a full assessment using the 9-point Beighton scale may be appropriate (Beighton et al 1999). A side-to-side comparison is also important to make sure one is not just dealing with laxity from a previous injury to the ligaments on one side.

VARIANTS OF THE SYNDROME SEEN WITH ROTATIONAL MALALIGNMENT

Malalignment of the pelvis, spine and extremities can result from a number of interacting causes. Postural

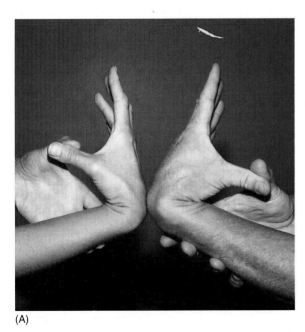

(A)

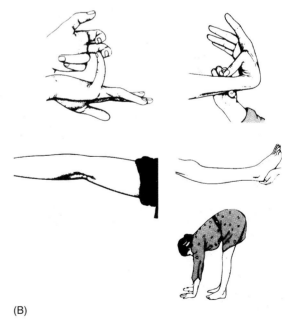

(B)

Figure 3.1 Test for degree of overall joint mobility. (A) Mobility is relatively decreased in the athlete on the left, whose thumb actually points away, compared with the athlete on the right, whose thumb ends up parallel to the forearm (the usual finding with normal mobility). (B) 9-point Beighton scale for hypermobility: passive finger dorsiflexion past 90 degress (R/L); passive thumb apposition to the flexor surface of the forearm (R/L); hyperextension of the R/L elbow, the R/L knee beyond 10 degrees; trunk flexion to rest the palms on the floor (with the knees extended). (From Beighton 1999, with permission.)

distortion, for example, may result in a muscle imbalance, but the distortion may itself be the result of such an imbalance. As Maffetone (1999) indicates, potentially more than one postural distortion can result from the same muscle imbalance. He gives the example of psoas major, indicating that inhibition of tension in this muscle for whatever reason typically causes the pelvis to tilt. The pelvis usually rises on the opposite side, where psoas major is now in relative 'overfacilitation', the tension in the muscle being increased compared with that on the inhibited side (Fig. 3.2). Maffetone, however, goes on to say that:

in many cases, the reverse is true and the psoas inhibition is found on the side of the elevated pelvis. This may depend

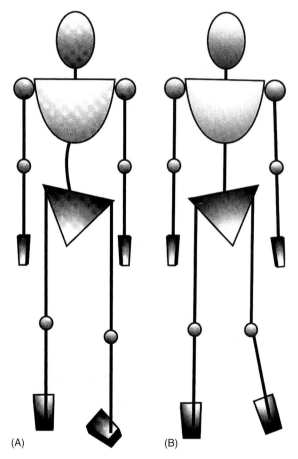

Figure 3.2 Assessing static posture. (A) Psoas inhibition on the right may allow medial rotation of the ipsilateral foot with excess pronation. The lumbar spine is convex on the contralateral side (tight psoas). The pelvis may be lower (sometimes higher) on the ipsilateral side. (B) Right sartorius or gracillis inhibition may cause a posterior rotation of the pelvis, seen as an elevation of the ipsilateral side and genu valgum. (From Maffetone 1999, with permission.)

on which problem was primary and which secondary, how the foot reacts, what other muscles are compensating, and other factors. (p. 88)

The reader is referred to works such as that by Maffetone (1999) for a detailed discussion of the postural imbalances that can result with the inhibition and facilitation of various muscles. The present book will concentrate on two variants of the malalignment syndrome that are of particular significance in the evaluation of athletes:

1. the *'left anterior and locked'* presentation (Fig. 3.3A):
– athletes who present with the left leg rotated externally (outwards from the midline) and the right rotated internally (inwards toward midline), with a pattern of weight-bearing tending to left pronation and right supination. This relatively rare presentation can result from a combination of factors, usually including anterior rotation and outflare of the left innominate and locking of the left SI joint. It will therefore be referred to as 'left anterior and locked'
2. *alternate* presentations (Fig. 3.3B): athletes who present with the right leg rotated externally and the left internally, with a pattern of weight-bearing tending to right pronation and left supination. This is a much more common presentation on examination and can result from any combination of anterior rotation of the right or left innominate, and locking of the right or left SI joint (other than the 'left anterior and locked' pattern mentioned above). Such presentations will therefore be referred to as 'alternate' presentations.

These two variants differ primarily from each other in terms of the associated pattern of:

● asymmetry of joint ranges of motion
● asymmetry of weight-bearing
● asymmetry of strength.

The difference will be highlighted in the discussion of these specific asymmetries. Otherwise, the descriptions of the clinical findings encountered with rotational malalignment pertain to both variants.

ASYMMETRY OF PELVIC ORIENTATION IN THE FRONTAL PLANE

Pelvic obliquity, suggesting rotation in the frontal plane, is one of the most consistent findings with both rotational malalignment and upslip.

As indicated in Chapter 2, rotational malalignment results in a complete asymmetry of the major landmarks, both side to side and front to back, because of an

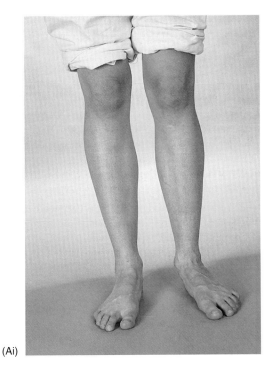

(Ai)

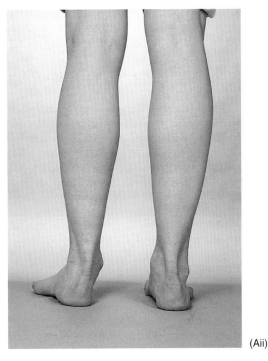

(Aii)

(B)

Figure 3.3 Two variants of the malalignment syndrome (see also Figs 3.18 and 3.19). (A) With the rare left anterior and locked presentation – the left foot turned outwards from the midline and pronating, the right in towards the midline and supinating: (i) standing and (ii) walking view. (B) With the more common 'alternate' presentations and upslip: the right foot is turned out and pronating, the left faces towards the midline and is supinating. The left foot may even cross the midline – see Fig. 3.16Bii.

asymmetry of the sacrum and the innominates in all planes: frontal, transverse and sagittal (see Figs 2.6, 2.29 and 2.46). Given the predominance of right anterior innominate rotation, one is more likely to find elevation of the right than the left lateral iliac crest – approximately 80% versus 20%. It can, however, be the left crest that is elevated with a right anterior rotation. Which iliac crest is higher is determined not only by the direction of innominate rotation, but also by factors such as:

- the position in which the athlete is examined: with a right anterior rotation, for example, the right iliac crest may be higher or lower in standing but will usually be higher in sitting and prone-lying (see Figs 2.43C and 2.46B)

- a coexisting anatomical leg length difference (LLD), upslip or downslip (see Figs 2.42B, 2.43A, B and 2.44)
- the direction of sacral torsion, if present (see Figs 2.7, 2.11, 2.29 and 2.57)
- the side of SI joint 'locking', if present (see Figs 2.86, 2.87 and 2.90).

As an example of these variations, an athlete with right anterior rotation may have elevation on the left iliac crest in standing because of a true LLD, left leg long. In sitting and in lying prone, however, the right side may be elevated because the effect of the LLD has been eliminated in these two positions. Alternatively, an athlete with no LLD and a left anterior and locked presentation typically has elevation of the right iliac crest in standing and sitting but elevation of the left side when lying prone (see Figs 2.43D and 2.55).

Clinical correlation

The difference in the elevation of the iliac crests is sometimes strikingly obvious and may be accentuated by the cut of a costume. The visual effect of this may distract from the aesthetic appearance. In disciplines such dancing and figure-skating, this could conceivably affect the perception and judgement of style. For the athlete, there may be more mundane problems related to clothing or belts repeatedly slipping down or even completely off on one side, just as objects carried over the 'lower' shoulder will tend to slip off (see Fig. 2.64A).

Sitting is likely to present problems. The ischial tuberosities are at different levels: raised on the side of the anterior, and lowered on the side of the posterior, rotation (see Figs 2.46D and 3.69A). With a right anterior rotation, the right ischial tuberosity can easily end up 1 cm off the sitting surface, the weight now being borne primarily by the left tuberosity. The athlete often talks of 'sitting more on one buttock than the other' and may get relief simply by putting a hand or a small pillow under the raised tuberosity for relief when sitting for longer periods of time and when driving.

Sitting increases the pressure on the lower tuberosity and creates a shearing force on the ipsilateral SI joint by pushing the innominate upward relative to the sacrum. In addition, the ischial tuberosities serve as the insertion of the sacrotuberous ligament and the origin of the hamstrings. These structures are particularly vulnerable to direct pressure at this site on the side of the posterior rotation, especially when sitting in a slouched position or on a hard surface. Slouching or sitting in a bucket seat allows the innominates and sacrum to rotate posteriorly as a unit, further increasing pressure, particularly on the ischial tuberosity and posterior superior iliac spine (PSIS) on the side of the exaggerated posterior rotation. Aside from using a hand or cushion between the raised ischial tuberosity and the seat, to actually fill in the gap created by the anterior rotation, the athlete may also get comfort by:

- increasing the general amount of cushioning under the buttocks
- placing a cushion under the thighs, ahead of the ischial tuberosities, or in the small of the back, in order to stop any tendency to further posterior rotation of the pelvis
- continuously shifting weight-bearing from side to side.

None of these methods may work very well, especially when the athlete has to remain seated for a longer period of time in a confined space or when the seating area is small and hard, such as in a rowing shell or on a bicycle.

In riding, the lowered ischial tuberosity may increase pressure on the horse's ipsilateral paravertebral musculature, by digging into the muscle directly (bareback) or through the saddle. This can cause a reflex increase in tension in these muscles and may make the horse appear 'stiff' on that side in its movements (see Ch. 6).

ASYMMETRY OF PELVIC ORIENTATION AND MOVEMENT IN THE TRANSVERSE PLANE

With rotational malalignment, the pelvis often appears rotated counterclockwise in the transverse plane some 5–10 degrees, rarely more. This probably relates to the fact that right anterior, left posterior rotation, which tends to twist the pelvic ring in a counterclockwise direction and bring the right ASIS forward and the left backward, is by far the most common presentation. Therefore, the pelvis is more likely to jut out at the front on the right side and recede on the left when the athlete is standing (Fig. 3.4A). Rotation in this plane will, however, also be influenced by the position of examination. Consider the example of the athlete who has obvious right forward rotation in standing. When he or she goes to lie prone on a hard plinth, the protruding right anterior superior iliac spine (ASIS) will be the first to contact the plinth and will be forced posteriorly. In this position, therefore, the pelvis could now look level in the transverse plane, or may even end up protruding backwards on the right side.

> In the presence of rotational malalignment, active and passive rotation of the pelvis in the transverse plane is restricted into the side of the posteriorly rotated innominate.

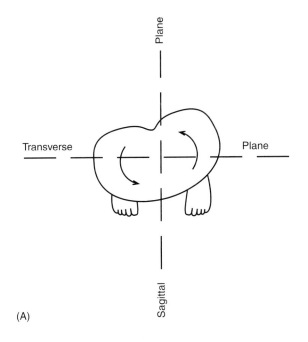

(A)

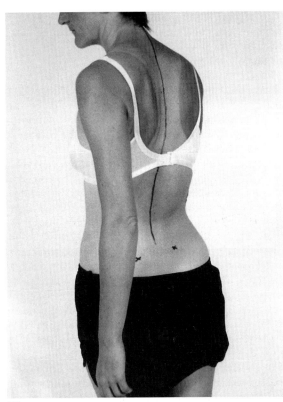

(C)

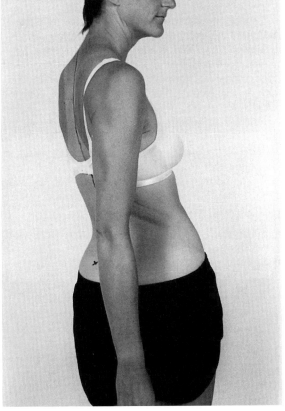

(B)

Figure 3.4 Asymmetry of pelvic rotation in the transverse plane typically seen with rotational malalignment. (A) Standing – asymmetry with right anterior, left posterior rotation of the pelvis on a superior view; the trunk may rotate in the opposite or the same direction, with compensatory rotation of the head and neck. (B) Clockwise rotation to 45 degrees. (C) Counterclockwise rotation decreased to 30 degrees (note the decreased facial profile compared with Fig. 3.4B).

Restriction is independent of the side of SI joint movement dysfunction and direction of sacral torsion. Restriction into the side of the posterior rotation occurs for the following reasons.

First, counterclockwise rotation of the pelvis in the transverse plane that occurs normally with walking requires the simultaneous contrary rotation of the innominates, posteriorly on the right and anteriorly on the left (see Figs 2.9, 2.17 and 2.28). The pattern is reversed with clockwise rotation.

Second, when there is rotational malalignment with the right innominate in anterior, and left in posterior rotation, clockwise rotation is increased by the fact that the malaligned innominates can rotate further from their resting position into the directions needed to allow this particular movement (Fig. 3.4B). The left innominate, which starts off rotated posteriorly, can rotate anteriorly through more degrees until it reaches the end of available range than if it had started from its normal position. Similarly, the anteriorly rotated right innominate can rotate posteriorly through more degrees until it reaches the end point of available range in that direction. Overall, this translates into more degrees of clockwise rotation.

In addition, counterclockwise rotation is limited by the fact that the innominates are already rotated part way in the directions required for them to move into with this manoeuvre (Fig. 3.4C). Namely, the right is already rotated anteriorly and the left posteriorly, restricting any further rotation into these directions required for counterclockwise rotation.

To assess rotation in the transverse plane, ask the athlete to stand with the inside of the legs or feet just touching. Sit behind the athlete, feet planted on either side of the athlete's feet and, using the pressure of your knees and calves press the lower part of the athlete's legs gently together in order to decrease the amount of rotation that can occur through the lower extremities. Instruct the athlete to let the trunk, head, neck and upper extremities follow the movement of the pelvis, that is, not to twist these parts of the body relative to the pelvis. Then passively rotate the pelvis in the transverse plane, first to one side and then the other. There is often the feel of a sudden, hard stop to rotation of the pelvis into the side of the restriction, which the athlete may well sense. Note the amount of rotation possible from neutral.

A rotation of 45 degrees to the right and only 30 degrees to the left would, for example, not be unusual in someone with posterior rotation of the left innominate (Fig. 3.4B, C). Discrepancies of greater magnitude can occur, the degree of limitation appearing to be proportionate to the degree of difference in anterior

versus posterior innominate rotation. However, correction of the malalignment immediately removes this restriction and allows for an equal amount of rotation. The fact that this would be 45 degrees to both right and left in the example given suggests that other factors are probably operative, such as restriction of sacral torsion/rotation, asymmetry of muscle tension, and asymmetry of the hip ranges of motion (see below).

Clinical correlation

This asymmetry interferes with the ability to execute turning manoeuvres that require pelvic rotation in the transverse plane. The prime example is downhill skiing, in which turns are initiated in large part by movement of the pelvis in the transverse plane, combined with shifting weight onto the appropriate edges. The skier is likely to experience more difficulty making a turn into the side of the posterior rotation.

> Forced active or passive rotation of the pelvis into the side of the limitation is more likely to lead to soft tissue or even bony injury because the anatomical barrier will now be exceeded earlier.

The anatomical barrier defines the terminal range of joint motion, movement past that point resulting in disruption of tissue. The athlete (e.g. skier or wrestler) presenting with malalignment is, therefore, at increased risk of injury whenever an opponent, a change in direction, or a collision forces the pelvis to rotate into the restriction.

Rotation of the spine occurs primarily through the thoracic segment. Whenever rotation of this segment is impaired, rotational stresses on the lumbar spine and the pelvic region are increased. Injury is then more likely should the pelvis be rotated actively or passively into the direction of the restriction. This can occur, for example, whenever:

- the thorax is pinned to the floor, such as in wrestling
- a gymnast spins or twists the rest of the body while holding on to the apparatus with both hands.

Conversely, a restriction of rotation in one direction at the pelvic level may require a compensatory increase in the amount of rotation of the thoracic spine. This is most likely to happen in sports requiring a simultaneous rotation of both the pelvis and trunk while standing upright: golf, baseball, court sports and certain field events (discus, hammer, shot and javelin). The increase in the rotational stress being placed on the thoracic segment, in particular the thoracolumbar junction, may account for the onset or aggravation of mid-back pain with these sports. This issue is discussed further under 'Curvatures of the lumbar, thoracic and cervical segments' below.

ASYMMETRY OF SACROILIAC JOINT MOBILITY

Between 80 and 90% of those presenting with right or left anterior rotation show SI joint mobility dysfunction, which may take any of the forms shown in Box 3.2.

The athlete who had rotational malalignment with locking or decreased mobility of one SI joint on initial examination may present for reassessment with malalignment still evident even after having undergone a course of manual therapy treatments. At this time, possible findings include the following:

- The previously noted locking or decreased mobility may still be detectable on the same side; rarely, it may even have 'switched sides'.
- More likely than not, movement on lumbosacral flexion, extension and kinetic rotational tests will now be found to be normal.
- There may now be evidence of hypermobility not noted before, indicating a problem of joint laxity that was previously hidden by hypomobility or outright locking caused by the excessive rotation of an innomi-

---

Box 3.2 Sacroiliac joint dysfunction in anterior rotation

- 'Locking': jamming of the innominate and sacrum against each other on one side results in a lack of movement between the two so that they tend to move together; on the affected side, this results in:
  - excessive upwards and downwards movement of the PSIS on trunk flexion and extension respectively (see Figs 2.86A and 2.87)
  - a failure of the landmarks to separate on the kinetic rotational or Gillet test (see Fig. 2.90)
  - no movement being discernible on SI joint 'spring' stress tests (see Figs 2.77–2.79)
- Partial 'locking': which results in:
  - some upwards and downwards movement of the PSIS relative to the sacrum on trunk flexion and extension respectively, but less than that occurring on the normal side
  - some movement detectable on the kinetic rotational and stress tests, but relatively less than on the normal side
- 'hypermobility' or 'laxity': detectable on the stress tests and defined as excessive movement in the anterior–posterior, craniocaudal or rotatory planes (see Figs 2.81 and 2.82)

---

nate relative to the sacrum, a reflex increase in muscle tone or a combination of these.

Correction of the rotational malalignment usually re-establishes normal movement on flexion/extension and kinetic rotational tests, and also serves to expose an underlying problem of hypermobility.

CURVATURE OF THE LUMBAR, THORACIC AND CERVICAL SEGMENTS

In 1903, Lovett pointed out that:

1. the spine is a flexible rod that is already bent in one plane (sagittal) to create the lumbar lordosis and thoracic kyphosis
2. the rod therefore cannot be bent in another plane (e.g. frontal) without twisting at the same time.

Therefore, in the absence of congenital or traumatic abnormalities of the vertebrae (e.g. hemivertebrae or stress fractures), the curves of the spine are formed by a rotation of the vertebrae of a respective segment: the lumbar, thoracic or cervical.

This feature has been explored further by Gracovetsky and Farfan (1986), who note that, when one tries to superimpose a lateral curve on the pre-existing lumbar lordosis and thoracic kyphosis, the following occur.

First, the components of the lumbar spine are twisted. For example, on side-bending the trunk to the left, the bodies of vertebrae L1–L4 inclusive rotate to the right, into the convexity formed. Their spinous processes therefore rotate to the left, towards the concavity (Fig. 3.5; see also Figs 2.29, 2.65, 4.6 and 4.22). This rotation is accompanied by simultaneous side flexion into the concavity, as well as forward flexion of the vertebrae.

In addition, the combined movement of flexion, side bending and rotation constitutes the so-called 'FSR movement'; should extension occur, the combination would be an 'ESR movement'; these patterns are delineated by the so-called 'laws' of Fryette (1954). A vertebra may become excessively rotated to the right or left and/or into extension or flexion, and become 'stuck' in that position. Movement in one facet joint will then be pathologically restricted, causing the vertebra to rotate around that facet on flexion or extension (see Fig. 2.63A).

In other words, the overall effect is normally 'a locking one and so plays a safety role. Where the physiological limit has been exceeded, to reverse this mechanism will be the key to the treatment of one part of the lower back syndrome' (Richard 1986).

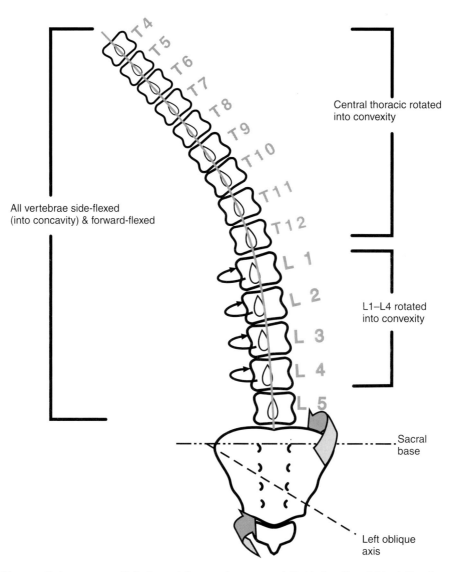

Central thoracic rotated into convexity

All vertebrae side-flexed (into concavity) & forward-flexed

L1–L4 rotated into convexity

Sacral base

Left oblique axis

Figure 3.5 Changes that occur normally in the vertebrae and sacrum on left side-bending: right rotation, forward flexion and left side flexion.

Second, it is harder to predict the direction of vertebral rotation in the thoracic segment, which is affected by the attaching ribs, the overlying scapulae and soft tissue attachments. The clear-cut correlation that exists in the lumbar segment is missing. The central thoracic vertebrae are more likely to rotate into the convexity (Fig. 3.5); the upper ones are less likely to do so (Lee 1992).

Third, during normal gait, there is rotation with possible formation of a convexity in the lumbar segment into one, and in the thoracic segment into the opposite direction, in order to balance body weight. For example, on right swing phase, lumbar vertebral rotation right and thoracic left occurs in response to torsion of the sacrum around the left oblique axis that occurs simultaneous with the posterior rotation of the right innominate as the right leg swings forward (see Fig. 2.28)

Effect of malalignment on the spine

The pelvic obliquity attributable to rotational malalignment results in compensatory curves of the spine or the accentuation of any pre-existing curves (the so-called 'normal' or 'intrinsic' curves). If the spine did not accommodate to the obliquity, the head would end up off centre, disturbing the visual and balancing mechanisms. As indicated above, the spine cannot accommodate without a rotation of the vertebrae in the thoracic and lumbar segments. The curve traced by the thoracic spinous processes is usually opposite in direction to that formed by the lumbar vertebrae (Figs 3.6A and 3.7; see also Figs 2.59, 2.60 and 2.64). X-rays also show this typical double curve, or so-called 'scoliosis', with a reversal at the thoracolumbar junction (see Figs 4.6 and 4.26).

If the cervical spine simply continued in the trajectory of the thoracic curve, the athlete would be walking about with the head and neck half-cocked, leaning towards the side of the thoracic concavity! Among other things, this would upset the balancing mechanism, which is dependent on visual and vestibular input and also, in large part, on proprioceptive signals arising from the muscles and joints in the neck region. The brain could have difficulty dealing with

sensory input derived if the head and neck were set at an angle.

There is therefore a further reversal in the curvature of the spine in order that the head will hopefully end up straight and in the midline. This reversal usually occurs at the level of the cervicothoracic junction (see Fig. 2.60A). It may, however, start as far down as T4 or T5 (see Fig. 2.60B), which accounts for a large number of those with a very obvious curvature of the lower and mid-thoracic segment convex, for example, to the right yet with the shoulder and scapula dipped down on the right side as well, or the reverse pattern. Reversal occurring in the upper thoracic region creates another stress point and may account for reports of interscapular and/or upper back discomfort.

The direction of the curves associated with rotational malalignment (or an upslip) may differ depending on whether the athlete is examined standing, sitting or lying prone. The curves are probably best regarded as an adaptation of the spine to the interaction of several factors, including the direction of sacral torsion, the lateralization of anterior/posterior innominate rotation

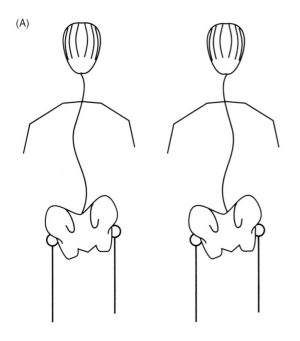

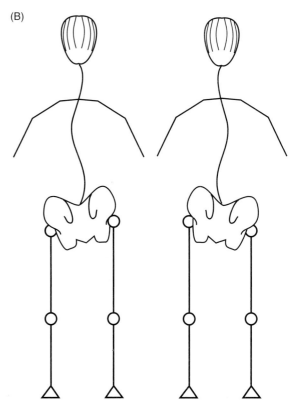

Right long leg   Left long leg

Figure 3.6 Typical patterns of scoliosis (standing). (A) Patterns seen with rotational malalignment and associated pelvic obliquity (up on the right side in the majority). (B) Scoliotic curves commonly seen with right and left anatomical leg length difference.

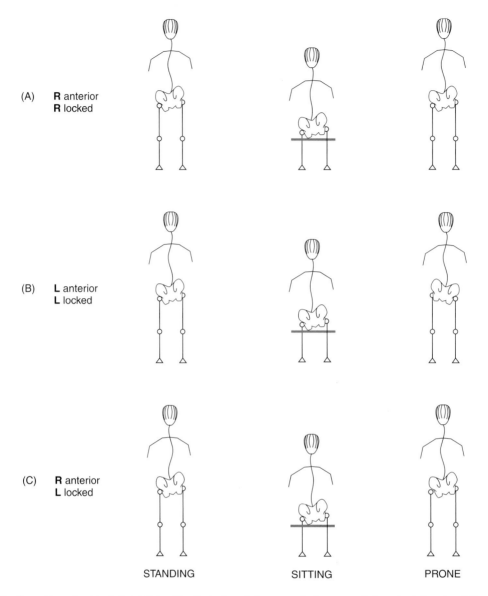

Figure 3.7 Common patterns relating pelvic obliquity and scoliotic curves to the presentation of rotational malalignment. NB. In (B), right pelvic crest is raised in standing and sitting, the left up in prone-lying; (C) shows a reversal of the scoliotic curves sometimes seen on moving from standing/sitting to prone-lying. (A) Right anterior, right locked. (B) Left anterior, left locked. (C) Right anterior, left locked.

and SI joint locking, and the presence of increased tension and/or contracture of the soft tissue attaching to the pelvis, ribs and spine.

When the athlete is lying prone or supine, there is also the passive torquing of the pelvis and/or thorax that results from the plinth pushing upward on any bony point that has been rotated in the transverse plane (e.g. shoulder, ASIS or PSIS). For example, the standing athlete not infrequently presents with 5–10 degrees of forwards rotation of the pelvis on the right side, and of the shoulder on the left. On lying prone, the contact of these protruding points with the surface results in a force that torques the pelvis clockwise and the thorax counterclockwise. This may account for the reversal of the curves sometimes noted in prone-lying compared with those seen in standing and sitting.

When one looks at the combination of pelvic obliquity and the pattern of the thoracic and lumbar curves, the pattern is least likely to change from standing to sitting to lying prone if the anterior rotation and the locking are both on the right side (Fig. 3.7A). With the 'left anterior and locked' presentation, the obliquity will change from the right side being high in standing and sitting, to the left being high in lying prone, whereas the curves will again usually remain unchanged (Fig. 3.7B). When the anterior rotation is on one side and the locking on the other, the curves are likely to change on lying prone, whereas the pelvic obliquity will probably stay the same (Fig. 3.7C).

Interestingly, the curves associated with an anatomical LLD in standing appear to be no less predictable than those associated with rotational malalignment, although clinical findings indicate that one is more likely to find a lumbar convexity into the high side, that is, into the side of the long leg (see Fig. 3.6B). This is in keeping with the literature, which suggests that the curve formed by the lumbar spine is usually convex to the long-leg side but which also warns of frequent exceptions.

Biomechanical effects of the curves

The normal movement patterns possible at the lumbar, thoracic and cervical segments of the spine are unique to each segment. They are determined, in large part, by the orientation of the facet joints. Contributory factors include the inherent lordosis and kyphosis of the segment, the attaching soft tissues, the thickness and diameter of the discs, and characteristics of the neural arch. In the thoracic spine, there is the limiting influence of the chest cage.

> Malalignment, be it rotational malalignment or an upslip or downslip, has the effect of superimposing lateral spinal curves, that is, curves in the frontal plane.

Needless to say, the overall effect is complex. What follows is a strictly biomechanical analysis that ignores the influence of muscles, ligaments and myofascial attachments. The reader is referred to Worth (1986), Grieve (1986a) and Gilmore (1986) for a more detailed analysis of movements of the cervical, thoracic and lumbar spine respectively, and to Lee (1993a, 1994a, 1994b) for an analysis of 'in vivo' thoracic spine movement.

Study results and clinical correlations for the lumbar and thoracic spine will be discussed together, in keeping with the fact that the spine should be considered as one unit and that pathology in one segment will also affect the other segments.

The lumbar segment of the spine

The lumbar facet joints are oriented almost in the sagittal plane. This allows primarily for the flexion and extension of this segment of the spine, with limited side-bending and rotation.

As indicated above, the 'laws' of Fryette (1954) dictate that the formation of a lumbar convexity to right on trunk flexion into the left is normally associated with:

- the rotation of L1–L4 inclusive into the convexity, that is, to the right (see Figs 2.65A, 3.5 and 4.22); there is a simultaneous opening of the facet joints on the right and a narrowing on the left
- forward flexion of the lumbar segment
- side flexion to the left.

Clinical correlation. The overall biomechanical effects of a lumbar convexity superimposed by malalignment, and possible clinical correlations, include the following.

Decreased movement, or even locking, of the lumbar segment. With time, this may exceed the safety role of the locking that occurs physiologically with normal side flexion of the trunk.

Narrowing of the facet joint space on the concave side. This might explain the not uncommon scenario of a history of low to mid-back pain coming on with activities requiring repeated rotation of the trunk on the pelvis (e.g. golf and court sports), and the finding on examination of a positive facet stress test, both of which disappear on correction of the malalignment. It might also be one reason why athletes with malalignment repeatedly report an increase in pain on attempting a posterior 'pelvic tilt': they are trying to flatten out a rotated lumbar segment whose overall flexibility is decreased and whose facet joints are already narrowed on one side and may therefore not tolerate the further compression that results with this manoeuvre (see Ch. 7, especially Fig. 7.2).

Narrowing of the disc and compression of the lateral vertebral margins on the side of the concavity. This constitutes a stress on both the disc and the vertebrae, with displacement of the nucleus pulposus and bulging of the annulus fibrosus toward the side of the convexity.

Widening of the joint margin on the side of the convexity. This widening, combined with the bulging of the annulus, puts the annular attachments to the vertebral margins under increased stress on the convex side.

Torsion of the annulus in a clockwise direction. This puts the oblique annular fibres and their nerve supply under increased stretch.

Narrowing of the disc anteriorly. This results from the forwards flexion of the lumbar vertebrae. There is an associated increase in pressure, forcing the disc contents posteriorly, which contributes to any posterior or lateral bulging of the disc and also increases the tension in the posterior longitudinal ligament.

The question is whether these individual stresses alone, or in combination, can initiate and/or accelerate the degeneration of the lumbar spine segment, including the deterioration of the annulus, with eventual disc protrusion. Certainly, the combination of axial rotation and simultaneous side flexion has been identified as the worst form of distortion to which the disc can be subjected in terms of precipitating the degenerative changes that eventually lead to disc protrusion (White & Panjabi 1978).

The thoracic segment of the spine

The more horizontal orientation of the facet joints allows primarily for rotation while limiting the side flexion and flexion/extension of this segment (Fig. 3.8). Movement in all three planes is restricted to some extent by the ribs and sternum.

There is disagreement over what exactly happens when one introduces a curve either by pure axial rotation or pure side flexion of the thoracic segment. Lee (1993a) feels that some of the disagreement may be the result of trying to study the problem with preparations of the thoracic spine that have had some or all of the ribs and sternum removed. In her clinical work, she has noted that:

1. rotation of the trunk results in simultaneous side flexion to the ipsilateral side
2. side flexion produces contralateral rotation of the mid-thoracic spine
3. the biomechanics of the lower thoracic region are more complex as a result of 'some significant differences in the anatomy of this region' (p. 20).

Clinical correlation. Given a thoracic convexity to right, the vertebrae are already side flexed to the left and may be rotated to the right, into the convexity, in the central segment of the thoracic spine (Lee 1992; see Fig. 3.5). In that case, there will now be a limitation of further side flexion to the left and of further clockwise rotation in the transverse plane. The reverse would apply with a thoracic convexity to the left.

Any limitation increases the risk of injury in sports in which the athlete carries out manoeuvres with a rotational component of the thorax, especially at a moment when pelvic rotation is either restricted (e.g. by standing

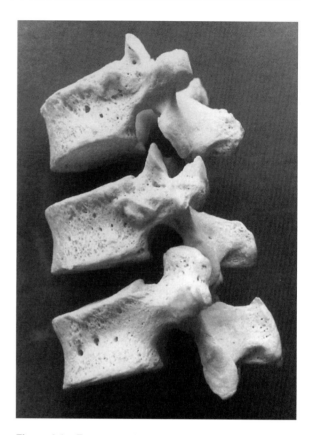

Figure 3.8 Transitional facet joints at the thoracolumbar junction. The inferior facets of T12 (central vertebra) have a coronal and sagittal component; articulation with L1 (on the left) allows mainly flexion/extension, restricting axial rotation. The change in the orientation of the proximal T12 facets allows for axial rotation but starts to restrict flexion/extension. (From Lee 1994, with permission.)

with both feet firmly planted on the ground) or made impossible (e.g. by sitting). These include:

- *court sports*: in particular tennis and other racquet sports
- *throwing sports*: with a rotational component of the trunk leading up to eventual release, while more or less supported on both feet (e.g. hammer throw, discus and shot put)
- *rowing and paddling sports*: from the symmetrical rotation of the thoracic spine required in open and flatwater kayaking to the more asymmetrical rotational strains imposed by canoeing, white-water kayaking and rowing (e.g. fours and eights).

In addition, the risk is increased in sports in which the athlete either voluntarily rotates the trunk or has it forced into the direction of limitation:

- *passive forced rotation*: by an opponent (e.g. wrestling, judo, karate; see Figs 5.29 and 5.30), as the result of an impact (e.g. falls or a collision in a vehicle) or from a collision with an opponent or a fixture (e.g. court sports, hockey and soccer)
- *in basketball*: excessive rotation of the trunk into the side of the limitation in the course of a lay-up, especially while the feet are still planted on the ground
- *in golf*: for example, with a thoracic convexity to right and some of the vertebrae already rotated clockwise (into the convexity), there will be less leeway for a back-swing to the right, and more for the stroke and follow-through to the left
- *in gymnastics*: increased rotational forces through the thoracolumbar junction with rotational manoeuvres carried out while the trunk is relatively fixed (e.g. rotations of the pelvis and legs while the trunk is supported by the arms; see Fig. 5.9).

The thoracic spine is particularly vulnerable in sports involving moving vehicles (e.g. bobsleds, the luge and cars), especially where safety restraints are limited to a lap belt with or without a strap across only one of the shoulders, the typical three-point system. This system permits the unrestrained shoulder to move forwards or backwards, resulting in rotation of the thoracic spine on the fixed pelvis and conceivably into the direction of limitation imposed by the coexisting malalignment.

The cervical segment of the spine

A number of athletes present with neck pain in association with pelvic malalignment. Sometimes there is a localizable increase in tension and tenderness in neck muscles, more commonly on the right side (e.g. right

upper trapezius). The curvature of the cervical segment is usually opposite in direction to that of the thoracic segment. As noted above, the point of reversal is sometimes as far down as T4 or T5 (see Fig. 2.60B). At the level of the reversal, wherever that may be, there is an associated rotation and side flexion of the adjoining vertebrae in opposite directions. Together, these factors create another site of increased stress, often tender to palpation even though the athlete may not otherwise be aware of pain from this site.

Neck rotation is most consistently limited to the right and side flexion to the left (Fig. 3.9). There are several factors that contribute to this asymmetry.

First, the malalignment of the pelvis and spine results in an asymmetry of tension in all the skeletal muscles (see 'Asymmetry of muscle tension' below). In the neck, there is more consistently evidence of increased tension in the right upper trapezius. This would by itself limit both right rotation and left side flexion. Asymmetry of tension in the cervical paravertebral and scalene muscles could also affect these ranges of motion.

Second, the direction of the cervical curve is likely to be an important determinant. The lateral curvature of the cervical spine superimposed on the cervical lordosis will make it easier to move in some directions than others.

Third, neck ranges of motion are also affected by the malrotation of individual cervical vertebrae and the direction of the thoracic and lumbar curves. Vertebral malrotation may be detected by:

- getting the athlete to lie prone, head and neck over the edge of the plinth, and comparing the level of the transverse processes; right rotation of the C5 vertebral complex, for example, elevates the process on the right and lowers it on the left side

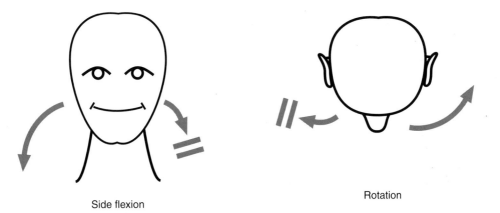

Side flexion

Rotation

Figure 3.9 Typical asymmetry of head and neck ranges of motion seen with rotational malalignment and upslip.

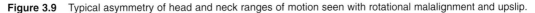

• palpating for deviation of the spinous processes in either prone- or supine-lying (see Fig. 2.65B); a right rotation of the C5 vertebral complex would, for example, deviate the process to the left, relative to the vertebrae above and below.

The neck ranges of motion usually become symmetrical again with correction of the malalignment. For example, right rotation may be limited to 50 degrees, compared with a left rotation of 70 degrees, giving a total of 120 degrees. Following realignment, and barring any other pathology, the values will usually become equal at 70 degrees. The overall increase in the total range to 140 degrees is probably a reflection of both the relaxation of the muscles and the realignment of the vertebrae.

Clinical correlation.   Athletes presenting with neck pain related to malalignment of the pelvis and spine sometimes have associated symptoms in the upper extremities. These include dysaesthesias and paraesthesias, which disappear with realignment only to recur as malalignment recurs. Possible causes for these arm symptoms include the following.

Referral from structures in the neck that are being irritated by the malalignment.   Curve reversal at the cervicothoracic junction, for example, indicates that there is a contrary rotation of C7 and T1, putting increased stress on the intervertebral, supraspinous and interspinous ligaments joining the two vertebrae, and the ligaments attaching to the C7 transverse processes. These ligaments can refer pain to the medial aspect of the forearm and the fourth and fifth fingers, in effect mimicking a C8 root problem and even angina (Fig. 3.10A, B4).

Rotation in the mid-cervical region can cause irritation of the C5 and/or C6 nerve roots, resulting in symptoms that may suggest a C5 or C6 radiculopathy (Fig. 3.10A, B2, B3). Evidence for root compression is usually lacking on neurological, electrodiagnostic or other investigations. The irritation of ligaments at the C5/C6 level can cause referred pain to the sclerotome region on the lateral aspect of the elbow, the symptoms often leading to futile treatments for a problem erroneously diagnosed as 'lateral' epicondylitis. Referral from the C8/T1 level can similarly mimic 'medial' epicondylitis.

The upper cervical and occipital region can refer to various areas of the skull (Fig. 3.10A, B1). Trigger points that develop in the neck muscles can refer to the shoulder girdle, the anterior and posterior chest regions and the upper extremities (Travell & Simons 1983). Interestingly, these trigger point referral patterns overlap with sclerotomal referral patterns originating from the ligaments attaching to the C7 transverse processes (Fig. 3.10A, B5).

Irritation of nerve tracts and vascular structures.   The cervical roots and brachial plexus exit the neck region running through the cervical paravertebral muscles and then in between the anterior and middle scalene muscles, together with the subclavian artery, whereas the subclavian vein runs anteriorly to the anterior scalene (Fig. 3.11). The vessels and nerves then proceed through the thoracic outlet, formed by the clavicle and first rib. A chronic increase in tension in the scalene and other surrounding muscles can narrow the space available to the exiting neurovascular bundle, both between the scalenes and in the thoracic outlet region, sometimes to the point of exerting direct pressure on these structures.

A rotation of the clavicle and the first rib caused by the malalignment can result in a further narrowing of the thoracic outlet (see Fig. 2.62). Irritation of the nerve fibres as a result of increased tension or direct pressure on the nerve tracts and/or a compromise of their blood supply can cause symptoms and clinical findings suggestive of a nerve root, brachial plexus or peripheral nerve lesion, or of a thoracic outlet syndrome. Adson's manoeuvre may provoke paraesthesia, occasionally with an associated diminution or obliteration of the radial pulse. In the absence of a neurological deficit on examination, electrodiagnostic studies are usually normal.

The symptoms may be abolished by correction of the malalignment, with particular attention to any co-existing malrotation of the cervical and upper thoracic vertebrae, the clavicle and the upper ribs (see Fig. 2.63). Realignment may help simply by increasing the space available for the neurovascular bundle by:

• relaxing the surrounding muscles and re-establishing the normal spatial relationship between the vertebrae, clavicle and first rib
• decreasing tension, and hence irritability, on nerves within ligaments and also on the autonomic fibres in this area.

In some sports (e.g. wrestling), the athlete is at risk if an opponent moves the head and neck passively into a direction that has a limitation of range imposed by the malalignment.

In shooting, sighting is a combined movement of rotation and forward and side flexion. A restriction of range in any of these directions may affect performance and provoke pain. In someone who rests the weapon against the right shoulder, for example, sighting requires right rotation, one of the ranges most likely to be restricted with malalignment (see Fig. 3.9).

The crawl, or freestyle swimming stroke, requires repeated head and neck rotation combined with some

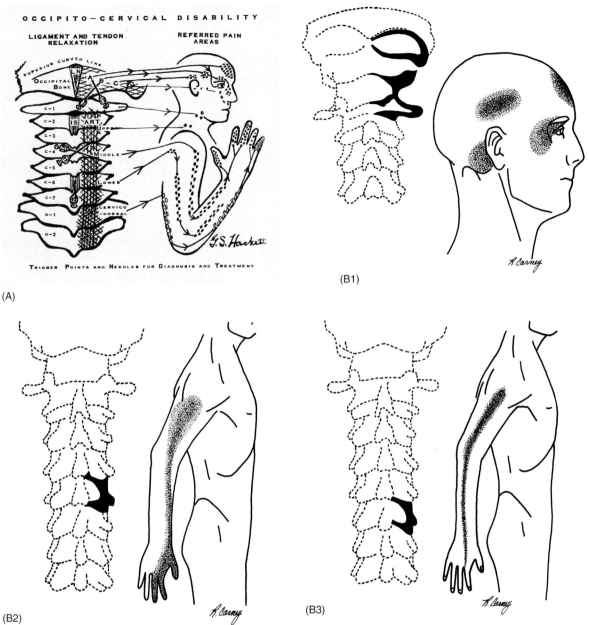

Figure 3.10 (A) Typical referral sites from ligament and tendon relaxation in the occipital region and cervical spine. Note the referral from the cervicothoracic junction area to the medial aspect of forearm and the fourth and fifth fingers, which can mimic a C8 root pattern and angina; there is also C5 and C6 sclerotomal referral to the area around the lateral epiphysis. ART, articular ligaments; IS, interspinous ligaments; IN = ligamentum nuchae. (From Hackett 1958, with permission.)
(B) Myofascial attachments to bone have characteristic patterns of referred pain when injured.

1. Upper neck sites (occipito-atlanto-axial).
2. The C5 sclerotome, the thumb, is usually involved.
3. At the C6 sclerotome, the pain does not usually spread into the hand.
4. The C7 sclerotome, the fifth and often the fourth fingers are involved.
5. The up, front and back of the transverse process of C7 have important patterns. (From Dorman & Ravin 1991, with permission.)

Fig. 3.10 (B4) and (B5), see overleaf

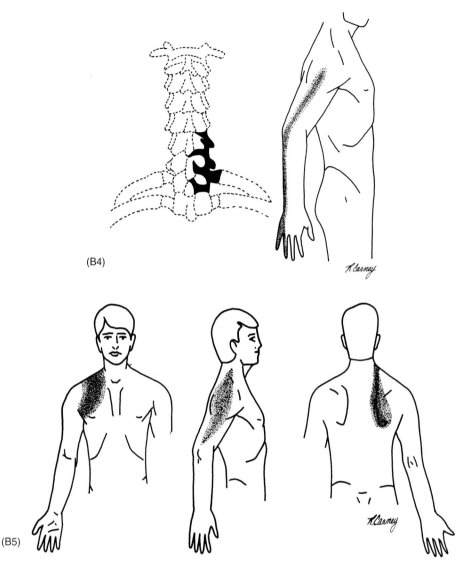

(B4)

(B5)

Figure 3.10   *Continued.*

ipsilateral side flexion, made even more demanding by breathing on alternate sides.

Sites of curve reversal

The sites of reversal of the curves in the frontal plane usually match the sites of reversal in the sagittal plane (Fig. 3.12A, B). A side view of the spine from a cranial to caudal direction usually shows a change from a cervical lordosis to a thoracic kyphosis at the cervicothoracic junction, to a lumbar lordosis at the thoracolumbar junction, and a further reversal to a sacral kyphosis at the lumbosacral junction. The stress at these normal sites of reversal in the sagittal plane is therefore compounded by the fact that reversal of any lateral curves present usually occurs at exactly the same sites.

Stress is further increased at these points of curve reversal by the fact that the adjoining vertebrae are actually rotated in opposite directions. For example, with a lumbar curve convex to right and thoracic to left, L1 is rotated to the right, whereas T12 is rotated to the left (Fig. 3.12C).

This twisting of vertebrae, combined with the changes in curvature, help to explain why tenderness

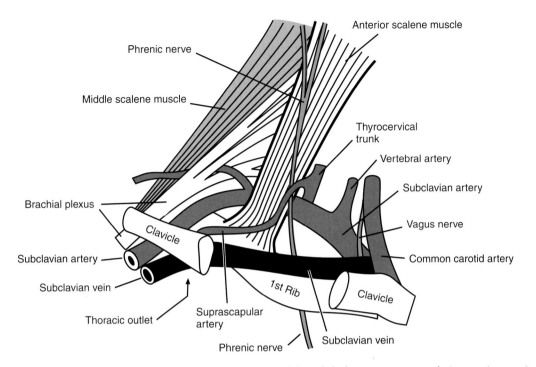

Figure 3.11 Compromise of the brachial plexus of nerves and the subclavian artery can occur between a tense anterior and middle scalene muscle, or as they exit through the narrow thoracic outlet between the clavicle and underlying 1st rib. (After Pansky & House 1975, with permission.)

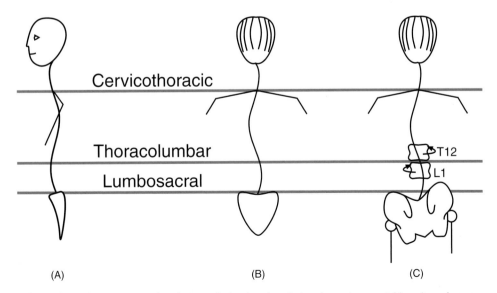

Figure 3.12 Sites of spinal curve reversal and stress. Lateral and posterior views show matching sites of curve reversal in the sagittal and frontal planes respectively. Reversal at the thoracolumbar junction results in the rotation of T12 and L1 in opposite directions. (A) Lateral view; (B) posterior view; (C) thoracolumbar (T/L) junction.

and pain so often localize to the thoracolumbar and cervicothoracic junctions. The other high-stress area is the lumbosacral junction, in large part as a result of the stress placed on:

- the L5–S1 level, by rotation of the sacrum relative to L5, in both the frontal and transverse planes
- the L4–L5 level, by the rotation of L1–L4 inclusive into the convexity of the curve.

Stress at sites of curve reversal may be further aggravated by the frequent occurrence of a malrotation of vertebrae near these sites of reversal: C7, T1, T12, L1, L4 and L5. An involvement of vertebrae at these levels often makes the immediate vicinity of the curve reversal feel stiff and unyielding. Palpation is likely to reveal increased tone and tenderness in the paravertebral muscles running alongside. This increase in tension may be reflex, in reaction to pain originating from the spine. Other mechanisms may, however, also be operative (see 'Asymmetry of muscle tension' below).

Pressure applied to the spinous processes repeatedly elicits a report of pain localizing around T11–T12–L1, L4–L5–S1 or both areas, even though the athlete may not otherwise be aware of pain from these sites. However, if athletes actually do report discomfort from the spine, this is most likely to localize to:

1. a site of curve reversal, and hence of high stress
2. a site where one or more vertebrae have rotated excessively.

Because of the altered biomechanics, these sites are not only more likely to be symptomatic, but also more vulnerable to injury from either an acute sprain or strain of the area, or the stress of the repetitive twisting and bending required for some athletic activities.

Clinical correlations. Activities that demand increased motion of the spine in all three planes are more likely to precipitate or aggravate pain from:

- sites of vertebral malrotation
- those sites already put under increased stress as a result of the compensatory curves formed with malalignment, in particular where these curves reverse – the cervicothoracic, thoracolumbar and lumbosacral junctions.

Increased tension in the paravertebral muscles restricts those trunk ranges of motion which put these muscles under further stretch. Forward flexion is affected by the involvement of the paravertebral muscles on one or both sides of the spine (e.g. in cycling and sculling). Side flexion in isolation, or combined with rotation (e.g. canoeing, rowing and kayaking), is limited in particular by increased tension in the

contralateral paravertebral and/or shoulder girdle muscles, affecting the right upper trapezius, infraspinatus and teres minor with increased frequency (see 'Asymmetry of muscle tension' below).

Thoracolumbar curve reversal may result in the 'thoracolumbar syndrome': the irritation of cutaneous sensory fibres from T12 and L1 giving rise to low back pain, with possible radiation to the buttock, abdomen and lateral thigh regions (see Ch. 4, particularly Fig. 4.21).

ASYMMETRY OF THE THORAX, SHOULDER GIRDLES AND ARMS

Side flexion of the trunk will normally have the effects listed in Box 3.3.

There is also an element of rotation of the vertebrae in the transverse plane. Whether this is directed into the convexity or the concavity seemingly depends on whether the initiating motion was either a pure side flexion or a trunk rotation (Lee 1993a, 1994a, 1994b). Vertebral rotation in the transverse plane automatically rotates each set of attaching ribs in the same plane, posteriorly on one side and anteriorly on the other.

The malrotation of a vertebra could result in similar effects on the ribs but in an exaggerated way. For example, left rotation and side flexion of T5 (see Fig. 2.63) can result in a rotational stress on the fifth ribs:

- at the back, anterior rotation of the left, and posterior rotation of the right, rib caused by the orientation of the costotransverse joints (Fig. 3.13B); this stress can be transmitted anteriorly to the costochondral junction (see Fig. 2.63B)

Box 3.3 Effects of side flexion of the trunk

1. Brings the ribs together on the concave side (Fig. 3.13A)
2. Causes some rotation of each pair of ribs in opposite directions – anteriorly on the concave side, posteriorly on the convex side – a movement that appears to be determined by the fact that:
   - after the motion of the ribs on the concave side has stopped, the thoracic vertebrae continue to side flex slightly into the concave side
   - this continued motion of the vertebrae causes the ribs on the concave side to glide upwards, and the ribs on the convex side to glide downwards, at the costotransverse joint
   - the direction of this movement of the ribs is guided by the orientation of the costotransverse joint surfaces, translating into anterior rotation on the concave and posterior on the convex side (Fig. 3.13B)

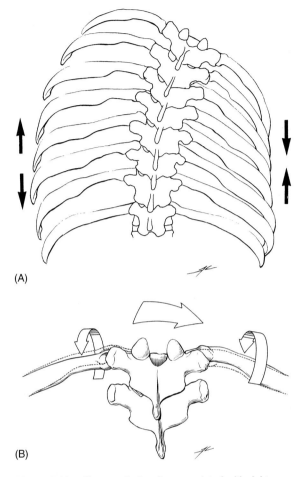

(A)

(B)

Figure 3.13 Changes in the ribs associated with right trunk side flexion. (A) As the thorax side-flexes to the right, the ribs on the right approximate and those on the left separate at their lateral margins. The costal motion stops first, the thoracic vertebrae then continuing to side-flex slightly to the right. (B) In the vertebrosternal region, the superior glide of the right rib at the costotransverse joint induces anterior rotation of the same rib as a result of the curvature of the joint surfaces. The inferior glide of the left rib at the costotransverse joint induces posterior rotation of the same rib. (From Lee 1994, with permission.)

- counterclockwise rotation in the transverse plane so that there is some displacement outwards of the left and inwards of the right rib relative to the ribs above and below.

Typical changes associated with rotational malalignment

When the vertebrae are side-flexed into the concavity of a thoracic curve because of malalignment, there

results a narrowing of the space between the ribs on this side; sometimes the lowest ribs actually touch the lateral iliac crest, or they may do so more readily on active side flexion. A lateral curve of the thoracic spine usually causes depression of the shoulder and scapula on the concave side and elevation on the convex side (see Fig. 2.60A). When the thoracic curve begins to reverse as low as the T4 or T5 level, the shoulder may actually be lower on the side of the concavity formed by the proximal part of the thoracic spine (see Fig. 2.60B). In addition, in most athletes standing at ease, one may note some rotation of the entire thorax in the transverse plane.

The overall effect is a combination of forward flexion, side flexion and axial rotation of the thoracic vertebrae, maximal at the apex of the curve. The attaching pairs of ribs are rotated in opposite directions at each level in the frontal, sagittal and transverse planes. This puts the rib attachments, both anteriorly and posteriorly, under some torsional stress and may lead to the development of tenderness and/or overt pain at these sites: the sternocostal and costochondral junctions anteriorly, and the costotransverse, costovertebral and facet joints posteriorly (Fig. 3.14).

The coexisting malrotation of one or more vertebrae, especially in the upper thoracic spine, will compound the torsional stress on these sites at specific levels (see Fig. 2.63A, B). Malalignment also creates a torsional

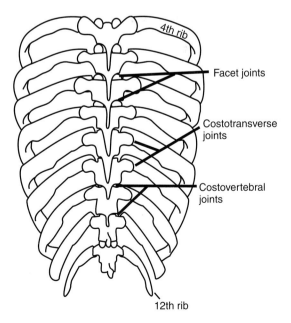

Figure 3.14 Posterior rib cage structures put under stress by malalignment and vertebral/rib rotation (see also Fig 2.63A).

force on the clavicles, increasing the stress on the acromioclavicular and sternoclavicular joints (see Fig. 2.63B). Typical complaints and findings include:

- anterior chest pain, which can sometimes mimic angina, tenderness localizing to the sternoclavicular joint and/or the sternocostal or costochondral junction of the rib(s) involved
- posterior chest, intercostal and/or 'mid-back' pain, recreated by stressing specific costovertebral and costotransverse joints
- shoulder pain localizing to the acromioclavicular joint
- tenderness over the lowest ribs, especially when these impinge on the lateral iliac crest.

In the absence of a history of trauma or evidence of an inflammatory process, these symptoms and signs are probably the result of increased torsional stresses. Resolution on the correction of pelvic malalignment and any thoracic vertebral malrotation confirms the diagnosis.

A common presentation in standing is with a counterclockwise rotation of the pelvis in the transverse plane (right side forward) and a thoracic curve convex to left. The most frequent associated findings on examination are as follows:

- There is clockwise *rotation of the thorax* in the transverse plane, bringing the left shoulder forwards as if to compensate for the pelvis being forward on the right side. Simultaneous counterclockwise rotation of the thorax is, however, almost as common and results in both the pelvis and the shoulder being rotated forwards on the right.
- The *right shoulder girdle* is retracted and depressed, the left protracted and elevated.
- The *right scapula* is rotated clockwise, sometimes to the point that the medial border 'wings' and studies are initiated for a suspected weakness of mid-trapezius, the rhomboids or serratus anterior and a possible long thoracic nerve injury.
- Depression of the right shoulder and clockwise rotation of the right scapula reorients the *glenoid fossa* downwards and posteriorly, whereas, on the elevated left side, the fossa ends up pointing more upwards and anteriorly.
- Reorientation of the thorax and shoulder girdles and asymmetries of muscle tension (see below) alter the *ranges of motion possible at the shoulder joints*. The typical pattern includes:
  – a decrease in right internal, left external rotation (Fig. 3.15A)
  – a decrease in left extension (Fig. 3.15B).

- Malalignment can also result in an obvious *asymmetry of some other upper extremity ranges of motion*. For example, a typical finding is a 5–15 degree limitation of left forearm pronation (Fig. 3.15C) and right supination (Fig. 3.15D).
- Malalignment usually results in an *asymmetry of strength* in the shoulder girdle and upper extremity muscles. The detection of weakness is dependent on the position of examination (Maffetone 1999) and may not be as easily or as consistently apparent as the asymmetrical weakness noted in the lower extremities (see 'Asymmetry of lower extremity muscle strength' below). Differences are usually more obvious in the proximal muscles, especially the arm flexors and particularly the anterior deltoid, and can disappear dramatically with realignment.

Clinical correlation

The asymmetry of thoracic and shoulder girdle alignment, and of the strength and tension of the muscles in this area, increases the stress on the shoulder joint and rotator cuff complex bilaterally. This stress increases the likelihood of developing shoulder pain and may predispose to impingement, acute or chronic sprain, and other injury to this region.

For example, the downwards slant of the glenoid shelf on the side of the depression decreases the passive support that the shelf usually provides for the humeral head. The capsule and cuff are now constantly subjected to increased gravitational traction forces which may be offset by the chronic reflex contraction of the shoulder girdle muscles attempting to stabilize the humeral head in the socket.

Supraspinatus is particularly well suited for this task, which may explain the frequent report of pain from the right supraspinatus on neck rotation and the localization of 'neck spasms' and tenderness to this muscle. These mechanisms may also play a role in the development of a complicating supraspinatus tendonitis, impingement, calcific tendonitis and subacromial bursitis.

Asymmetrical shoulder ranges of motion may affect performance, particularly in throwing sports and those requiring a normal range of motion in combination with full and symmetrical muscle strength (e.g. weight-lifting or the symmetrical strokes of swimming). The effect may be favourable or unfavourable, as illustrated by the athlete showing the typical asymmetry in extension (Fig. 3.15B).

If extension is increased on the dominant side, it may help in certain of the throwing sports in which the ability to generate velocity is dependent on an initial

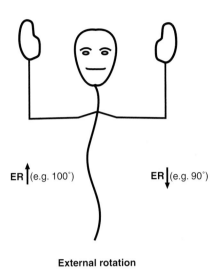

ER ↑ (e.g. 100°)   ER ↓ (e.g. 90°)

IR ↓ (e.g. 80°)   IR ↑ (e.g. 90°)

(A)   **External rotation**   **Internal rotation**

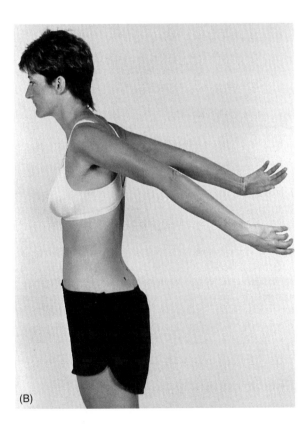

(B)

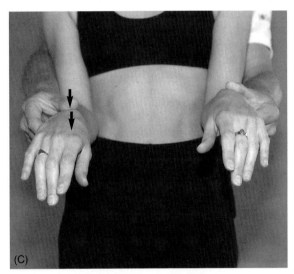

(C)

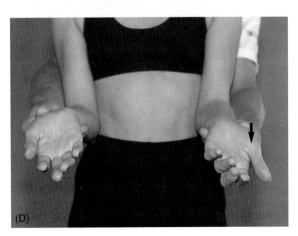

(D)

Figure 3.15 Typical changes in upper extremity ranges of motion with 'alternate' rotational malalignment and upslip. When testing forearm pronation and supination, the elbows are steadied against the side (Figs 3.15C, D). (A) Decrease of right internal rotation (IR) and left external rotation (ER). (B) Limitation of left extension. (C) Limitation of left forearm pronation. (D) Limitation of right forearm supination.

extension of the throwing arm (e.g. baseball, football and athletic events). The overhand throw, for example, begins with the throwing arm abducted, externally rotated and fully extended (see Fig. 5.25). An underarm throw begins with a backswing of the throwing arm, as far as extension at the shoulder will allow. In the side-arm throw used for the discus, the throwing arm is again initially extended.

A unilateral increase in extension may, however, be a drawback in sports in which symmetry of movement sometimes counts (e.g. gymnastics, synchronized swimming and diving).

The asymmetry may also be costly in sports that require symmetrical arm extension for propulsion. For example, if the left arm cannot extend as far as the right, the swimmer using the butterfly stroke can compensate by rotating the trunk counterclockwise to increase the amount of extension possible on the left side, to the point of creating symmetry of stroke force. Active trunk rotation, however, increases energy requirements and could introduce a wobble and increase resistance in the water, both factors that would result in a slowing.

ASYMMETRY OF LOWER EXTREMITY ORIENTATION

Most athletes who are in alignment have their lower extremities in some external rotation, both feet pointing outwards some 10–15 degrees relative to the middle (Fig. 3.16A). A small number have their legs in 'neutral', the feet pointing straight forwards, and some are 'pigeon-toed', both feet pointing inwards. Barring the effect of previous injuries, foot orientation relative to the midline is usually symmetrical with all three presentations.

> Rotational malalignment, on the other hand, results in an asymmetrical orientation of the lower extremities: one leg undergoes external and the other internal rotation.

There are many factors that can result in such a rotation. For example, facilitation of the right gluteus maximus, with simultaneous inhibition of tensor fascia lata, results in forces favouring outward rotation of the right leg. Inhibition of left gracilis and sartorius would favour internal rotation of that leg. The collapse of the right cuboid into eversion will cause the foot to collapse into pronation and create forces tending towards external rotation.

Whatever the underlying cause may be, we appear eventually to be left with some consistent patterns of malalignment relating to lower extremity orientation and weight-bearing and associated asymmetries, as discussed in this chapter. For ease of recognition, the pattern related to the presentations of rotational malalignment have been divided into:

- the *'alternate'* presentations: the right lower extremity has rotated externally and the left internally (see Fig. 3.3B):
  - athletes typically show an outward rotation of the right foot relative to midline to a varying degree; it is not unusual to see the right foot pointing out as much as 30–45 degrees from the midline
  - the left leg will have rotated towards the midline, sometimes so far that the foot has actually crossed the midline and ends up pointing to the right side (Fig. 3.16B).
- the *'left anterior and locked'* presentation: the left lower extremity has rotated externally and the right internally (see Fig. 3.3A):
  - athletes typically show an outward rotation of the left foot relative to the midline to varying degree
  - the right foot will have rotated towards or even across the midline.

The exaggerated external and internal rotation is usually even more readily apparent with the athlete relaxed and lying supine (Fig. 3.16C). On gait examination, the final pattern will be influenced by other factors that affect weight-bearing, such as a natural tendency to pronation or supination. The amount of external and internal rotation may become more obvious on having the athlete walk on the heels and toes, hop on one foot at a time or run at increasing speed on a treadmill. At the extreme, if the leg that has rotated internally has gone so far that the foot actually crosses the midline, the athlete may almost appear to be walking sideways, alternately leading with the inside of one foot and the outside of the other (Fig. 3.16B).

Clinical correlation

The asymmetrical orientation of the lower extremities seen with the malalignment syndrome is one of the major factors contributing to the asymmetry of lower limb biomechanical function. Other factors – including asymmetry of weight-bearing, muscle strength and tension – also affect orientation and influence the biomechanics of standing and walking. These are discussed in more detail below.

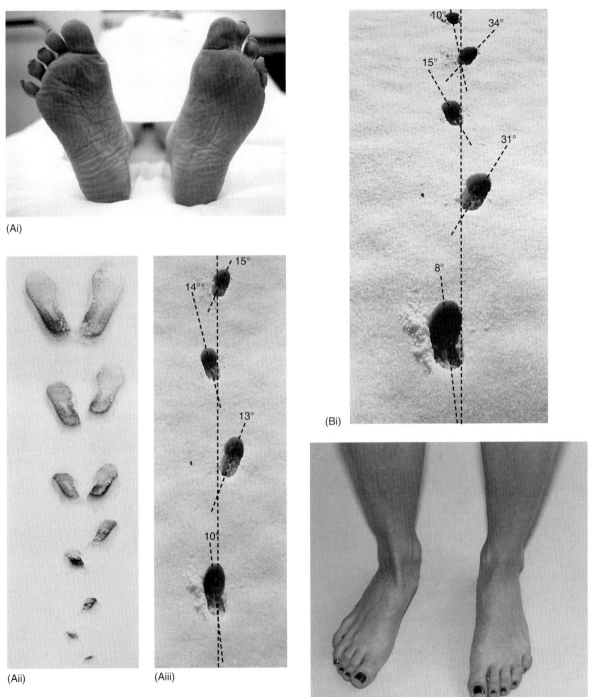

Figure 3.16   Lower extremity rotation associated with malalignment. (A) Aligned: legs externally rotated to a near-equal extent relative to the midline: (i) lying supine; (ii) walking on snow; (iii) running on snow. (B) Malalignment present ('alternate' rotational or upslip): the right leg undergoes external, the left internal rotation: (i) running on snow (the same athlete as in Fig. 3.16Aii and iii but before realignment): the right foot turned out considerably more than the left; (ii) left internal rotation to the point at which the left foot actually crosses the midline and points to the right. (C) Typical right external rotation evident in relaxed supine-lying.

Fig. 3.16 (C), see overleaf

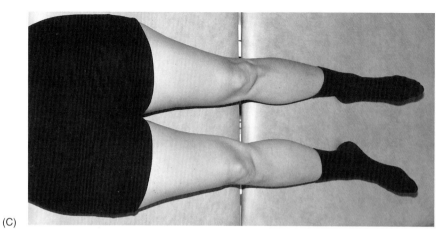

(C)

Figure 3.16 *Continued.*

In those with the 'alternate' presentations and a clockwise rotation of the lower extremities, the heel of the out-turned right foot can now more easily strike against the inside of the left foot or calf, usually just above the medial malleolus (Fig. 3.17A). Similarly, the toes or the tip of the shoe of the in-turned left foot can catch more easily against the medial aspect of the right shoe or the posteromedial aspect of the right calf (Fig. 3.17B).

Proof of such contact becomes more readily apparent when playing or running on a wet surface, when dirt and water tend to mark these sites. Contact may briefly upset the athlete, or even cause the athlete to trip and fall at times. Tripping as a result of malalign-

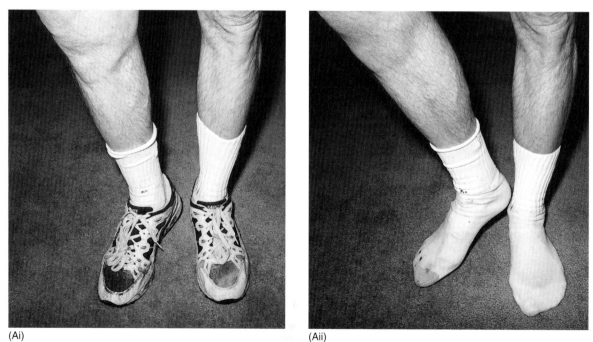

(Ai)　　　　　　　　　　　　　　　　　　(Aii)

Figure 3.17 Malalignment with increased right external, left internal rotation. (A) Right heel (i) strikes at or above the left medial malleolus, (ii) marking the inside of the left sock. (B) The tip of the left foot catches the posteromedial right Achilles/calf.

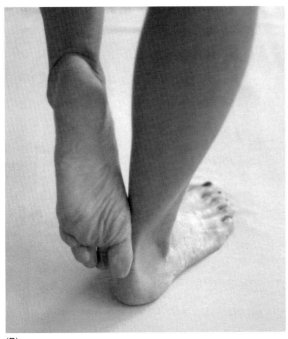

(B)

Figure 3.17 *Continued.*

ment may, however, pose more of a problem for children given their general decrease in coordination and balance compared with adults.

Compared with the pattern just described, the reverse pattern and associated problems are seen with the 'left anterior and locked' presentation.

ASYMMETRY OF FOOT ALIGNMENT, WEIGHT-BEARING AND SHOE WEAR

It cannot be stressed enough that malalignment causes a shift in weight-bearing that often results in a striking asymmetry of the weight-bearing pattern. The direction of this shift is related to the pattern of lower extremity rotation (Fig. 3.18; see also Figs I.1, 3.3 and 7.1):

- inwards on the side that has rotated externally; this may be into obvious pronation
- outwards on the side that has rotated internally; this may be into obvious supination.

Which leg rotates inwards or outwards is in turn related to the presentation of malalignment: left outwards and right inwards with the 'left anterior and locked', the reverse with the 'alternate', presentation.

Given the fact that most athletes show one of the 'alternate' presentations, with external rotation of the right and internal of the left lower extremity, the most common weight-bearing pattern is that of pronation on the right and supination on the left side (Fig. 3.18A). The opposite pattern will be apparent in those with the less common 'left anterior and locked' presentation (Fig. 3.18B).

Gradations between these extremes are possible, but the same trend will be apparent, for example in the athlete with one of the 'alternate' presentations who is noted to:

- pronate on both sides: the degree of pronation will be more marked on the side of external rotation (Fig. 3.19A)
- supinate on both sides: the degree of supination will be more marked on the side of the internal rotation (Fig. 3.19B).

In other words, the actual weight-bearing pattern depends in large part on the presentation of the malalignment but continues to be influenced by the athlete's inherent tendency towards pronation or supination. The examiner must therefore look at the attitude of the feet both at rest and on weight-bearing.

The detection of asymmetry can be improved by having the athlete walk on the heels and toes, hop on one foot, and walk or run at increasing speed on a treadmill. When the athlete with one of the 'alternate' presentations toe-walks or hops, the right heel will typically be noted to 'whip' inwards as the foot tends to collapse into pronation, whereas the left heel will stay vertical as the foot maintains a neutral position, or may actually whip outwards as the foot collapses into frank supination (Fig. 3.20A).

On an analysis of a pair of day shoes or running shoes, the asymmetry can often be verified by the pattern of midsole compression, of wear on the heels and soles, and of collapse of the heel cup and uppers. A quantitative assessment of side-to-side differences is also possible. For example, the asymmetry of weight-bearing that occurs in an athlete with one of the 'alternate' presentations and a tendency to right pronation and left supination, can be noted on:

- a static topographical map of the soles made standing (Fig. 3.21A)
- a dynamic pressure pattern made when walking or running (Fig. 3.21B).

These methods can show the right medial and left lateral shift: the left medial longitudinal arch will be deeper because of the tendency to supination, whereas

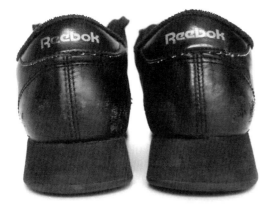

(Ai)

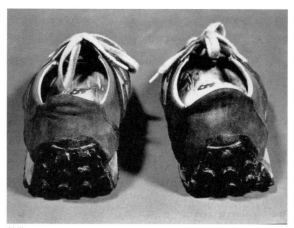

(Aii)

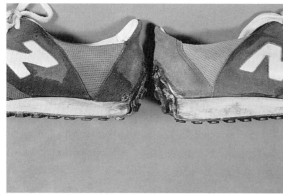

(Aiii)

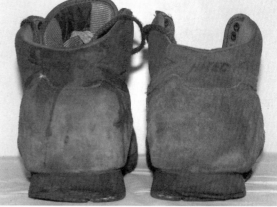

(Aiv)

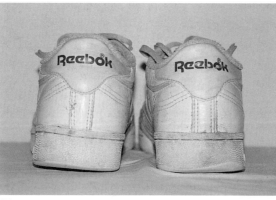

(B)

Figure 3.18 Heel cup collapse reflecting a shift of weight-bearing with malalignment. (A) 'Alternate' presentations and upslips: heel cups collapse towards the left side with right pronation, left supination: (i) walking shoes; (ii) running shoes after 6 weeks of 100 miles per week; (iii) the same running shoes; note the compression of the right medial heel material; (iv) boots. (B) 'Left anterior and locked': the heels are shifted to the right with left pronation and right supination.

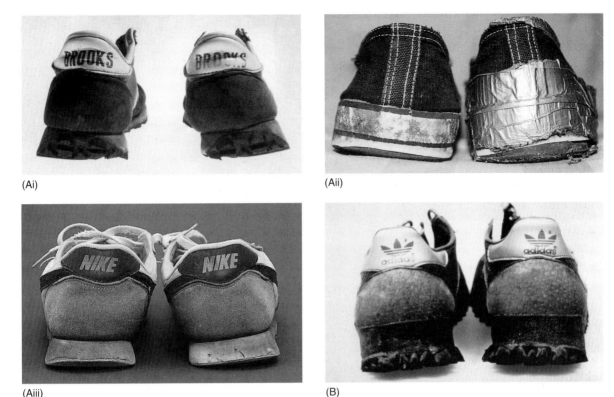

(Ai)

(Aii)

(Aiii)

(B)

Figure 3.19   Patterns of heel cup collapse reflecting the shift in weight-bearing seen with 'alternate' presentations and upslips. (A) With bilateral pronation: (i) worse on the side of external rotation (right); (ii) marked right pronation leading to desperate measures with duct tape; (iii) typical running shoes (see also Fig. 3.28B). (B) With bilateral supination: worse on the side of internal rotation (left).

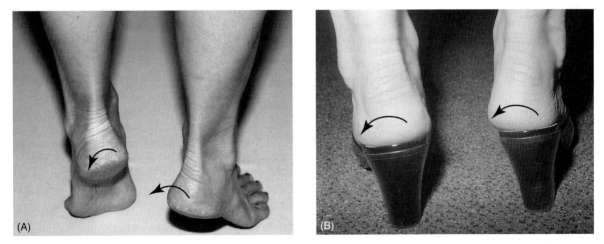

(A)

(B)

Figure 3.20   Toe-walking accentuates the asymmetry of weight-bearing in the athlete with an 'alternate' presentation or upslip. (A) Inward whip and collapse of the right heel (calcaneal eversion) on the pronating side; positioning in neutral or even a whipping outward of the left heel (calcaneal inversion) on the supinating side; note the markedly increased external rotation of the right leg compared with the left. (B) A similar pattern evident walking on high heels: the right heel pronates to the point of falling inwards off the heel support, the left leaning slightly outwards.

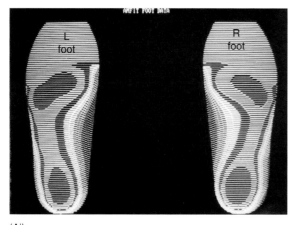

(Ai)

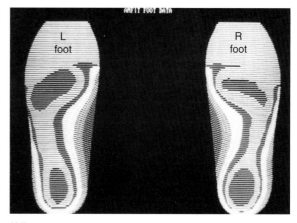

(Aii)

BEFORE   AFTER

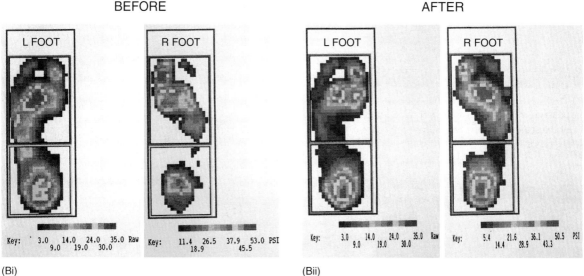

(Bi)   (Bii)

Figure 3.21 Quantitative assessment of wear pattern. (A) Static topographical pattern of the sole of the foot on weight-bearing, recorded by air pressure sensors (Amfit Inc. CAD/CAM orthotic fabrication system). (i) Malalignment – an asymmetrical pattern: in particular, increased width of the left grey bar (denoting the highest part of the medial longitudinal arch), in keeping with the tendency towards left supination; the width of the right bar has, however, decreased with the collapse of the arch as a result of pronation. (ii) Realignment – increased symmetry of pattern: note the almost identical width of the right and left grey and white bars at the midsection of the arch. (B) Dynamic pattern of weight distribution, recorded by 960 electronic measuring points within a 'sensor mat' in the shoe, which scans the foot in motion 30 times per second throughout stance (Footmaxx TM); the weight borne is indicated by shading – maximal being black. (i) Malalignment – asymmetrical weight-bearing pattern reflecting the tendency towards right pronation and left supination: the right transfer of weight from the heel to the forefoot is 'disconnected' and overall less forceful; the left foot pattern shows more weight-bearing laterally and on the ball of the foot. (ii) Realignment – the pattern is much more symmetrical: the right foot now shows the weight being transferred from heel to forefoot in a 'connected' pattern, with increased concentration on the heel, midfoot and ball of the foot regions; the left shows shift medially (especially in the midfoot and first toe region), considerable weight-bearing now being evident in the heel and medial midfoot areas.

the right arch will tend to flatten with pronation. These methods also offer one way of recording the return to a more symmetrical weight-bearing pattern that occurs with realignment (Fig. 3.21A, B).

Attitude of the feet

When non-weight-bearing, the feet of most athletes who are in alignment are suspended with the heels in varus and the inside border of the foot up relative to the outside (Fig. 3.22Ai). This is true even for most of those who turn out to be supinators when weight-bearing; in only approximately 5% of these are the feet in neutral or actual valgus angulation at rest.

With malalignment, the attitude of the non-weight-bearing feet becomes asymmetrical. The most common finding, then, is an increase in the amount of varus angulation on the side of the externally rotated lower extremity compared with the side of internal rotation (Fig. 3.22Aii). With right external rotation, for example, the varus angulation of the right foot may be 30 degrees but that on the left only 15 (Fig. 3.22B). Factors contributing to this asymmetry at rest include:

- the asymmetrical orientation of the foot and ankle joints
- the increased amount of inversion possible on passive movement of the subtalar joint on the side of external rotation (Fig. 3.23)
- the asymmetrical tone in the right versus left ankle invertors and evertors (see 'Asymmetry of muscle tension' below).

This varus angulation seen when the feet are non-weight-bearing results in the following findings on weight-bearing. In those who are in alignment, all of the non-weight-bearing foot is in varus and all of the lateral border therefore in a position to touch the ground immediately after heel strike. However, shoe wear occurs primarily on the posterior and posterolateral aspect of the heel, and then centrally underneath the ball of the foot, in a fairly symmetrical pattern (Figs 3.24A, B; see 'Asymmetry of shoe wear' below). This wear pattern reflects the fact that, in preparation for weight-bearing, the feet are most often suspended not only in a varus attitude, but also in neutral or slight dorsiflexion at the ankle.

Therefore, contact at heel strike is more likely to occur first with the posterolateral edge of the heel, and that contact immediately initiates a force to torque the foot and ankle into valgus, that is, towards medial weight-bearing and often frank pronation. This sequence of events, with the foot rolling inwards, occurs so quickly that wear usually tends to be more obvious along the posterior rather than the posterolateral aspect of the heel (Fig. 3.24C).

In those with rotational malalignment, weight-bearing typically tends to be more posterolateral on the side of the externally rotated and more posterior on the side of the internally rotated lower extremity. In those with one of the 'alternate' presentations:

- on the *right side*, the increased varus angulation of the heel at heel strike results in:
  - initial contact and wear at the posterolateral to lateral aspect of the heel (Fig. 3.25A, B)
  - an accentuated medial torquing of the foot with increasingly more medial weight-bearing on progressing anteriorly from the heel
  - tendency to pronation
- on the *left side*, initial contact is more uniform across the back of the heel, and the medial torquing force is diminished. Heel wear may be less obvious, and there is usually less wear posterolaterally, or involving more the posterior aspect of the heel, compared with the right side (Fig. 3.25A, B). Weight-bearing on the sole remains relatively more lateral, reflecting the tendency towards supination.

The tendency to right pronation and medial weight-bearing appears to be a strictly passive phenomenon, the result of a number of factors and initiated at heel strike in most.

First, because of the varus angulation of the non-weight-bearing foot, the lateral edge of the heel is first to contact ground on weight-bearing; this has an outrigger effect, forcing the foot into neutral, or even valgus, on impact.

In addition, the more the right leg is in external rotation, the more the medial border of this foot comes to lie ahead of the lateral one. On weight-bearing, there results a passive rolling from the lateral onto the medial aspect of the foot as it progresses from heel strike to foot-flat.

Pronation and the associated eversion of the subtalar joint are accompanied by internal rotation of the tibia, which, through a 'hinge-like' effect (Mann 1982), forces the calcaneus into further eversion (Fig. 3.26Ai). The initial varus angulation of the non-weight-bearing calcaneus changes to valgus. This allows for more movement of the transverse tarsal joint by bringing the axes running through the talonavicular and calcaneocuboid joints more into parallel (Mann 1982). An unlocking of the metatarsals occurs, allowing the medial longitudinal arch to collapse as the foot simultaneously pronates, abducts and dorsiflexes (Fig. 3.26Bi).

A further collapse of the medial longitudinal arch may occur because of the malalignment-related functional weakness, or inhibition, of the right ankle

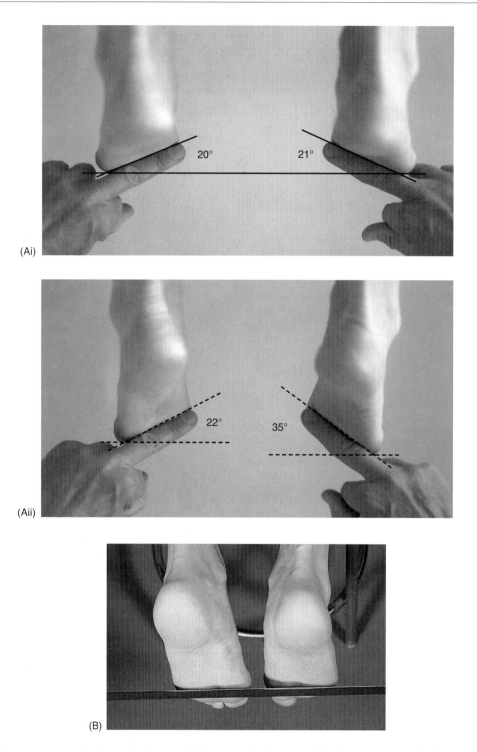

Figure 3.22 Angulation of the feet at rest (non-weight-bearing). (A) Athlete 1: (i) in alignment: symmetrical varus angulation (20 degrees); (ii) with malalignment: the varus angulation is increased to 35 degrees on the right (the side of external rotation) compared with 22 degrees on the left (the side of internal rotation). (B) Athlete 2: with malalignment, varus angulation on the right is 30 versus 15 degrees on the left.

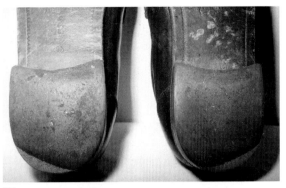

(A)

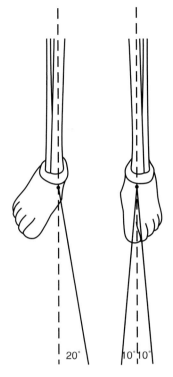

Figure 3.23 Asymmetry of subtalar ranges of motion with 'alternate' presentations or upslips. With the athlete lying supine and the ankle 'locked' at 90 degrees, passive movement of the calcaneus here shows typical: decreased right eversion (here 0 degrees versus left 10) and decreased left inversion (10 degrees versus right 20). The combined range remains the same bilaterally: 20 degrees. The right leg has rotated externally, the left internally.

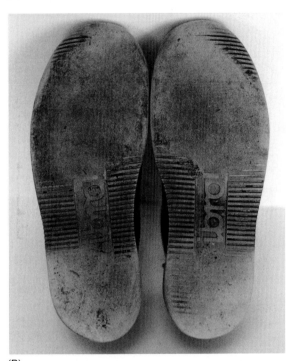

(B)

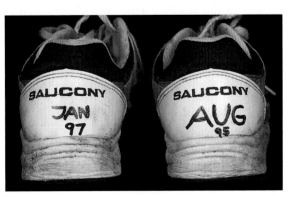

Figure 3.24 Typical shoe wear pattern when in alignment. (A, B) View of heels and soles: heel wear is even and more posterior than lateral. (C) Posterior view: symmetrical width of heel and sole; bilateral 5 degrees pronation of the heel cup (after 19 months wear!).

(C)

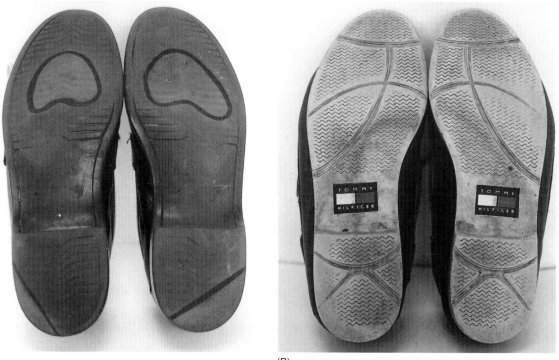

(A)   (B)

Figure 3.25 Typical asymmetrical wear pattern with malalignment evident in the soles of shoes (A) and (B). The right shoes both show increased wear: posterolaterally in the heel (reflecting the increased varus angulation at contact), and medially in the forefoot (reflecting the tendency towards pronation). The left shoes both show increased wear: posterolaterally, but less so than on the right (reflecting the decreased varus angulation – see also Fig. 3.22), and more laterally in the forefoot (reflecting the tendency towards supination).

invertors – tibialis anterior and posterior (see 'Asymmetry of muscle strength' below).

Finally, the limitation of right subtalar eversion noted in supine lying (see Fig. 3.23) may play a role, provided this is still operative when the athlete is weight-bearing. If eversion continues to be restricted, any further shift towards medial weight-bearing will, as soon as all available eversion has been exhausted, have to occur through the ability of the foot to pronate, as well as by allowing the tibia to tilt inwards, predisposing to valgus angulation at the knee (see Fig. 3.33).

The shift towards supination and lateral weight-bearing on the side of the internally rotated left leg is, for several reasons, probably also a strictly passive phenomenon, similar to the shift towards pronation on the side of external rotation.

The first reason is that the tendency to torquing from varus to valgus is decreased, abolished or reversed in part by the fact that the non-weight-bearing foot is in less varus angulation at rest, rarely even neutral or in a valgus attitude.

Second, the internal rotation of the lower extremity orients the foot more in the line of progression. If internal rotation has caused the foot actually to cross the midline so that it points inwards (see Fig. 3.16Bii):

- the lateral border will come to lie, relatively speaking, ahead of the medial one
- the foot will passively roll from the inner to the outer border on progressing from heel strike to foot-flat.

Because of the internal rotation of the femur, the tibia undergoes external rotation, and the subtalar joint is reoriented so that the calcaneus is passively forced into further inversion on weight-bearing. The axes of the transverse tarsal joint diverge; motion at this joint is decreased, locking the metatarsals and increasing the stability of the longitudinal arch (Fig. 3.26Bii). Weight is transferred forwards either in a direct line from the heel to the toes, consistent with a neutral pattern of weight-bearing, or along the outside border of the foot if the pattern is one of frank lateral weight-bearing and supination (see Fig. 3.21A, B).

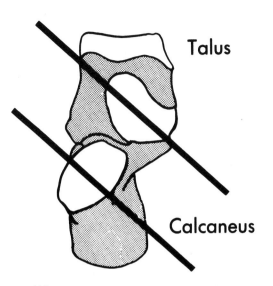

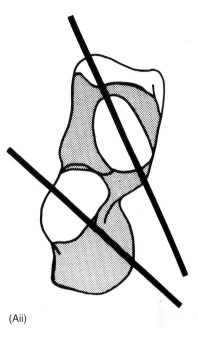

Talus

Calcaneus

(Ai)   (Aii)

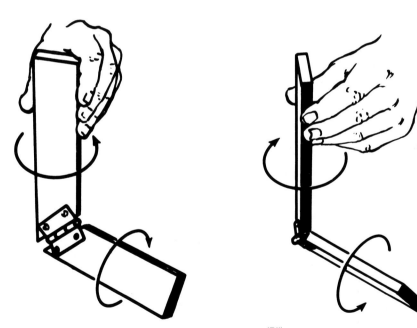

(Bi)   (Bii)

Figure 3.26 Mobility of the foot and ankle. (A) Related to the axes of the transverse tarsal joint. (i) When the calcaneus is in eversion (e.g. pronation), the conjoint axes between the talonavicular and calcaneocuboid joints are parallel to one another so that increased motion occurs in the transverse tarsal joint. (ii) When the calcaneus is in inversion (e.g. supination), the axes are no longer parallel, and there is decreased motion and increased stability of the transverse tarsal joint. (B) Model of function of the subtalar joint as it translates motion from the tibia above to the calcaneus below: (i) inward rotation of the tibia causes outward rotation of the calcaneus (= eversion), (ii) outward rotation of the tibia causes inward rotation of the calcaneus (= inversion). (From Mann 1982, with permission.)

Next, the limitation of subtalar inversion on this side would reinforce the tendency to lateral weight-bearing once the available range of inversion had been exhausted. The tibia, which rotates externally, would be forced outwards proximally, and the knee towards genu varum, increasing stress on the lateral aspect of the knee.

Last, a further collapse of the lateral longitudinal arch may occur because of the malalignment-related weakness of the left ankle evertors – peroneus longus, brevis and tertius.

As a result of these factors, the shift in weight-bearing commonly seen in association with the 'alternate' presentations is one tending inwards on the right and outwards on the left. In 15–20% of athletes, the right foot will actually end up overtly pronating, and the left supinating (see Figs I.1 and 3.18A). If bilateral pronation persists, it will probably be worse on the right (see Fig. 3.19A); if bilateral supination persists, it will most likely be worse on the left (see Fig. 3.19B). The reverse of these findings is seen with the left anterior and locked presentation.

Sloping of the supporting surface will dramatically affect the shift in weight-bearing. The more common shift to right pronation, left supination (Fig. 3.27A) will, for example, be accentuated whenever the right foot is raised relative to the left; for example, when running against traffic in Canada and the USA, or with the traffic in the UK (Fig. 3.27B). The athlete will often have learned to appreciate that this shift is decreased,

and the stability of the feet increased, by running or walking with the right foot on the 'down side' relative to the left (Fig. 3.27C).

Asymmetry of shoe wear

The shoes are just as important an indicator of the weight-bearing pattern as is watching the athlete walk up and down the hallway, barefoot or wearing shoes. If possible, look at a pair of both day shoes and running shoes, or other athletic shoewear that has been worn for several months. The running shoes will help to determine what happens at higher speeds, when the athlete is actually participating in sports, and will also help to pick out the occasional athlete who pronates when walking and changes to neutral or even progressively increasing supination on running, or the reverse.

High-heeled shoes may not be very helpful because the heel cups, sitting up on a pedestal, may too easily sway in either direction along with the heel itself; in addition, the point of the heel is often too small to determine the true impact wear pattern. Observing the athlete walking in high heels may, however, still reveal the asymmetry typical of malalignment, with the heel on the pronating side tending to fall inwards over the edge, similar to toe-walking (see Fig. 3.20B). The stiff ankle section of a boot will sometimes yield enough to reflect accurately the asymmetry of weight-bearing forces (see Fig. 3.18Aiv).

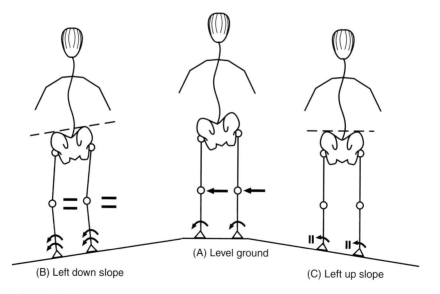

(B) Left down slope   (A) Level ground   (C) Left up slope

Figure 3.27 The effect of a slope on the malalignment-related tendency towards right pronation, left supination on level ground (A). The shift towards both is accentuated on a slope banked down on the left (B) and decreased on a slope banked up on the left (C).

Heel cups and uppers

The pattern of heel cup collapse will often allow one to deduce:

- that malalignment is or is not present
- whether the malalignment is likely to be:
  - the left anterior and locked presentation
  - one of the 'alternate' presentations or an upslip (although it cannot distinguish between these)
- the athlete's inherent weight-bearing pattern: pronation or supination.

Patterns of wear associated with rotational malalignment are given in Box 3.4.

Other commonly seen patterns still in keeping with this shift are:

- bilateral inwards collapse, worse on the left
- bilateral outwards collapse, worse on the right.

These patterns reflect the effect of this presentation on what may turn out to be the athlete's inherent weight-bearing pattern on realignment, namely pronation and supination respectively.

> In summary, the heel cup and upper of the shoes of an athlete with rotational malalignment have a wind-swept apearance.

Box 3.4 Patterns of shoe wear typically associated with rotational malalignment

- **'Alternate' presentations**: the classical pattern associated with these presentations reflects the tendency to right pronation and left supination, with frank inwards collapse of the right and outwards collapse of the left heel cup and upper respectively (see Figs I.1 and 3.18A). Other commonly seen patterns that are still in keeping with this shift are:
  - bilateral inwards collapse, worse on the right (Fig. 3.19A)
  - bilateral outwards collapse, worse on the left (Fig. 3.19B).
  These patterns reflect the effect of the malalignment on what may turn out to be the athlete's inherent weight-bearing pattern on realignment, namely bilateral pronation and supination respectively.
- **Left anterior and locked**: the classical pattern associated with this presentation is one of frank inwards collapse of the left and outwards collapse of the right heel cup and upper as a result of the forces tending towards pronation on the left and supination on the right respectively (see Fig. 3.18B).

With *'alternate' presentations*, a force from the right appears to have displaced them towards the left side (see Fig. 3.18A). With *left anterior and locked* presentations, a force from the left appears to have displaced them towards the right side (Fig. 3.18B). The final pattern will depend on the effect of the malalignment-related forces on the athlete's inherent weight-bearing pattern.

Heel, sole and midsole wear patterns

Wear of the heel, sole and midsole often reflect the shift in weight-bearing. The following pattern is typical of the 'alternate' presentations.

Heel (see Fig. 3.25A, B). Right heel wear tends to involve primarily the posterolateral aspect. As discussed above, this reflects the combined effect of the right external rotation and increased varus angulation, which, in essence, lowers the posterolateral part of the heel so that it is first to contact the ground. The greater the external rotation and varus angulation, the more lateral the wear and the more quickly the foot will torque into a medial weight-bearing position. Left heel wear, in contrast, tends to be less pronounced and likely to involve more the posterior than the posterolateral aspect.

Sole (Fig. 3.25A, B). Right sole wear is more medial under the ball of the foot, reflecting the rapid switch from varus at heel strike to valgus by foot-flat. Depending on the degree of supination, the wear of the left sole may be relatively less medial, more probably central or even lateral at the ball of the foot.

Midsole (Fig. 3.28). Because the foot can switch from lateral impact to medial weight-bearing so quickly, a compression of midsole material on the medial aspect can occur as far back as the heel and go on from there to involve the mid and forefoot. In contrast, the left midsole material tends to compress and deteriorate more on the lateral aspect, usually most markedly in the heel.

Predicting weight-bearing following realignment

In athletes who are in alignment, the heel cups and uppers tend to collapse inwards bilaterally to some extent in those who are pronators and outwards in those who are supinators, remaining undisplaced in those with a neutral pattern of weight-bearing. Sometimes the hindfoot pronates and the forefoot supinates, or vice versa, in which case the direction of collapse of the heel cups is opposite to that of the uppers.

When malalignment is present, the amount and direction of collapse of the heel cups and uppers can

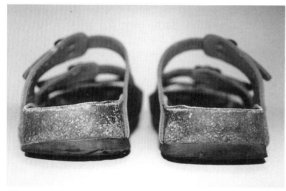

(A)

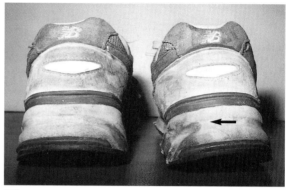

(Bi)

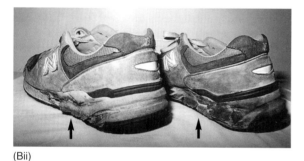

(Bii)

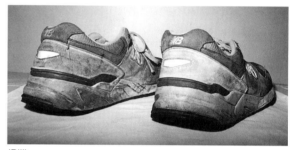

(Biii)

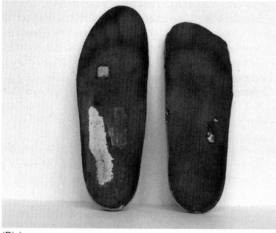

(Biv)

Figure 3.28 Asymmetry of midsole compression and wear caused by malalignment (the right medially from a tendency towards pronation, the left laterally from a tendency to supination) may be evident from heel to forefoot.
(A) Birkenstock sandals: compression of the right medial and left lateral heel. (B) Running shoes: (i) pronation more marked on the right, with a deterioration (compression) of the right heel medially (arrow); (ii) view from the left: deterioration of the right inner and left outer midsole (arrows); (iii) view from the right: the left inner and right outer midsoles are both intact; (iv) the top of the insoles shows marked wear of the left shoe on its lateral aspect.

sometimes be a fairly reliable indicator of the inherent pattern of weight-bearing that will emerge on correction. When both shoes show an inwards collapse, the athlete may well turn out to be a true pronator; when both show outwards collapse, a true supinator (see Fig. 3.19). These assumptions do not, however, always hold true. For example, some athletes who pronate bilaterally – albeit asymmetrically – when out of alignment

turn out to have a neutral or even lateral weight-bearing pattern with frank supination following realignment (Fig. 3.29). The athlete's true weight-bearing pattern may therefore not become evident until the malalignment has been corrected. The author has, however, yet to see an athlete who supinates asymmetrically when out of alignment but turns out to be a pronator on realignment.

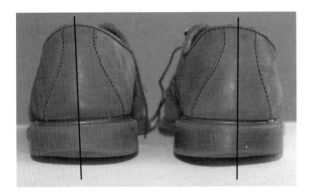

Figure 3.29 This athlete has a pattern of right pronation, left supination evident when malalignment is present (see Fig. 3.18A). On realignment (shown here), the athlete has reverted to his natural weight-bearing pattern of bilateral symmetrical supination.

Pitfalls

It must be remembered that the shoe itself may influence the weight-bearing pattern or may be worn down in a certain way for reasons other than malalignment. This may interfere with the assessment.

Increased heel and sole width. Increased heel and sole width may predispose to pronation. Assuming that the non-weight-bearing foot is in a varus attitude, the more the sole flares out and extends past the margins of the heel cup and upper, the earlier it makes contact with the ground. In effect, it comes to act like an outrigger that can quickly flip the foot into pronation. The Nike LDV-1000 serves as an unfortunate reminder of this (Fig. 3.30).

The intent of the especially wide, outflaring heel and sole of this running shoe was to provide a larger base to

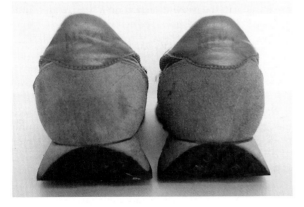

Figure 3.30 Nike LDV-1000 running shoe with an 'outrigger-type' heel and a sole intended to counteract pronation.

land on, thereby improving the stability of the foot and countering any tendency towards pronation. Instead, the heel extending outward created an 'outrigger' effect that had exactly the opposite result in many: it increased the tendency to pronation because the foot itself was not positioned in neutral at heel strike but actually held in a varus attitude (see Fig. 3.22A, B). The lateral border of the shoe, which served as an extension of the foot, merely came to touch the ground earlier and flipped the foot into pronation even sooner and more forcefully than would have occurred without the shoe.

A wide heel and sole could conceivably also aggravate a problem of supination if the medial border made contact with the ground first. For this to happen, the non-weight-bearing foot would have to be in a valgus attitude, something that occurs less frequently.

'Pronator' shoes with a 'double-density midsole' and 'straight' last (left shoe, Fig. 3.31A, B). There are now numerous running shoes on the market made specifically for pronators. Most of these have a medial reinforcement in the form of high-density midsole material, or so-called 'double-density midsole', to help to counteract excessive pronation (the grey and black material in the left shoe of Fig. 3.31A). A 'straight last sole', one with the sole filling in the space underlying the medial arch, provides further support to prevent medial longitudinal arch collapse (left shoe, Fig. 3.31B).

These concepts were first incorporated in the Brooks Chariot in the 1970s. In the presence of malalignment, running shoes conceived along these same lines may be helpful if the athlete still pronates to some extent bilaterally (see Fig. 3.19A). If, however, the athlete actually pronates on one side and supinates on the other, this type of shoe could create problems on the side that supinates because:

- the medial reinforcement will further increase the tendency towards supination by acting like a medial raise and countering any inward collapse of this foot
- the ability to absorb shock and deal with ground reaction forces is further impaired as the foot is maintained in a more rigid, supinated position by the increased density of the medial midsole material and by the inability of the medial longitudinal arch to collapse.

Excessive shoe wear. Excessive wearing down of the medial or lateral part of the heel and sole, and/or excessive inwards or outwards collapse of the heel cup and upper for whatever reason (e.g., breakdown attributable to prolonged use), will predispose the athlete to an exaggerated degree of medial or lateral weight-bearing respectively. It may also hide the actual weight-bearing pattern, asymmetrical though this may be.

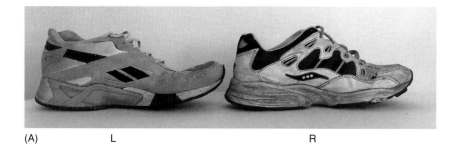

(A)   L   R

(B)   R   L

Figure 3.31 Running shoes: modifications of the (A) midsole and (B) last. The shoes on the left are for a pronator: 'double-density' (medially reinforced) midsole and straight last (the medial arch filled in for extra support) to counteract medial arch collapse. The shoes on the right are for a supinator: uniform 'single-density' or 'neutral' extra-thick midsole and curved last (with an indent or 'waist' at the medial arch level), which allows for some collapse of the medial arch to increase the flexibility of the foot and its ability to absorb shock.

Factory-related changes. The way in which shoes leave the factory may sometimes be misleading. A common variant is the pair that has the heel cups set in 5–10 degrees of varus; this could mistakenly suggest that the athlete is a supinator (Fig. 3.30). The angulation may be greater on one side than the other, which may suggest that malalignment is present when this is not even the case.

Habits and ergonomics. Wear of the shoe may reflect a habit or way of using the shoe in a vocational or avocational setting rather than forces attributable to malalignment. The right shoe may, for example, have collapsed outwards from operating a car pedal with the foot in a varus attitude while pivoting with the heel on the car floor. Seeing such a lateral drift of the right shoe in an athlete with one of the 'alternate' presentations would be completely out of keeping with the direction of the asymmetrical forces associated with these presentations, that is, towards pronation. In such cases, an examination of shoes not worn for

driving is likely to show the changes in keeping with those predicted for the presentation of malalignment at hand.

Walking or running on a slope. Repeatedly walking or running in the same direction on a road with a pronounced downslope from the centre, or parallel to the side of a hill, will eventually collapse the uphill shoe inwards and the downhill shoe outwards in someone who is in alignment (Fig. 3.32). This pattern may erroneously suggest that malalignment is present (see Fig. 3.18).

Walking versus running. Remember that the athlete may pronate when walking but supinate with running or vice versa! Therefore, always ask to see both a pair of day shoes and those worn for athletic activities.

Rotational versus straight-line sports. The asymmetry of malalignment expresses itself differently in those sports with a rotational component compared with those involving straight-line progression. The pattern of weight-bearing may therefore be different with one

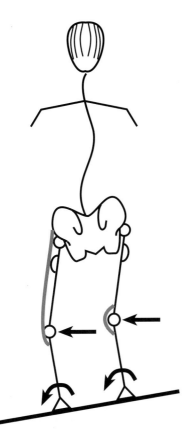

Figure 3.32 In someone who is in alignment, repeated walks/runs on a slope banked upwards to the right can eventually result in: (A) a pattern of heel cup collapse that mimics that seen with upslips and 'alternate' presentations of malalignment (see Figs 3.18 and 3.27); (B) increased tension in the soft tissue structures – left lateral (e.g. tensor fascia lata/iliotibial band complex), right medial (e.g. medial collateral ligament) – to the point at which these become symptomatic (see Figs 3.33 and 3.38).

athletic activity than with another. The wear pattern of the shoes worn for these different activities may reveal these different stresses and hold the clue to an injury.

Remember that if the examination findings and the impression gained from looking at the shoes do not seem to correlate, ask to see some day shoes worn for different activities and a pair of running shoes.

A final observation on weight-bearing

Over the years, the author has been struck in clinical practice by the fact that a neutral to supination pattern of weight-bearing seems to be almost as prevalent as pronation in those who are in alignment. In one study

(W. Schamberger, unpublished data, 1994), he looked at 120 athletes as they presented consecutively at the office and subsequently for follow-up after treatment. On the initial examination, 96 (80%) of these athletes proved to be out of alignment and 24 (20%) in alignment. The results of this study as they relate specifically to the examination of weight-bearing on walking, heel- and toe-walking, and hopping were as follows:

1. Of those with initial malalignment ($n = 96$):
   - 35% had bilateral pronation
   - 8% had bilateral supination
   - 35% had a neutral pattern of weight-bearing bilaterally, with no evident tendency to pronation or supination
   - 17% had the right pronation, left supination pattern
   - 5% had the left pronation, right supination pattern
2. On the initial reassessment following realignment ($n = 96$):
   - 45% had bilateral pronation
   - 11% had right pronation and left supination
   - 11% had bilateral supination
   - 33% had a neutral weight-bearing pattern.

In other words, with realignment there was an increase in the number of those with bilateral pronation, from 35% to 45%, whereas the total of those in a neutral position or supination remained relatively unchanged at 44%. Asymmetry was still apparent in 11%, which could be expected to decrease as a more symmetrical gait pattern was gradually re-established by maintaining realignment.

Time and time again, athletes have presented with 'lateral' symptoms (e.g. tensor fascia lata/iliotibial band [TFL/ITB] tenderness, trochanteric pain and recurrent ankle inversion sprains) but had previously been diagnosed as being 'pronators' and had therefore been provided with double-density running shoes, medially posted rigid or semi-rigid orthotics, or both. They were usually being referred because their symptoms had persisted or worsened. An appropriate course of ankle strengthening exercises and lateral stretches combined with a simple change to a running shoe with a thicker, neutral (single-density) midsole and a curved last (right shoe, Fig. 3.31A, B), with or without the addition of a soft-shell orthotic and a lateral raise, proved adequate therapy for most.

'Pronation' became a powerful buzzword in the 1970s and 80s, to the point at which it probably prevented or delayed recognition of the supination pattern. Indeed, as recently as the 1993 American College of Sports Medicine annual meeting, a top executive of one of the major manufacturers of athletic shoewear, when asked what his company was doing to accommodate those with neutral weight-bearing or supination, flatly stated that 'there is no such thing as a supinator'. Luckily, a number of appropriate shoes are now available for these athletes.

Since the mid-1970s, there has been an over-emphasis on the recognition of pronation and on the problems associated with it. As a result, pronation became more eagerly sought for – and probably more readily recognized – than supination. Given this back-ground, and the fact that excessive pronation on one side is not an uncommon feature with rotational malalignment and also upslips:

1. the pronation pattern on one side has probably often caught the eye more easily
2. the coexisting neutral or supination pattern on the other side could easily be ignored as attention is diverted towards the pronating side
3. in those athletes who pronate bilaterally, any asymmetry of pronation (another feature of malalign-ment) has probably tended to go unrecognized.

As stated before, some 10–20% of those who pronate bilaterally when out of alignment actually end up supinating once in alignment. It should therefore come as no surprise that study results (W. Schamberger, unpublished data, 1994) have shown, on realignment, as many as 44% adopting either a neutral or a supin-ation pattern (33% and 11% respectively), a number equivalent to the 45% who proved to pronate bilaterally.

Clinical correlation

The shift in weight-bearing that occurs with malalign-ment results in an asymmetry of forces in the lower extremities that predisposes to the injuries typically associated with pronation and supination.

On the side of external rotation and pronation

Increased tension in structures on the medial aspect of the leg (Fig. 3.33);
- groin pain and/or medial thigh pain (irritation or sprain of the pectineus/adductor origin muscle mass or insertions)
- medial collateral ligament and medial plica
- snapping of the medial plica and vastus medialis tendon across the medial condyle
- medial shin splints from irritation and periosteal inflammation along the tibialis posterior origin
- medial ankle ligaments (especially anterior tibiotalar).

Peripheral nerve involvement (Fig. 3.34A):
- traction injury to the posterior tibial, saphenous and distal (medial) deep peroneal nerves
- compression injury of the sural nerve

Increased valgus tendency at the knee, with:
- increased pressure in the lateral joint compartment
- increased Q-angle and lateral tracking of the patella, pressure in the patellofemoral compartment and tension in the patellar tendon
- irritation of the saphenous nerve.

Increased weight-bearing on the medial aspect of the foot:
- aggravation of problems relating to a hallux valgus, rigidus and limitus
- acceleration of first metatarsophalangeal bunion formation and degeneration
- sesamoiditis
- plantar fasciitis on the basis of excessive traction attributable to calcaneus eversion and collapse of the medial longitudinal arch
- posterior tarsal tunnel syndrome, with irritation or compression of the posterior tibial nerve
- in the case of bilateral Morton's toes, a unilateral aggravation of stress on the second and third metatarsal heads with callus formation (Fig. 3.35), tenderness and/or outright pain (metatarsalgia) or even stress fracture.

Achilles tendonitis on the basis of excessive traction, attributable to:
- the separation of origin and insertion that occurs because of the calcaneus collapsing into valgus (Fig. 3.36)
- the increased ankle dorsiflexion usually possible on this side (see Figs 3.68 and 3.77).

On the side of internal rotation and supination

Increased tension in the lateral structures of the leg (see Fig. 3.33):
- sprain of the hip abductors (gluteus medius/minimus) and the TFL/ITB complex
- bursitis (greater trochanter and lateral femoral condyle; Fig. 3.37)
- lateral shin splints (tibialis anterior and/or peroneal muscle group tendonitis or sprain)
- lateral ankle ligaments.

Peripheral nerve involvement (see Fig. 3.34B):
- traction injury to the common and superficial peroneal nerves, the sural nerve and the lateral

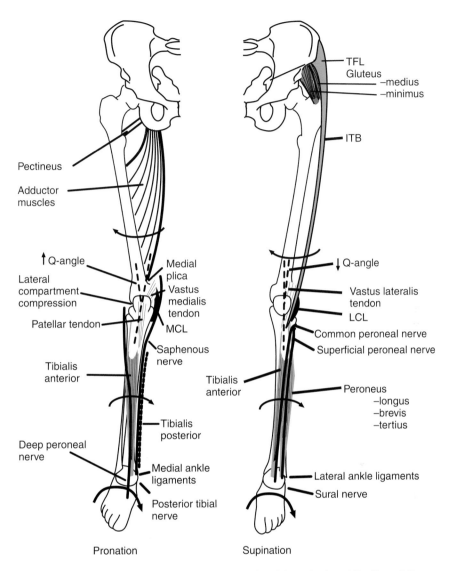

Figure 3.33   Structures put under stress by a right pronation, left supination shift with malalignment.

femoral cutaneous nerve (not shown – see Fig. 4.13)
- compression injury of the posterior tibial nerve.

Tendency to varum at the knee, with:

- increased pressure in the medial joint compartment
- traction on the vastus lateralis insertion and lateral collateral ligament
- snapping of the vastus lateralis across the lateral femoral condyle.

Increased rigidity of the foot and ankle:

- an impaired ability to dissipate ground forces, predisposing to the development of plantar fasciitis, Achilles tendonitis and stress fractures.

Increased weight-bearing on the lateral aspect of the foot:

- painful callus formation, fourth and fifth metatarsalgia, and metatarsal stress fractures (see Fig. 3.35)

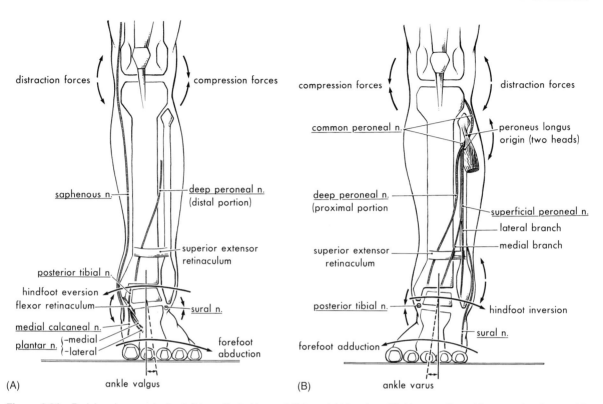

Figure 3.34 Peripheral nerves in the left leg affected by a shift in weight-bearing. (A) Nerves affected by pronation forces. (B) Nerves affected by supination forces. (From Schamberger 1987, with permission.)

- Morton's neuroma
- ankle inversion sprains.

Problems relating to pronation and supination will be discussed in further detail, as appropriate, in other sections of this and the other chapters.

ASYMMETRY OF MUSCLE TENSION

Normally functioning muscle is relaxed and non-tender when at rest. On gentle palpation, the tips of the fingers can sink into the muscle easily, and the pressure elicits no pain. Concentrate on the feel of the muscle being palpated and compare this with that of the muscle(s) immediately adjacent, and of its partner on the opposite side. In addition, look for reactive muscle tensing, a tell-tale sign that the muscle, its nerve supply or the vertebral segment to which they both belong is in trouble.

Muscles are meant to contract and relax. Relaxation results in an increase in blood flow, allowing for the optimal clearance of waste and the delivery of oxygen and nutrients. Contraction results in a decrease in

blood flow and an impaired clearance of waste. A contraction of only 60% of maximum has been shown to stop blood flow into and out of the muscle completely (McArdle et al 1986).

A constant increase in muscle tension means that the muscle is always to some extent working; there is a continuous increase in energy consumption and production of waste occurring at a time of diminished blood flow. At the same time, a constant traction force is being exerted on the muscle's origin and insertion. Given this persistent increase in tension, the muscle bulk proper and/or its points of attachment will eventually become tender to palpation or outright painful. The term 'chronic tension myalgia' seems appropriate because the pain itself is myofascial in origin, involving the muscle itself, the neurovascular bundle, the enveloping fascia and the fibro-osseous junctions.

The athlete with chronic tension myalgia may not even be aware that he or she is constantly tensing these muscles. A vicious cycle often ensues. The pain causes a reflex increase in tension and splinting of the painful area; this reaction, in turn, results in more pain. At this stage, it is often still possible to interrupt the cycle

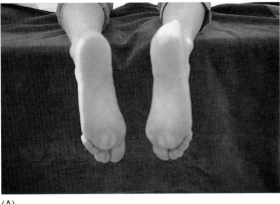

(A)

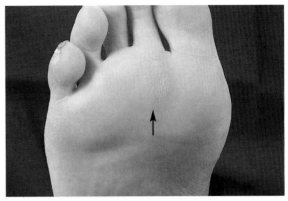

(Bi)

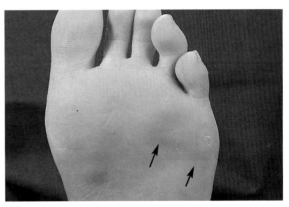

Figure 3.35   Callus formation under metatarsal (MT) heads.
(A) Aligned: bilaterally under 2nd and 3rd reflects weight-
transfer with short 1st (Morton's) toe and collapse of the
anterior arch of the foot (see Fig. 4.16, lower A,B).
(B) asymmetrical callus formation reflects malalignment-
related shift in weight-bearing: (i) more medially on the right
(under the 2nd) and (ii) more laterally on the left (4th and 5th)
MT heads.

(Bii)

Figure 3.36   Increased tension in
the right Achilles tendon, reflecting
external rotation of the right leg,
heel collapse inwards (pronation)
and increased knee valgus
angulation; the narrowing of the
right tendon compared with that on
the supinating left side is
accentuated by toe-walking (see
also Fig. 3.20).

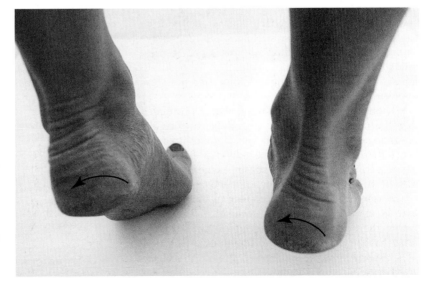

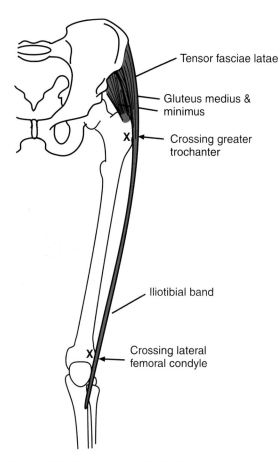

Figure 3.37 Tensor fascia lata/iliotibial band complex spanning the greater trochanter and lateral femoral condyle – common sites of irritation and 'bursitis'.

Labels in figure: Tensor fasciae latae; Gluteus medius & minimus; Crossing greater trochanter; Iliotibial band; Crossing lateral femoral condyle

simply by relaxing the muscle and/or temporarily stopping the pain. Frequent stretching and progressive strengthening, in conjunction with massage, electrical modalities (e.g. transcutaneous electrical nerve stimulation, acupuncture or trigger point injection) are appropriate.

Whatmore & Kohli (1974) have, however, postulated that the chronic contraction eventually fatigues the physiological mechanisms that sustain the contraction. When the energy reserves of the individual fibres drop below a critical level, 'fatigue spasm' ensues: the fibres remain involuntarily shortened. Persistent fatigue spasm can lead to a fixed shortening of muscle fibres that is maintained by 'physicochemical processes' within the fibres. Muscle fibres atrophy at the same time that the fibrous content of the muscle increases. This can sometimes be appreciated as tender, localized areas of crepitus on palpation. Once the condition has

reached this stage it becomes much harder, sometimes impossible, to reverse.

Myofascial pain associated with chronic tension myalgia is not to be confused with myofascial trigger points. Trigger points are, by definition, very localized areas of hyperirritable tissue usually found within a taut band of skeletal muscle or the fascia surrounding or invaginating the muscle. A trigger point can, for example, localize to an excessively active muscle spindle. Trigger points are painful to compression and can give rise to characteristic referred pain patterns, tenderness and autonomic phenomena (Travell & Simons 1983, 1992). Chronic tension myalgia and trigger points can coexist, but trigger points in a muscle are not felt to result from a chronic increase in tension (Travell & Simons 1983).

Malalignment-related increase in muscle tension

In the presence of malalignment, a chronic increase in muscle tension can result for four main reasons (Box 3.5).

These points will now be discussed in some detail. The prevalence and distribution of increased tension and tenderness in the athletes presenting with malalignment in the 1992 and 1993 studies are summarized in Tables 3.1 and 3.2 respectively.

Increased distance between origin and insertion

In association will malalignment, such an increase can result for two main reasons:

A spatial reorientation of the bones has occurred. This point is best illustrated by anterior and posterior rotation of the innominates in the sagittal plane and the effect of such rotation on the hamstrings, iliacus and rectus femoris (Fig. 3.38).

Anterior rotation of the right innominate moves the right ischial tuberosity posteriorly and upwards effec-

---

Box 3.5 Causes of a chronic increase in muscle tension in malalignment

- The malalignment has increased the distance between the muscle's origin and insertion
- The malalignment *per se* is associated with an automatic increase in tension or 'facilitation' of specific muscles
- The increase in muscle tension is an attempt to splint
    - an area that is painful
    - an area that is unstable

Table 3.1 1992 Study: prevalence of increased muscle tone and tenderness

Structure	Overall involved (%)	Right (%)	Left (%)	Bilateral (%)
Piriformis	56	57	6	37
Hip abductors	42	10	50	40
Iliotibial band	44	13	50	37
Thoracic paravertebral muscles	44	13	15	72
Lumbar paravertebral muscles	26	19	9	72

Right, left and bilateral involvement have been calculated as a percentage of 'overall' prevalence.

Table 3.2 1993 Study: prevalence of increased muscle tone and tenderness

Structure	Overall involved (%)	Right (%)	Left (%)	Bilateral (%)
Piriformis	44	19 (43)	3 (7)	22 (50)
Hip abductors	30	4 (15)	13 (44)	12 (41)
Iliotibial band	43	5 (13)	9 (21)	29 (67)
Thoracic paravertebral muscles	45	13 (29)	4 (10)	27 (61)
Lumbar paravertebral muscles	11	3 (30)	3 (30)	4 (40)

Calculations reflect the percentage of the total ($n = 92$) involved in each category; in parentheses is a breakdown of each as a percentage of the 'overall' category.

tively separating the hamstring origin from the insertions into the proximal tibia, and increasing tension in this muscle complex.

Anterior rotation effectively moves the anterior aspect of the innominate shell downwards, moving the iliacus origin towards its insertion into the lesser trochanter and decreasing tension in that muscle; it has a similar effect on rectus femoris.

Posterior rotation of the innominate has the reverse effect by depressing the ischial tuberosity and elevating the anterior aspect of the innominate shell, thereby helping to relax the hamstrings while increasing tension in iliacus and rectus femoris.

The distance between origin and insertion can increase as a result of the pattern of weight-bearing (see Fig. 3.33). Pronation, as discussed above, increases the distance along the inner part of the leg, from foot to groin, and increases the tension in the muscles on the medial aspect. Supination increases the distance along the outer part of the leg, from the foot to the iliac crest, and increases the tension in the muscles on the lateral aspect. The shift in weight-bearing typically associated with malalignment can actually result in symptoms and signs related to the stresses of pronation on one side and supination on the other (see 'Asymmetry of foot alignment, weight-bearing and shoe wear' above).

The remarks regarding the increase in muscle tension related to the separation of origin and insertion also apply to ligaments (see 'Asymmetry of ligament tension' below).

Automatic increase in tension, or 'facilitation', of specific muscles

Both rotational malalignment and upslips cause an automatic increase in tension in certain muscles, in a pattern that cannot be attributed simply to a separation of origin and insertion (Fig. 3.39). On examining the athlete lying down, muscles most consistently involved are:

- on the right side, the upper trapezius, infraspinatus/teres minor, piriformis and the hamstrings
- on the left side, the hip abductors and TFL/ITB complex, iliopsoas and gastrocnemius/soleus.

The increase in muscle tension often reverts to normal as soon as the malalignment has been corrected, suggesting that it may be related to an asymmetry of signals arising from structures that are affected by the malalignment. The TFL/ITB complex serves as a good example of this. When rotational malalignment or upslip is present, the right complex remains relaxed and will usually allow the knee to come down on the plinth on Ober's test (Fig. 3.40Ai), whereas the complex on the left is tense and holds the knee at a variable distance up in the air (Fig. 3.40Aii). Following realignment, the tension in the left complex

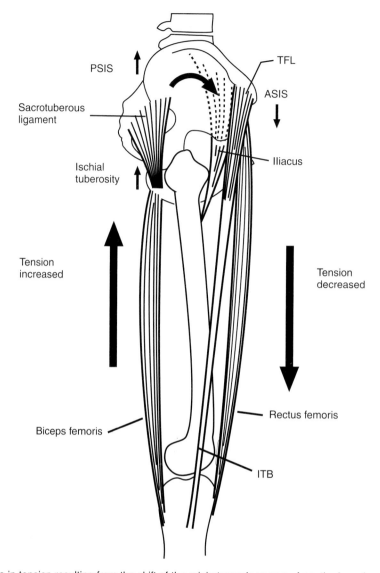

Figure 3.38 Change in tension resulting from the shift of the origin towards or away from the insertion with right innominate anterior rotation (e.g. tension increased in rectus femoris and decreased in iliacus). The reverse changes occur with right posterior rotation. PSIS, posterior superior iliac spine; ASIS, anterior superior iliac spine; TFL, tensor fascia lata; ITB, iliotibial band.

immediately decreases, allowing the left knee to come down as far as the right (Fig. 3.40B).

The following are some possible mechanisms to consider. First, malalignment results in an asymmetry of proprioceptive signals arising from the joints. However, as with muscle weakness (discussed below), the muscles showing the increase in tension tend to be consistently the same regardless of the presentation of malalignment. For example, the increase in tension consistently involves the left hip abductors and

TFL/ITB complex (Fig. 3.40A), regardless of whether the malalignment is in the form of an upslip or anterior rotation, has associated SI joint 'locking' or is on the right or left side. Asymmetry of proprioceptive signals, therefore, does not seem to offer a plausible explanation for this phenomenon.

Second, the above findings argue more for a cause at the spinal segmental or cortical level (Korr 1978). The increased tension may reflect segmental muscle 'facilitation' or 'inhibition'. The pelvic malalignment could

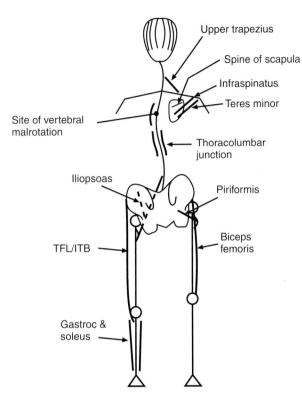

Figure 3.39 Typical sites of increased muscle/tendon tension and tenderness resulting with malalignment. The drawing also indicates the typical lateralization; if the structure is involved bilaterally, the one indicated here is usually affected more severely. TFL/ITB, tensor fascia lata/iliotibial band.

cause an increase or decrease in excitatory or inhibitory signals to muscles; alternatively, the malalignment may itself have evolved as a result of such signals to the muscles arising from some other cause.

T12 or L1 vertebral malrotation, for example, is usually associated with an increase in tension (facilitation) in the psoas on one side, and a relaxation (inhibition) of the muscle on the other side; this would result in asymmetrical forces capable of causing not only malalignment of the pelvis, but also more distal effects that influence the alignment of the lower extremities and weight-bearing (see Fig. 3.2). The segmental dysfunction may act on the muscle directly or affect muscle tone (and strength) indirectly by interfering with cortically mediated motor control.

Third, some of the central effects of articular mechanoreceptor stimulation pointed out by Wyke (1985) may be operative. These include the nociceptor afferent activity arising from the type IV receptor system within the joint capsule and the fibres of the intrinsic joint and spinal ligaments. A pain-suppressive effect normally occurs with 'activation of the apical spinal interneurons', producing 'presynaptic inhibition of [this] nociceptor afferent activity' (p. 75). Perhaps with the distortion of joint surfaces, ligaments and capsules associated with malalignment, there is an excessive stimulation of type IV receptors to the point at which activation of interneurons becomes inadequate, resulting in a failure of pain suppression at a segmental level. The increased tension in the paravertebral and more distal muscles may therefore reflect a problem at the spinal segmental level.

Finally, the malalignment, whatever its presentation, may induce rather non-specific signals related, for example, to stretching or irritation of the dura. These signals in turn have a general effect of stimulating or suppressing cortical motor signals to certain motor spindles, and inducing facilitation or inhibition, respectively.

Tension increased in an attempt to splint a painful area

The muscles in the vicinity of a painful area usually show an increase in tension. This may occur as a reaction to irritation of the nociceptive fibres. It may also reflect a reflex attempt to splint the painful area in order to prevent the aggravation that would otherwise occur with movement. Malalignment automatically stresses a number of structures, in particular the joints of the spine and pelvis. These sites can eventually become a source of irritation or pain that is aggravated by movement or further stress imposed by activity. It is not unusual to find increased tension (and tenderness) in the muscles capable of decreasing or preventing the movement of these painful areas. There is, for example, often splinting of the paravertebral muscles immediately adjacent to a malrotated vertebra and at sites of curve reversal, particularly the thoracolumbar junction.

Tension increased in an attempt to stabilize an area

Malalignment is frequently associated with joint instability for various reasons (see Ch. 2). Laxity of the ligaments, which allows for a recurrent malrotation of one or more vertebrae, results in a recurrent or chronic increase in tension in the paravertebrals and any other muscles that span that segment. The instability of SI joints that can occur with sacral and innominate rotation and upslips typically increases tension in the prime muscles that can stabilize the joint by wedging

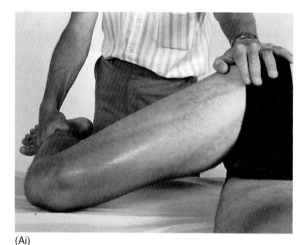

(Ai)

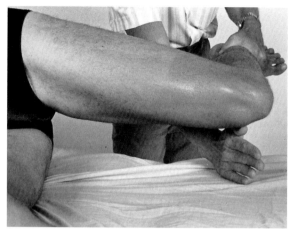

(Aii)

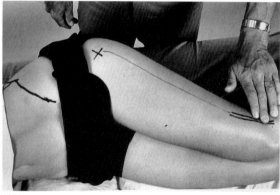

(Aiii)

(B)

Figure 3.40 Ober's test for limitation of hip adduction: tight tensor fascia lata/iliotibial band (TFL/ITB). (A) With malalignment: (i) the right adducts to touch the plinth; (ii) left adduction is limited compared with right; (iii) the facilitated left TFL/ITB complex proves consistently tense (and usually tender along part or all of its length). (B) Following realignment: left adduction equals right.

the sacrum against one or both innominates: piriformis by pulling the sacrum backwards relative to an innominate, iliacus by pulling the innominate forwards against the anteriorly widening sacrum (see Fig. 2.31).

In summary, in the presence of malalignment, one sees an increase in tension in certain muscles. This may be in response to pain or instability, a mechanical increase in the distance between origin and insertion, or some other mechanism, segmental or cortical, that affects the muscle spindle setting and results in facilitation.

As long as the malalignment is present, the muscles involved are unlikely to respond to stretching attempts or will do so only temporarily. With time, these muscles, their tendons and points of attachment can become tender to palpation or overtly painful. The

myofascial pain that results may remain localized, have a referred component or both. A persistent increase in tension secondary to malalignment increases the risk of sprain or strain of the affected muscles with athletic activity. Conversely, realignment may greatly benefit the recovery of those who have suffered a sprain or strain, simply by removing that component of the increase in tension and pain which is attributable to the malalignment (Cibulka et al 1986).

Studies of those presenting with malalignment give an indication of the prevalence of the muscles typically noted to show an increase in tension and/or tenderness to palpation, as illustrated in Fig. 3.39 above. This figure also reflects the predilection for involvement of muscles on either the right or the left side. The following are the muscles most consistently affected.

The right piriformis muscle

Fifty-eight per cent of the 96 athletes presenting with malalignment in the 1994 (W. Schamberger, unpublished data) study had increased tone in the piriformis; the right was six times more likely to be affected in isolation and even more likely to be tender to palpation than the left. Those with one of the 'alternate' presentations of rotational malalignment were noted to have external rotation of the right lower extremity, the majority also showing torsion of the sacrum around an oblique axis, almost as often to the right as to the left (see Figs 2.7, 2.11, 2.29 and 2.35).

Both external rotation and torsion around the left oblique axis would bring the piriformis origin (from the anterior aspect of the sacrum) closer to its insertion (into the upper, posterior aspect of the greater trochanter) and should therefore relax this muscle (see Fig. 2.31). The increased involvement of right piriformis with malalignment therefore appears more likely to be a reflection of the facilitation of that muscle, an attempt to splint an unstable or painful right SI joint or a combination of these.

The separation of the piriformis origin and insertion could be expected as a more probable cause for the involvement of this muscle on the left side. The commonly noted internal rotation of the left lower extremity, combined with sacral torsion around the left oblique axis, would certainly increase the distance between its origin and insertion. However, the athletes who presented with this combination ($n = 28$ in the 1994 study) failed to show any correlation to whether the left or right piriformis was involved. Study results relating to sacral torsion would also argue against a separation of origin and insertion being the cause of any increase in tension on the left side. The less frequently noted involvement of the left piriformis is probably also more likely to be attributable to facilitation, an attempt to stabilize the left SI joint or a combination of these factors.

It also appears doubtful that it is the increased tension in piriformis that is actually responsible for the external rotation of the right leg consistently noted with the 'alternate' presentations and right or left upslip. In the 1994 study, of the 96 athletes who presented with malalignment, all of the 37% who had increased tension in piriformis bilaterally showed an outwards rotation of one leg and an inwards rotation of the other, in a pattern in keeping with whether they were left anterior and locked (left outwards) or had one of the 'alternate' presentations (right outwards). In addition, the right piriformis showed an involvement in isolation three and six times as often as the left with the left anterior and locked and the 'alternate' presentations respectively.

In another study (W. Schamberger, unpublished data, 1993), 12 athletes presented with the left anterior and locked pattern and associated external rotation of the left leg, yet four showed increased tone only in the right piriformis, four bilaterally and one in the left alone. These findings argue against the increased tone in piriformis being directly responsible for the external rotation of one or other leg noted in association with these different presentations.

In summary, given the lack of correlation to the pattern of malalignment present, the increased involvement of right piriformis probably reflects an automatic increase in tone through a facilitation triggered by the malalignment, an attempt by this muscle to help to stabilize the right SI joint (see Fig. 2.31) or a combination of these. Piriformis involvement does not appear to correlate with the side of lower extremity external rotation.

Clinical correlation

Increased tone and recurrent spasm in one or other piriformis muscle is often blamed for a failure to correct the malalignment initially or for the recurrence of malalignment following correction. Its oblique attachment to the sacrum normally plays a vital role in stabilizing the SI joint on the side of single leg stance but has also been implicated as a cause of SI joint locking and sacral torsion (see Ch. 2).

Lying and sitting, especially when slouching or sitting in bucket seats, can put direct pressure on the piriformis muscle bulk and insertion, creating problems for those in whom these sites are already tender.

The increased tension in piriformis can result in buttock and lower extremity pain on the basis of:

- referred pain, felt primarily in the posterior thigh region (Fig. 3.41)
- compromise and irritation of the sciatic nerve or its components; the problem of 'piriformis syndrome' and 'sciatica' are discussed separately in Chapter 4.

Piriformis involvement can contribute to the deep pain associated with pelvic floor dysfunction, with increased tension and acute tenderness noted on palpation of piriformis per rectum or vagina (see Ch. 4).

The left hip abductors and TFL/ITB complex

Gluteus medius, gluteus minimus and TFL, with its continuation as the ITB, show an involvement in practically all athletes with malalignment regardless of the pattern of presentation (see Fig. 3.40Aii, iii). Pain in the

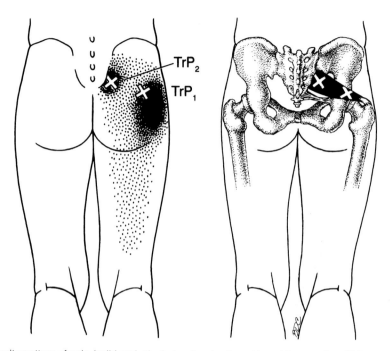

Figure 3.41 Composite pattern of pain (solid and stippled pattern) referred from trigger points (TrPs; marked by X) in the right piriformis muscle. The lateral X (TrP1) indicates the most common TrP location. The stippling locates the spillover pattern that may be felt as less intense pain than that of the essential pattern (solid black). Spillover may be absent. (From Travell & Simons 1992, with permission.)

region of the left hip, greater trochanter and lateral thigh and knee is certainly one of the more common presenting complaints. Increased tone and tenderness to palpation are usually evident on the left side. Tenderness is most likely to be found over the distal part of the left ITB, and less often, along the full length of the ITB, the TFL and the hip abductor origin and gluteus medius/minimus muscle mass. Any increase in tension in the left hip abductors will of course contribute to the limitation of left hip adduction found in almost 100% of the athletes (see 'Asymmetry of lower extremity ranges of motion' below, and Figs 3.40Aii, 3.44 and 3.70).

The TFL/ITB complex flexes, abducts and internally rotates the thigh. Therefore, one is most likely to reproduce the pain by first passively extending, adducting, and externally rotating the leg, to put the complex under tension, and then resisting the athlete's attempt to internally rotate that leg. Any increase in tension applies TFL and gluteus medius/minimus more tightly against the greater trochanter, and the distal ITB against the lateral femoral condyle, increasing the chance of developing painful inflammation and/or bursitis at these sites (see Fig. 3.37). The frequent lateralization of symptoms to the left seen with

malalignment is the result of a combination of factors, including:

1. the apparently automatic increase in tension in the left hip abductor muscles through facilitation (see Fig. 3.40Aiii)
2. these muscles tensing up in reaction to an underlying source of pain on the left side: local (e.g. pain from the SI joint, or from rubbing against the greater trochanter) or referred (e.g. the iliolumbar ligament referring pain to the sclerotome involving the greater trochanteric region; Fig. 3.42)
3. in athletes with one of the 'alternate' presentations, a lateral shift of weight-bearing on the left (sometimes to frank supination), which increases the traction on these lateral structures (see Figs 3.33, 3.39)
4. in athletes with the left anterior and locked presentation, a simultaneous external rotation of the left lower extremity, which increases tension by separating the TFL/ITB complex origin and insertion
5. the functional weakness of the left hip abductors consistently found in association with malalignment (see 'Asymmetrical functional weakness of lower extremity muscles' below); weak muscles fatigue more easily, causing them to tense up.

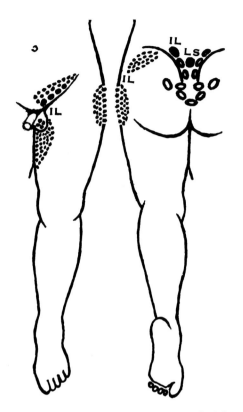

Figure 3.42 Typical sites of referred pain from the left iliolumbar ligaments (IL), which are being irritated as a result of lumbosacral (LS) joint instability: the groin, the anterior medial upper two-thirds of the thigh, the lower abdomen above Poupart's ligament, the testicle in the male, the vagina in the female, the upper buttock beneath the crest of the ilium and the upper outer thigh. (From Hackett 1958, with permission.)

The study results show that increased tension and tenderness in the left hip abductors, and tenderness over the left greater trochanter and ITB, are all more prevalent with right anterior innominate rotation and with the 'alternate' presentations, whereas bilateral involvement or no involvement at all is more likely to be associated with the left anterior and locked presentation (W. Schamberger, unpublished data, 1993, 1994). The presence of a bilateral increase in hip abductor and/or ITB tone and tenderness should trigger a search for other factors capable of increasing tension in these lateral structures Fig. 3.43).

First is contracture of the TFL/ITB complex on the side on which the origin and insertion have been brought closer together (e.g. on the right side during the time an 'alternate' presentation is present). When contracture of the right complex is present, tenderness and outright pain may result with walking on a slope with the right leg on the down side or with any other

activities that further increase tension in this complex (Fig. 3.43A).

Second, one should look for conditions that increase the distance along the lateral aspect of the lower extremity:

- the athlete having a natural tendency towards a neutral to supination pattern of weight-bearing bilaterally, which is evident even when not in alignment (Figs 3.19B, 3.43B)
- genu varum, which also predisposes to supination (Fig. 3.43C)
- genu valgum, in which the acute inward angulation of the femur effectively strings the TFL across the greater trochanter (Fig. 3.43D)
- orthotics with an unnecessary or excessive medial raise on the side that tends to supinate (see Fig. 5.33)
- a supinator wearing shoes intended for a pronator (see Fig. 3.31).

Following realignment, tightness and/or discomfort of the previously 'normal' (usually right) hip abductors and TFL/ITB complex is not unusual and may reflect:

1. this complex having undergone contracture by being put in a relaxed position by the decrease in distance between the origin and insertion while malalignment was present; on realignment, the shortened complex is now being put under increased tension and needs to stretch out to regain its normal length
2. the athlete's true weight-bearing pattern actually being one of supination (see Fig. 3.29).

The athlete should be advised that symptoms related to an increase in tension and tenderness precipitated by realignment are self-limiting, usually lasting no more than 3 or 4 weeks, as the contracted soft tissues gradually adapt to the symmetrical stresses inherent to realignment.

Clinical correlation

Problems in sports related primarily to a limitation of left hip adduction may arise either because of the actual physical limitation to adduction associated with malalignment or because attempted adduction past a certain point provokes pain by further increasing tension in a TFL/ITB complex and hip abductors that are already tight. Particularly affected will be those activities requiring crossing or 'scissoring' of the legs.

Given the uniform limitation of left hip adduction, it will usually be harder to cross the left leg over the right when sitting on a chair (Fig. 3.44B) or sitting cross-legged on the floor.

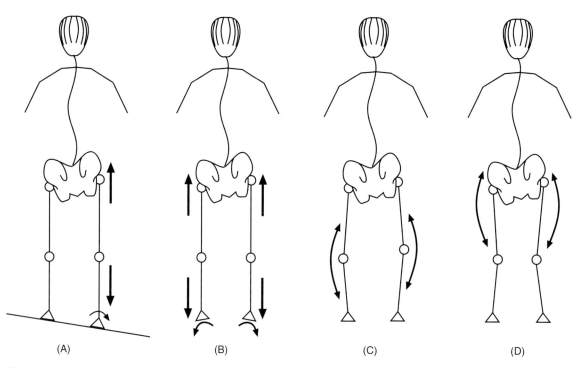

Figure 3.43 Factors that can further aggravate a malalignment-related increase in tension and/or contracture in lateral structures. (A) Right leg 'downhill', contracture of the right tensor fascia lata/iliotibial band (TFL/ITB). (B) Tendency to bilateral supination. (C) Genu varum. (D) Genu valgum.

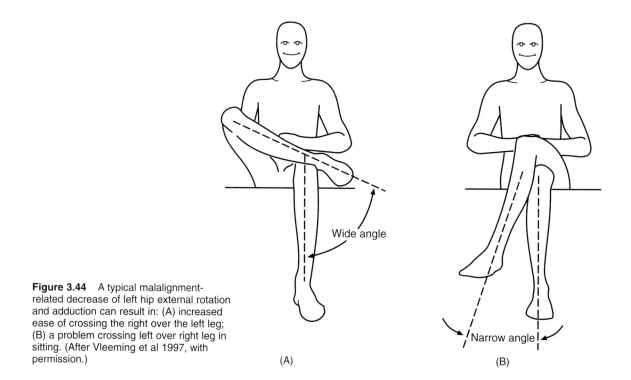

Figure 3.44 A typical malalignment-related decrease of left hip external rotation and adduction can result in: (A) increased ease of crossing the right over the left leg; (B) a problem crossing left over right leg in sitting. (After Vleeming et al 1997, with permission.)

This limitation is in part also caused by the loss of left external rotation noted in those with one of the 'alternate' presentations and upslips (see 'Asymmetry of lower extremity ranges of motion' below, and Fig. 3.72).

Other activities that may be affected by a limitation of adduction include:

- lateral movement of the body, as in running sideways or with cutting movements
- certain steps in ballet and dance, and a number of routines in synchronized swimming, floor exercises and on the balance beam and other pieces of gymnastic apparatus
- figure skating, particularly whenever the trailing left leg has to be brought forward and acutely adducted to become the leading leg, such as when executing a clockwise circle
- horseback riding, in which a limitation of adduction may interfere with the ability to apply pressure against the flank with the inside of the thigh or knee in order to control and guide a horse; inability to symmetrically adduct the thighs to secure one's seating may compromise the ability to maintain stability and form (see Ch. 6).

The thoracic paravertebral muscles

Increased tone and tenderness to palpation most consistently involve the paravertebral muscles on either side of the lower half of the thoracic spine, in particular the erector spinalis and semispinalis thoracis, and less often iliocostalis and longissimus thoracis (see Fig. 2.26). Most often affected is the segment running from around the level of T3, T4 or T5 down to T12 or L1. Less frequently, the involvement is limited to one or both sides of the mid-thoracic (T3–T7) spine or the thoracolumbar junction area, sometimes immediately adjacent to a malrotated vertebra or vertebrae.

The tense muscles are usually palpable like thick ropes under the skin, and there may be obvious crepitus. Tenderness is more likely to be found alongside the thoracolumbar junction but may involve other isolated sections (especially at sites of vertebral malrotation) or the full length of the tense muscle segment.

Clinical correlation

On clinical examination, the athlete may complain of tightness and pain in the affected paravertebral muscles whenever the tension in these muscles is increased further as they are stretched with flexion and/or rotation, or whenever reflex contraction is triggered by these manoeuvres. Symptoms are less frequently precipitated by triggering reactive splinting on extension.

The range of motion examination should be carried out not just in standing, but also in sitting, the latter to stabilize the pelvis and more selectively stress the thoracic and lumbosacral regions (Fig. 3.45). The most common finding, in sitting, is a restriction of trunk rotation by some 5–15 degrees, usually into the direction of the thoracic convexity (Fig. 3.45B).

The restriction may be a reflection of the fact that there is probably already a rotation of the central vertebrae into the convexity (see Fig. 3.5). In the presence of an underlying thoracic convexity to the left, for example, this restriction of left rotation may reflect the fact that the central thoracic vertebrae are already rotated counterclockwise into the convexity, limiting their ability to rotate further in that direction.

Other factors must, however, be involved, given that the limitation to the left may also be seen in association with a thoracic convexity to the right. There is, for example, often an element of a uni- or bilateral increase in tension involving segments of the thoracic paravertebral muscles, for whatever reason (e.g. as a reaction to vertebral malrotation).

Athletes frequently experience discomfort and a sensation of pulling in tense and tender contralateral paravertebrals on side flexion, on trunk rotation while sitting or on first bending forwards and then twisting the trunk to the right or left. This tightness and discomfort is most likely to become a problem with activities requiring repeated trunk flexion and/or rotation (e.g. kayaking, canoeing, gymnastics, martial arts, golfing and throwing sports). Typical of soft tissue, the symptoms will be maximal at the beginning of an activity, particularly after having rested or maintained one position for a longer period of time. The symptoms may gradually subside as the muscles warm up with use and lengthen to accommodate to any stretching, but they may recur again as persistence with the activity precipitates muscle fatigue and a further increase in tension.

Range of motion will be limited in any direction of movement that causes a further increase in tension in these already tense and tender structures. Movement past the anatomical barrier imposed by the increase in tension can result in paravertebral muscle spasm, sprain or strain. This may happen inadvertently in the course of executing a manoeuvre that requires movement into one of the restricted ranges (e.g. a lay-up twist in basketball) or if the trunk is passively forced past the restriction (e.g. as in wrestling; see Fig. 5.29).

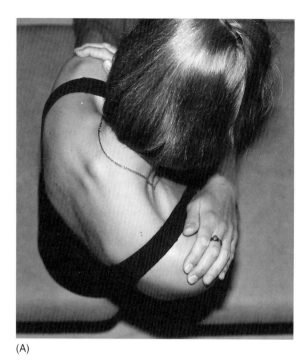

(A)

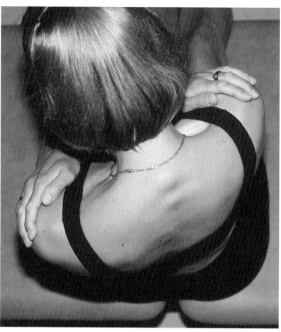

(B)

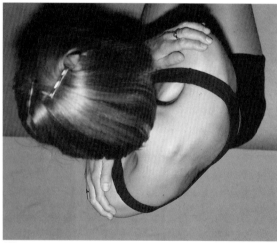

(C)

Figure 3.45 Trunk rotation in sitting to stress the thoracic structures. Restriction to the left may relate to the fact that the athlete has a left thoracic convexity (see Fig. 2.64) with a counterclockwise rotation of the central thoracic vertebrae into the convexity, limiting further rotation into that direction (see also Figs 3.5 and 4.26B). (A) Right rotation to 45 degrees. (B) Left rotation limited to 35 degrees. (C) Left rotation actually increased to 55 degrees with realignment, the left now being equal to the right.

The lumbar and sacral paravertebral muscles

Distal to L1, the paravertebral muscles are more likely to be relaxed and non-tender, even in the presence of malalignment, pelvic obliquity and compensatory scoliosis. Increased tension and/ or tenderness, if present, should raise the suspicion that one might be dealing with splinting in reaction to some underlying pathological condition. The following need to be considered:

- malrotation of any of the lumbar vertebrae
- instability, often involving L4 and/or L5
- pain attributable to facet joint or disc degeneration, spondylolisthesis, partial lumbarization or

sacralization with pseudo-joint formation, disc protrusion or lateral recess stenosis
- irritation of the posterior root fibres, from whatever cause.

Quadratus lumborum

Increased tension in quadratus lumborum has frequently been implicated in the recurrence of an upslip, rotational malalignment, vertebral rotation or combinations of these.

First, attachments to the twelfth rib and the posterior iliac crest allow this muscle to pull the innominate upwards (see Fig. 2.40).

Second, attachments to the posterior iliac crest and the iliolumbar ligament together exert an anterior rotational force on the innominate.

Third, attachments to the tips of the transverse processes of L1 to L4 inclusive exert a lateral and rotational force on these vertebrae and may play a role in determining the direction that a compensatory curve of the lumbar spine will assume. Alternatively, a malrotation of any of these vertebrae may facilitate the muscle on one side and inhibit its partner on the other. The frequently noted left rotation of the L1 vertebral complex (spinous process to the right) facilitates the left quadratus lumborum and inhibits that on the right (Fig. 2.40).

The iliopsoas muscle

The three components that make up this conjoint muscle are all strategically placed (see Fig. 2.40). Psoas minor originates from the sides of the vertebral bodies of T12 to L5 and inserts into the superolateral aspect of the superior pubic ramus. Psoas major originates from the transverse processes of L1 to L5 and inserts into the lesser trochanter. Iliacus comes off the upper iliac fossa, iliac crest, anterior sacroiliac ligament and base of the sacrum; it inserts in part into the tendon of psoas major and in part directly into the lesser trochanter (see Fig. 2.37).

A side-to-side difference in tension in the individual components can result in the effects described in Box 3.6.

Increased tension in iliopsoas is felt to be one of the main reasons for the recurrence of malalignment after correction (Grieve 1983). Traction forces on the innominate could, for example, predispose to:

- anterior rotation (e.g. increased tension in iliacus)
- posterior rotation (e.g. increased tension in psoas minor)
- upslip (e.g. increased tension in psoas minor in particular, but also psoas major and iliacus)
- simultaneous rotational malalignment and upslip.

Box 3.6   Effects of tension in the iliopsoas muscle

1. *Psoas major*: the rotation, forwards flexion and side-bending of one or more vertebrae
2. *Psoas minor*: an upwards shift of the ipsilateral pubic bone with or without posterior rotation of the innominate
3. *Iliacus*: anterior rotation of the innominate in the sagittal plane, and rotation of the sacrum around the contralateral oblique axis
4. *Conjoint iliopsoas*: External rotation, adduction and flexion of the femur, as well as upwards traction force on the ipsilateral innominate
5. *Psoas major and minor*: an increase in the lumbar lordosis

---

Intermittent spasm of the iliopsoas probably accounts for the frequent report of a lancinating pain felt in the groin, often so severe that the athlete stops the activity in which he or she is engaged until the pain subsides (Wells 1986). Frequent findings on clinical examination involving iliopsoas include the following.

First, active or passive adduction of the femur may be limited because it provokes pain by compromising the space available for an already tender iliopsoas.

Second, iliopsoas is more often tender on the left than the right side, or is worse on the left. This finding frequently occurs in the presence of left innominate posterior rotation and left lower extremity internal rotation (noted in 80% and 95% of those with rotational malalignment respectively), both of which can increase tension in the components of iliopsoas by separating their origin and insertion: posterior rotation in iliacus, internal rotation in iliopsoas. The fact that iliacus inserts in part into the tendon of psoas major will increase tension in that muscle as well.

Third, passive left hip abduction is limited in nearly 100% of those with rotational malalignment. An increase in tension in iliopsoas may be one factor contributing to this limitation, but it does not explain why this limitation occurs regardless of the particular presentation of rotational malalignment at hand. Nor does it explain why tenderness is also more common in the left iliopsoas with the left anterior and locked pattern, which would be expected to relax iliopsoas on the basis of bringing its origin and insertion closer together (see Fig. 3.38).

Possible explanations for these findings include the following:

1. Malalignment frequently appears to result in an automatic increase in tension in the left iliopsoas (facilitation). Alternately, the malalignment of the pelvis may itself be the result of a facilitation of the components

of iliopsoas, such as can be triggered by T12, L1 or L2 malrotation (Maffetone 1999; see Fig. 3.2).

2. The increase in left iliopsoas tension may occur in reaction to the increase in stress on the left SI joint caused by coexisting right anterior rotation and locking of the right SI joint, which is by far the most common presentation. The left SI joint may actually become hypermobile as a result of this increased stress, and left iliopsoas is simply contracting in an attempt to stabilize this joint.

3. Reorientation of the acetabula is less likely to play a role, given that the limitation of passive left hip abduction in supine lying occurs with both right and left anterior rotational malalignment. Similarly, a limitation of left hip abduction is also noted with both right and left upslip, even though there is no acetabular reorientation and an increase in tension in any component of iliopsoas is unlikely for biomechanical reasons with either type: with a right upslip the distance between the left origin and insertion does not change, and with a left upslip the insertions of psoas major and minor are actually moved up towards the origins.

Again, the facilitation of iliopsoas on a spinal segmental or cortical basis seems a more probable explanation. With either an upslip or a rotational malalignment, increased tension and tenderness can be found in iliopsoas bilaterally, in which case it is usually significantly worse on the left than the right side. Bilateral involvement may be attributable to attempts to stabilize both SI joints and to cope with the increased workload that results from the change in weight-bearing stresses with pelvic and femoral reorientation.

Clinical correlation

The increased tension in the left iliopsoas noted in conjunction with left posterior innominate rotation increases the chance of sustaining a sprain or strain of this muscle and/or avulsing the lesser trochanter (Fig. 3.46). Injury is more likely with quick abduction manoeuvres, such as occur in ice hockey when the goalie does the 'splits' or hyperabducts the leg on the side of the restriction.

The muscle is also more vulnerable to any increase in tension that results with activities calling for internal rotation of the left lower extremity when the foot is fixed on the ground. This occurs, for example, just as a right-handed pitcher wearing cleats unwinds to release the ball (Fig. 3.47; see Figs 5.24 and 5.25) and when a speed or figure-skater circling counterclockwise starts to adduct the right leg while balanced on the outer edge of the left skate (see Fig. 5.15).

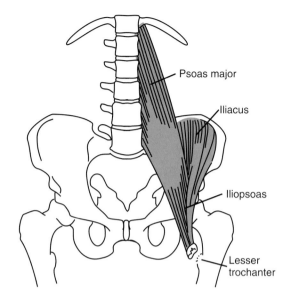

Figure 3.46 Avulsion of the left lesser trochanter.

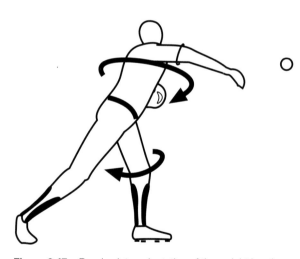

Figure 3.47 Passive internal rotation of the weight-bearing left leg as the right-handed pitcher unwinds counterclockwise to release the ball (see also Figs 5.24 and 5.25).

Anterior innominate rotation depresses the superior pubic ramus, increasing tension in the attaching psoas minor and exerting a traction force on its origins from T12 to L5. The result is a rotational stress on these vertebrae, augmenting the lumbar lordosis and limiting trunk extension.

Rectus femoris

Rectus femoris originates from the anterior inferior iliac spine and the rim of the acetabulum; it inserts into the base of the patella and indirectly into the tibial tubercle by way of the patellar tendon. This muscle therefore can act to flex the hip and/or extend the knee, allowing it to be used for the correction of rotational malalignment by the muscle energy technique (see Ch. 7). Anterior innominate rotation will decrease the tension by bringing its origin closer to its insertion; whereas posterior rotation will increase the tension by separating these sites (see Fig. 3.38).

Clinical correlation

Increased tension in the rectus femoris results in an ipsilateral limitation of hip extension (Wells 1986b). This restriction can be compensated for by:

- decreasing the stride length
- increasing the lumbar lordosis/anterior rotation
- increasing the amount of pelvic rotation in the transverse plane, for example counterclockwise toward the side of a restriction on the left side as

that leg moves into extension during the stance phase of the gait cycle (see Fig. 2.9)
- increasing plantar flexion of the ankle and foot to increase the length of that leg.

Rectus femoris on the side of a posterior innominate rotation is at increased risk of sprain or strain with sudden or excessive hip extension, particularly if there is a simultaneous eccentric or concentric contraction of the quadriceps. This occurs, for example, when coming out of the blocks on a sprint start. Extension of the hip is coupled with an initial eccentric contraction of the quadriceps to help to extend and stabilize the knee of the driving leg (Fig. 3.48A). A concentric contraction is superimposed at a time when the rectus femoris is already under maximal tension at the extreme of hip extension in order to help initiate hip flexion (Fig. 3.48C).

The upper trapezius muscle

As noted above in the discussion on the neck region, there is usually an asymmetrical and apparently automatic increase in tone involving the right upper trapezius alone or the right more than the left. Clinical

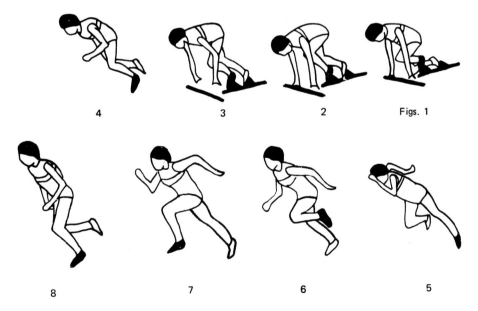

Figure 3.48 Sprint start. The athlete who has increased resting tension in the left rectus femoris because of left posterior innominate rotation (see Fig. 3.38) is at increased risk of injuring this muscle on a sprint start as tension is increased further with: (A) initial eccentric contraction to help to advance the pelvis and simultaneously steady the knee as it extends to provide the force for pushing off from the blocks (1–4); (B) superimposed passive stretching with acceleration as the pelvis (origin) continues to move forwards and the hip extends, further separating origin and insertion (5); then concentric contraction (hip flexion–6) (C) eccentric contraction to help to stabilize the knee as the foot comes to weight-bear again and the hamstrings contract to straighten the knee for the next push-off (8). (From Paish 1976, with permission.)

correlations have been cited above under 'The cervical segment of the spine' above.

ASYMMETRICAL FUNCTIONAL WEAKNESS OF LOWER EXTREMITY MUSCLES

In those presenting with malalignment, manual assessment of muscle strength will usually reveal weakness in some upper and lower extremity muscles, which may be attributable to :

- an asymmetrical 'functional' weakness
- a reorientation of the muscle fibres
- a loss of muscle bulk
- pain (perceived or subconscious).

An example of the latter is a giving-way of rhomboids and infraspinatus, often even wrist flexors/extensors and triceps, usually bilaterally, as a result of subconscious pain relating to T4 or T5 malrotation.

Weakness of the lower extremity muscles noted in association with malalignment presents in a surprisingly consistent, asymmetrical pattern (see Appendix 3). This weakness has been referred to as a 'pseudo-weakness' but is probably more appropriately called a 'functional weakness', one that usually disappears at once on realignment. With few exceptions, a consistent pattern of this functional weakness is seen in association with the SI joint upslips and 'alternate' presentations; a similar pattern of asymmetrical weakness has also been noted with the left anterior and locked presentation. In other words:

1. the presence of the functional weakness appears to correlate with the fact that malalignment of the pelvis is present
2. the pattern of this functional weakness appears to be determined primarily by factors other than the actual presentation of malalignment: spinal segmental and/or cortical inhibition need to be considered.

The athlete should be standing, sitting or lying in the same way in order to test specific muscles. Whenever

In order to establish the presence and the extent of a functional weakness, muscles must be tested in a consistent way to ensure validity of comparison by:
- testing each pair of muscles with the athlete in the same position
- applying resistance
  - to the same location in reference to the bony landmarks
  - with the same hand or number of fingers
  - at the same angle

possible, the examiner should be standing the same way in relation to each one of the pair of muscles being tested and use the same hand or fingers. The ankle evertors (peroneus longus and brevis) are, for example, tested with the athlete supine and ordered to move the foot 'down and out'. The examiner preferably stands opposite the side being tested (Fig. 3.49A, B). Initial resistance is applied with the hand and all the fingers hooked around the lateral border of the foot; if that can overcome the evertors on one or both sides, resistance can then be applied with 4, 3, 2, or sometimes only 1 finger for an accurate side-to-side comparison. For some muscles (e.g. hip abductors and hamstrings), the accuracy of comparison can be increased by applying resistance progressively more proximally or distally to find the breaking point.

The side-to-side difference can sometimes be surprising: 1–1.5 grades on the Oxford scale of 5 is not unusual. Right tibialis posterior (ankle inversion) might, for example, show a weakness graded at 3.5

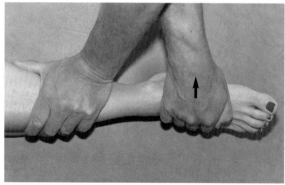

(A)

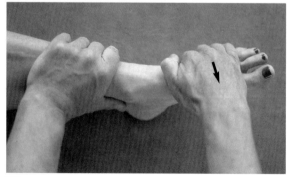

(B)

Figure 3.49 Testing the strength of peroneus longus and brevis (ankle evertors). NB. Whenever possible, the same hand (here the right) is used to test both sides. (A) Right (consistently strong). (B) Left (consistently weak).

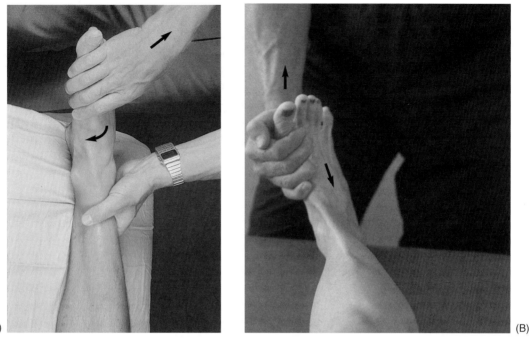

(A)   (B)

Figure 3.50   Testing the strength of the ankle invertors. Both the right tibialis posterior (down and in – being tested in A) and right tibialis anterior (up and in – being tested in B) are consistently weak, whereas their left counterparts are strong.

or 4, whereas its counterpart on the left tests at full strength (Fig. 3.50A). Peroneus longus (ankle eversion) will show a similar weakness but on the left side, whereas its right counterpart is considerably – and consistently – stronger.

Clinical and research findings

The full pattern of this functional weakness seen in association with 'alternate' presentations and upslips is described in Box 3.7.

Box 3.7   Patterns of functional weakness seen with 'alternate' presentations and upslips

- *Left ankle evertors* (peroneus longus and brevis): tested lying supine; foot 'down and out' (see Fig. 3.49A, B)
- *Right ankle invertors* (tibialis posterior and anterior): tested lying supine; foot 'down and in' and 'up and in' respectively (Fig. 3.50A, B)
- *Right extensor hallucis longus*: tested lying supine; 'first toe up'; tested simultaneously on both sides, with the arms crossed and with resistance applied to the first toe, using the left index finger hooked around the left one, and right index finger hooked around the right (Fig. 3.51A)
- *Left hip abductors* (gluteus medius and minimus, and TFL): tested in side-lying, with the hip joint in neutral alignment so that the leg is in line with the body, and the knee straight; resistance applied using a hand placed at, or just above or below, the knee joint (Fig. 3.51B)
- *Left hamstrings*: tested in prone-lying with the knee flexed to 90 degrees, against a resistance applied to the calf muscles or more distally (Fig. 3.51C)

- *Right hip flexors* (iliopsoas, rectus femoris, pectineus (Figs 2.31B & C, 2.40, 3.33, 4.2)): tested in sitting, with legs over the edge of the plinth and the knee flexed 90 degrees, against a resistance applied to the distal thigh (Fig. 3.51D)
- *Right hip extensors* (primarily gluteus maximus): tested in prone-lying, with the knee 90 degrees flexed, against a resistance applied initially to the distal thigh (Fig. 3.51E)
- *Right hip adductors*: tested by resisting adduction in right side-lying, the knee straight and the leg in line with the body, against a resistance applied at or around knee joint level
- *Left hip external rotators*: tested lying supine, the hips and knees both flexed to 90 degrees, against a resistance applied to the leg distally
- *Left hip internal rotators*: the initial position is as that for testing the external rotators (neutral)

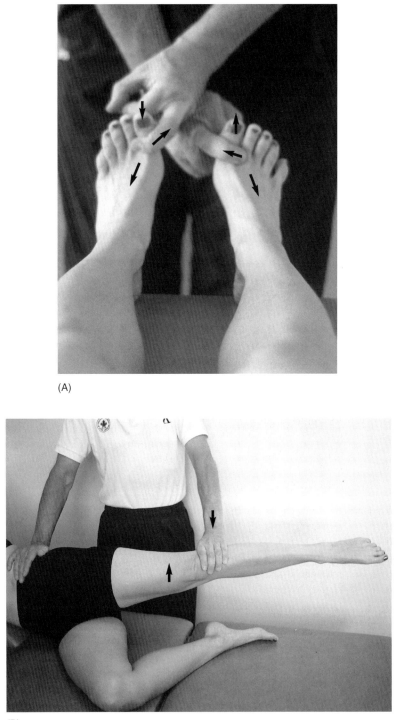

(A)

(B)

Figure 3.51 Other muscles typically weak when rotational malalignment or upslip is present: (A) extensor hallucis longus: note the weakness on the right side; (B) the left hip abductors and tensor fascia lata/iliotibial band complex; (C) the left hamstrings; (D) the right hip flexors; (E) the right hip extensors.

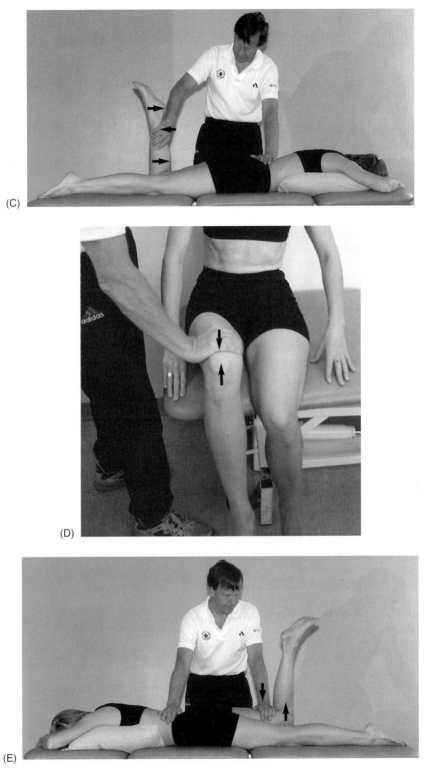

Figure 3.51 *Continued.*

Athletes with malalignment may display a functional weakness in all, some or (rarely) none of the muscles within the pattern outlined above. The muscles that most consistently prove weak are, however:

- on the right side, the hip flexors, ankle invertors and extensor hallucis longus
- on the left side, the hip abductors and ankle evertors.

The weakness is consistently most pronounced in the right ankle invertors, left ankle evertors and right extensor hallucis longus (e.g. 3+ to 4 out of 5). The right hip extensors and left hamstrings are more likely to show full strength, but weakness, when evident, is frequently in this lower range of 3+ to 4.

Some muscles (e.g. quadriceps and triceps surae) are consistently strong on manual testing, but this may be more a reflection of the inherent strength of these muscles, which the examiner just cannot overcome. Clinically unapparent quadriceps weakness, for example, could sometimes be detected only on dynamometry studies (Sweeting et al 1989). These same studies showed that:

- both the endurance and the power of the 'involved' leg muscles can be reduced in the presence of malalignment, and both can increase immediately following realignment
- the increase in strength post-manipulation may be greater for an eccentric than a concentric contraction; the latter will frequently not change at all.

Other dynamometer studies have also shown a significant asymmetry in quadriceps strength on a side-to-side comparison before realignment, the right being weaker than the left (C. Hershler et al, unpublished data, 1989). The same effects noted in the above studies were recorded immediately following correction of the malalignment. Clinically, previously weak muscles will also show an appreciable increase in strength on manual retesting immediately following correction. Any side-to-side difference will either have disappeared completely or have decreased significantly. Ankle invertors and evertors, hamstrings and hip flexors and extensors usually retest at 5 out of 5 bilaterally.

The left hip abductors are more likely to show persistent weakness, sometimes of the same degree as before. Interestingly, they will usually show a gradually increasing strength on repeat examinations until finally testing at 5 out of 5 some weeks or sometimes months after the initial correction, provided that alignment is being maintained.

Improvement has been recorded on dynamometry studies in an athlete who had shown an increase in left hip abductor force and endurance on an isometric fatigue test immediately after correction, a further increase in strength being noted on retesting after having maintained alignment for 4 months; the left hip abductors were, however, still weaker than the right, even after that length of time (C. Hershler et al, unpublished data, 1989). Herzog et al (1988) have reported a significant difference in force results on comparing gait trials conducted early and late in the rehabilitation process aimed at the correction of sacroiliac dysfunction.

> In other words, the changes relating to strength and weight-bearing that are attributable to the correction of malalignment are not all necessarily apparent on initial post-realignment testing.

The time it takes for these changes to materialize may relate to the time it takes:

1. for the body to adapt fully to the realignment, with the elimination of any residual asymmetries in tension, for example the resolution of any contractures
2. to achieve full pelvic and spinal alignment, with the elimination of any change in tension attributable to facilitation and inhibition. Of note in this respect is the fact that the achievement and maintenance of pelvic realignment and stability are, unfortunately, often marked by the onset of recurrent vertebral malrotation at various levels in the thoracic and cervical spine, which may persist and require ongoing treatment for some weeks or even months.

Any residual bilateral ankle weakness will usually occur in keeping with the true weight-bearing pattern that becomes evident on realignment. This will usually respond to selective strengthening. More specifically:

- in those who turn out to be true pronators when aligned, there is weakness of ankle invertors bilaterally (e.g., tibialis posterior)
- in those who turn out to be true supinators when aligned, the weakness of the ankle evertors will be bilateral (e.g., peroneus longus).

Theoretical considerations

The following are some points to consider when trying to explain the pattern of asymmetrical functional weakness seen in association with malalignment.

The pattern cannot be attributed to laterality. With laterality, the increase in right or left upper and lower limb strength, muscle bulk and circumference are fairly consistently noted to be on the dominant side.

The pattern does not correspond to a nerve root or peripheral nerve lesion. There is usually a weakness involving the muscles in both lower extremities, but in an asymmetrical pattern that consistently involves muscles supplied by different nerve roots and/or peripheral nerves. In addition, nerve conduction and electromyographic studies are normal.

The pattern may relate to the relative leg length. Dorman et al (1995) consistently found a weakness in the hip abductors on the side of the long leg, which corresponded to the side of the anterior innominate rotation. The side could be changed simply by using a manual therapy manoeuvre to change the side of the anterior and posterior rotation. The fact that the strong abductors were found on the short leg (i.e. posteriorly rotated) side seemed to correspond to the facilitation of these muscles at the time of initial stance during the gait cycle, thereby enhancing 'force closure' when this was crucial to ensure the stability of the SI joints.

Given the amount of movement possible at the SI joints in various studies, the anterior rotation of one and the posterior rotation of the other innominate were calculated to result in as much as 7.22 mm of difference in leg length. The weakness could be the result of a combination of abductor facilitation and shortening of the lever arm. This author has, however, consistently noticed the weakness in the left hip abductors regardless of whether there is a left anterior or posterior rotation, or a left short or long leg in supine lying. The athlete is admittedly tested only once before and after realignment, and the isometric resistance is applied to the leg at the knee level, so that any difference in length would be less pronounced than if resistance were applied down at the ankles (Fig. 3.51B).

In addition, the inhibitory effect on the muscles on the left side may be more established if the malalignment has been present for some time, whereas facilitation and inhibition may be more easily reversible by repeated manual measures carried out within a short span of time.

The pattern may relate to impaired proprioception or kinaesthetic awareness. The pattern may be, as proposed by Guymer (1986), an expression of a 'proprioceptive adaptation' that has occurred as a result of the asymmetry of the joints. One manifestation of this could be the frequently noted inability of the athlete to contract one of the weak muscles on command. This happens, for example, quite often when requesting an isolated contraction of the left peroneal muscles in order to evert the left ankle. The athlete may eventually muster a fairly good contraction when given some tactile, visual and/or verbal feedback. The term 'functional weakness' has been used because the weakness

is noted to disappear immediately on correction of the malalignment (Janda 1986, Sweeting et al 1989). Janda has suggested some mechanisms to explain what has also been termed a 'pseudoparesis', including:

- the impaired 'facilitation' of a muscle segment
- an impaired sequencing of muscle contraction
- an asynchrony of muscle contraction
- an asymmetrical proprioceptive input from the muscles and joints.

It is this last suggestion that is the most appealing as an explanation of why the strength, and perhaps also the tone, should be affected so readily by simple realignment procedures. The blatant weakness in the right extensor hallucis longus may, for example, be reversed simply by squeezing the right tibia and fibula together at the level of the ankle; the weakness recurs as quickly as the pressure is released (D. Grant, personal communication, 2000).

If, however, an asymmetry of joint proprioceptive signals was the cause, one would expect the pattern of this functional weakness to differ depending on the presentation of malalignment, but this does not appear to be the case. For example, even though the asymmetry of the joints of the pelvis, the lower extremities and the lumbar spine could be the complete opposite for a left anterior and locked than for an 'alternate' presentation, the pattern of asymmetrical weakness was not consistently and completely reversed in one compared with the other. The left hip abductors were the most obvious exception, being weak in 84% of those with left anterior and locked and 82% of those with one of the 'alternate' presentations or upslips (W. Schamberger, unpublished data, 1994).

> Asymmetry of the joints, and hence asymmetry of the proprioceptive signals arising from the joints, does not seem to offer a full explanation for the difference in the pattern of asymmetrical functional weakness seen in association with the most common presentations of malalignment.

The pattern may reflect dysfunction at the level of the spine or cranium. More specifically, the dysfunction may involve a spinal segment and its associated dermatome, myotome and sclerotome, a theory advanced by Korr (1978). Segmental dysfunction could cause muscle weakness by interfering with centrally mediated motor control, which depends on the appropriate inhibition or facilitation of the segment and in turn affects muscle tone. Decreased tension is associated with weakness, increased tension with increased strength.

The pattern may reflect impaired cerebrospinal fluid circulation. The answer may well lie in the hands of those therapists using the craniosacral release method for the treatment of alignment-related disorders (see Chs 7 and 8). It is postulated that the malalignment reflects a disturbance of the normal pulsating flow of cerebrospinal fluid anywhere along its course. The disturbance, it is felt, comes in large part from an imbalance of tension affecting the dural sheath or theca, which surrounds the cord and the individual nerve roots and is in reality an extension of the meninges running from the foramen magnum down to the filum terminale inserting into the coccyx.

The fact that asymmetries of the spine, pelvis and lower extremities can be corrected with therapy restricted to working on the dural attachments at the foramen magnum and/or the insertions into the coccyx, without ever touching these distant structures, certainly lends some strength to the argument that the asymmetries seen are in large part the result of changes in tension involving the dura and meninges and the neural tissues that they enclose. Those skilled in craniosacral release are adept at sensing even minor changes in muscle tension that occur in tandem with the pulsations of the rhythmic flow of cerebrospinal fluid, for example the palpable waxing and waning of tension in the external and internal rotators of the extremities.

Finding a persistent increase or decrease in tension in any of the peripheral muscles is abnormal. An asymmetrical, as opposed to the normal symmetrical, increase in tension could also reflect a disturbance of this rhythmic flow. The malalignment and associated asymmetrical weakness could simply be the end result of a persistent, pathological increase in tension in some muscle groups. If the disturbance of the cranial rhythm can result in asymmetrical tension involving the external and internal rotators, a similar mechanism might perhaps account for the asymmetry of muscle strength from head to foot. Treatment is aimed at re-establishing the cranial rhythm and the normal, symmetrical cycle of tension in the muscles.

The pattern may reflect a lateralization of motor dominance. Approximately 70% of us are left and 15% right motor cortex dominant, the other 15% having about an equal representation bilaterally. Could this asymmetry in motor control at the cortical level result in the asymmetry in muscle strength? If that were so, one might expect a different pattern of weakness in those who are right rather than left motor dominant, but so far only one consistent pattern of weakness has been noted in the positions of testing. The prevalence of the rare exception, found in association with the left anterior and locked malalignment pattern, amounts to nowhere near the figure of 15% given above.

An asymmetry of motor dominance conceivably could, however, explain why one athlete goes out of alignment in consistently the same pattern (e.g. left anterior and locked) and a second consistently in another pattern (e.g. a right or left 'alternate' presentation or upslip), whereas a third appears with a completely different presentation of malalignment at different times. Rather than being the cause of a uniform pattern of weakness, an asymmetry of motor dominance seems, however, more likely to be just another possible cause that can contribute to asymmetry in muscle tension.

The pattern may be a combination of some of the factors postulated above. Segmental or cortical factors may, for example, decrease the strength in left hamstrings by decreasing the spindle setting or inhibiting the firing of the spindle, whereas they have the opposite effect on the right hamstrings, which consistently show increased tension to palpation and prove strong. The actual degree of weakness could be modified by:

- a change in the length-to-tension ratio, which occurs with any change in the distance between the origin and the insertion (see Fig. 3.38)
- subliminal pain that interferes with mustering a full contraction.

Clinical correlation

Athletes sometimes complain of one leg being weaker or feeling unstable on weight-bearing, fatiguing more easily or feeling sore after activity. Cyclists, for example, may note a decreased strength in one leg when pushing down on the pedal. Weightlifters doing a dead lift from a squatting position report a weakness in one leg compared with the other (see Fig. 5.27), whereas runners may be aware of one leg fatiguing more readily and the muscles on that side feeling sore as if from overuse (see the 'Introduction'). Swimmers may feel that one leg is not as effective as the other when kicking. Ice skaters and gymnasts may mistrust one leg because of a recurring sensation of giving way or unsteadiness on single-support activities and when landing on that leg (usually the right).

In the author's experience, these reports have involved primarily the right leg in athletes who on examination presented with one of the 'alternate' patterns or an upslip and had their right leg rotated outward. The author is aware of only two athletes with similar problems affecting the left leg. Both had a left anterior and locked pattern. The preponderance of athletes with complaints relating to the right leg may just be a reflection of the increased prevalence of 'alternate' presentations and upslips, as opposed to the less frequently seen left anterior and locked pattern.

The pattern of functional weakness associated with malalignment is not in keeping with an injury to a specific root or peripheral nerve. Certainly, any weakness out of keeping with this asymmetrical pattern should trigger a closer search for an underlying neurological lesion. Otherwise, if there are no suggestions of such a lesion by history or on clinical examination, and examination findings are limited to the asymmetrical weakness, the approach should be:

- to correct the malalignment first
- then to re-examine the strength to see if the elimination of the malalignment-related functional weakness has unmasked a residual 'true' weakness confined to muscles supplied by a specific root or peripheral nerve
- if so, to initiate appropriate further investigations.

The following case history serves to illustrate this point.

Case history

A 42-year-old recreational runner presented with a history of gradually increasing, non-radiating low back pain aggravated by lifting, bending and running. On examination, malalignment with a right anterior and locked presentation was noted, with outward rotation of the right leg and pronation of the right foot and ankle. Weakness (4 to 4+ or 5) was confined to the right tibialis anterior and posterior, extensor hallucis longus and hip extensors, as well as the left peroneus longus and hip abductors.

Left root stretch tests (Lasegue's, bowstring and Maitland's or slump testing – see Fig. 3.68) were questionably positive; otherwise neurological examination was normal. An examination of the back was unremarkable except for localized soft tissue tenderness and a report of pain with posterior–anterior pressure to the spinous processes in prone-lying, this being confined to the L5 and S1 level. X-rays showed a moderate L5–S1 disc space narrowing.

A correction of the malalignment was easily achieved but failed to decrease the back pain even temporarily and could never be maintained for more than a few days. More importantly when the athlete was re-examined while in alignment, the weakness was limited to the left hip abductors and ankle evertors, the previously weak muscles on the right side now all possessing full strength. Further investigations were prompted by:

- the persistent weakness when in alignment, restricted to the muscles on the left side with both L5 and S1 root innervation

- the questionably positive left root stretch tests
- the failure to respond symptomatically to a correction of the malalignment
- the failure to maintain realignment.

A computed tomography scan showed a large L5–S1 posterolateral disc protrusion impinging on the left S1 root, and electromyography studies were in keeping with a left S1 radiculopathy. Denervation activity, which one can see with ongoing axon degeneration, was restricted to muscles in the left S1 anterior myotome and the left paravertebral muscles at the level of S1 and S2, consistent with anterior and posterior S1 root involvement respectively. Following a resection of the protrusion, the back pain resolved completely, realignment was now maintained, and full strength returned eventually to the left muscle groups as well.

ASYMMETRY OF STRENGTH RELATED TO MUSCLE REORIENTATION AND BULK

In the presence of malalignment, asymmetry of bulk in the lower extremities has been noted most easily in the quadriceps, and specifically in vastus medialis. It is usual for quadriceps bilaterally to test at full strength manually, which is not surprising given that this probably ranks as the strongest muscle in most people (see 'Asymmetrical functional weakness of lower extremity muscles' below).

Obvious wasting of the vastus medialis appears to correlate to the side of anterior innominate rotation. In addition, those with one of the 'alternate' presentations, and hence external rotation of the right lower extremity, are more likely to show relative wasting of the right and hypertrophy of the left vastus medialis (Fig. 3.52), whereas those with the left anterior and locked presentation are more likely to show equal muscle bulk (W. Schamberger, unpublished data, 1994).

A difference in bulk of vastus medialis can be readily documented objectively using techniques such as the laser scanner for mapping the surface topography (Fig. 3.53A). The difference has usually decreased dramatically, or may no longer be apparent, on reassessment after alignment has been maintained for some 4–6 months and with no attempt aimed specifically at strengthening the wasted vastus medialis (Fig. 3.53B).

Differences in the bulk of quadriceps components may reflect the fact that malalignment results in an asymmetry of both the tension and the orientation of the fibres in these muscles. The strength of contraction will conceivably be affected by the following.

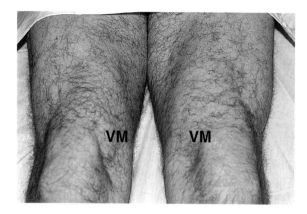

Figure 3.52   Quadriceps asymmetry in an athlete with malalignment (right anterior and left posterior innominate rotation): wasting of the right and hypertrophy of the left vastus medialis (VM).

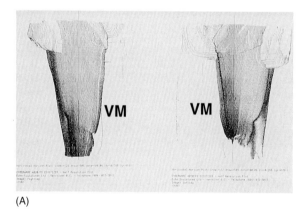

(A)

(B)

Figure 3.53   Quadriceps bulk delineated with a laser scanner. (A) Asymmetry of vastus medialis (VM) with malalignment (right anterior, left posterior rotation): right wasted, left hypertrophied. (B) Almost symmetrical VM bulk within 4 months of maintaining alignment and return to normal activities.

Changes in tension

Anterior rotation of the innominate, for example, approximates the rectus femoris origin and insertion, inhibiting muscle spindle firing and thereby decreasing tension and hence the strength of the contraction that the muscle can muster (see Fig. 3.38). Vastus medialis could be affected secondarily because of its invaginations with rectus femoris. Posterior rotation would have the opposite effect by increasing tension in the rectus femoris. Facilitation and inhibition would also affect tension.

Orientation of muscle fibres

The fibres in the various components of the quadriceps muscle are oriented at different angles to the midline (Fig. 3.54). Changing the angulation of these fibres by externally or internally rotating the lower extremity will in turn affect the ability of each component to contribute to the strength of a contraction aimed at extending the knee and advancing the leg in the sagittal plane.

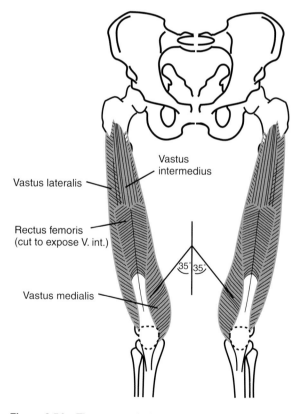

Vastus intermedius

Vastus lateralis

Rectus femoris (cut to expose V. int.)

Vastus medialis

35 | 35

Figure 3.54   The symmetrical angulation of vastus medialis fibres relative to the sagittal plane when the athlete is in alignment.

External rotation (Fig. 3.55, right leg). The quadriceps muscle as a whole is oriented away from midline, decreasing its ability to contribute to forward progression.

The fibres of some of the quadriceps components are oriented at an increasing angle to the line of progression, which further impairs their ability to contribute during the gait cycle. This effect will be maximal for muscles whose fibres are already running outwards at a more oblique angle to the sagittal plane (e.g. vastus medialis), as opposed to those more in line with this plane of progression (e.g. rectus femoris and vastus intermedialis). Increasing external rotation, for example, causes the bulk of vastus medialis to face more and more forwards. The fibres of the muscle then come to pull at an increasing angle to the sagittal plane, decreasing their ability to contribute to this movement.

There also results an increased tendency to pronation at the foot and hence to inwards (valgus) collapse at the knee. Vastus medialis is placed at a further biomechanical disadvantage as the stability of the knee is impaired now that it no longer sits directly over the foot (see Ch. 5). Increased valgus angulation also puts the muscle under increased tension.

Internal rotation (Fig. 3.55, left leg). The quadriceps complex, specifically the fibres of vastus medialis, are oriented more favourably relative to the line of progression by bringing the foot and leg more in line with the sagittal plane.

The foot and knee are stabilized somewhat during the weight-bearing phase, the knee sitting more directly over the foot (see Figs. 5.8 and 5.11D).

When wasting of vastus medialis is present, one must always be sure to rule out other pathology, given that this muscle is notorious for being the most likely, and usually the first, to show wasting with painful afflictions of the knee in particular and of the lower extremity in general.

Clinical correlation

The reorientation of the components of the quadriceps muscle away from the sagittal plane on the side on which the lower extremity rotates externally with malalignment may:

- decrease their ability to contribute to advancing the leg in the sagittal plane
- result in a more rapid fatiguing of these muscles, which in turn would contribute to:
  - the muscles becoming sore as with overuse, even on running shorter distances than would normally cause them to feel this way (e.g. feeling it on the side of the external rotation after running only 20 km, whereas it might take a marathon to provoke the same feeling on the side of internal rotation; see the 'Introduction').
  - that leg feeling weak and/or unstable
  - an increasing tendency to valgus angulation at the knee, attributable in part to vastus medialis being weaker and fatiguing more rapidly
  - these changes, in combination with other factors cited, such as the tendency to pronation on that side and an increased tendency to lateral tracking of the patella, predisposing to the development of patellofemoral compartment syndrome and patellar tendonitis, which are typically much more common, or more severe, on the right side, given the preponderance of right lower extremity external rotation (see Fig. 3.33).

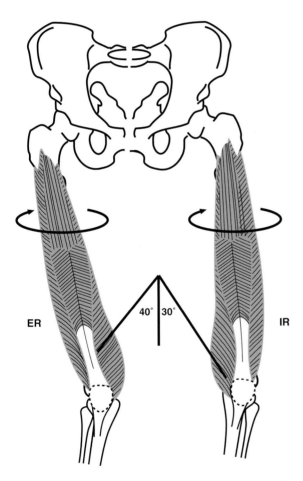

Figure 3.55 The asymmetrical angulation of vastus medialis fibres with 'alternate' presentations and upslips: the right increased with external rotation and valgus angulation, the left decreased with internal rotation and varus angulation.

Unilateral quadriceps wasting will cause or worsen an imbalance of strength involving the right versus the left quadriceps, and of the quadriceps versus the hamstrings on the same side. Imbalances involving these strong muscles are probably best detected using dynamometric studies (Sweeting et al 1989). If such imbalances are present, they put the athlete at increased risk of sustaining a muscle sprain or strain.

The question is whether malalignment affects the other muscles of the extremities, pelvis and trunk in a similar way, changing their orientation and therefore their ability to muster an optimal contraction and maintain their bulk. Are there, for example, differences in bulk involving the muscles around the buttock and hip girdle regions that may be hard to appreciate on examination but which are nevertheless present and could be contributing to the feeling that one hip girdle or leg is just not as strong as, feels more unstable than or fatigues more easily than the other?

A difference in the bulk and strength of piriformis, iliopsoas or any of the gluteal components could certainly have these effects. Anterior innominate rotation, for example, changes the orientation of iliacus and decreases the tension in it, which could in turn result in a decreased ability of that muscle to contribute to hip flexion, possibly wasting and fatiguing more readily as a result (see Fig. 3.38).

The wasted muscle(s) may or may not respond normally to efforts at selective strengthening as long as they are placed at a disadvantage by the malalignment. Following correction, muscle bulk increases with just normal use of the lower extremities during daily activities and may come to equal that on the opposite side without selective strengthening exercises (see Fig. 3.53B). The addition of symmetrical strengthening may help to maintain bulk on the hypertrophied side and speed up its return on the wasted side (where this may not have been possible with selective exercise prior to realignment).

ASYMMETRY OF LIGAMENT TENSION

Ligaments should feel neither lax nor excessively taut, and they should not be tender. A side-to-side comparison is invaluable for determining any differences. Malalignment can increase tension by:

1. increasing the distance between the origin and insertion (see Fig. 3.38)
2. increasing tension in a muscle that attaches to, or is in continuity with, the ligament.

As an example of the latter, Pansky & House (1975) note the sacrotuberous ligament to be one of the origins of the long head of biceps femoris. Previous reference has been made to Vleeming et al (1989C), who reported attachments running to the sacrotuberous ligament:

- from the dorsal fascia
- in the form of muscle fibres from piriformis and gluteus maximus
- as partial or complete continuity with the lateral head of biceps femoris in 50% of cases (see Figs 2.4, 2.17 and 2.26).

Traction applied to the gluteus maximus and biceps femoris thus increased tension in the sacrotuberous ligament (see Figs 2.26 and 2.37).

A persistent increase in tension in a ligament has four undesirable consequences. First, the ligament eventually *lengthens* and fails to provide adequate support (see Fig. 3.60B).

Second, the ligament ultimately *becomes painful*. Pain most consistently localizes to the ligament origin and insertion, which probably relates to the fact that histological studies show the highest concentration of neurological structures (e. g. pressure-sensitive corpuscles, proprioceptive sensors and pain fibres) to lie in the region of the fibro-osseous junctions (Hackett & Henderson 1955). Chronic tension results in elongation, irritation and inflammation, particularly of the nerve structures within the ligament. The nerve fibres cannot elongate as much as the elastic components of the ligament and are therefore put under excessive stretch long before elongation of the elastic elements has reached its limit (Hackett 1958).

Prechtl & Powley (1990) have shown how lumbosacral ligaments and other connective tissues are innervated by small-calibre, primary afferent fibres that can send nociceptive stimuli to the spinal cord. When irritated, these same fibres can also secrete proinflammatory neuropeptides capable of initiating peptide release and a chain of events leading to eventual tissue inflammation and oedema. Connective tissue structures in this region are also supplied by sympathetic efferent axons capable of releasing catecholamines.

A balance between these two neutral systems is thought to be important to the 'maintenance of the integrity of the lumbosacral ligamentous structures' (Willard 1995, p. 53). The balance can presumably be upset with chronic excessive tension in the ligaments, which may help to explain why ligament inflammation and pain often fail to settle down until normal tension has been re-established by correction of the malalignment; the posterior pelvic ligaments are a prime example of this phenomenon (see Fig. 2.3).

In addition, the blood supply to the ligaments is already poor in comparison to that of other tissues and would be further compromised by any increase in tension and the associated catecholamine release with irritation of the sympathetic system.

Third, an elongated, irritated and inflamed ligament can become a source of aberrant proprioceptive signals and *referred pain* symptoms (Hackett 1958). Trigger points can also develop in ligaments (Travell & Simons 1983, 1992).

Finally, pain from the ligaments results in a *reflex splinting* of muscles in the vicinity in an attempt to prevent further irritation of the ligaments. If the splinting is asymmetrical, it will predispose to the recurrence of malalignment. Chronic splinting eventually results in chronic tension myalgia and myofascial pain.

Ligaments typically affected by malalignment

Rotational malalignment (and upslip) most consistently affects the sacrospinous and the four major posterior pelvic ligaments on each side: the sacrotuberous, the iliolumbar, the posterior SI joint ligaments and the long posterior (dorsal) sacroiliac ligament (Table 3.3; see Figs 2.3 and 2.16). Also involved are the interosseous ligaments (see Figs 2.2B and 2.10Aiii) and those surrounding the symphysis pubis (see Fig. 3.61). The altered biomechanics can increase tension in specific lower extremity ligaments as well, sometimes to the point that they too become tender and even symptomatic. Typical of these are the lateral ligaments of the knee and ankle on the supinating side, and the medial ligaments on the pronating side (see Fig. 3.33). What follows is a discussion relating to specific pelvic ligaments as they are affected by rotational malalignment and/or upslip.

The iliolumbar ligaments

The iliolumbar ligaments originate from the transverse processes of L4 and L5 (see Fig. 2.2). They insert by way of:

- a superficial portion on the medial aspect of the posterior iliac crest at the level of L5 and S1

- a deep portion with a fairly broad attachment along the anterior part of the ilium.

Overlying muscle and fat preclude any palpation of the origin and midpart in most, but the superficial insertion is usually directly palpable. The ligaments can be put under increased tension by separating origin and insertion through:

- a rotation of either L4 or L5 or both (see Figs 2.2 and 2.35A)
- anterior rotation of the innominate
- sacral counternutation.

Involvement of the iliolumbar ligaments is suggested by:

1. tenderness to direct palpation of the tips of the L4 and L5 transverse processes, the ligaments themselves and the superficial insertions
2. pain on selective stress tests:
   - contralateral side flexion of the trunk alone, or in combination with simultaneous trunk extension and rotation, into the side of the ligament
   - passive anterior innominate rotation or sacral counternutation (see Fig. 2.71B).

A referral of pain from the iliolumbar ligaments to the greater trochanter and lateral thigh can easily lead to a misdiagnosis of trochanteric bursitis (see Fig. 3.42). The following may be of help when contemplating this differential diagnosis.

A normal bone scan, and a failure of an injection of local anaesthetic around the trochanter to bring even temporary relief, should suggest the possibility that one is dealing with pain on a referred basis. The iliolumbar ligaments refer to the sclerotome around the greater trochanter; if this is the case, the injection of local anaesthetic into the ligament itself should resolve the pain completely. The 'thoracolumbar syndrome' (see Ch. 4) can result in hypersensitivity of the skin overlying the trochanter, which may be decreased with an injection of local anaesthetic into the skin itself but is completely abolished by blocking the posterior cutaneous fibres

Table 3.3 1992, 1993 Studies: sites of ligament tenderness

Ligament	1992 study (%)	1993 study (n = 92) Rotation (n = 80) (%)	Upslip (n = 12) (%)	All (n = 92) (%)	Right side (%)	Left side (%)	Bilateral (%)
Sacrotuberous ligament	83	61	66	63	10	13	37
Posterior SI joint ligaments	82	50	25	46	19	8	24
Iliolumbar ligament	41	14	None	12	5	4	5

originating primarily at the T11, T12 and L1 level (see Fig. 4.21).

If there is an actual component of trochanteric bursitis, injection around the area of the trochanter will probably bring only partial relief limited to the duration of the anaesthetic. In that case, cortisone injection around the bursa needs to be coordinated with realignment, and possibly also injection into the ligament itself, in order to achieve complete relief.

If realignment alone fails to bring relief, cortisone injection into the tender ligament origins and insertions is advisable. The deep insertions may be difficult to reach other than with a 75–90 mm needle under fluoroscopic control. Surgery around the greater trochanter plays absolutely no role if the problem is one of pain referred to this region (see Ch. 7).

The sacrotuberous ligament

The sacrotuberous ligament has an extensive origin from the PSIS of the ilium, the 4th and 5th transverse tubercles of the sacrum, and the lateral border of the sacrum and coccyx (see Figs 2.3, 3.57 and 3.59). It inserts into the superior rim of the inner ischial tuberosity but may be in direct continuity with biceps femoris or, indirectly, by way of fascial connections with the hamstring origin (Pansky & House 1975, Vleeming et al 1989b, 1989c; see Fig. 2.4). The sacrotuberous origin is particularly vulnerable in that:

1. anterior rotation of the innominate, sacral torsion and nutation, and coccygeal rotation not only increase the distance between its origin and insertion, but can also separate its points of origin on the sacrum and innominate from each other (see Figs 2.16 and 2.17)

2. an upslip can similarly increase tension in the long dorsal sacrotuberous ligament, the part of the ligament that originates from the PSIS and interdigitates with that originating from the sacrum, by moving the PSIS upwards and away from the sacrum (see Figs 2.4 and 2.16B)

3. tension in the ligament will be increased by active contraction of the hamstrings, gluteus maximus and/or piriformis, depending on the amount of continuity or fascial interconnection present between the ligament and these muscles. The ligament is also put at increased risk of injury by any passive increase in tension in these muscles, such as can occur with straight leg raising, stretching, squatting and jumping.

It is therefore not surprising that the sacrotuberous ligament is tender to palpation in 70–80% of those presenting with malalignment. In some 90% of these, the tenderness localizes to the origin alone; a small number

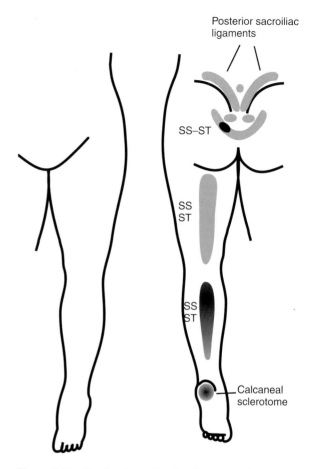

Figure 3.56   Overlapping pain referral patterns of the sacrotuberous (ST) and sacrospinous (SS) ligaments. (After Hackett 1958, with permission.)

(5–10%) have tenderness localizing along the length of the ligament and/or to its insertion or to all three sites, but rarely just to the insertion (W. Schamberger, unpublished work, 1994). The referred pain pattern overlies primarily the posterior thigh and calf and the area around the heel – the calcaneal sclerotome – and overlaps to large extent that of the sacrospinous ligament (Fig. 3.56; see Fig. I.2). A side-to-side difference in tension is usually readily apparent on palpating the ligament with the athlete lying prone (Fig. 3.57A).

The sacroiliac ligaments

The downwards and medial slant of a large part of the sacroiliac ligaments makes them particularly well suited for:

- helping to transfer weight between the sacrum and the innominates

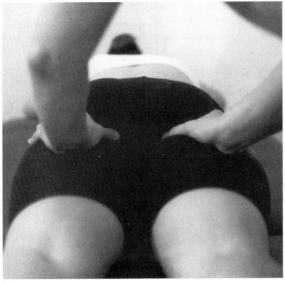

(A)

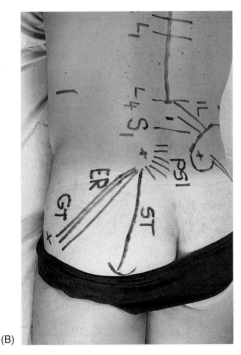

(B)

Figure 3.57 Sacrotuberous ligament tension (see also Figs 2.3, 2.4, 2.16 and 2.17). (A) Comparative assessment of tension and tenderness in the right and left sacrotuberous ligaments. (From Lee & Walsh 1996, with permission.) (B) Surface outlines showing the position of the left sacrotuberous (ST) ligament and other structures (L4–Sl, vertebrae; IL, iliolumbar ligaments; PSI, posterior sacroiliac joint ligaments; ER, external rotator (pirifomis); GT (x), greater trochanter).

- absorbing the shock associated with any downwards movement of the sacrum relative to the innominates, such as occurs with landing on one or both feet.

Specific ligaments in this complex include the following.

The posterior sacroiliac joint ligaments. These ligaments span the upper, middle and lower parts of the SI joint. Their origin from the ilium sweeps from the PSIS to the posterior inferior iliac spine (PIIS), the insertion being onto the first three transverse tubercles of the sacrum (see Figs. 2.3 and 2.16A). They are most easily palpated deep to the contours of the posterior pelvic rim (Fig. 3.57B). Tension in these ligaments is increased with any displacement of the ilium relative to the sacrum. Referred pain patterns from the superior and inferior segments are shown in Fig. 3.58.

The long posterior or 'dorsal' sacroiliac ligament. This distinct ligament has its origin primarily on the PSIS, running caudally to insert onto the posterolateral aspect of the sacrum at about the S3 level (see Figs 2.3 and 2.16B). The S1, S2, and S3 posterior root fibres, which help to innervate the posterior SI joint ligaments, are at risk of irritation or even compression with any increase in tension in the medial and lateral components of the ligament as these fibres run laterally, traversing between the two components. This ligament may play a particular role in helping to limit:

- counternutation of the sacrum (see Figs 2.8 and 2.16B)
- torsion of the sacrum around the oblique axes: torsion around the right oblique axis, for example, results in nutation of the left side with relaxation, and counternutation of the right side with tightening, of the long dorsal ligament (see Fig. 2.11)
- anterior rotation and upslip of the innominate (see Fig. 2.16B).

Excessive movement in these directions probably accounts for the fact that the origin of this ligament is typically one of the most tender sites when malalignment is present. Pain attributable to excessive counternutation can sometimes be temporarily relieved by applying pressure to the base of the sacrum with the heel of the hand, forcing the sacrum into nutation and decreasing the tension in this ligament; pressure on the sacral apex to effect sacral counternutation typically aggravates the pain (see Fig. 2.71).

The interosseous sacroiliac joint ligaments. These are short fibres running between the tuberosities of the sacrum and the ilium. They lie deep to the posterior SI joint ligaments and cannot be directly palpated (see Figs 2.2B and 2.10Aiii). They will, however, be put

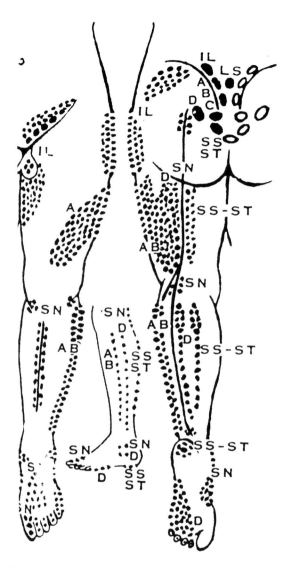

Figure 3.58 Referral patterns from the posterior sacroiliac ligaments. From the superior segments: 'Relaxation of the ligaments of the lumbosacral (LS) and upper portion of the sacroiliac articulations (A and B) occur together so frequently that their referred pain area from the iliolumbar ligament and AB are combined in one dermatome.' From the inferior segments (C and D): 'Relaxation occurs together so frequently that their referred pain areas from ...D and ...SS–ST [sacrospinous–sacrotuberous] are combined in one dermatome.' SN, sciatic nerve. (From Hackett 1958, with permission.)

under increased tension, and may become a source of pain, with any displacement of the sacral and iliac joint surfaces relative to each other, as in rotation, upslip or downslip, shear injury or excessive nutation or counternutation.

The anterior sacroiliac joint ligaments. These cross the anterior part of the joint, running from the antero-lateral sacrum to the ilium (see Figs. 2.2B and 2.10Aiii).

The sacrospinous ligament

The sacrospinous ligament originates from the pos-terolateral aspect of the sacrum and coccyx, and inserts into the ischial spine so that the greater sciatic foramen lies superiorly and the lesser one inferiorly (Fig. 3.59; see Figs 2.2, 2.3 and 2.16A). It is covered in large part by the sacrotuberous ligament and the buttock muscles and is therefore most easily palpated in its entirety by way of the rectum or vagina. Its origin and insertion are approximately equidistant bilaterally in someone who is in alignment (Fig. 3.60A).

Posterior rotation of the innominate separates the origin and the insertion, increasing tension and often resulting in marked tenderness; anterior rotation brings the origin and insertion closer together, relaxing the ligament on this side by putting it into a shortened position (Fig. 3.60B). Hesch et al (1992) note that sacrospinous tenderness and hypotonus are often seen in association with ipsilateral symphysis pubis dys-function. The involvement of these ligaments con-tributes to the 'deep' pain associated with pelvic floor dysfunction (see Ch. 4).

Ligaments spanning the pubic symphysis

The superior pubic ligaments connect the upper aspect of the pubic rami, the arcuate ligaments connect the rami inferiorly, and the interpubic ligaments run trans-versely across the fibrocartilaginous disc that is part of this amphiarthrodial joint (Fig. 3.61; see Fig. 2.2). A dis-placement and/or torsion of one pubic bone relative to the other creates stress on the ligaments and the disc (see Figs. 2.29, 2.45 and 2.46C).

In summary, because of their attachment to the sacrum on one side and the ilium on the other, tension is increased in some or all of these sacroiliac ligaments by:

● upwards or downwards translation
● anterior or posterior rotation of one bone relative to the other
● outflare and inflare (discussed below)
● trunk rotation and simultaneous flexion or extension
● sacroiliac joint gapping and other selective stress tests (see Ch. 2)

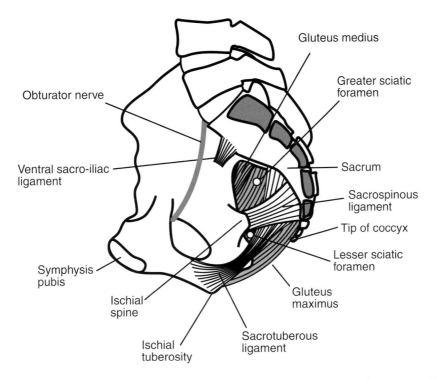

Gluteus medius

Greater sciatic
foramen

Obturator nerve

Ventral sacro-iliac
ligament

Sacrum

Sacrospinous
ligament

Tip of coccyx

Lesser sciatic
foramen

Symphysis
pubis

Gluteus
maximus

Ischial
spine

Sacrotuberous
ligament

Ischial
tuberosity

Figure 3.59   Sacrospinous ligament on a lateral view from the inside of the pelvis. (After Grant 1980, with permission.)

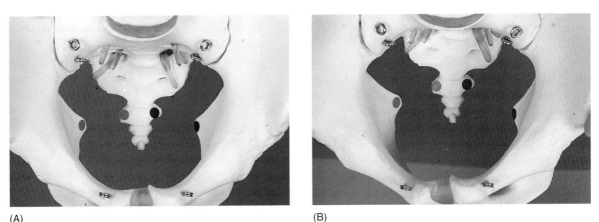

(A)   (B)

Figure 3.60   Sacrospinous ligament origins and insertions on an anterior–posterior view of pelvis. (A) Pelvis aligned: the distance between the right origin and insertion (light dots) is equal to that on the left (black dots). (B) Rotational malalignment with right innominate anterior, left posterior rotation: the origin and insertion are brought closer together on the right (light dots) and separated on the left (black dots).

The inguinal ligaments

One or both inguinal ligaments may be tense and tender in the presence of pelvic malalignment. Pain is usually felt in the groin region, tenderness being most acute at the insertion into the pubic tubercle (see Fig. 2.2).

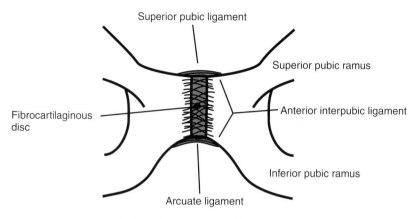

Figure 3.61 Ligaments around the symphysis pubis.

The hip joint ligaments

The iliofemoral and pubofemoral ligaments (see Figs 2.2A and 4.3) and the capsule are particularly stressed by internal and external rotation of the lower extremities. Excessive tension can result in a 'deep' pain in the hip joint region. Pain is referred primarily to the medial and posterior thigh, the lateral knee, the anterior shin and ankle, and the first toe (Fig. 3.62).

The intervertebral ligaments

The vertebral rotation that occurs with the formation of the compensatory curves of the spine, in particular with vertebral malrotation, predictably increases tension in specific ligaments and their nerve supply while relaxing others. The ligaments that connect one vertebra to another include those running:

- from one body to another
- between the posterior elements: the lamina and the transverse and spinous processes
- across the facet joints (Fig. 3.63).

Ligaments of the knee

The medial plica and medial collateral ligament. These are likely to be under stress on the side of medial

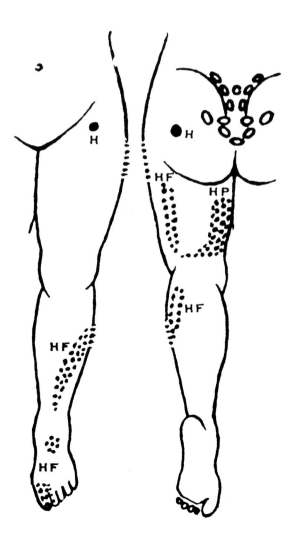

Figure 3.62 Referred pain patterns from the iliofemoral and pubofemoral ligaments of the hip joint noted with hip joint instability (see also Fig. 2.2A). H, location of the hip joint; HP, referral from the pelvic attachments; HF, referral from the femoral attachments. (From Hackett 1958, with permission.)

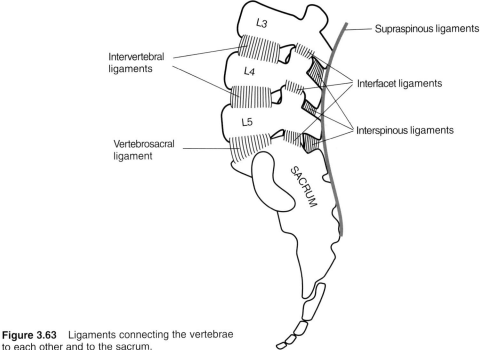

Intervertebral ligaments

L3

L4

L5

SACRUM

Vertebrosacral ligament

Supraspinous ligaments

Interfacet ligaments

Interspinous ligaments

Figure 3.63   Ligaments connecting the vertebrae to each other and to the sacrum.

weight-bearing and pronation, and with any tendency to genu valgum as a result of these or any other causes (see Figs 3.27 and 3.33). The problem will be on the right side in those with 'alternate' presentations and upslips.

The lateral collateral ligament. The lateral collateral ligament is likely to be involved on the side of lateral weight-bearing or supination, the tendency to genu varum more likely to be a problem on the left side.

TFL/ITB complex. Tightness of this complex, typically seen on the left side, may restrict knee flexion because of connections between the ITB insertion and the anterior capsule (see Figs 3.33, 3.37 and 3.40).

Ankle ligaments

Tenderness of these ligaments in the absence of injury may relate to a chronic or repetitive increase in tension. This is more likely to involve the lateral ligaments on the left side, in keeping with the increased prevalence of 'alternate' presentations and the associated tendency to left lateral weight-bearing and supination (see Figs 3.3B, 3.18A and 3.33). There may be simultaneous peroneus longus and brevis tendonitis, and rarely sural nerve involvement (see Fig. 3.34B).

The medial ankle ligaments are more likely to be involved on the pronating side, where there may also

be associated tibialis posterior tendonitis with irritation of the posterior tibial nerve or even a frank posterior tarsal tunnel syndrome (see Fig. 3.34A).

Clinical correlation

Rotational malalignment results in a predictable increase in tension in a number of ligaments, which, with time, makes these ligaments more likely to become tender to palpation, to elongate and eventually to compromise joint stability and/or become a source of local as well as referred pain.

Ligaments that have undergone contracture because of having been temporarily placed in a shortened position by malalignment are now at increased risk of suffering a sprain or strain in the event of any sudden or unexpected superimposed stress.

Reflex muscles splinting, intended to minimize the pain and to protect the ligament against further abuse or injury, can unfortunately impair athletic style by limiting freedom of movement, can result in complicating myofascial pain and puts the muscles at increased risk of injury.

In addition, a ligament may fail in its role as an appropriate source of proprioceptive signals. The concept of ligament malfunction and recurrent injury is explored further under 'A problem with balance and recovery' below and in Ch. 5.

A common problem associated with malalignment is the limitation of standing and sitting tolerance – also described as the 'cocktail party syndrome' – which is often attributable, in large part, to the painful posterior pelvic ligaments, in addition to the related biomechanical problems previously discussed (see 'Asymmetry of pelvic orientation in the frontal plane').

Sitting in a slouched position tends to make matters worse by further increasing the tension in some of these ligaments or by exerting direct pressure on a painful ligament (e.g. the sacrotuberous origin and insertion and/or the sacrococcygeal ligaments). Side-lying with the upper leg adducted and flexed at the hip puts the uppermost iliolumbar and posterior sacroiliac ligaments under increased tension; limiting adduction with a pillow between the knees helps to counter these stresses.

In some, the ligament pain resolves with time as alignment is maintained. In others, realignment alone fails to bring relief. This failure is probably a reflection of the length of time required for these tissues to heal after what often amounts to months or even years of insult. While the pain persists, it can severely limit the athlete's ability to participate in sports that:

- require prolonged standing (e.g. archery or court sports) or sitting (e.g. cycling and rowing)
- repeatedly put the ligaments under increased stretch by squatting (e.g. weight-lifting), bending forward (e.g. cycling), twisting (e.g. kayaking) or a combination of these (e.g. rowing and canoeing).

ASYMMETRY OF LOWER EXTREMITY RANGES OF MOTION

One of the findings associated with rotational malalignment is a consistent pattern of asymmetry of the lower extremity joint ranges of motion (Box 3.8; see Appendix 3).

Some of these asymmetries can be explained on a purely mechanical basis. The example of hip extension and flexion (with the knee bent) in Box 3.8 will help to illustrate this point.

Reorientation of the joint. Anterior rotation of the right innominate brings the anterior acetabular rim forwards and down so that the mechanical blocking of hip joint flexion that occurs when the femur contacts this rim now occurs earlier (Fig. 3.65B). The posterior acetabular rim on this side will have moved backwards and up, allowing increased extension before the mechanical blocking occurs. If there has been com-

---

Box 3.8 Lower extremity ranges of motion in rotational malalignment

- Movement in any one plane of motion is restricted in one and increased in the opposite direction. A typical finding with right anterior and left posterior innominate rotation, for example, would be:

	Right	Left
passive hip flexion (supine)	110 degrees	120 degrees
passive hip extension (prone)	30 degrees	20 degrees

The findings would be reversed with left posterior, right anterior rotation (Figs 3.64 and 3.65).

- The total range of motion possible in a particular plane is, however, the same on both sides, that is, provided there is no underlying pathology that could affect movement in that plane, such as ligament or joint deterioration, soft tissue contracture or impairment of neural control (see Figs 2.18 and 2.19). In the example above, the total range possible in the sagittal plane with either presentation would be the same:

	Right	Left
total hip flexion and extension	140	140

---

pensatory posterior rotation of the left innominate bone, repositioning of the left anterior and posterior rim allows for increased flexion but decreases extension by an equivalent amount (Fig. 3.65C). The findings will be reversed with left anterior, right posterior rotation. In both cases, the total of flexion/extension range of motion remains the same (90 degrees) on the right and left sides.

Displacement of origins and insertions. Right hip flexion, for example, is decreased by the increase in tension in the right gluteus maximus and hamstrings that results when right anterior innominate rotation increases the distance between their origin and insertion. Simultaneous posterior rotation of the left innominate will limit left hip extension by increasing tension in iliacus and rectus femoris via the same mechanism (see Figs 2.37 and 3.38).

Interaction between muscles, tendons and myofascial tissue. Right hip flexion can, for example, be decreased by any increase in tension in the sacrotuberous ligament, which can in turn result in an increase in tension in:

- the hamstrings, when these are in continuity with the ligament
- a muscle such as piriformis or gluteus maximus that is attached to the ligament directly or by way of fascial tissue (see Figs 2.4 and 2.16).

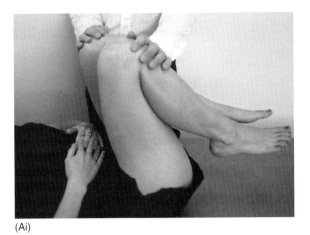

(Ai)

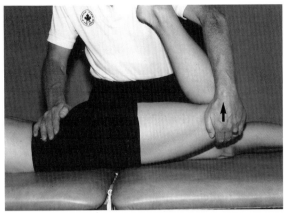

(Aii)

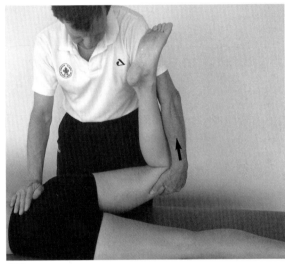

(Aiii)

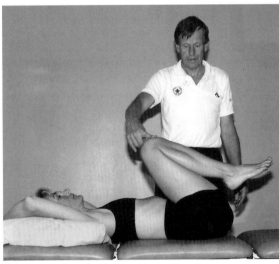

(B)

Figure 3.64   Effect of alignment on passive hip flexion and extension. Note that there may be an overall increase in flexion/ extension range with realignment that cannot be explained just by realignment of the acetabula but probably relates in part to the re-establishment of normal muscle tension. (A) With rotational malalignment (right innominate anterior, left posterior): (i) limitation of right flexion (105 degrees) compared with left (115 degrees); (ii) limitation of left extension (10 degrees), compared with right (iii); (iii) right hip extension full (25 degrees). (B) In alignment: hip flexion is now equal, increased to 130 degrees (and extension is equal at 25 degrees).

The asymmetry of some ranges of motion cannot be explained on a purely mechanical basis. Other factors, such as the automatic increase in tension or facilitation that occurs in certain muscles, help to determine the differences noted (see 'Asymmetry of muscle tension' above and Fig. 3.39). There is, for example, the typical malalignment-related increase in tension in:

- *the left TFL, gluteus medius and minimus*, which would account for the almost universal restriction of passive left hip adduction (see Figs. 3.40 and 3.70B)

- *the right hamstrings and piriformis*, which would contribute to the limitation of right hip flexion (see Fig. 3.64Ai)

- *left gastrocnemius*, which is one factor that limits dorsiflexion of the left foot and ankle and probably helps to limit passive left straight leg raising (Fig. 3.66A), although rotation of the femur may also play a part (E.H. Larsen, personal communication, 1999).

A distinctly different pattern of asymmetrical passive lower extremity joint ranges of motion can be

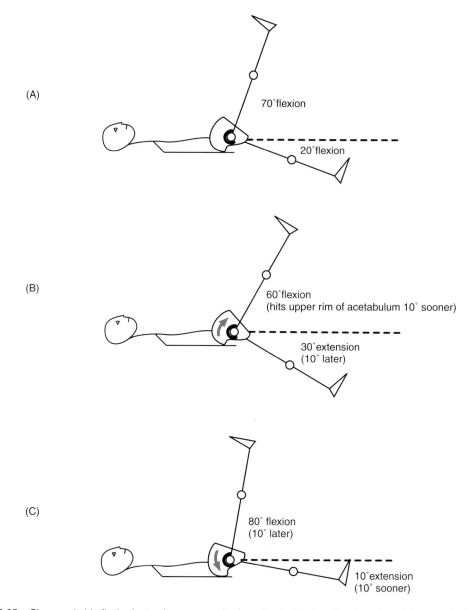

Figure 3.65 Changes in hip flexion/extension as a result of mechanical factors (reorientation of the acetabulum with pelvic rotation: (B) Anterior. (C) Posterior.), the total range remaining 90 degrees throughout.

documented with the different presentations of rotational malalignment:

1. *'Alternate' presentations.* The one variation to be found within this group is a restriction of passive hip flexion on the right side in those with right anterior rotation, and on the left in those with left anterior rotation; hip extension is affected in a reverse fashion (see Figs 3.64 and 3.65).

2. *Rotational malalignment: 'left anterior and locked'.* The pattern is the reverse of that seen in those with the 'alternate' presentations having 'right anterior' rotation except that the limitation of left hip adduction is evident in both groups.

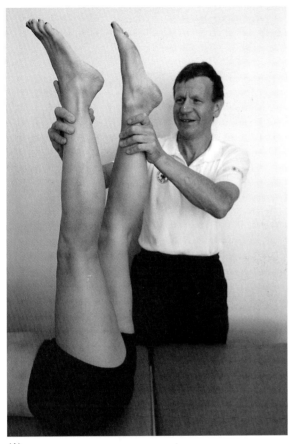

(A)

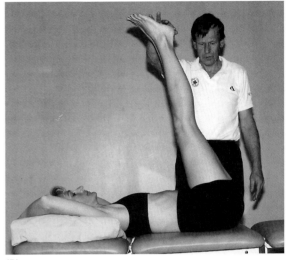

(B)

Figure 3.66 Effect of multiple factors associated with malalignment resulting in asymmetrical passive straight leg raising. (A) With malalignment (right anterior, left posterior rotation): right 95, left limited to 80 degrees. (B) In alignment: right and left now equal at 100 degrees.

Hip flexion and extension

As indicated above, right anterior and left posterior innominate rotation results in a restriction of passive right hip flexion and left hip extension on carrying out these ranges of motion with the knees flexed and lying supine (see Figs 3.64 and 3.65). The reverse pattern of restrictions is seen with left anterior, right posterior innominate rotation. Malalignment also affects active movement in these directions. The actual restrictions are in part determined by whether the pelvis is 'fixed' or free to move.

In the athlete who is in alignment, all of the pelvis is free to rotate around one of the transverse axes to increase the amount of hip flexion possible, as illustrated by the following examples:

- The athlete is standing and kicks upwards at a bag or opponent while keeping the knee straight. Simultaneous posterior rotation of the entire pelvis increases ipsilateral hip flexion and allows the athlete

to kick higher. There is no limitation of range on the right compared with the left side.

- The athlete, sitting on the floor with the legs out in front and abducted, reaches forwards alternately to the right and left side to stretch the hamstrings and back extensor muscles. The pelvis is relatively 'fixed' by the floor. However, as the trunk flexes towards the right or left foot, the pelvis as a whole can still rotate anteriorly, increasing flexion at the hip joints to approximately the same extent on forwards reaching to either foot or to both simultaneously (Fig. 3.67A).

The corresponding findings in the athlete presenting with right anterior, left posterior innominate rotation are as follows. The athlete probably cannot kick as high with the right as with the left leg (see Fig. 5.12A). Factors that can contribute to this block to right hip flexion include:

- rotation of the anterior acetabular rim forwards and downwards (see Fig. 3.65B)

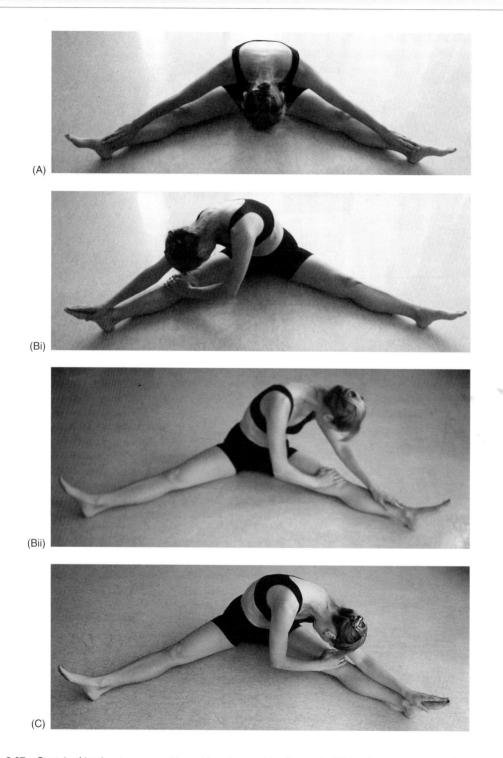

Figure 3.67 Stretch of back extensors and hamstrings by reaching forwards. (A) In alignment: symmetrical reach to both ankles/feet simultaneously, and to the right and left sides individually (not shown here). (B) With rotational malalignment (right anterior, left posterior), the reach to the left is impaired: (i) forehead 5 cm off right knee; (ii) forehead 25 cm off left knee. (C) On realignment: the left reach now equals that to the right.

- increased tension in the right hamstrings relating to a separation of their origin and insertion, and to the automatic increase (facilitation) commonly seen on this side in association with malalignment (see Figs 2.37 and 3.39)
- a failure of the pelvis to rotate posteriorly as a unit; the left innominate is already 'fixed' in a position of posterior rotation and can rotate only a little or no further in that direction; the right may be 'locked' in anterior rotation.

In the athlete with left anterior, right posterior rotation, the restriction will be on attempting a left high kick.

The athlete sitting on the floor with legs abducted cannot bring his or her forehead as close to the left knee as to the right (Fig. 3.67B). The athlete is often under the impression that the left hamstrings are tighter than the right ones, limiting this movement. In reality, with the left being the side of the posterior rotation, one might expect more hip flexion to be possible because the anterior acetabular rim has rotated backwards and upwards, out of the way, and tension in the hamstrings should decrease as the origin and insertion have been brought closer together.

The problem, however, actually relates to the fact that the pelvis has been 'fixed' with the left innominate in a posteriorly rotated position. On attempted trunk and left hip flexion, the left innominate can no longer accommodate by rotating anteriorly around one of the transverse axes along with the rest of the pelvis, limiting hip, and thereby also trunk, flexion on the left side.

A further limitation of left hip flexion occurs because of the common automatic increase in tension in the left gastrocnemius (see Fig. 3.39). This facilitation accounts for some of the limitation of passive straight leg raising and ankle dorsiflexion on this side; there is frequently a report of tightness, sometimes even pain, which tends to be maximal near the gastrocnemius origins from the distal femur, just above the popliteal region (Fig. 3.68; see Fig. 3.66).

On the right side, the innominate is 'fixed' in an anteriorly rotated position. This simulates the anterior rotation of the pelvis that would normally occur with trunk flexion and allows the trunk to bend further forwards.

This side-to-side difference in trunk flexion can also be seen on the slump or Maitland's test for detecting possible nerve root and/or dural irritation (Fig. 3.68). The athlete sits on the plinth, one leg out in front and supported at the ankle by the examiner in order to keep the hip approximately 90 degrees flexed and the knee in extension. The athlete then proceeds to flex the

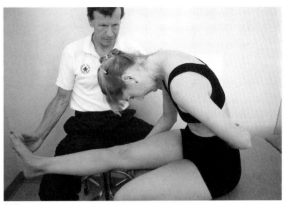

(Ai)

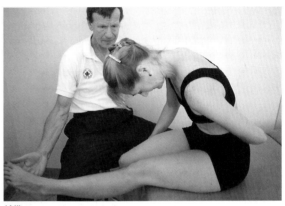

(Aii)

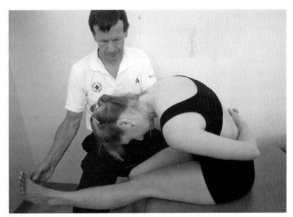

(B)

Figure 3.68 Maitland's slump test for dural, root and peripheral nerve irritation. (A) With malalignment present (right anterior, left posterior rotation). (i) Right: relatively unrestricted trunk and head flexion (forehead 20 cm off knee); ankle dorsiflexion within 30 degrees short of neutral. (ii) Left: limitation of trunk and head flexion (forehead 28 cm off knee) and of dorsiflexion (45 degrees short of neutral). (B) In alignment: left trunk and head flexion improved and equal to the right; dorsiflexion increased bilaterally (15 degrees short of neutral).

trunk and then the head. On the side of the posteriorly rotated innominate, there is usually a noticeable restriction of trunk and head flexion. The athlete may complain of tightness in the posterior thigh (hamstrings).

Tightness in the gastrocnemius also limits passive ankle dorsiflexion on this side and frequently provokes discomfort in the popliteal region and the calf (Fig. 3.68Aii). 'Back pain' often localizes to the hamstrings up to the origin but may also be felt in the ipsilateral buttock or lumbosacral region, most probably from an excessive stretching of already tense and tender buttock muscles and ligaments. However, whenever tightness, irritation or inflammation of the meninges, spinal cord, dura, nerve root or peripheral nerve structures is present, head flexion superimposed on the already flexed trunk, and the subsequent ankle dorsiflexion, may provoke pain and/or dysesthesias (e.g. an electric shock sensation) from the low, middle or even upper back and neck region, and possibly down into the extended leg.

Clinical correlation

Athletes in sports that require running, jumping and high kicking may be aware of restrictions of hip flexion and extension which is in fact attributable to innominate rotation.

Restriction of hip flexion on the side of anterior rotation.
In standing. This restriction is unfortunately often mistakenly attributed to 'hamstring tightness' when in fact the problem is actually the result of a combination of increased tension and biomechanical restriction secondary to the malalignment. Stretching is, therefore, unlikely to result in other than a temporary improvement until one corrects the malalignment.

The high kick is more likely to be restricted on the side of the anterior rotation for the reasons cited above. The combined effect of these restrictions is to make these athletes more vulnerable to injuring the sacrotuberous ligament or the hamstrings, gluteus maximus or gastrocnemius when attempting a high kick, or when the athlete tries to clear an obstacle, such as a hurdle, with the 'wrong' leg leading.

In squatting. The restriction of hip flexion may be noted on a full squat, so that the right thigh appears lower than the left (Fig. 3.69A) but more often the right thigh ends up higher, probably a reflection of a combination of factors such as spasm in right iliopsoas and any pelvic rotation in the frontal plane. The right knee also appears to protrude further forwards, as if the right thigh were longer than the left (Fig. 3.69B). Such asymmetry can prove costly in sports (e.g. some gymnastics and weight-lifting events) that reward the ability to squat fully and symmetrically (Fig. 3.69C).

Restriction of hip extension on the side of posterior rotation when standing. Posterior innominate rotation creates a mechanical block to hip extension with the anterior shift of the inferior acetabular rim (see Fig. 3.65). The rotation also increases tension in the rectus femoris, as well as in iliacus and its conjoint tendon with psoas major, by separating the origins and insertions (see Fig. 3.38). The athlete may notice a decreased ability to extend the hip when the pelvis is supposedly free to move.

There may be associated discomfort, possibly felt just as a pulling sensation, localizing to the groin and/or anterior thigh region on that side with hip extension and on attempting to stretch these so-called 'tight' muscles. The back may become painful because of an increase in the lumbar lordosis to accommodate for the limitation of hip extension. Passive hip extension will be decreased and may provoke the athlete's symptoms of back and/or hip pain (see Fig. 3.64Aii).

A repeated or chronic increase in tension can result in myofascial pain and make these muscles more irritable, predisposing to spasms or 'cramping', which is sometimes felt as if someone had plunged a knife into the groin or the lateral aspect (the so-called 'gutter') of the abdomen. There is an increased risk of tearing the iliopsoas complex on excessive hip extension, abduction or combined manoeuvres. Rectus femoris is at increased risk of tearing in the following situations:

- when the muscle is subjected to a further increase in tension by simultaneous hip and knee extension. When accelerating out of the blocks, for example, rectus femoris on the side of the driving leg is put under increased tension both passively as the hip extends, and actively as the muscle contracts eccentrically to help to control extension of the knee (see Fig. 3.48)
- when there is a demand for a sudden increase in stride length, such as occurs with any increase in speed and with jumping activities
- when the muscle undergoes a lengthening (eccentric) contraction to control knee flexion as the hip extends. This can occur, for example, when jumping and landing on one leg. The lengthening contraction of the quadriceps allows for controlled knee flexion to help to absorb ground forces. At the same time, the trunk may be thrown backwards to help deceleration, increasing the extension of the hip joint on the weight-bearing side and separating the muscle's origin from its insertion.

In walking or running events, rotational malalignment can result in an asymmetry of stride and a limitation of stride length for the same reasons that cause restrictions in stretching. A restriction of hip extension or flexion

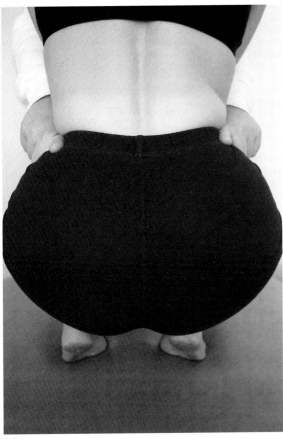

(A)

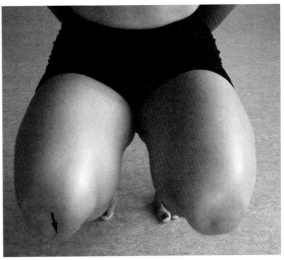

(Bi)

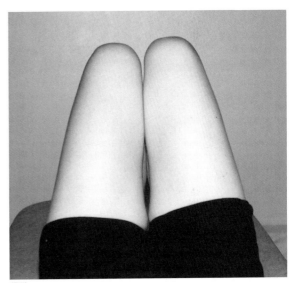

(Bii)

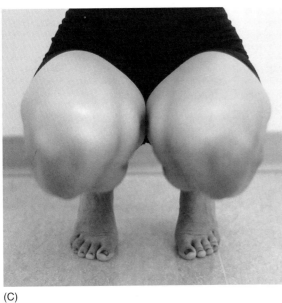

(C)

Figure 3.69 Asymmetries with right anterior rotation noted on squatting. (A) Right iliac crest (and ischial tuberosity) up on the right. (B) Thigh asymmetry: (i) right knee forwards compared with the left one and lower because of a decreased ability to flex the right hip (see also Fig. 3.64Ai; (ii) right knee higher than the left one (= forwards on Bi). (C) Following correction, the pelvis is now level and the knees match in length and height.

can theoretically be compensated for in part by increased plantar flexion of the foot and ankle, or by a supination pattern of movement on weight-bearing, to increase the length of the respective extremity. Both methods, however, raise the centre of gravity and therefore also increase the workload and decrease stability.

In an attempt to maintain a uniform stride length, compensation is more likely to come about as a result of increased pelvic rotation in the transverse plane: forwards to counter the restricted flexion on the swing-leg side, and backwards to counter the restricted hip extension on the stance-leg side (see Fig. 2.9). Unfortunately, this adjustment:

- comes at the cost of increased counter-rotation of the trunk, simultaneous active external rotation of the swing-leg to keep it in the sagittal plane, and passive internal rotation of the stance-leg
- may not be possible in the first place, or may be severely restrained, as with outflare and inflare, in which the pelvis tends to rotate towards the side of the outflare (see Ch. 2, Figs 2.10Aiii, 2.14).

In jumping events, malalignment may be a factor determining the take-off leg in events such as pole vaulting and the long, triple and high jumps. These events all involve a high kick and require an unrestricted range of hip flexion and extension.

Hip adduction

Hip adduction is found to be restricted on the left side in practically all regardless of the presentation of malalignment. The restriction may occur primarily on the basis of the asymmetry in muscle tension that results with malalignment, a larger number of athletes showing a palpable increase in tension (facilitation) in the left hip abductors and the TFL/ITB complex.

The decrease in left hip adduction is evident on:

- passive hip adduction carried out with the athlete supine, the hip being flexed to 90 degrees (Fig. 3.70)
- Ober's test:
  - in the majority, adduction is adequate to allow the right knee to touch the plinth (see

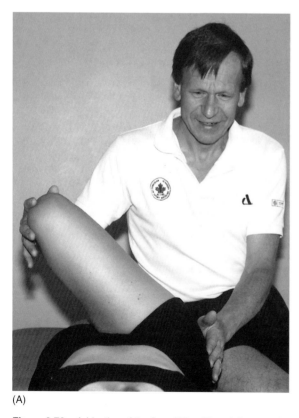

(A)

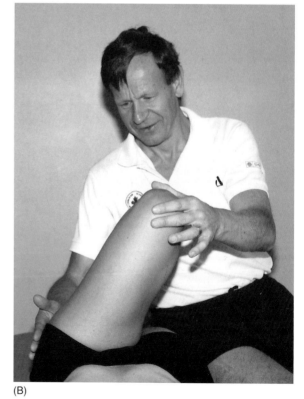

(B)

Figure 3.70 Adduction of the flexed hip with malalignment (upslips and 'alternate' presentations). (A) Right normal at 45 degrees. (B) Left decreased to 30 degrees.

Fig. 3.40Ai); in a minority, the right knee ends up a short distance off the plinth

– left hip adduction is decreased relative to the right, so that the left knee comes to rest a variable distance up in the air but consistently further off the plinth than the right one (Fig. 3.40Aii).

Successful correction of the malalignment restores the symmetry of right and left hip adduction. The actual amount is then usually the same as that noted on the right side prior to realignment (45 degrees in Fig. 3.70). In the majority therefore, both knees will now touch the plinth on Ober's test (see Fig. 3.40B). Persistent asymmetry may indicate that:

1. the correction was incomplete
2. there is a true element of tightness or contracture involving the hip abductors and/or TFL/ITB complex
3. adduction is limited because it results in:
   – excessive pressure on a tender iliopsoas muscle
   – an excessive stretching of painful posterior pelvic ligaments, in particular the iliolumbar and sacrospinous ligaments and those crossing the posterior SI joints.

If (3) is the case, the athlete will often report pain from the groin region or the lumbosacral and/or sacroiliac region when passive adduction is carried out in supine-lying (see Fig. 2.73).

Clinical correlation

This has been discussed in detail under 'left hip abductors' in the section on 'Asymmetry of muscle tension' above; in particular, relating to problems with control and seating when horseback riding, circling in skating, crossing the legs, turning corners and cutting.

Hip abduction

Abduction is, interestingly, also limited on the left side in the majority of athletes. The limitation may be caused by a number of factors, including:

- the asymmetrical reorientation of the hip sockets
- the fact that, in the majority, this is the side of the posterior rotation, which effectively increases the tension in iliacus and the adductor group by increasing the distance between their origin and insertion
- possibly a facilitation of iliopsoas and the adductor group mediated via the autonomic nervous system (see 'Asymmetry of muscle tension' above).

Clinical correlation

Goalies, especially in ice hockey, repeatedly use a rapid abduction of one or both lower extremities in the course of guarding a goal crease. On the side of the posterior rotation, they are at particular risk of spraining or straining the iliopsoas or avulsing the lesser trochanter (see Fig. 3.46).

An asymmetrical abduction range may prove a limiting factor in speed-skating (see Fig. 5.15) and ski-skating (see Fig. 5.20A), in which full abduction is required to generate maximum symmetrical propulsion forces.

In gymnastics and synchronized swimming, sports that repeatedly require a greater than normal amount of abduction, asymmetry may be costly in terms of performance and awards for style.

In horseback riding, the thigh on the side of internal rotation (usually the left) will be more closely applied to the flank, whereas on the side of external rotation the thigh tends to fall away (see Fig. 5.31). This could result in misleading signals and interfere with control of the horse. The rider may compensate by sitting asymmetrically in the saddle, but this may interfere with control in other ways, puts more strain on the rider and may be costly in terms of style (see Chs 5 and 6).

Hip external and internal rotation

When the athlete is in alignment, external and internal rotation of the right and left hip joints are symmetrical (Fig. 3.71A). The 'alternate' presentations and upslips show a restriction of right internal (Fig. 3.71B) and left external rotation (Fig. 3.72A); barring underlying pathology, however, the total combined external and internal range available on the right and left sides is nearly the same. The left anterior and locked presentation results in the opposite pattern, with a restriction of left internal and right external rotation.

One might think that these restrictions are determined by the asymmetry in muscle tension. The pattern noted with the 'alternate' presentations, for example, could easily result from the frequently noted increase in tension in the right piriformis, an external rotator, and the left hip abductors and TFL/ITB complex, which are internal rotators. It is, however, these same muscles which most often show an increase in tension not just with the 'alternate', but also with the 'left anterior and locked' presentation and upslips.

An asymmetrical orientation of the hip joints also fails to explain these limitations, given that the pattern of limitation is the same regardless of whether the right or left innominate is rotated anteriorly. The exception is when left anterior rotation is combined

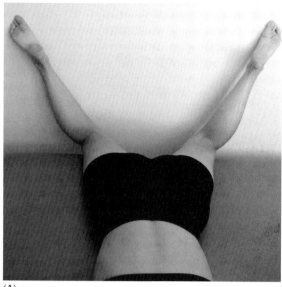

(A)

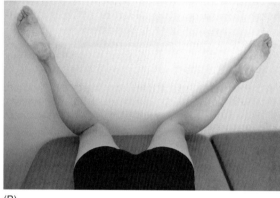

(B)

Fig. 3.71 Internal rotation (IR) of the hip. (A) In alignment: symmetrical at 40 degrees. (B) With malalignment: right 30 versus left 50 degrees.

with locking of the left SI joint. The combination of innominate orientation and SI joint mobility may therefore be a major determining factor.

Clinical correlation

A limitation of external rotation on one side allows the athlete to use a modified Patrick's or FABER's test (see Fig. 2.74A) for a quick self-check on whether or not he or she is out of alignment: lying supine, the athlete lets the knees fall outwards on either side while maintaining contact between the soles of the feet (see Fig. 3.73). The test combines hip flexion, abduction and external

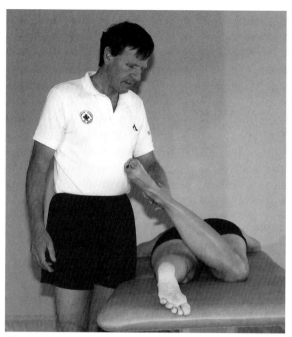

(A)

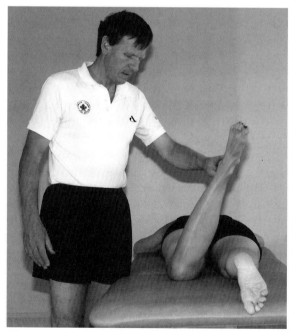

(B)

Fig. 3.72 External rotation (ER) of the hip with malalignment. (A) Right of 45 versus (B) left of 25 degrees. Prior to realignment, the total of right internal rotation (IR; 30 degrees) and ER (45 degrees) equals the total of left IR (50 degrees) and ER (25 degrees), i.e. 75 degrees (compared to 85 degrees bilaterally when in alignment).

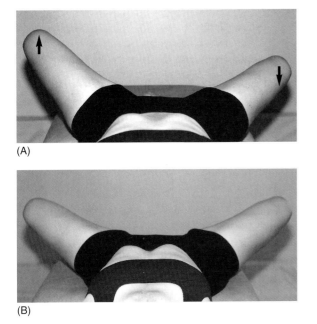

(A)

(B)

Fig. 3.73 Simultaneous bilateral flexion, abduction and external rotation (see also Fig. 2.74A). (A) With malalignment: there is a restriction of ranges on the left compared with the right side, so the left knee ends up higher than the right. (B) In alignment: the left ranges now equal those on the right, and the knees end up level.

rotation to stress the hip and SI joints. A restriction of movement in any of these directions for whatever reason, for example, contracture of any of the muscles or of the hip joint capsule, will affect the results.

Assuming no underlying pathology other than malalignment, and given that malalignment will affect all three ranges of motion in an asymmetrical way, one knee will usually end up higher than the other (see Fig. 3.73A). The most common finding is that the left knee ends up higher than the right, reflecting the restriction of left hip abduction and external rotation seen with the 'alternate' presentations and upslips.

Unfortunately, the test gives no indication of the exact nature of the underlying malalignment, seeing that left external rotation is decreased by right or left anterior rotation and upslips; the only obvious exceptions are those with the left anterior and locked presentation, who show the opposite pattern of restriction. On realignment, the knees will again end up at equal height (Fig. 3.73B).

External rotation is part of the lower extremity action in ski-skating, which is a part of traditional cross-country skiing, and has more recently become a separate nordic event (see Fig. 5.20). It occurs in the

trailing leg in speed-skating and is maximal as the blade reaches the terminal point of push-off (see Fig. 5.15). In those with one of the 'alternate' presentations or an upslip:

- push-off in these events may be impaired on the left side by the limitation of external rotation, compounded by the limitation of abduction and the impaired ability to dig in the inside of the ski or blade. The latter can occur in association with malalignment because a left neutral to supinating pattern of weight-bearing will make it difficult to get onto the inside edge on this side (see Figs 3.18 and 3.33)
- the right, usually pronating, side may be able to dig in the inside edge but may run into problems holding this position because of a weakness and early fatiguing of the ankle invertors – tibialis anterior and posterior.

A restriction of external rotation can contribute to difficulty with crossing one leg over the other while sitting, an action that requires simultaneous adduction and external rotation of the crossing leg. This becomes a particular problem with the 'alternate' presentations and upslips, in which adduction and external rotation are both restricted on the left side, making it harder to cross the left leg over the right (see Fig. 3.44B). With the left anterior and locked presentation, adduction is also restricted on the left, whereas external rotation is restricted on the right, so that crossing the legs may or may not be more difficult on one or other side.

A restriction of internal and external rotation of a lower extremity may impair sweeping and kicking actions in soccer and a number of other sports. When the hip and knee are flexed, sweeping or kicking the ball with the inside of the foot occurs in the direction of external rotation; with the outside of the foot, it occurs in the direction of internal rotation.

Problems arise too when horseback riding. Limitations of left external and right internal rotation, in combination with a tendency towards left internal and right external rotation, interfere with the ability to achieve a secure seating position, or 'deep seat', and to use the thighs, knees and calves appropriately for signalling (see Chs 5 and 6). Typically:

- on the side of increased external rotation, and with the hip and knee flexed, the hip and knee will tend to move away from the horse's flank and the stirrup sweep inwards
- on the side of increased internal rotation, the knee and thigh will come to be more closely applied, whereas the stirrup moves outwards (see Fig. 5.31).

The knee

> The knee appears to be an innocent bystander, subjected to stresses that arise from the various asymmetries associated with malalignment.

The most common finding in sitting and lying is that the patella rides high and squints outwards on the side on which the leg has rotated outwards (see Fig. 3.33). When standing, an athlete with one of the 'alternate' presentation or an upslip may be noted to flex the knee on the side of the 'high' pelvis, as if subconsciously trying to level the pelvis (see Fig. 2.59). The knee flexion may also be a reflection of the tendency to pronation on the side of external rotation, increasing both the knee valgus and flexion strain (see Fig. 3.33).

Unfortunately, flexing the knee when the foot is planted on the ground increases tension in the quadriceps mechanism, tending to pull the patella upwards and increasing the pressure within the patellofemoral compartment. Problems relating to weight-bearing include the following (see Fig. 3.33).

Pronation results in internal rotation of the tibia relative to the femur at the same time that the patella itself is being displaced upwards by the increase in quadriceps tension and laterally by the relative external rotation of the femur and the increase in the Q-angle. The combined effect is to increase the tension in the patellar tendon by separating the origin and insertion, and to offset the position of the patellar tendon relative to the groove, thereby further increasing the pressure within the patellofemoral compartment. The increased tendency to pronation predisposes to valgus angulation of the knee, with:

- increasing traction on the medial soft tissue structures (e.g. the medial collateral ligament, medial plica, vastus medialis tendon and saphenous nerve)
- increased pressure within the lateral knee joint compartment (Figs 3.74 and 3.75).

Supination results in external rotation of the tibia relative to the femur and predisposes to varus angulation at the knee, increasing traction on the lateral soft tissue

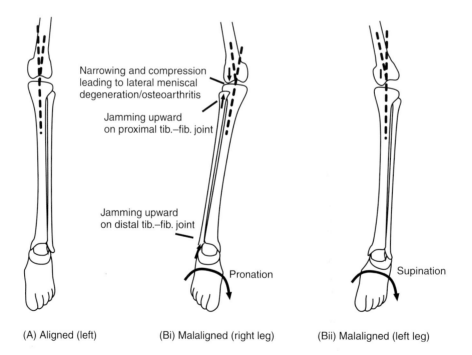

Narrowing and compression leading to lateral meniscal degeneration/osteoarthritis

Jamming upward on proximal tib.–fib. joint

Jamming upward on distal tib.–fib. joint

Pronation

Supination

(A) Aligned (left) (Bi) Malaligned (right leg) (Bii) Malaligned (left leg)

Figure 3.74 Effect on Q-angle, pressure distribution in the knee joint compartments and tibiofibular joints with a malalignment-related shift to right pronation and left supination. (A) Aligned: there is a fairly uniform weight distribution through the medial and lateral knee compartments bilaterally (only the left being shown). (B) With malalignment. (i) Right: increased pressure on the lateral compartment with the tendency towards pronation and knee valgus angulation. The Q-angle is increased. Excessive pronation can result in a forceful upward movement of the fibula and a jamming of the proximal tibiofibular joint (similar to an ankle eversion sprain). (ii) Left: increased pressure on the medial compartment with the tendency towards supination and knee varus angulation. The Q-angle is decreased.

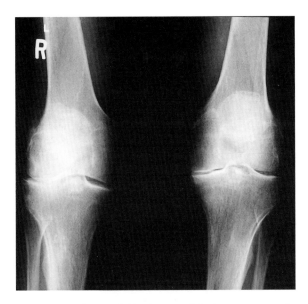

Figure 3.75 Osteoarthritic changes of the knees as a result of a long-term pressure redistribution similar to that occurring with malalignment: accentuated wear of the right lateral and left medial knee joint compartments (see Fig. 3.74B).

structures (e.g. the lateral collateral ligament and common peroneal nerve) and increasing the pressure within the medial knee joint compartment (Figs 3.74 and 3.75).

Rotation of the tibia relative to the femur associated with pronation and supination results in a torsional stress on the menisci, the cruciate ligament, and the collateral and interosseous ligaments, as well as the proximal and distal tibiofibular joints.

Clinical correlation

In the athlete with one of the 'alternate' presentation, the pelvis being high on the right side, with a tendency to partly flex the right knee in standing, and right pronation, left supination on weight-bearing (see Fig. 3.33 and Appendix 5), typical complications include the following.

On the side of the externally rotated right lower extremity:

● patellofemoral compartment syndrome
● an increased risk of patellar subluxation or even dislocation
● patellar tendonitis
● right traction epiphysitis (Osgood–Schlatter's epiphysitis): if the tibial tubercle and tibia are not yet completely fused at the time they are being subjected to this increased stress, the irritation can stimulate increased bone turnover, which may result in an enlarged right

tibial tubercle by the time growth has been completed; a chronic increase in tension in the tendon and/or direct pressure on the vulnerable epiphysis (e.g. with kneeling or contusion) can make this site an ongoing source of pain

● increased traction on the right medial collateral ligament, which may lead to tenderness, pain and eventual elongation and joint instability, with increased medial opening on valgus stress
● inflammation of the medial collateral ligament, medial plica and vastus medialis, these sometimes snapping across the medial femoral condyle on flexion/extension movements of the knee
● increased traction on the pes anserinus
● paraesthesia or pain from irritation of the saphenous nerve (see Fig. 3.34A)
● accelerated degeneration of the lateral knee joint compartment cartilage and meniscus (Figs 3.74 and 3.75).

On the side of the internally rotated left lower extremity:

● left lateral collateral ligament tenderness, pain, elongation and eventual joint laxity, with lateral joint line opening on varus stress
● increased traction in the distal ITB, biceps femoris and tendinous insertions of vastus lateralis lying between the two; when under tension, one or all three structures may snap across the lateral femoral condyle on repeated knee flexion and extension. ITB bursitis can also occur
● upwards traction exerted by the biceps femoris on its insertion into the proximal fibula, which can disturb the movement normally possible at the proximal and also the distal tibiofibular joint
● irritation of the common peroneal nerve or its branches (see Fig. 3.34B)
● accelerated degeneration of the medial knee joint compartment cartilage and meniscus (Figs 3.74 and 3.75).

In addition to the possibility of pain having been referred to the knee, always keep in mind abnormal or exaggerated stresses resulting from malalignment as an underlying cause of knee pain, instability or degeneration, especially when the athlete presents with unilateral knee problems in the absence of a history of trauma. Right patellofemoral compartment syndrome is the most frequent complication.

Tibiofibular joints

Normal movement at the proximal and distal tibiofibular joints is required to allow proper movement of

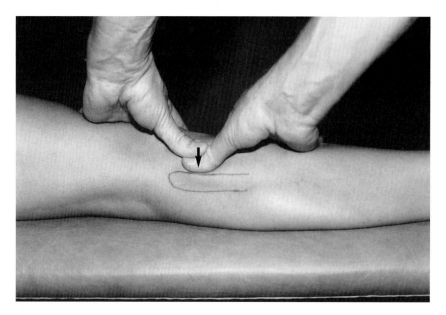

Figure 3.76 Springing test for anterior–posterior movement of the proximal tibiofibular joint.

the tibia, ankle and foot. There should be some glide possible in the anteroposterior and vertical (cephalocaudal) planes, with a sensation of giving way on passively moving or 'springing' these joints, usually more easily detectable in the proximal joint (Fig. 3.76).

A failure of one or both of these joints to move, or decreased movement on side-to-side comparison, usually indicates a problem. The anterior– posterior glide of either joint can, for example, be impaired by a direct blow to the anterior or posterior aspect of the proximal or distal fibula; an acute ankle sprain or the repetitive excessive dorsiflexion associated with malalignment on the side of the pronating foot can force the fibula upward and cause it to jam proximally (see Fig. 3.74B).

Attempts at passive movement may elicit pain from the joint itself, the ligaments or both. Proximal joint pain calls for a check for undue tenderness or irritability of the common peroneal nerve, which innervates the joint and is at increased risk of either entrapment or traction injury as it winds around the fibular neck (see Fig. 4.11B).

The proximal tibiofibular joint

At this joint, the fibula normally glides anteriorly and upwards on ankle dorsiflexion, and posteriorly and downwards on plantar flexion. It can get 'stuck' in an excessive upwards or downwards position with an ankle eversion and inversion sprain respectively.

Upwards traction forces can jam the fibula against the outflare of the proximal tibia. Mechanisms include an excessive traction force through biceps femoris or the lateral collateral ligament (both of which insert into the fibular head), excessive valgus angulation at the knee, or dorsiflexion/eversion at the ankle pushing the fibula proximally.

Aggravating factors such as these are frequently operative in the presence of malalignment; with 'alternate' presentations, there is, for example, an increase in tension in right biceps femoris and increased dorsiflexion with pronation. The proximal end of the fibula may be displaced upwards and posteriorly, and get jammed in that position. Anterior jamming may occur if the increased dorsiflexion and eversion displaces the distal tibia posteriorly and interferes with function of that joint.

The distal tibiofibular joint

Movement at this joint is closely related to movement of the tibiotalar and, to lesser extent, subtalar joints. Varus or valgus angulation of the tibiotalar joint, for example, can result in some splaying of the space between the fibula and tibia, increasing tension on the tibiofibular ligaments and the interosseous membrane. Dorsiflexion at the tibiotalar joint has a similar effect because of the wedge-shaped talus, wider inferiorly. Supination and increased ankle varus pull the fibula downwards.

If the distal tibiofibular joint gets 'stuck', the amount of calcaneal varus and valgus angulation, as well as of ankle dorsiflexion, is automatically decreased. The ankle becomes 'stiff'. The loss of ankle mobility, especially if associated with a downwards displacement of the distal fibula, will also impair the internal and external rotation of the tibia that normally occurs with pronation and supination respectively. A number of these factors are likely to be operative in the presence of malalignment.

The ankle (tibiotalar) joint

Ankle dorsiflexion and plantar flexion reflect primarily movement of the tibiotalar joint in the sagittal plane, with contributions from the subtalar and distal tibiofibular joints. With any of the 'alternate' presentations of rotational malalignment and upslip, the right side shows increased dorsiflexion and decreased plantar flexion relative to the left (Fig. 3.77). These patterns are in keeping with the tendency towards right pronation (calcaneal eversion, forefoot abduction and dorsiflexion) and left supination (calcaneal inversion, forefoot adduction and plantarflexion). These findings are reversed with the left anterior and locked presentation: dorsiflexion increased on the left and plantar flexion on the right, reflecting the tendency towards left pronation and right supination respectively.

When there is an exception to this pattern, consider (1) a previous ankle injury that may have resulted in unilateral restriction of dorsi- and/or plantarflexion and often also limitation of subtalar eversion and/or inversion, or (2) cuboid subluxation, which results in a stiff ankle with restricted motion in all four directions.

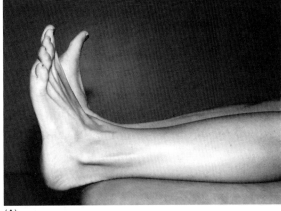

(A)

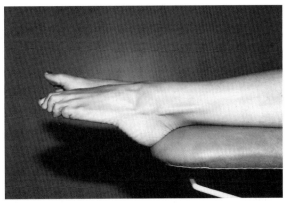

(B)

Figure 3.77 Effect of 'alternate' presentations and upslips on ankle movement. (A) Relatively restricted left dorsiflexion. (B) Relatively restricted right plantar flexion.

Clinical correlation

Propulsion with the flutter kick depends in part on the ability to plantarflex the foot. The asymmetry of plantar flexion seen with malalignment is probably one reason why some swimmers are unusually slow, fail to move forwards or may actually move backward on doing the flutter kick while holding on to a board. Other factors, such as the rotation of the lower extremities in opposite directions and the asymmetry of lower extremity muscle strength, probably also play a role (see Ch. 5).

Deep squats require a full range of ankle dorsiflexion, especially if the heels are to stay on the floor (e.g. some gymnastics and weight-lifting routines). With malalignment, dorsiflexion will be decreased on one side. Once the limit of available dorsiflexion has been reached on that side, the following sequence occurs:

1. Tension in the Achilles tendon complex on that side increases to the point at which attempts at further dorsiflexion begin to tighten up the plantar fascia and activate the 'windlass' mechanism sooner than normal.

2. The heel will now begin to lift, weight being increasingly transferred to the forefoot as the foot and ankle are passively plantarflexed by this mechanism.

The athlete who is stationary (e.g. a weight-lifter) may end up lifting the heel right off the floor. The athlete who is in motion (e.g. a floor gymnast) may end up:

- vaulting over the ball of the foot from mid-stance to toe-off
- or collapsing into medial weight-bearing and pronation with that foot in an attempt to counter the tendency for the heel to come off the floor, that is, to counter the increasing plantarflexion and the associated rise of the centre of gravity.

Both ways of compensation decrease stability and affect style. The increase in tension that results in the tendo Achilles complex and in the plantar fascia with the windlass mechanism being activated prematurely increases the chance of causing painful inflammation (Achilles tendonitis or plantar fasciitis), or even sustaining a tear of these structures.

The limitation of hip extension seen on the side of the posterior innominate rotation decreases the ability to lengthen that leg by extending the hip in late stance. The athlete can compensate by increasing the plantarflexion of that foot in order to increase the leg length, but this option will be limited on the side on which plantarflexion is restricted.

Dance routines calling on a maximum range of dorsiflexion or plantarflexion will be affected by any limitation(s).

A decrease in dorsiflexion range may become a limiting factor in cross-country skiing and especially telemarking, in which acute dorsiflexion accompanies knee flexion and hip extension of the back or inside leg when assuming the 'telemark' stance to execute a turn (see Fig. 5.21).

In sports that require full dorsiflexion, the decrease of this motion seen on one side will cause an earlier transfer of weight to the metatarsal heads and an earlier impingement of structures on the dorsum of the foot (Fig. 3.78). Stress would be maximal in activities requiring controlled ankle dorsiflexion, such as occurs when landing on the feet during or at the end of a floor routine or on a dismount. Anterior impingement of the ankle is also known as 'footballer's ankle'; it particularly affects those playing American football, soccer or rugby on dry, hardened playing fields or artificial surfaces such as astroturf (O'Brien 1992). With time, the repeated stress can lead to problems: pain from irrita-

tion of the capsules, ligaments and bone, and from an acceleration of degenerative changes. The increased transfer of weight-bearing to the forefoot region may also contribute to the development of plantar fasciitis, metatarsalgia and metatarsal stress fractures.

The limitation of plantarflexion can result in contracture of the capsules, ligaments and tendons on the dorsum of the foot. In activities that repeatedly require maximum available plantarflexion range (e.g. dancing and gymnastics), contracture can result in the eventual formation of dorsal traction spurs (osteophytes) and other degenerative changes. Injuries such as marginal avulsion fractures are then more likely to occur with activities that impart a sudden or excessive stress to the dorsum of the plantarflexed foot (e.g. kicking a ball, or an opponent with the top of that foot, as in karate). The increase in plantarflexion seen on the opposite side could exert traction forces on the dorsal aspect.

The subtalar (talocalcaneal) joint

The subtalar joint primarily permits calcaneal inversion and eversion relative to the talus. Some degree of abduction and adduction, as well as dorsi- and plantarflexion, is also normally possible. When examined lying supine and with the tibiotalar joint locked by holding the ankle at 90 degrees, athletes presenting with the left anterior and locked pattern show a restriction of passive right inversion and left eversion, whereas those with one of the 'alternate' presentations or an upslip show a restriction of passive right eversion and left inversion (see Fig. 3.23).

Compared with the findings at rest, a gait examination of these athletes shows the tendency to pronate to be increased on the side that has the restriction of

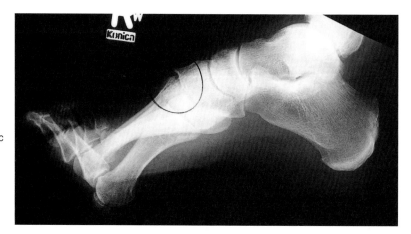

Figure 3.78 Degenerative changes on the dorsum of the foot with an osteophytic spur projecting superiority at the cuneiform–2nd metatarsal articulation, which can be precipitated/aggravated by malalignment: increased dorsiflexion can cause impingement, and increased plantar flexion excessive traction, at this site.

passive subtalar eversion, and the tendency to supinate to be increased on the side that shows the restriction of passive subtalar inversion. These changes suggest that:

- pronation and supination may occur mainly through the transverse tarsal joints and the mid and forefoot section
- restrictions of calcaneal inversion and eversion may differ, depending on whether the athlete is examined at rest (as described) or when weight-bearing.

Clinical correlation

Injury is more likely to result if either subtalar joint is forced into the direction of limited range, either passively or actively, because the anatomical barrier will be exceeded earlier than usual.

Weight-bearing probably reverses the restrictions at the subtalar joint so that the previously noted limitations of passive eversion and inversion at rest may not be of much consequence when the athlete is up and about (see 'Asymmetry of foot alignment, weight-bearing and shoe wear' above). On the gait examination of those with an upslip or an 'alternate' presentation, there is certainly usually a very noticeable calcaneal eversion on the right pronating side and an inversion on the left supinating side (see Figs 3.3B and 3.36), the reverse being seen with the left anterior and locked pattern. With weight-bearing, however, there occur other changes that might make up for the restrictions of passive calcaneal eversion and inversion seen on non-weight-bearing with the ankle at 90 degrees to lock the tibio-talar joint.

First, there is the change in the axes running through the transverse tarsal (calcaneocuboid and talonavicular) joints (Mann 1982; see Fig. 3.26), with:

1. divergence on the side of the internally rotated lower extremity:
- this decreases the motion possible in these joints, locks the metatarsals and increases the stability of the longitudinal arch
- the end result is a tendency of this foot towards supination, adduction and plantarflexion, in other words, calcaneal inversion
2. more parallel alignment on the side of the externally rotated lower extremity:
- this increases the motion possible in these joints, unlocks the metatarsals and allows for a collapse of the medial longitudinal arch
- the end result is a tendency of this foot towards pronation, abduction and dorsiflexion, with calcaneal eversion (see Figs 3.3B, 3.16 and 3.20).

Second, a certain amount of inversion and eversion can occur at the tibiotalar joint. There is also the effect of the knee collapsing into valgus on the pronating side and into varus on the supinating side.

APPARENT LEG LENGTH DIFFERENCE

Unless otherwise indicated, the discussion that follows will be based on the premise that the athlete does not have an anatomical LLD. The basis of the 'sitting–lying' test has been discussed in Ch. 2 (see Figs 2.47–2.55). Typical examination findings with anatomical LLD are noted in Appendix 6, and findings relating to LLD in combination with upslips and rotational malalignment in Appendixes 7 and 8.

With rotational malalignment and upslips, the most common finding is that the right iliac crest is higher than the left when the athlete is standing (Fig. 3.79A; see Figs 2.43, 2.46B, D, and 3.7) which is not unlike the case of an athlete with an anatomically long right leg (see Fig. 2.42B). The pelvic obliquity will, however, persist in sitting (Fig. 3.79B), which is unlike the situation in the athlete with an anatomical LLD, whose pelvis would now be level (see Fig. 2.42B). The obliquity may now rarely be the reverse of that seen in standing, but it will usually still be up on the right side, as in standing (see Figs 2.43B, C and 2.46B). The fact that an obliquity persists in sitting indicates that:

- the obliquity noted in standing is not simply caused by an anatomical LLD (although a concomitant anatomical LLD could not be ruled out at this point)
- malalignment (rotational or upslip) is most probably present.

A persistence of the obliquity as a result of asymmetrical growth of the right compared with the left innominate is a possibility. When one examines athletes who are in alignment, however, it is extremely rare to find developmental changes in the pelvic region that result in side-to-side differences of the magnitude of the 1.0–2.0 cm that one commonly sees when malalignment is present (Fig. 3.80).

A knowledge of which iliac crest is higher when standing is not helpful for predicting which leg will be longer in long-sitting or supine-lying. Nor does it help to determine the side of an anterior rotation or upslip, although the odds are statistically around 5:1 to 6:1 in favour of finding the former on the right side.

Diagnosing leg length difference

From a diagnostic point of view, the actual length of the legs, as noted in standing or in long-sitting and

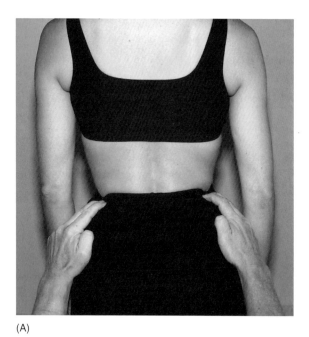

(A)

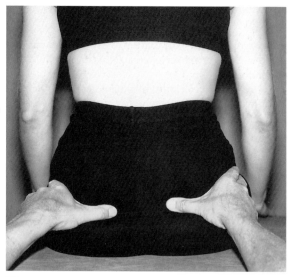

(B)

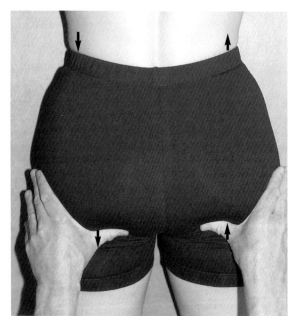

(C)

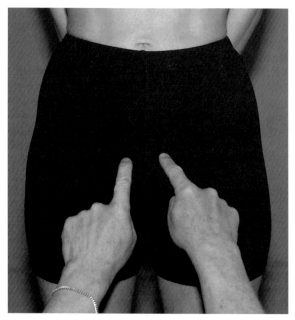

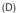

(D)

Figure 3.79 Athlete with an anatomically equal leg length presenting with pelvic malalignment (right anterior, left posterior rotation). Compare with the left side: (A) standing – right iliac crest up; (B) sitting – right posterior superior iliac spine (and iliac crest) up; (C) lying prone – right ischial tuberosity (and iliac crest) up; (D) standing – right pubic bone down.

supine-lying, is of little importance in the presence of rotational malalignment. The right leg may, for example, be longer than the left in long-sitting and even longer in supine-lying (Fig. 3.81), but all this means is

that there is probably an anterior rotation of the right innominate that should then be verified by an assessment of the pelvic landmarks. It does not presuppose that the right leg is anatomically longer than the left!

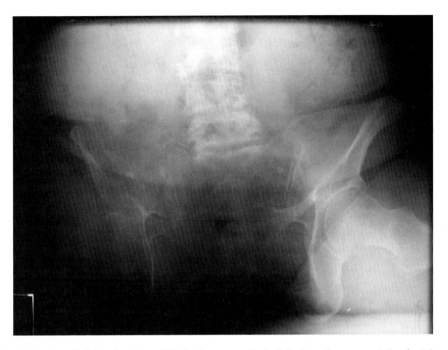

Figure 3.80 Underdeveloped left hemipelvis and hip joint as a result of a left above knee amputation for tuberculosis at age 12. (The athlete is in alignment; when sitting, the left iliac crest appears 1 cm lower than the right.

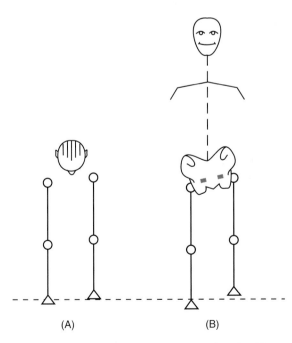

(A)   (B)

Figure 3.81 Sitting–lying test: a change in functional leg length difference indicating probable right anterior rotation. (A) Right leg longer in long-sitting. (B) Right leg even longer in supine-lying.

A typical example is that of the runner described in the case study (p. 184).

The 'long-sitting to supine-lying' test serves as an easy indicator of the probable presence of rotational malalignment and helps to differentiate it from an anatomical LLD and an upslip, although a co-existing upslip or anatomical LLD cannot be ruled out. It also affords the clinician and the athlete an easy way of determining which side has rotated anteriorly or posteriorly. This knowledge is essential in order to carry out properly some of the techniques used to correct a rotational malalignment (see Chs 7 and 8).

Other factors to consider

It must again be emphasized that leg length *per se* is influenced by other factors, including whether there is a concomitant anatomical LLD, sacral torsion, upslip/ downslip, contracture or asymmetry of tension in the muscles and ligaments of the pelvic and hip girdle region.

Differences in leg length of 2, 3 or even 4 cm can be caused entirely by the presence of rotational malalignment.

Case study

A runner presented initially with low back pain. She was noted to be in alignment but had an anatomical (true) LLD, the right leg being 1 cm longer than the left (Fig. 3.82A). The back pain cleared with exercise and the provision of an appropriately tapered right heel lift, initially of 5 and then of 10 mm. Eight months later, she returned complaining of pain in both the mid and the low back region that had developed following a fall on ice. She was now found to have a rotational malalignment, with a left anterior and locked presentation. Despite the fact that she was known to have an anatomically longer right leg, the left leg was now 5 mm longer than the right in long-sitting; on lying supine, the left leg lengthened even more and ended up being 1 cm longer than the right (Fig. 3.82B). These findings were consistent with the left anterior rotation, confirmed by an examination of the pelvic landmarks, and obviously said nothing about the true anatomical length of either leg.

In fact, differences as great as that may be observed to reverse on changing from the long-sitting to the supine-lying position and yet, with realignment, most of these athletes will turn out to have legs of equal length! Remember that although 80–90% of athletes present with an apparent LLD, only about 6–12% actually have evidence of a true anatomical LLD once in alignment (Armour & Scott 1981, W. Schamberger, unpublished data 1993, 1994).

The following basic approach is appropriate when dealing with a possible LLD:

1. As long as rotational malalignment is present, a functional LLD will be present; there is therefore no point measuring leg length using the bony landmarks on the pelvis. Measurement from the ASIS or PSIS to the medial malleoli, for example, will be incorrect on both sides. The ASIS and PSIS, and for that matter any other pelvic landmark, will have changed position on one side compared with the other, not only in the sagittal, but also in the transverse and frontal planes. At the same time, the asymmetrical reorientation of the right and left acetabulum has pushed the leg down on one side and pulled it up on the other. In other words, all the measurements will be inaccurate. Measuring from the greater trochanters to the floor in standing ignores any differences in the femoral head and neck and those due to displacement of the greater trochanters in opposite directions with the internal/external rotation of the legs (see Effect on lesser trochanter, Fig. 2.45).
2. If an anatomical LLD is suspected, one must first correct the rotation (and any coexisting malalignment) and then carry out the measurements, using the appropriate landmarks.
3. If the malalignment just cannot be corrected in a symptomatic athlete, the following approach

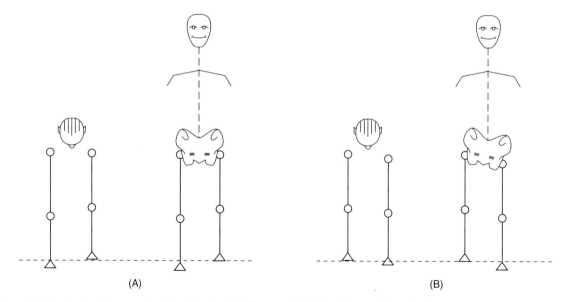

(A)   (B)

Figure 3.82 Anatomical versus functional leg length difference (LLD) (see the case history). (A) Aligned: anatomical LLD with right leg longer than left by 1 cm sitting and lying. (B) Left anterior rotation: the left leg is now longer than the right by 0.5 cm in long-sitting and 1 cm supine-lying.

should be considered before trying to make up the functional LLD with a lift:

- Check the standing X-rays to see whether they show any evidence of levelling of the sacrum having occurred in an attempt to counter the pelvic obliquity and compensate for the LLD.
- If the sacrum is still unlevel, compensation either has not yet occurred or is incomplete. A lift to decrease or eliminate the residual pelvic obliquity may then be of help by levelling the sacral base, decreasing the stress on the lumbosacral junction and lessening any compensatory curves of the spine (Fig. 3.83A). The assessment of the LLD for the purpose of providing an appropriate lift should be made with the athlete standing, measuring from the lateral pelvic crest to the floor itself in order to minimize any error.
- If sacral levelling (compensation) has occurred, correction of the persistent pelvic obliquity with a lift under the apparently 'short' leg will actually unlevel the sacral base again, increasing the compensatory curves and the

stress on the lumbosacral junction and the rest of the spine (Fig. 3.83B).

Clinical correlation

Athletes are frequently told that one of their legs is 'long' or 'short'. This is usually based on an examination in which the leg length was assessed in one position only, for example looking at the iliac crest levels when standing or comparing leg length in long-sitting or when lying prone or supine. Lifts are sometimes prescribed on the basis of such a limited assessment. Problems may arise when the conclusions regarding leg length are based only on the following.

A comparison of the pelvic crests in standing alone. The examiner might presuppose that the leg is short on the side on which the pelvis is low. A lift on the 'short' side might possibly be helpful because it will level out the pelvis and decrease the compensatory curves of the spine. If a compensatory levelling of the sacrum has, however, already occurred, the addition of a lift on the side on which the pelvis appears low will only aggravate matters (Fig. 3.83B).

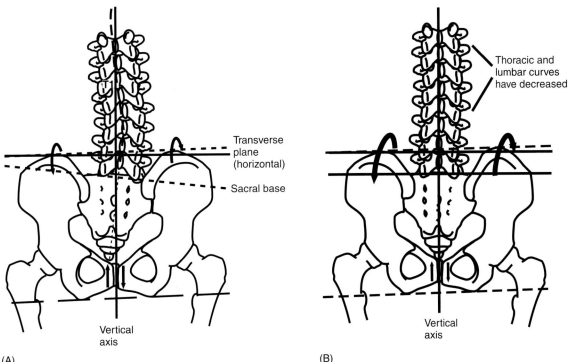

(A)   (B)

Figure 3.83   Sacral adjustment to functional leg length difference caused by malalignment. (A) Uncompensated: the sacral base and iliac crest are oblique (-----), and there is an accentuated compensatory scoliosis. (B) Compensated: although the obliquity of iliac crests persists, the sacral base is now level and the degree of scoliosis decreased.

Examination in either supine-lying or long-sitting only.
Prescribing a lift on the basis of such a limited examination invites disaster. It completely ignores the fact that when there is a concomitant malalignment of the pelvis, what seems to be the 'short' leg in one or both of these positions may actually become the 'long' leg in standing. It is, for example, not unusual to see the right leg shorter than the left in long-sitting and also shorter, but less so, when lying supine, yet to find the right iliac crest higher than the left when standing (Fig. 3.84).

This relative lengthening of the 'short' right leg on going from sitting to lying is probably indicative of a right anterior rotation being present. The right leg will also be short in both long-sitting and supine-lying with a right upslip, yet the right side of the pelvis will turn out to be higher than the left in these and the standing positions. In both of these cases, prescribing a right heel lift on the basis of having looked at leg length only in the sitting or lying position will inadvertently result in a further increase of the pelvic tilt and the compensatory curves, thereby increasing the stress to which the system is already being subjected by the malalignment.

Following realignment, the prevalence of those with an anatomical LLD noted in the author's clinical studies (12% in 1993, 10% in 1994) is in line with study findings based on a comparison of the height of the femoral heads on anteroposterior pelvic X-rays taken while standing. Using this more accurate technique, for example, Armour & Scott (1981) found a prevalence of 10% in an adult population.

The tendency to pronate on one or other side is sometimes felt to be an attempt to compensate for a 'long' leg on that side. This may be true on the side of an anatomically long leg in someone who is in alignment. In those presenting with malalignment, however, the tendency to pronate does not always correspond to the side on which the pelvis is high in standing but is more likely to be part and parcel of the presentation noted: on the right side in those with an upslip or one of the 'alternate' presentations and associated external rotation of the right lower extremity, and on the left side in those with the 'left anterior and locked' pattern and associated left external rotation.

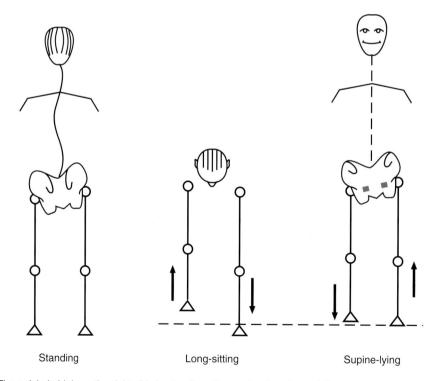

Standing   Long-sitting   Supine-lying

Figure 3.84   The pelvis is high on the right side in standing. On moving from long-sitting to supine-lying, there is a relative lengthening of the short right leg, although it still ends up shorter than the left. This lengthening suggests right anterior rotational malalignment. A true (anatomical) leg length difference, with the left longer than the right, or even the right longer than the left, cannot be ruled out from these findings.

Pronation that results in leg length shortening may also occur on the basis of:

- isolated lower extremity muscle facilitation or inhibition, for example, the facilitation of peroneus longus/ brevis and the inhibition of tibialis anterior/posterior (whereas an inhibition of the peroneal and a facilitation of the tibial muscles would predispose to supination and leg lengthening)
- the malalignment of specific bones (e.g. cuboid subluxation).

The reader is referred to material specific to the topic of facilitation and inhibition relating to malalignment (e.g. Maffetone 1999). The emphasis here is on the fact that LLD seen in association with malalignment is usually part of a larger picture that can be readily divided into those with the conglomeration of findings typical of either the 'left anterior and locked' or the 'alternate' rotational presentation (and upslips). LLD is one feature that allows for the ready detection and classification of these presentations (see the 'sitting–lying test', Figs. 2.47–2.55).

In summary, it is of the utmost importance that the examiner assess leg length in all positions – standing, sitting and lying – to see whether a difference is consistently present and whether it is consistently the same. If the difference varies from one position to another, the diagnosis of rotational malalignment must be considered and further clarified by correlation to the pelvic landmarks.

A PROBLEM WITH BALANCE AND RECOVERY

The asymmetries affecting the muscles, joints and lower extremities influence the ability to recover after having accidentally misplaced a foot, 'overshot' the mark or upset the balance in some other way. Impaired balance and recovery may become strikingly obvious as a problem *per se* on taking the history or during the course of the examination.

Problems on static testing

On strength assessment of the ankle invertors and evertors, the athlete is instructed to move the foot 'up and in' (tibialis anterior), 'down and in' (tibialis posterior) and 'down and out' (peroneus longus and brevis). There is sometimes an obvious hesitation on trying to move the foot into one or more of these directions on command. The muscle or muscles that present a problem on attempting to initiate a specific movement are usually those which ultimately turn out to be weak, in particular the left ankle evertors and right ankle invertors.

Not infrequently, the athlete cannot even muster a contraction of these muscles until given some tactile and/or visual feedback, repeated verbal cues and encouragement. One might therefore argue that impaired proprioception plays a role in the causation of this functional weakness.

Facilitation and inhibition are another factor; the athlete often cannot, for example, initiate a right gluteus maximus contraction in proper sequence with that of the hamstrings when gluteus maximus is inhibited – and weak – and the hamstrings facilitated – and strong (as well as being 'set to fire', so to speak). The question of 'causation' has already been discussed at some length in relation to the findings of asymmetry of lower extremity muscle strength and tension.

> A problem with balance is most often noted while carrying out the kinetic rotational or Gillet test for SI joint mobility, in which the athlete alternately ends up standing on only one leg.

When asked to bring the right knee up to the horizontal, there is usually not a moment's hesitation as the right thigh moves upwards in the sagittal plane, the body weight being balanced over a fairly straight left leg and minimal Trendelenburg sign being evident. In a small number of athletes, the attempt to carry out the same manoeuvre on the left side causes a problem. Most often, the weight-bearing right leg is noted to adduct, the trunk and pelvis simultaneously swaying, the trunk usually shifting to the left as the pelvis shifts outwards to the right (a compensated Trendelenburg gait; Fig. 3.85). Equilibrium is reached when the weight of the body is balanced over the right hip, with the leg somewhat adducted.

These changes may indicate a problem of transferring weight through the right SI joint, with impaired form and/or force closure (see Fig. 2.20). The system compensates by shifting the centre of gravity outwards to the right; shear stresses through the right SI joint are minimized by having vertical forces now run more directly down through the hip joint.

In some athletes, however, the sway may turn into an unmistakable wobble. They may even reach for support, suggesting that the right leg is weak or possibly that they are disorientated in terms of their position in space. A few are actually unable to carry out the manoeuvre at all. They may fail on repeated attempts and express the fear that they will lose their balance or that their right hip or knee will buckle and cause them to fall. This problem of imbalance on attempts to stand

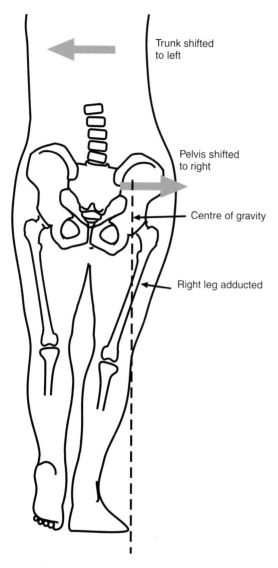

Trunk shifted
to left

Pelvis shifted
to right

Centre of gravity

Right leg adducted

Figure 3.85 Compensated right Trendelenburg gait. A problem with transfer of weight through the right sacroiliac joint as a result of impaired form or force closure is reduced or prevented by having the pelvis abduct and shift to the right so that the centre of gravity moves towards or directly over the right hip joint, thereby minimizing the vertical shear stress through the right sacroiliac joint.

on the right leg alone has so far been seen only in association with the 'alternate' presentations.

The author has to date seen only two athletes who had difficulty with stability when attempting to stand on the left leg alone without evidence of other pathology. One had a very abnormal gait pattern and even felt insecure during the left stance phase when walking.

The other noticed problems particularly when coming downstairs, the left knee feeling 'wobbly' as that leg started weight-bearing. Both had the left anterior and locked presentation.

The clinical findings suggest that the side of the instability may be determined by the pattern of malalignment, involving the left leg with 'left anterior and locked' and the right with 'alternate', presentations. The limited number of times this phenomenon has been observed with the 'left anterior and locked' presentation may reflect the fact that this pattern is so much less prevalent than 'alternate' presentations and that only a small number of those with rotational malalignment actually admit to a problem or show evidence of instability.

This instability cannot be explained on the basis of the functional weakness, given that the pattern of asymmetrical weakness involves muscles in the hip girdles and legs on both sides. Other factors to consider include:

- asymmetry of the lower extremity joint ranges of motion
- a probable asymmetry of proprioceptive input from the pelvic and lower extremity joints and soft tissues
- deficient kinaesthetic sensitivity of the ankle on the side of the instability (as discussed below); the knee and hip joint on this side could conceivably be affected in the same way
- an asymmetry of weight-bearing, the instability being on the side where the athlete tends towards pronation so that:
  - the foot and ankle are 'unlocked' and more mobile
  - the knee is placed under valgus stress and is not located directly over the foot
- instability of the SI joint due to ligamentous or osteoarticular damage, muscle weakness or impaired neural control, with a history suggestive of the 'slipping clutch' phenomenon (see below)
- deficient segmental or even central nervous system control.

Needless to say, a feeling of instability when weight-bearing on only one leg while participating in an athletic activity could invite disaster. Athletes probably learn to decrease the chance of this happening by tailoring their style to suit their specific problem. That still, however, leaves them open to mishap should they accidentally be forced to lead with, take off from or land on the 'shaky' leg. Consider the predicament of the ice hockey player who inadvertently ends up having to bear all the weight on the 'wrong', or unstable, leg while making a turn or attempting to shoot the puck.

All of us have patterns of movement that we can carry out feeling strong and confident; other patterns we perform feeling weak and insecure. Some of that may be caused by laterality, but the vast majority of the athletes who have a problem balancing on the right leg happen to be right-handed and right-footed, and might be expected to have a slightly stronger leg on that side. Following correction of the malalignment, the single-stance test is performed by most without hesitation or evidence of instability. This immediate improvement argues against the problem being one of laterality but makes it much more likely to be attributable to one or more of the changes seen in association with malalignment.

Problems on dynamic testing: gait examination

Regular walking, including heel- or toe-walking, rarely presents a problem. Attempting to hop on one foot while staying up on the toes may, however, prove difficult, if not impossible, when out of alignment.

The problem usually occurs on the side that tends to pronate; the foot and ankle feel insecure and collapse inwards. A definite medial whip of the heel is often evident on the pronating side (see Figs 3.20 and 3.36). In contrast, the foot on the side that tends to supinate provides a more stable base, hopping being carried out with greater ease; the heel usually remains in the midline (neutral) but sometimes actually whips outwards. The tendency for the pronating foot to whip inwards and the supinating foot to whip outwards, which may already have been evident on toe-walking, can usually be accentuated by hopping (see Fig. 3.20).

Instability of isolated joints on walking or running

When asked about 'weakness', athletes presenting with malalignment may recall a sensation of the hip or knee giving way, but examination usually fails to show any evidence of pathology of the hip or knee joint itself. The giving way is sometimes preceded by a sharp pain, possibly originating from one of the soft tissues or nerves that is already in trouble as a result of the malalignment:

- in the immediate vicinity of the knee joint (see Fig. 3.33)
- distant from the knee joint but able to refer to this area, for example, a referral from the femoral attachments of the hip articular ligaments (see Figs 3.62 and 4.3).

The pain causes a reflex relaxation of muscles responsible for supporting the joint, and the feeling of the joint 'giving way'. Reflex relaxation of the quadriceps, for example, makes the knee buckle; temporarily shutting down piriformis or gluteus maximus would have a similar effect on the hip joint, allowing it to collapse into flexion. The athlete may actually fall.

The 'slipping clutch' syndrome refers to the experience of an episodic giving way of one leg without any preceding pain (Dorman 1994, 1995, Dorman et al. 1998, Vleeming 1995a). The giving way occurs as the patient first puts weight on the affected leg, often on getting up after sitting for a while, but also as that side enters the stance phase during the walking cycle. The problem is felt to relate to a 'slight slippage due to failure of the force closure mechanism of the joint, which should occur normally at this moment' (Dorman 1997, p. 512) (Fig. 3.86). Although 'force closure' is mentioned, the problem is probably caused by a combination of:

1. a failure of the muscles that normally would help to stabilize the joint (force closure), in that the contraction is inadequate (e.g. muscle weakness) or occurs in an uncoordinated manner (e.g. impaired neural control)
2. a failure of the supporting ligaments, with a loss of the normal elasticity in the posterior sacroiliac ligaments (form closure).

Recovery is achieved through the combination of muscle strengthening and retraining for coordinated contraction, prolotherapy injections to tighten up the ligaments and ongoing efforts at achieving and maintaining realignment (see Ch. 7).

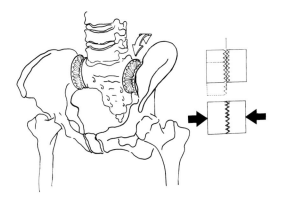

Figure 3.86 Whimsical depiction of sacroiliac joints with friction device. Failure can result in what has been called a 'slipping clutch' phenomenon, with a sensation of something giving way in the hip girdle region. (From Vleeming et al 1997, with permission.)

Athletes with a history of recurrent ankle sprains may not experience any preceding pain, or the pain may occur only rarely. If tenderness is present, it is usually limited to the lateral ankle ligaments and is hardly ever found in the peroneal muscles or tendons. There is sometimes an obvious precipitating event, such as stepping off a curb or onto a pebble, that causes inversion or eversion to occur, but the history often suggests that the ankle 'just gives way'. Ankle inversion sprains tend to be more common than eversion sprains, the left ankle being involved more often than the right.

The athletes are usually diagnosed as having a 'chronically unstable ankle', lengthening of the ligaments having occurred as a result of the previous sprains or strains; ligament lengthening and ankle instability may certainly be evident on clinical examination. In this author's experience, however, this is very often not the case. In those athletes with one of the 'alternate' presentations, passively moving the subtalar joint consistently reveals an actual limitation of left inversion, and an increase in left eversion compared with right side (see Fig. 3.23).

As previously indicated, in addition to an inability to muster a full-strength contraction of the right ankle invertors and left evertors, there is sometimes actually a problem with knowing how to move the right foot 'down and in' and the left 'down and out' on command. The problem can usually be overcome by providing tactile and other types of feedback. This suggests that, in the absence of any obvious ligament laxity, it is the functional weakness, possibly in combination with impaired proprioception and kinaesthetic awareness, that is responsible for the feeling of instability and results in a problem of insecure placement of the foot and ankle and a tendency to recurrent sprains.

This conjecture is supported by Lentell et al (1992), whose studies on subjects with chronically unstable ankles indicate that impaired balance is more of a problem than weakness of the ankle invertors and evertors. They report that strength studies failed to show a significant difference between the involved and the uninvolved side. A modified Romberg test, however, revealed differences in gross balance between the two extremities in the majority of subjects. These authors concluded that:

muscular weakness is not a major contributing factor to the chronically unstable ankle [and that] the findings do support the presence of proprioceptive deficits associated with this condition. (p. 85)

Their advice was to make proprioceptive activities a primary consideration in the management of this condition.

Reports by others (Freeman et al 1965, Garn & Newton 1988, Glencross & Thornton 1981) have all remarked on the apparent proprioceptive deficits and the need to improve kinaesthetic awareness in these individuals. It does not appear that the subjects were classified according to alignment status in any of these studies.

> Unfortunately, if a coexisting problem of malalignment is responsible for the functional weakness and apparent proprioceptive impairment, activities to improve ankle strength and kinaesthetic awareness, without a simultaneous correction of the malalignment, may fail to improve matters significantly, if at all.

Given that the ligaments often do not show instability in those presenting with malalignment, how can they 'malfunction' – in terms of impaired proprioception and kinaesthetic awareness – in order actually to lead to recurrent ankle inversion sprains? Suppose that the medial part of the runner's left foot has just landed on a rock or curb that inadvertently tilts the left foot into increased lateral weight-bearing. This results in a sudden increase in tension in the lateral ankle ligaments and would normally trigger a barrage of proprioceptive signals to quickly activate the ankle evertors. The timely, strong contraction of these muscles would usually counter any further inversion and avert possible injury. For some reason, however, the sequence fails, and an ankle inversion sprain or strain results. The following are some explanations to consider:

1. There may be a malalignment-related *functional weakness of the peroneal muscles*.

2. *A failure or delay of peroneal muscle contraction may be occurring*. Perhaps the tendency to supination on the left, resulting from the malalignment, puts these ligaments constantly under stretch and 'fatigues' the stretch receptors so that when they are suddenly put under an even greater load, they fail to respond appropriately. Some of the mechanoreceptors may no longer respond, or they may respond at varying rates, so that the duration of the signal is increased but its strength (amplitude) decreased. The signal generated may be too weak to trigger an 'all or none' contraction of the ankle evertors. Alternatively, the formation of the signal may be delayed so that by the time it finally triggers a muscle contraction, it is too late to be of use. The strength of the actual contraction achieved may be inadequate because of the functional weakness.

3. There is *temporary ligament deafferentation*. In those athletes presenting with malalignment who do not have any evidence of ligament laxity, the feeling of

instability and the weakness of the left ankle evertors usually disappears with realignment. The 'kinaesthetic deficit' in these athletes may be occurring on the basis of a temporary deafferentation.

4. There is some *joint instability* related to the malalignment. With malalignment, there is frequently a detectable instability of the right SI joint that is abolished or decreased with realignment. This phenomenon may affect other joints as well but may not be as easily detectable, or it may just not be looked for on the examination.

The problem of recurrent right ankle inversion sprains, relating to the increased varus angulation just as the foot touches the ground, has been discussed above (see Fig. 3.22).

Clinical correlation

Balance plays a major role in ensuring a stable landing from a jump or dismount. When the athlete sways momentarily, or even has to take a small step to aid recovery, we talk in terms of the athlete having lost his or her 'footing'. Could it be that often the problem is actually caused by an unstable leg, the one the athlete may also prove to have trouble standing on when carrying out the kinetic rotational or single-leg stance test? Maybe this leg sometimes simply 'gives way' when suddenly having to bear weight on landing.

The 'slipping clutch' phenomenon offers another possible explanation. This 'loss of balance' may often be just another manifestation of how the changes associated with malalignment can interfere with athletic performance. It would be more of a problem in those sports in which the athlete has to land on one leg (e.g. figure-skating). In order to avoid the mishaps that might otherwise occur, this 'instability' could conceivably lead to a leg preference and/or a habit of approaching the task repeatedly from the same side.

Sports such as fencing, karate and judo involve 'lunging' or rapidly moving one foot forward in a straight line (see Figs 5.8 and 5.11D). Maximum stability derives from the placement of the knee directly over the advancing foot. A malalignment-related shift off centre to right or left decreases stability and may prove costly at a time when this foot is supporting most of the athlete's weight (see Ch. 5).

Some moves in sports such as karate and judo require a rapid rotation of the body while supported on just one leg. The roundhouse kick, for example, requires balancing on one foot at a time when the body is rotating to develop the momentum required to deliver a good blow with the other leg (see Fig. 5.12B,

C). Many athletes find it easier to make the turn supported on the one rather than the other leg. This may relate to a feeling of stability when supported on that leg (usually the left), rather than leg dominance. Other factors may be the asymmetries of pelvic and lower extremity ranges of motion.

UPSLIP AND DOWNSLIP OF THE SACROILIAC JOINT

> Apart from rotational malalignment, the other common presentation of asymmetric malalignment is that associated with sacroiliac joint displacement in the vertical plane.

In one of the author's studies of 122 athletes seen in succession at the office, none presented with a downslip (W. Schamberger, unpublished data, 1992). Twelve per cent presented with an upslip alone, whereas in another 9%, an upslip became evident following the correction of a rotational malalignment; that is, in 9% the presence of the upslip was masked by a coexisting rotational malalignment. Therefore, the combined total of those presenting with an upslip was 21%. The upslip was on the right in 85% of cases and on the left in 15%. On initial examination, 13% in the 1993 and 6% in the 1994 study presenting with malalignment had an upslip only, all being on the right side. The number of upslips masked by a coexisting rotational malalignment is not known for the 1993 and 1994 cohorts because the initial correction of the rotational malalignment was not performed by the author.

Downslips obviously occur less frequently than upslips and will not be discussed further other than to note that they are usually diagnosed when the athlete fails to respond to treatment that would normally be appropriate for a supposed 'upslip' on one side, eventually raising doubts about the diagnosis, leading to a reassessment and then treatment aimed at correcting the downslip present on the other side (see Ch. 2).

MALALIGNMENT SYNDROME ASSOCIATED WITH SACROILIAC JOINT UPSLIP

The malalignment syndrome seen in association with an upslip is in large part the same as that seen with the 'alternate' presentations of rotational malalignment. Similarities and salient differences will be discussed briefly at this time under the same headings as for rotational malalignment. Unless otherwise stated, it is assumed that there is no associated anatomical LLD.

Asymmetry of pelvic orientation in the frontal plane. Upwards translation of the innominate relative to the sacrum results in an elevation of all the anterior and posterior bony landmarks – PSIS, ASIS, pubic rami and pelvic crest – on the side of the upslip relative to the other side (see Fig. 2.39). This shift, which includes a 2–3 mm step deformity at the symphysis pubis, is best observed in supine- and prone-lying (see Fig. 2.43A, B).

The upslip is associated with rotation of the pelvis in the frontal plane. With a right upslip, the iliac crest is high on the right side in standing, sitting and lying prone. With a left upslip, the right iliac crest is, interestingly, also usually high in both standing and sitting, and the left crest high in lying prone (see Fig. 2.43B).

With an upslip in isolation, there is no rotation of the innominates in the sagittal plane, nor is there torsion of the sacrum. When the upslip coexists with a rotational malalignment, the asymmetries caused by the rotation will be evident on examination. The step deformity of the pubic bones, with the usual downwards displacement on the side of the anterior rotation, may, however, be decreased or not even discernible when there is a coexisting upslip on the side of the anterior rotation. Similarly, the downwards placement of the ASIS may be less obvious, but the upwards movement of the PSIS accentuated, on this side. Correction of the rotation will reveal the underlying upslip.

Pelvic orientation and movement in the transverse plane. On standing, there may be some minimal rotation in the transverse plane evident, causing the pelvis to protrude slightly forward, on the right or left side (see Fig. 3.4A). The actual range of motion in the transverse plane is, however, symmetrical on right and left (unlike those with rotational malalignment, who show a restriction into the side of the posterior rotation; see Fig. 3.4C).

Sacroiliac joint mobility. The innominate moving upwards relative to the sacrum may have 'jammed' the SI joint upwards in the vertical plane. There is, however, usually no restriction of mobility noted on the sacral flexion and extension, kinetic rotational (Gillet) and SI joint stress tests.

Curvature of the lumbar, thoracic and cervical segments. The pelvis will be high on the right side in standing and sitting. The combined results of 17 athletes presenting with a right upslip in the 1993 and 1994 study showed the curve in the lumbar segment to be convex to the high side in 53% and to the low side in 47%. Data from those presenting with a left upslip seem to indicate a similar 50/50 distribution.

In all cases, the lumbar curve reverses at the thoracolumbar junction to give rise to a thoracic curve convex in the opposite direction, with a further reversal that can happen anywhere in the upper thoracic spine, usually at the cervicothoracic junction. As with rotational malalignment, any asymmetry of head and neck movement usually involves a limitation of right rotation and left side-bending (see Fig. 3.9).

Asymmetry of the thorax, shoulder girdle and arms. The findings are similar to those noted with the 'alternate' presentations of rotational malalignment (see Fig. 3.15).

Asymmetry of lower extremity orientation. The pattern is similar to that noted with the 'alternate' presentations: external rotation of the right, and internal rotation of the left, lower extremity.

Asymmetry of foot alignment, weight-bearing and shoe wear. This is the same as seen with the 'alternate' presentations, with a shift usually to right pronation and left supination.

Asymmetry of lower extremity muscle tension. The asymmetry that results with an upslip appears to be in the same pattern as that associated with rotational malalignment. There is, for example, increased tension in the left gluteus medius/minimus and TFL/ITB complex, limiting left hip adduction on Ober's test (see Fig. 3.40). This would support the conjecture that the asymmetry of tension is not determined by the actual presentation of pelvic malalignment but by spinal segmental or cortical factors.

The upslip itself may be the result of an asymmetry in muscle tension. A left upslip may, for example, result from an increase in tension in the left quadratus lumborum or iliopsoas (see Fig. 2.40). This increase in tension may in turn be attributable to:

- muscle injury
- increased irritability, injury or irritation of the nerve supply with vertebral malrotation (commonly involving L1 and less often L2 or L3) and secondary facilitation
- a protective splinting reaction, such as occurs in reaction to pain from the SI joints themselves or from ligaments (e.g. iliolumbar) put under strain by malalignment.

Asymmetry of lower extremity muscle strength. The asymmetry is similar to that noted in association with the 'alternate' presentations (see Appendix 4).

Bulk. Numbers are insufficient to comment regarding bulk.

Asymmetry of ligament tension. Tenderness of one or more of the posterior pelvic ligaments (iliolumbar, posterior SI joint and sacrotuberous) can be seen on one or both sides in association with a right or left upslip. Some ligaments will end up in a shortened position, for example, the ipsilateral iliolumbar ligaments: if these ligaments contract with time, they may become a problem on correction of the upslip until their proper length has finally been restored.

The tension in several ligaments will increase because:

- the upwards shift of one innominate relative to the sacrum separates their origin and insertion; in particular, the ipsilateral sacrospinous ligament, central and inferior parts of the anterior and posterior SI joint ligaments, and the long dorsal SI ligament are affected in this way (see Figs. 2.2, 2.3 and 2.16).
- there is an element of rotation in the frontal plane, which can affect the posterior pelvic ligaments on either side.

Asymmetry of lower extremity ranges of motion. Hip flexion and extension are usually both symmetrical, but passive hip extension is occasionally decreased on the side of the upslip. This may reflect the increase in tension in the ipsilateral rectus femoris. The other hip ranges of motion, and those at the ankles, are asymmetrical in the same pattern as with 'alternate' presentations of rotational malalignment.

Apparent leg length difference. On the side of the upslip, the leg is drawn upwards along with the innominate. Assuming an anatomically equal leg length, the athlete will now have a short leg evident on that side. The difference in length may amount to no more than 3–5 mm but is usually easily discernible in both long-sitting and supine-lying, the difference remaining the same in both positions (see Fig. 2.52). Since an anatomical LLD in isolation will also present with one leg short by the same amount in both positions, the pointers in Box 3.9 should be remembered.

MALALIGNMENT SYNDROME AS SEEN WITH OUTFLARE AND INFLARE

As previously indicated, only some features of the malalignment syndrome are seen with outflare and inflare (see Figs 2.10 and 2.14).

Asymmetry of pelvic orientation in the frontal plane. The pelvis is level.

Pelvic orientation and movement in the transverse plane. The pelvis rotates toward the side of the outflare so that the ASIS on that side moves backwards and that on the side of inflare forwards as observed in standing and lying supine. The PSIS will, however, have rotated in the opposite direction.

> **Box 3.9** Effect of leg length difference on the diagnosis of upslip
>
> - The diagnosis of an upslip should never be based on the finding of a leg length difference (LLD) on the long-sitting and supine-lying test alone; always check the position of the pelvic landmarks as well, which will:
>   - all be up, both anteriorly and posteriorly, on the side of an upslip
>   - all be in their normal positions and symmetrical when one is dealing with an anatomical LLD.
> - An anatomical LLD, long on the side of the upslip, could compensate for, or even exceed, the shortening of the leg that has occurred because of the upslip; the pelvic landmarks will, however, all still be raised on the side of the upslip, and the pelvic obliquity will persist in sitting and lying.
> - Other than by way of a comparison of the height of the femoral heads on an X-ray taken in standing, the presence or absence of an anatomical LLD is best established accurately after correction of the upslip.
> - The right iliac crest is high in standing and sitting, both with a right and a left upslip, suggesting that some rotation in the frontal plane is common to both.

The trunk may rotate with the pelvis, backwards on the side of the outflare and forwards on the side of the inflare but more often faces straight forward and thereby makes the rotation of the pelvis more easily evident even during walking and running.

The athlete may report that when walking, and particularly when running, there is a sensation of the pelvis and trunk constantly rotating towards the side of the outflare, which they are in fact actually doing. It seems easier to swing the leg forwards on the inflare and stride backwards on the outflare side, as a result of the reorientation of the acetabula. The athlete may actually be aware of a persistent 'block' to the pelvis rotating towards the side of the inflare and of a problem achieving the same unhindered swing phase on the outflare side.

Sacroiliac joint mobility. No locking and no instability relating simply to the outflare and inflare are observed (unlike rotational malalignment, in which the displacement of the joint surfaces alone results in some instability even in the absence of actual ligament laxity or muscle weakness).

Curvature of the lumbar, thoracic and cervical segments. There is a torsional effect on the spine as a result of rotation of the lumbar and thoracic spine in one direction, with reversal at the cervicothoracic junction (see above).

Asymmetry of the thorax, shoulder girdle and arms. The thorax usually compensates by rotating in the opposite direction to the pelvis (see above) to the point that the trunk, neck and head of the athlete ends up facing forward. Shoulder and arm ranges of motion are symmetrical.

Asymmetry of lower extremity orientation. Right outflare and left inflare result in a reorientation of the acetabula, creating a block primarily to:

- right hip flexion, adduction and straight leg raising
- left hip extension and abduction.

The clockwise rotation of the pelvis results in passive external rotation of the right leg and internal rotation of the left, as observed in supine-lying. The reverse findings are seen with an inflare.

Asymmetry of foot alignment, weight-bearing and shoe wear. Those will be influenced by the position of the legs on weight-bearing and any passive internal or external rotation during the stance phase.

Asymmetry of lower extremity muscle tension. There is no indication of the asymmetrical pattern of tension seen with rotational malalignment and upslip.

Asymmetry of lower extremity muscle strength. There is no evidence of the asymmetrical pattern of weakness seen with rotational malalignment and upslip.

Bulk. Numbers are insufficient to comment regarding muscle bulk.

Asymmetry of ligament tension. Tension in most of the pelvic ligaments is affected by the following.

Outflare. The pelvis on this side 'opens up', so to speak: the innominate, 'hinged' at the SI joint, moves outwards and opens the SI joint anteriorly while closing it posteriorly. Posterior landmarks, such as the PSIS and PIIS, move medially, whereas anterior landmarks, such as the ASIS, move laterally.

The shift results in increased tension in the ipsilateral anterior SI joint capsule and ligaments, the deep iliolumbar ligaments, and across the symphysis pubis in particular (see Figs 2.2A, B, 2.3, 3.59 and 3.61), whereas tension is decreased in the sacrospinous ligament, the ipsilateral posterior SI joint ligaments, interosseous ligaments and long (dorsal) sacrotuberous and long (dorsal) sacroiliac ligaments (see Figs 2.3, 2.4, 2.10Aiii and 2.16).

Inflare. The front of the innominate moves inwards, opening the SI joint posteriorly while closing it anteriorly. Posterior landmarks move laterally, anterior ones medially. Tension decreases in the ipsilateral anterior SI joint capsule and ligaments, the deep iliolumbar ligaments and across the symphysis pubis, whereas tension increases in the sacrospinous ligament, long (dorsal) sacrotuberous and ipsilateral long (dorsal) sacroiliac ligaments, interosseous ligaments and posterior SI joint ligaments.

The more common presentation of a right outflare, left inflare would therefore result in an associated increase in tension primarily in right anterior and left posterior ligaments (see Fig. 2.10A).

Asymmetry of lower extremity ranges of motion. See 'Asymmetry of lower extremity orientation' above.

Apparent leg length difference. Leg length is equal, provided there is no anatomical LLD.

COMBINATIONS OF ASYMMETRIES

Athletes not infrequently present with combinations of asymmetries, and the findings on examination may at first be confusing. The choice of treatment and the prognosis are very much dependent on an accurate assessment. Keep in mind the following:

- Between approximately 10% and 20% of athletes have a coexisting rotational malalignment and upslip.
- Rotational malalignment is much more common than an isolated upslip (5:1 to 6:1), approximately 80–90% of these being right, and 10–20% left, innominate anterior. Clinically, a left upslip appears more common than a right one. About 5–10% can switch sides, so that an upslip, anterior or posterior rotation, or outflare/inflare may be evident on one side at one time, on the opposite side at another time or split between the two sides in varying patterns on different occasions (e.g. right anterior innominate, left upslip).
- Approximately 10% have an anatomical LLD that will affect the findings associated with a coexisting malalignment.

The following approach should make it relatively easy to sort out any combination.

1. First establish whether there is any pelvic obliquity in standing. If there is, and if it is abolished in sitting, the obliquity is most likely to be caused by an anatomical LLD.

2. If the obliquity is not abolished in sitting, malalignment is probably present. Persistent obliquity attributable to a difference in the development of the two sides of the pelvis is a rather rare cause, one which could be confirmed by X-ray studies if that is felt to be necessary.

3. Next, examine the athlete in both the long-sitting and supine-lying positions.

- The leg on the side of an upslip will be short in both positions to an equal extent, and all the pelvic landmarks will have been moved upwards on this side. Remember that a right and left upslip both show

the pelvis high on the right side in standing (and sitting). Therefore, the short leg on the long-sitting and supine-lying test is actually ipsilateral to the side that is high in standing in the case of a right upslip and contralateral in the case of a left upslip.

- An anatomical short leg will also be short in both positions to an equal extent. The short-leg side, however, corresponds to the side on which the pelvis is low in standing, and the pelvic landmarks will be symmetrical in sitting and lying.

- If there is a combination of an upslip and an anatomical LLD, one may cancel the other so that there may or may not be an evident leg length difference. The pelvic obliquity in standing may be similarly affected. Whatever the resulting length of the legs, it will remain the same in the long-sitting and supine-lying positions. Any persistent pelvic obliquity will continue to be evident in both sitting and lying, with persistent elevation of all the pelvic landmarks on the side of the upslip.

- With an outflare/inflare, the pelvis will be level and the leg length equal. When lying supine, however, the ASIS will appear down and out from midline on the side of the outflare, and up and in towards the midline on the side of the inflare. The findings will be reversed for the PSIS in prone-lying.

- If the difference in leg length changes on moving from the long-sitting to the supine-lying position, one is most likely dealing with a rotational malalignment (which may or may not be hiding a coexisting upslip, anatomical LLD or both). Barring complicating factors (see Ch. 2), the leg that lengthens on supine-lying probably indicates the side of the anterior innominate rotation, but this needs to be confirmed by finding a complete asymmetry of all the pelvic landmarks. Which leg actually ends up being the longer or shorter one on this test is irrelevant. The true leg length will not become apparent until any malalignment (rotational or upslip) present has been corrected.

4. Examine the relative position of the pelvic landmarks in supine- and prone-lying.

- With an anatomical LLD, the anterior and posterior landmarks on the right and left side will be symmetrical.

- An upslip results in an elevation of all the ipsilateral landmarks.

- Rotational malalignment results in a complete asymmetry of landmarks on anterior/posterior and right/left comparison.

- The landmarks for outflare/inflare will appear as described in 3 above.

The next chapter will explore some of the pain phenomena and medical problems commonly associated with the malalignment syndrome.

4

Related pain phenomena and medical problems

One facet of the malalignment syndrome is the asymmetrical stress on soft tissues and joints that can eventually result in predictable sites of tenderness to palpation. With time, or as the result of a superimposed acute insult, overt localized and/or referred pain symptoms may arise from these tender structures. The altered biomechanics also results in some commonly recognized pain patterns, injuries and 'syndromes' being seen with increased frequency in association with malalignment; right patello-femoral compartment syndrome is just one example (see below).

Treatment is unfortunately often limited to the specific site of tenderness or pain, or to the particular pain syndrome, because of a failure to realize that these are but part of a greater entity: the malalignment syndrome. Correct the malalignment and the associated pain phenomena will often disappear spontaneously or with little need for additional treatment. Some common clinical conditions (e.g. idiopathic scoliosis) are unfavourably affected by coexisting malalignment. In addition, symptoms resulting from malalignment can sometimes mimic clinical problems typically related to one or more of the major systems of the body. The confusion that can result when trying to establish a diagnosis may result in needless and sometimes costly and even dangerous investigations, and can lead to inappropriate treatment.

PAIN CAUSED BY AN INCREASE IN SOFT TISSUE TENSION

A malalignment-related increase in tension involving muscle, ligament, capsule or fascia can occur by different mechanisms. To summarize, these include:

- an increase in the length-to-tension ratio with any increase in the distance between the origin and insertion

- the torsion of a vertebral, pelvic or appendicular bone relative to another
- facilitation and inhibition, noted to occur in specific muscles in an asymmetrical pattern
- an attempt to splint a painful or unstable area
- the associated functional leg length difference (LLD).

The first four mechanisms have been discussed in detail in Chapter 3 under 'Asymmetry of muscle tension' (see Figs 3.38–3.48). An LLD affects tension in both static and dynamic situations. Take the example of an athlete whose right side of the pelvis is higher than the left when standing. There may be a static increase in tension in right hip abductor muscles and the tensor fascia lata/iliotibial band (TFL/ITB) complex because the downwards drop of the pelvis on the left side increases the distance between the origin and insertion of these structures on the right (Fig. 4.1A). When weight-bearing on the short left leg during a walk or run, the left hip abductors have to work harder in order to minimize any drop of the pelvis on the right, perhaps even to raise the pelvis further on the right side, in order to allow the long right leg to clear the ground without hindrance on swing-through (Fig. 4.1B).

The structures that most consistently show an increase in tension and/or tenderness as a result of these various mechanisms relating to malalignment are shown in Box 4.1.

With time, any soft tissue subjected to an increase in tension because of malalignment is likely to become tender to palpation (DonTigny 1986, Midttun & Bojsen-Moller 1986). That structure may eventually develop an aching discomfort or outright pain often characterized as a deep, achy bone pain. Mechanisms that can precipitate pain include:

1. a chronic increase in tension (particularly as it affects the muscles, which are supposed to contract

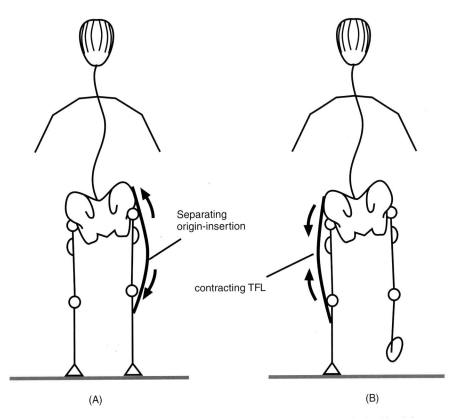

Figure 4.1 Effect of functional leg length difference (right leg long in standing) on tension in the hip abductors and tensor fascia lata/iliotibial band complex. Tension increases on right in standing (A) as the origin and insertion are separated and muscle contraction counteracts the drop of the pelvis to the left side; the athlete can compensate by shifting the pelvis to right (see Fig. 3.85). Tension increases on left side when walking or running (B) as the abductors contract to keep the right side of pelvis elevated and to help with clearance of the 'long' right leg. (A) Static – stand (tense right). (B) Dynamic – walk, run (tense left).

> **Box 4.1** Structures showing an increase in tension and/or tenderness
>
> - **Muscles** (see Fig. 3.39)
>   - right infraspinatus and/or teres minor
>   - the thoracic paravertebral muscles, especially adjacent to sites of vertebral malrotation and curve reversal (e.g. the thoracolumbar junction)
>   - piriformis, particularly the right one with right anterior rotation
>   - iliopsoas, particularly the left one with left posterior rotation
>   - the left hip abductors and the TFL/ITB complex
>   - the right hamstrings
>   - the left gastrocnemius/soleus complex
> 2. **Ligaments** (see Figs 2.2, 2.3, 2.16 and 3.57–3.63)
>   - the iliolumbar and sacrotuberous ligaments, and those crossing the posterior sacroiliac joint (often bilaterally)
>   - the long dorsal (or posterior) sacroiliac ligaments (see Fig. 2.16B)
>   - the lumbosacral intervertebral ligaments and facet joint ligaments

> **Box 4.2** Causes of pain on palpation in joint upslip and rotational malalignment
>
> - A chronic increase in tension in a specific soft tissue structure (e.g. joint capsule, muscle, tendon or ligament)
> - Unevenly distributed or excessive pressure within and around the joints, particularly those which are weight-bearing and/or subjected to a torsional stress by malalignment (e.g. the hip and knee joints; Fig. 4.3 and see Figs 3.33, 3.74 and 3.75)
> - An irritation or injury of the nerve roots and peripheral nerves as a result of a chronic increase in traction, compression or a combination of these forces (see Fig. 3.33 and 'Implications for neurology and neurosurgery' below).
> - A referral of pain to sites distant from the affected structure (see Figs I.2, 3.10, 3.41, 3.58, 3.62 and 4.10)

and relax, and ligaments, whose nerve supply cannot elongate as well as the elastic components can)

2. a further increase in tension:
– acute, such as with a sudden movement
– chronic, such as with increased demand during athletic activity (e.g. running longer distances or up and down hill)

3. the tense structure being 'strung' over a bony or other elevation, possibly even 'snapping' across that prominence (e.g. the TFL over the greater trochanter and the ITB over the lateral femoral condyle – see Fig. 3.37; or iliopsoas/pectineus over the anterior aspect of the hip joint – Fig. 4.2; see Figs 2.31, 2.40 and 3.38).

The long-term resolution of the pain from these structures will depend primarily on the resolution of the abnormal tension, which in turn depends on the correction of the malalignment and the maintenance of realignment.

SPECIFIC SITES OF PAIN RELATED TO MALALIGNMENT

The sometimes very specific and often predictable patterns of pain and tenderness to palpation seen in association with sacroliac (SI) joint upslip and rotational malalignment are primarily the result of the four factors outlined in Box 4.2.

Therefore, even though the athlete may be asymptomatic, examination will usually reveal tenderness localizing to specific structures that are put under stress by the malalignment. This athlete must be considered at increased risk of developing an overtly painful condition with any activity that inadvertently results in an additional stress on any of these sites.

Acutely. Even a minor lifting or twisting action that exerts a further traction or compression force on such an asymptomatic but tender structure may convert it into one that is now frankly painful. The athlete is often diagnosed as having sustained a 'sprain' or 'strain'.

On a chronic or repetitive basis. The athlete may also become symptomatic when even a minor increase in stress is superimposed on such a site on a chronic or repetitive basis. An athlete with one of the 'alternate' presentations may, for example, be asymptomatic but on examination show increased tension and tenderness in the left hip abductors and TFL/ITB complex, attributable to the combined effect of the malalignment-related:

- automatic increase in tension in this complex on the left side through facilitation
- shift to left lateral weight-bearing.

If the athlete now increases the number of miles walked or run on surfaces with a slope banked down to the left (e.g. running against the traffic in Canada or the USA, or with the traffic in the UK; or walking clockwise on a hillside), the left lateral shift, and the tendency towards supination and genu varum on this side, will be accentuated (Fig. 4.4A; see Figs 3.27 and 3.32). The increase in mileage added to these increased left lateral traction forces may, with time, make the already tender left hip abductors and TFL/ITB

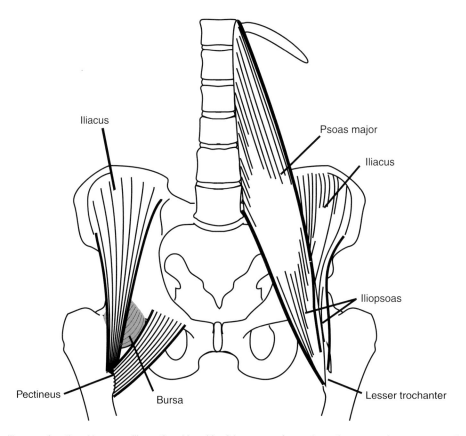

Figure 4.2 Iliopsoas/pectineal bursa or iliopectineal bursitis. A bursa can form where these muscles run across the prominence of the anterior hip joint. An increase in muscle tension can result in a painful bursitis and/or the feeling of something (the muscles) snapping across the anterior hip joint area. For example (A) repetitive hip flexion/extension, or (B) tightening of the iliopectineal complex, either (i) actively when they contract to externally rotate the leg, or (ii) on passive internal rotation of the leg.

complex overtly symptomatic. Increasing the amount of up and downhill running also puts more demand on this complex, but bilaterally; the more susceptible left complex is, however, again more likely to become symptomatic.

In essence, one is dealing with a type of 'overuse' injury. The athlete may get some relief running on a slope banked upwards to the left (Fig. 4.4B). Understandably, lateral traction forces are decreased with the left foot now on the upside and a straightening of the legs, possibly as well as some levelling of the pelvis if it is high on the right side because of the malalignment. This practice should not, however, be encouraged if it means going with the traffic (e.g in Canada and the USA).

Standard treatment measures that would be appropriate for a sprain or strain or an overuse injury are usually instituted. The injury in both cases may respond to

such treatment, and the pain subside with healing. Unfortunately, if the malalignment is not corrected at the same time, the athlete remains at increased risk of having the same injury recur on resuming the activity.

These injuries may also actually fail to respond to standard treatment measures as a result of ongoing malalignment.

> It appears that the persistence of chronic tension or compression forces attributable to malalignment can interfere with the ability of the tissue to heal following a superimposed acute or chronic injury.

In other words, recovery is slowed or may fail to occur until the stress caused by these forces is removed by realignment. Box 4.3 lists some ways in which the persistence of this stress could affect healing unfavourably.

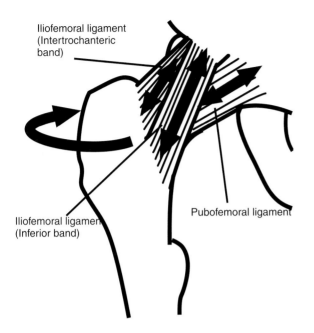

Iliofemoral ligament
(Intertrochanteric band)

Iliofemoral ligament
(Inferior band)

Pubofemoral ligament

Figure 4.3 Anterior hip joint capsule and iliofemoral and pubofemoral ligaments subjected to a torsional stress with malalignment-related external rotation of the right lower extremity (see also Figs 2.2 and 2.3).

Box 4.3 Negative effect of malalignment stresses on healing

- It interferes with the flow of blood needed for:
  - the delivery of oxygen, nutrients and scavenger and repair cells
  - the removal of damaged tissue and the clearance of waste.
- It perpetuates the inflammatory response (Willard 1995).
- Stretching a ligament results in excessive tension on the nerve fibres long before the connective tissue components because the nerve fibres have relatively less elasticity (Hackett 1956, 1958). The stretching can result in nerve irritation and eventually frank neuralgic pain and/or hypersensitivity. The insult to the nerves can then be perpetuated by even relatively minor ongoing traction or compression forces.
- Constant compression of the joint surfaces accelerates degeneration by interfering with cartilage nutrition and repair.

In summary, the recognition of the specific sites of tenderness and of the pain patterns typically associated with malalignment should:

1. raise the suspicion that malalignment is indeed present
2. prompt a search for other features of the malalignment syndrome

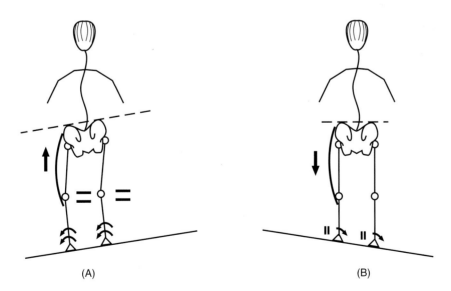

(A)   (B)

Figure 4.4 Effect of a slope on the increased tension in the left hip abductors and tensor fascia lata/iliotibial band complex that has already resulted with malalignment through facilitation and the shift in weight-bearing (right pronation and left supination). (A) A left downslope increases the tension by accentuating supination. (B) A left upslope decreases the tension by countering supination.

3. help to ensure appropriate treatment, the key component of this being realignment to remove any abnormal tension and/or compression forces and to promote healing.

COMMON PAIN SYNDROMES CAUSED OR AGGRAVATED BY MALALIGNMENT

A syndrome is a constellation of signs and symptoms attributable to a unifying cause. Although we may identify the syndrome and even recognize the cause, we must, however, always ask ourselves whether the syndrome or that cause may not be part of an even larger entity. A typical example is that of the athlete who presents with right knee pain of unknown origin. We may quickly arrive at a diagnosis of 'patellofemoral compartment syndrome' (PFCS) on the basis of the outward tracking of the patella on knee extension, a positive apprehension test and tenderness of the patellar tendon origin and the medial and lateral patellar facets. We have established patellofemoral compartment syndrome as the 'cause' of the pain, but it may really amount to no more than having established the 'location'. We have not answered the questions of 'what caused the PFCS to develop in the first place?', 'why at this time?' and 'why on the right side and not the left, or bilaterally?'

If we look further, we might note that this athlete pronates markedly with the right foot, causing the right knee to collapse into valgus on weight-bearing, whereas the left foot pronates less so, remains in neutral or may actually supinate. The right lower extremity is in obvious external rotation relative to the left.

By looking beyond the right knee and at the kinetic chain, we have established the reason for the pain: excessive external rotation coupled with right pronation and increased valgus stress on the right knee, with an increase of the Q-angle and lateral patellar tracking (Fig. 4.5; see Figs 3.33 and 3.74). The combined effect is to increase the tension in the patellofemoral complex, increasing the pressure with which the patella is forced onto the underlying femoral groove and condyles, and to decrease the accuracy with which the patellofemoral surfaces match as the patella tends to track laterally on extension.

Looking at the larger picture, we might find that this athlete actually presents with an upslip or one of the 'alternate' patterns of rotational malalignment, with the associated right external rotation, pronation and valgus stress (Fig. 4.5; see Figs 3.33 and 3.74). If the right side of the pelvis were higher than the left – which it is in about 80% of those with a rotational pre-

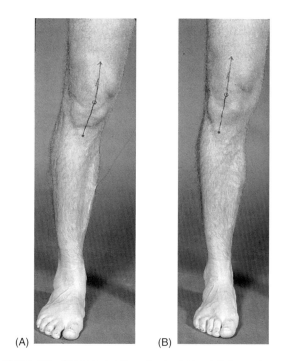

(A)   (B)

Figure 4.5   Stresses predisposing to right patellofemoral compartment syndrome. (A) With malalignment: the tendency towards pronation and knee valgus has increased the Q-angle to 10 degrees; the right patella now tracks more laterally on knee extension, increasing the stress on the compartment. (B) On realignment: the Q-angle is reduced to almost 0 degrees; improved patellar tracking (relatively straight up and down) decreases the stress on the compartment.

sentation and 100% with an upslip – the increase in pressure within the patellofemoral compartment could be compounded by keeping the right knee slightly flexed in an attempt to lower the pelvis on that side (see Fig. 2.59). Problems in the right knee may be further aggravated by a secondary wasting of vastus medialis (see Figs 3.52 and 3.53) and by the weakness attributable to an inhibition of the right hip flexors. Inhibition, for example, can result as right anterior innominate rotation decreases the tension in iliacus and rectus femoris by bringing their origins and insertions closer together (see Fig. 3.38).

MALALIGNMENT: IMPLICATIONS FOR MEDICINE

The patellofemoral syndrome discussed above did not represent just an isolated phenomenon but was an integral part of a larger entity, the malalignment syndrome, and so can it be with a number of other well known medical conditions. Malalignment is of significance for the following reasons.

1. Some clinical presentations may be unfavourably affected by coexisting malalignment. For example, those with idiopathic scoliosis may become sympto-

matic only whenever malalignment recurs (Fig. 4.6A). These symptoms presumably result from their attempts to compensate for the malalignment-related pelvic obliquity and the additional stresses that they now have to cope with, in particular the increased stress on:

– the thoracolumbar and lumbosacral junctions, which probably accounts for their frequent complaint

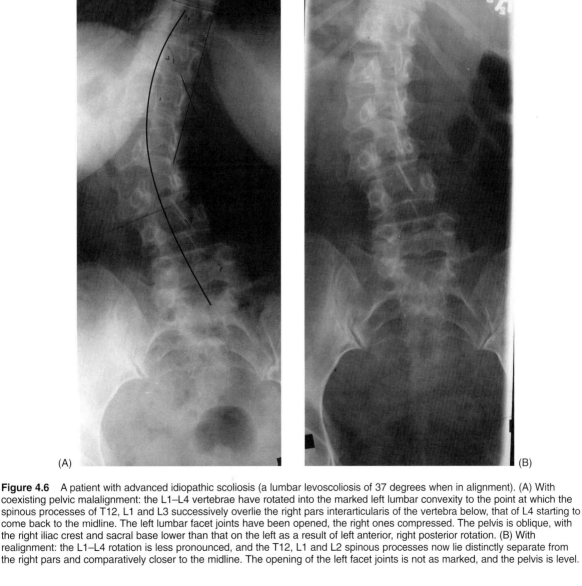

(A)   (B)

Figure 4.6   A patient with advanced idiopathic scoliosis (a lumbar levoscoliosis of 37 degrees when in alignment). (A) With coexisting pelvic malalignment: the L1–L4 vertebrae have rotated into the marked left lumbar convexity to the point at which the spinous processes of T12, L1 and L3 successively overlie the right pars interarticularis of the vertebra below, that of L4 starting to come back to the midline. The left lumbar facet joints have been opened, the right ones compressed. The pelvis is oblique, with the right iliac crest and sacral base lower than that on the left as a result of left anterior, right posterior rotation. (B) With realignment: the L1–L4 rotation is less pronounced, and the T12, L1 and L2 spinous processes now lie distinctly separate from the right pars and comparatively closer to the midline. The opening of the left facet joints is not as marked, and the pelvis is level.

of mid- and low back pain when they are out of alignment

– the facet joints and discs as a result of aggravation of L1–L4 rotation into the exacerbated lumbar convexity (Fig. 4.6A; see Figs 2.65 and 4.28).

2. Some of the structures that become tender and/or painful as a result of being put under increased stress, and some of their common referral sites, i.e. in close proximity to areas classically identified with problems in major organ systems. Both the deep ilio-lumbar and the anterior SI joint ligaments, for example, are capable of referring to McBurney's point and mimicking appendicitis.

3. Malalignment-related symptoms may mimic some common pain phenomena.

A failure to recognize these facets of the malalignment syndrome runs the risk of causing confusion, which may result in investigations that are at best harmless, albeit perhaps not required, and at worst costly or dangerous and may lead to misdiagnosis and inadequate or even inappropriate treatment. The following discussion will concentrate on more common pain phenomena and syndromes that may be attributable to malalignment or can be affected by the presence of malalignment, and on how these conditions may overlap with problems typically dealt with by some of the medical specialties.

IMPLICATIONS FOR CARDIOLOGY AND CARDIAC REHABILITATION

Chest pain of musculoskeletal origin is a complaint that can be related to malalignment, one that a cardiologist may have to differentiate from angina and other symptoms typical of coronary artery disease. In cardiac rehabilitation, musculoskeletal symptoms caused by malalignment are:

- responsible for some of the more frequently encountered complaints that staff have to deal with in exercise classes on a day-to-day basis
- one of the more common reasons for the temporary or permanent interruption of a patient's exercise programme.

As the following case studies of patients enrolled in a cardiac rehabilitation programme show, malalignment:

1. may not be a problem until the patient begins to exercise
2. may not be evident on initial examination but may develop with exercise

3. can result in needless investigation and ongoing patient discomfort as a result of failure to suspect malalignment in the first place.

Case study

Mrs O.J.

- *History*: two myocardial infarcts in 1994; five-vessel coronary artery bypass graft in 1995; since then, occasional angina, brought on by effort and relieved by nitroglycerine spray
- *On referral*: in alignment; no musculoskeletal problems noted
- *Course*: 4 weeks after starting the programme, complained of interscapular pain when using the rower
- *Findings*: T8 vertebral body rotated to the right; acute pain on trunk extension, flexion and especially rotation while sitting, as well as with direct pressure on the T8 spinous process
- *Treatment*: realignment of T8 resolved the problem

Case study

Mr D.S.

- *History*: myocardial infarcts in 1997 at age 49; going on to five-vessel coronary artery bypass graft
- *On referral*: no musculoskeletal complaints; malalignment of the pelvis and spine, but no indication of tenderness anywhere
- *Course*: has to date managed to increase the exercise level without a problem; the malalignment has not therefore needed correction

---

Case study

Mrs M.M.

- *History*: myocardial infarct 1995, one-vessel coronary artery bypass graft in 1996
- *Discharge clinic* (1997): note made that programme had been started in August 1996 but was interrupted from 18 December to 29 January 1997 because of 'low back pain', now localized to the right sacroiliac joint
- *Findings*: pelvic malalignment (right anterior rotation); also rotation of T7; tenderness localizing to the left 7th costochondral junction and the ligaments crossing the posterior aspect of the right sacroiliac joint
- *Course*: realignment of the pelvis and spine resolved the pain

---

Case study

Mrs K.M.

- *History*: pulmonary hypertension requiring the repair of an atrioseptal defect; for 3 months postoperatively, ongoing tightness of the sternotomy scar area and discomfort in the left anterior chest region, leading to $30 000 of repeat investigations (including cardiac catheterization), which were negative
- *Findings*: acutely tender bilateral 4th and 5th costochondral junctions (those on the left corresponding to her site of pain); left rotation of the T6 vertebra with displacement of the 4th, 5th and 6th ribs bilaterally (similar to the T5 malrotation in Fig. 2.63); malalignment of the pelvis and spine
- *Course*: 'cardiac' symptoms resolved on realignment combined with massage of the anterior chest and thoracic paravertebral muscles

Typical 'cardiac' presentations of malalignment

Those involved in the care of patients with coronary artery disease should bear in mind that malalignment may cause the following problems that may be confused with symptoms precipitated by coronary artery disease.

Back pain

Particularly important is back pain arising from the sites of stress caused by:

- curve reversal (see Fig. 3.12)
  - mid-back pain from reversal at the thoracolumbar junction
  - upper back pain from reversal that occurs most frequently at the cervicothoracic junction but may occur in the upper thoracic spine and is then more likely to become a problem, leading to confusion with the symptoms of coronary artery disease (see Fig. 2.60)
- malrotation of any of the thoracic vertebrae, T4 and T5 being most likely to be involved and to cause pain by stressing the costovertebral and costotransverse joints in particular (see Figs. 2.63, 3.13 and 3.14).

Anterior chest pain that can mimic angina

There may be anterior chest pain from the irritation of one or more of the costochondral junctions:

- irritation of a junction caused by rib rotation or subluxation that may occur in isolation (e.g.

following trauma or from a severe cough), but is also seen in association with malrotation of one of the thoracic vertebrae (see Fig. 2.63)
- in those who have undergone open heart surgery, the vertebral rotation may itself represent a complication of the rib displacement that occurred with the sternotomy; unfortunately, the vertebral rotation has persisted and now perpetuates the rib displacement and the rotational stress on the costochondral junction(s), long after the sternotomy has healed.

Anterior chest pain can arise as a result of the excessive rotation of a clavicle and increased stress on:

- the sternoclavicular joint (see Fig. 2.63B)
- the acromioclavicular joint and the ligaments connecting the distal clavicle to the coracoid process, resulting in chest pain that is more anterolateral (Fig. 4.7).

Pain may radiate straight through to the anterior chest from the irritation of a disc, facet joint, costovertebral or costotransverse joint, or any other structure stressed by malrotation of one of the upper or mid-thoracic vertebrae, such as the ligaments coming off the C7 transverse process (Grieve 1986b; see Fig 3.10A, B5).

Recurrent right, left or central mid-chest discomfort may be attributable to increased irritability of the thoracic diaphragm and 'cramping' or spasm of that muscle triggered, for example, by:

- irritation of the roots supplying the phrenic nerve (C3, C4 and C5) by malrotation of one of the mid-cervical vertebra, or irritation of the nerve anywhere along its course (see Fig. 3.11)
- irritation of the autonomic nerve supply (e.g. because of cervical vertebral rotation or paravertebral muscle spasm triggering a hyper- autonomic response by irritation of the parasympathetic outflow tracts)
- increased tension on the diaphragm muscle caused by the shift of its attachments to the seventh to twelfth ribs that can occur with malrotation of any of the lower thoracic vertebrae.

Pain referred into one or other arm or to the jaw

Referral may occur from cervical spine ligaments and joints:

- in the occipito-atlanto-axial region: to the jaw and skull (see Figs 3.10A, B1)
- at the cervicothoracic junction: mainly in a C8/T1 pattern, to the medial arm and forearm and the fourth and fifth fingers, more likely to occur when there is a malrotation of C7 and T1 in addition to the stress of curve reversal at this junction (see Fig. 3.10A, B4)

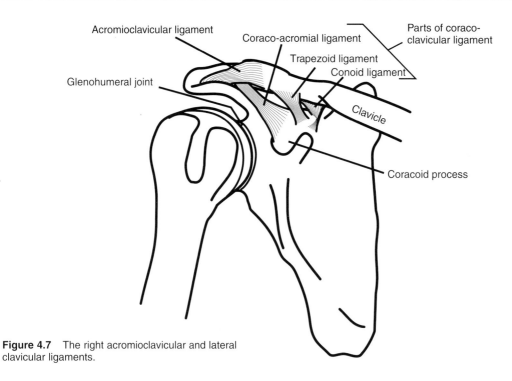

Figure 4.7 The right acromioclavicular and lateral clavicular ligaments.

There may be myofascial pain and trigger points in the neck and shoulder girdle:

- Localized pain from muscles, tendons, ligaments or fascia in this area can eventually develop with the chronic increase in tension that results with malalignment (e.g. pectoral or intercostal muscles splinting a painful costochondral junction), and with the development of trigger points in these tissues.
- A number of the shoulder girdle soft tissues that are put under increased stress by malalignment can give rise to pain referred to the areas classically associated with angina; for example, a trigger point in latissimus dorsi can also refer along the inner arm and forearm, down to the fourth and fifth fingers (Fig. 4.8).

As part of the 'T4 (or T3) syndrome' (see Ch. 5), malrotation of any of the vertebrae in the T3 to T7 region, but most often involving T3 or T4, can result in referred pain that typically involves the hand and fingers, and less often part or all of the arm, either uni- or bilaterally (in which case it is symmetrical) and/or parts of the head and neck (Fig. 4.9).

Angina coexisting with symptomatic malalignment

Typically seen is the patient with 'unstable' angina whose 'cardiac' symptoms may come on either at rest or with effort and may or may not respond to nitroglycerine spray, or may do so incompletely. One must always rule out the possibility that this is not someone whose symptoms at any one time may vary because:

1. recurrent angina triggers a further increase in muscle tension and precipitates symptoms related to the malalignment
2. angina may itself be triggered by the increase in the workload on the heart associated with the cardiovascular changes (e.g. the increase in blood pressure and heart rate) that occur as a result of pain caused by the malalignment.

When dealing with any cardiac patients, remember that symptoms that may be attributable to malalignment have to be considered in the differential diagnosis. Those who are already out of alignment on entering an exercise programme are at increased risk of becoming symptomatic or of aggravating their malalignment-related musculoskeletal symptoms. Becoming aware of malalignment, diagnosing it at the initial outpatient visit and treating it as if it were already symptomatic (or at least keeping an eye on it as the patient starts in the programme) would go a long way towards making participation in a cardiac rehabilitation programme more productive and enjoyable.

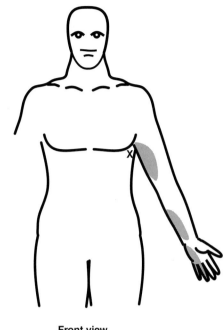

Front view

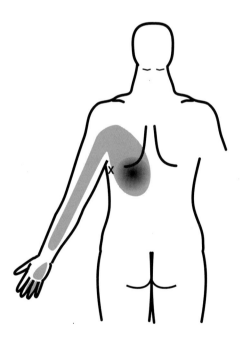

Back view

Figure 4.8 Referral pattern from trigger points (X) in latissimus dorsi. 'Spill-over' into the arm (light grey) can mimic a C8/T1 root problem or angina. (After Travell & Simons 1983, with permission.)

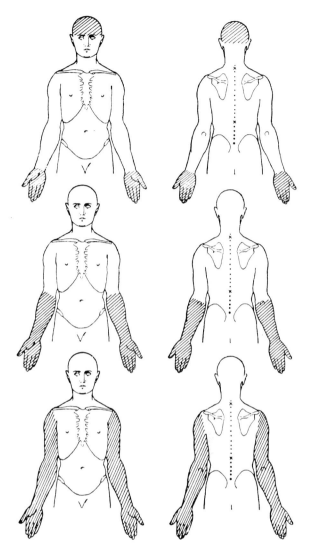

Figure 4.9 'T3' or 'T4' syndrome: common areas of upper limb symptoms. The upper diagram shows classical areas of head pain. (From McGuckin 1986, with permission.)

IMPLICATIONS FOR NEUROLOGY AND NEUROSURGERY

Malalignment can result in symptoms or signs that suggest an involvement of the neurological system, on the basis of:

- patterns of referred pain and paraesthesia that may mimic a root or peripheral nerve distribution
- nerve fibre traction or compression, caused mainly by shifts in weight-bearing and an asymmetry in muscle tension

- weakness of the lower extremity muscles in a pattern that may be confused with a root or peripheral nerve lesion
- seemingly positive root stretch tests, which, by further stressing structures already tender as a result of the malalignment (e.g. the SI joints and posterior pelvic ligaments) and by provoking back or buttock pain with radiation or referral to a leg, can mimic a root or plexus problem (Fig. 4.10; see Figs. I.2, 3.41 and 3.58).

These patients are frequently referred for neurological or neurosurgical consultation and for electrodiagnostic studies. However, unless the consultant is aware of the various presentations of malalignment and their 'neurological' implications, none of these examinations and investigations is likely to be very helpful other than to rule out a coexisting neurological lesion.

Once that has been done, the temptation is not infrequently to attribute the patient's problems to a catch-all diagnosis such as 'mechanical back pain'. Worse yet is to blame the patient of malingering, or to attach some unfavourable psychiatric associations, when in reality the patient's actual problem, namely symptoms and signs related to the presence of malalignment, has been overlooked because of a shortcoming in the clinician's diagnostic skills.

Referred patterns of pain and paraesthesias

Pain and paraesthesias can be referred to the dermatome, myotome and/or sclerotome that reflects the innervation of the structure that is the actual source of these symptoms. Hackett (1958) deserves special mention for his exquisite work of mapping these pat-

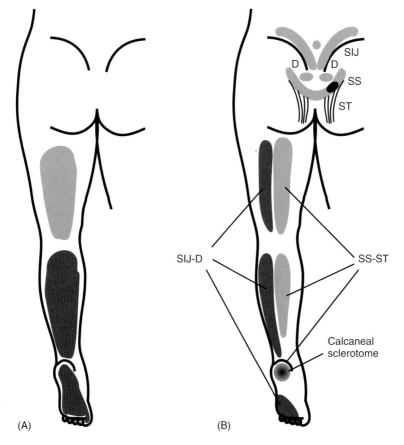

(A)   (B)

Figure 4.10 Nerve root versus referred pattern of dysaesthesias. (A) S1 radiculopathy pattern. (B) Referred pattern from lower posterior sacroiliac (SIJ-D), sacrotuberous (ST) and sacrospinous (SS) ligaments associated with sacroiliac joint instability. (After Hackett 1958, with permission.)

terns by injecting hypertonic saline into specific ligaments (see Fig. 3.10A). Travell & Simons (1983, 1992) did much to clarify the referral pattern of trigger points. Patterns originating from deteriorating discs, facet joints and inflamed or impinged tendons are also well documented (McCall et al 1979, Mooney & Robertson 1976, Travell & Simons 1992).

The stress imposed on numerous structures by malalignment frequently results in referred symptoms. Particularly common are paraesthesias in the form of altered sensation, in what may at first appear to be a 'non-anatomical' distribution in terms of not fitting a root or peripheral nerve pattern. An area often involved is the anterior aspect of one or other thigh, which can reflect a referral from the ligaments crossing the upper aspect of the posterior SI joint (see 'A' in Fig. 3.58A). The athlete may report feeling pins and needles or numbness, or sometimes just a sensation that something is 'off', for example, that the touch of clothes here just feels 'different' compared with the surrounding area or the other side.

More importantly, referral patterns can mimic a root or peripheral nerve problem. An S1 root injury can, for example, result in pain and/or paraesthesias in the posterior calf, the lateral aspect and sole of the foot and infrequently also the posterior thigh (Fig. 4.10A). The lower posterior sacroiliac, sacrospinous and sacrotuberous ligaments, which have mainly an S1, S2 and S3 root supply, are capable of referring to all three sites, and this may raise suspicions of an S1 root lesion when the real problem is one of irritation or injury affecting one or more of these ligaments (Fig. 4.10B).

The pain and paraesthesias represent referred symptoms involving the S1 myotome (muscles in the calf and posterior thigh, particularly the lateral hamstrings), dermatome (the skin overlying the posterior calf and the heel and sole) and sclerotome (which includes the weight-bearing part of the calcaneus). Symptoms are more likely to be on a referred basis, rather than from irritation or injury of the S1 root, when the neurological examination discloses the findings outlined in Box 4.4.

Significant points to appreciate when trying to differentiate between a nerve injury and referred symptoms include the following:

Location

Symptoms arising from a nerve injury tend to be more or less constant in location, coinciding with the area supplied by the compromised root or peripheral nerve. With referred symptoms, the location of the areas involved may also remain constant, but the number of these areas that are symptomatic at any one time may vary.

Box 4.4   Findings suggesting referred pain rather than nerve root irritation

- Full strength in the S1 myotome muscles, or the typical asymmetrical pattern of weakness that involves some S1 myotome muscles bilaterally (e.g. the right gluteus maximus and tibialis posterior, and the left hamstrings and peroneus longus)
- Normal pinprick and light touch sensation over the posterior calf and the sole, or responses to sensory testing that are somewhat variable or ill defined
- Preservation of the ankle jerk
- Negative root stretch tests, or symptoms that could be attributed to tender soft tissue or joint structures (e.g. the posterior pelvic ligaments, the posterior SI joint capsule or the joint itself) being put under further stress by these manoeuvres

---

In the example involving the lower posterior sacroiliac, the sacrospinal and sacrotuberous ligaments (Fig. 4.10B; see Fig. I.2), the athlete may report that there is sometimes no pain at all, or there may be just heel pain, whereas at other times dysaesthesias are felt just in the posterior thigh or the posterior calf region. All three sites are, however, likely to be involved when the pain is 'really bad'.

In others with an affliction of these ligaments, dysaesthesias may affect the posterior thigh first, and only if this gets worse will there eventually be pain also in the calf and finally on the heel and foot region – a domino-like effect. The ligaments that are the source of the referred pain may actually remain asymptomatic, but they are likely to prove tender to palpation.

Intensity

Referred pain is more likely to fluctuate in intensity from being very severe at one time to being just bothersome or not even present at another. Nerve pain is more likely to get gradually worse with the increasing nerve irritation and inflammation associated with a traction or compression injury, and may gradually get better as these factors resolve.

Relation to activity and rest

Referred pain from the irritation of ligaments, fascia and other connective tissue structures is a particular problem immediately on getting up from lying or sitting, tends to get better on moving about but may worsen again when the activity is continued for a longer period of time.

These tissues tend to shorten with rest and will, therefore, often be a source of pain on initially moving around until they have been stretched out again. Pain recurs as muscle fatigue sets in with continued activity: the muscles tire and tense up and, along with the ligaments and other connective tissues, are once more subjected to increased stress.

In contrast, pain arising from nerve tissue may settle somewhat with rest but may also worsen, often assuming a 'burning' quality at these times; the pain tends to get steadily worse with activity.

Pattern of weakness and wasting

Barring generalized disuse weakness and wasting in an extremity, a root or peripheral nerve injury usually results in weakness and wasting confined to the muscle(s) supplied by the affected root or nerve. A left S1 root lesion, for example, will result in weakness and wasting restricted to muscles in the ipsilateral S1 myotome.

In contrast, malalignment results in an asymmetrical pattern of weakness that involves muscles from multiple myotomes – L2 to S1 – on both sides in a pattern that is not consistent with either a root or a peripheral nerve injury (see Appendix 4). In the presence of malalignment, weakness not in keeping with this asymmetrical pattern should raise suspicions of an underlying neurological lesion and call for immediate further investigations. If, however, there is no good indication of a neurological lesion, and there is no apparent contraindication to mobilization, the best thing is to proceed with realignment.

The athlete is re-examined after the correction to determine whether there is any residual weakness and, if so, whether it conforms to a root or peripheral nerve pattern that may previously have been hidden by the functional weakness associated with the malalignment (see 'Asymmetry of muscle strength' in Ch. 3). Further investigations should be guided by these findings.

Response to block with local anaesthetic

A block will usually give temporary relief if a nerve root or peripheral nerve is the cause of the problem. Local anaesthetic should similarly give relief when injected into the structure that is the cause of any referred symptoms (e.g. the sacrospinal or sacrotuberous ligaments) but not when injected into the actual site of referral (e.g. the S1 sclerotome around the heel part of the calcaneus; see the 'Introduction').

Response to realignment

The correction of malalignment is not very likely to abolish the dysaesthesias associated with the irritation or injury of a nerve root or peripheral nerve, although it may decrease the pain by:

- relieving the tension on the root or nerve itself (e.g. bringing its origin and insertion back into a normal position)
- decreasing compression (e.g. relaxing the surrounding muscles by shutting off any facilitation)
- increasing the space available (e.g. increasing foraminal openings or decreasing disc bulging or protrusion by decreasing disc torsion and compression).

The abolition of pain and paraesthesias following realignment will help to confirm the referred nature of these symptoms. Abolition does not, however, always occur on realignment even when these symptoms are indeed malalignment-related. If a ligament has, for example, been stretched for a long period of time because of malalignment, simply restoring the tension to normal with realignment may no longer be adequate to stop this ligament from continuing to be tender and a source of referred symptoms. Similarly, trigger points may fail to disappear with realignment alone. Both can be an ongoing source of pain and referred symptoms until dealt with by additional means (Ch. 7).

Malalignment-related nerve injury

Malalignment particularly affects the peripheral nerves in the lower extremities by causing a shift in weight-bearing and accentuating the stresses relating to pronation and supination (Schamberger 1987). The shift in weight-bearing can result in excessive traction, compression or a combination of the two, which may be compounded by the functional LLD and a coexisting genu valgum or varum.

Peripheral nerves affected by medial shift (pronation)

A medial shift increases the tension primarily in the saphenous and posterior tibial nerves (see Fig. 3.34A). The deep peroneal nerve may also be affected as parts of it, in particular the sensory branch supplying the first web space, come to lie progressively more medially distal to the anterior tarsal tunnel (Figs 4.11B and 4.12A; see Fig. 3.34A). Posterior tarsal tunnel syndrome can result from the medial traction forces on the posterior tibial nerve and its branches, compounded

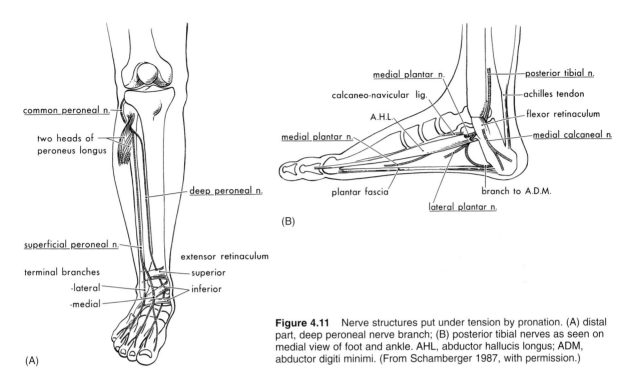

(A)

(B)

Figure 4.11 Nerve structures put under tension by pronation. (A) distal part, deep peroneal nerve branch; (B) posterior tibial nerves as seen on medial view of foot and ankle. AHL, abductor hallucis longus; ADM, abductor digiti minimi. (From Schamberger 1987, with permission.)

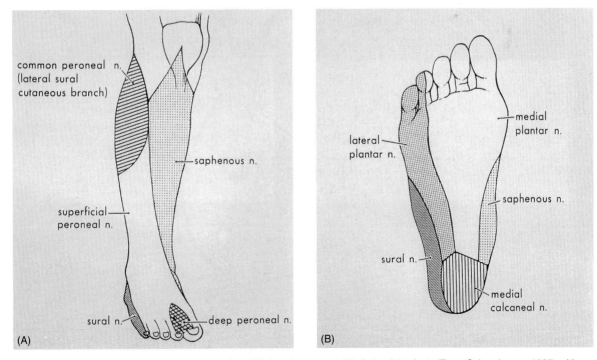

(A)

(B)

Figure 4.12 Sensory distribution in the lower leg. (A) Anterior aspect. (B) Sole of the foot. (From Schamberger 1987, with permission.)

by compression within the tunnel as the medial restraining ligament (flexor retinaculum) is also put under tension (Fig. 4.11B; see Fig. 3.34A). The sural nerve may be entrapped and compressed by excessive ankle eversion (Fig. 4.12A, B; see Fig. 3.34A).

Peripheral nerves affected by lateral shift (supination)

A lateral shift increases the traction forces distally on the sural nerve and the common peroneal nerve and its branches, especially the superficial peroneal nerve (see Fig. 3.34B), and proximally on lateral superficial sensory nerves such as the lateral sural cutaneous branch (Fig. 4.12A) and lateral femoral cutaneous nerve (LFCN – Fig. 4.13). The posterior tibial nerve can

be entrapped and compressed as the space available within the posterior tarsal tunnel is compromised by excessive varus angulation (ankle inversion) occurring with supination (see Fig. 3.34B).

Other mechanisms of injury to nerves

Malalignment can result in irritation, actual compression or compromise of the blood supply to the nerves in the upper and lower extremities by several mechanisms.

Narrowing of an outlet for the nerve fibres. Vertebral rotation into the convexity with a simultaneous flexion forwards and sideways, or frank vertebral malrotation, can accentuate a disc bulge or protrusion on one

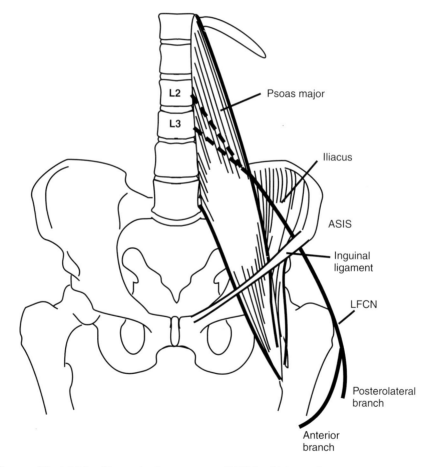

Figure 4.13 Course of the left lateral femoral cutaneous nerve (LFCN), which supplies sensation to the anterolateral thigh. Nerve irritation can occur: at its origin (the posterior roots of L2 and L3) and as it travels laterally between psoas and iliacus, down to the medial aspect of the anterior superior iliac spine (ASIS) and under the inguinal ligament, by: (i) compression with increased tension in the iliopsoas, left innominate posterior rotation and/or inflare; and (ii) traction forces caused by left innominate anterior rotation and/or outflare; below the ASIS or at the point 12 cm distally where it becomes superficial and divides into the anterior and posterolateral branches to the thigh (e.g. by being put under tension with excessive supination).

side and compromise the root exit by decreasing the size of the intervertebral foramen. Symptoms of root compromise may occur whenever malalignment is present, only to subside with realignment and a decrease in the size of the protrusion, and/or a reopening of the intervertebral foramen.

A malalignment-related rotation of the bones, muscle hypertonicity and contracture can compromise:

1. *the posterior triangle of the neck*: dysaesthesias may be attributable to an increase in tension in the anterior and middle scalene muscles, which narrows the outlet for the mid-section of the brachial plexus and subclavian artery (see Fig. 3.11)
2. *the thoracic outlet lying between the clavicle and first rib* (see Fig. 3.11): an increase in tension, particularly in the scalenes and subclavius muscle, and a rotation of the first rib and the clavicle relative to each other, can narrow the space available for the traversing lower section of the subclavian vessels and brachial plexus (especially the C8 and T1 fibres that constitute the lower cord of the plexus)
3. *the femoral triangle*: iliacus and psoas can push the exiting ilioinguinal, iliohypogastric or LFCN (Fig. 4.13) against the medial edge of the anterior superior iliac spine, the LFCN against the inguinal ligament or the fascia lata (which it pierces), or the femoral neurovascular complex anteriorly against the iliac fascia and inguinal ligament (Fig. 4.14)
4. *the greater sciatic foramen*: piriformis contraction can narrow the exit of the sciatic nerve or its tibial and/or peroneal nerve component (see 'Sciatica' and 'Piriformis syndrome' below and Figs 4.17 and 4.18)
5. *the pelvic floor*: tightness in the myofascial tissue compromises the space available for the lumbosacral plexus and the pudendal and genitofemoral nerves (Fig. 4.15)
6. *the long dorsal sacroiliac ligament*: the dorsal rami of S1, S2 and S3 can be compressed as they traverse laterally between the medial and lateral components of a tight ligament (see Fig. 2.16B).

Compression of the interdigital nerves of the foot. Pronation results in the collapse of the anterior transverse arch of the foot and angulation of the

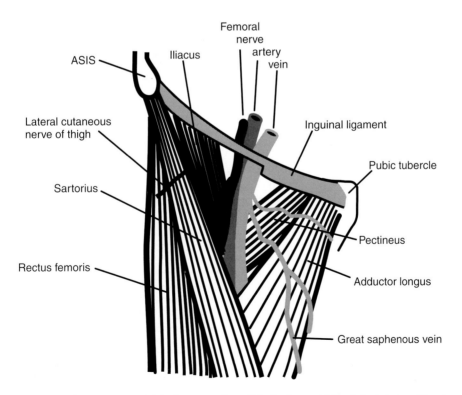

Figure 4.14 Neurovascular structures at risk of compromise within the femoral triangle by increased tension, particularly in iliacus, psoas and pectineus. ASIS, anterior superior iliac spine. (After Grant 1980, with permission.)

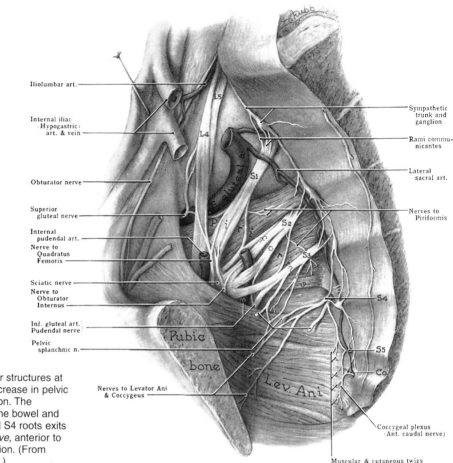

Figure 4.15 Neurovascular structures at risk of compromise by an increase in pelvic floor myofascial tissue tension. The autonomic nerve supply to the bowel and bladder from the S2, S3 and S4 roots exits as the *pelvic splanchnic nerve*, anterior to the sacrococcygeal joint region. (From Grant 1980, with permission.)

metatarsophalangeal joints into extension. Increased pressure is exerted particularly on the now acutely angulated plantar digital nerves by the edges of the deep transverse metatarsal ligaments, which, together with the superficial ligament underneath, sandwich the nerves at this site (Fig. 4.16).

A lateral shift in weight-bearing (supination) can activate a latent Morton's neuroma by narrowing the space between the third and fourth metatarsal heads. A neuroma on the left side is more likely to become symptomatic given that, in the vast majority with malalignment, the shift is towards left lateral weight-bearing and supination (Fig. 4.16B – lower).

All of these nerves become more vulnerable to a traction and/or compression injury on the basis of:

- activity-related repetitive minor increases in pronation or supination
- an acute injury, for example, the excessive supination that results with an ankle inversion

sprain acting on an already tense and irritable LFCN, peroneal or sural nerve.

IMPLICATIONS FOR ORTHOPAEDIC SURGERY

The biomechanics of malalignment should be of particular interest to those practising orthopaedic surgery.

Typical problems relating to the altered stresses that result with malalignment are mentioned throughout this text and relate primarily to:

- asymmetries of ranges of motion, especially those affecting the hip girdle, ankle and foot
- asymmetries of weight-bearing, specifically those resulting in excessive unilateral pronation or supination, alterations of the gait pattern and abnormal tension in the soft tissue structures
- asymmetries of muscle strength and bulk

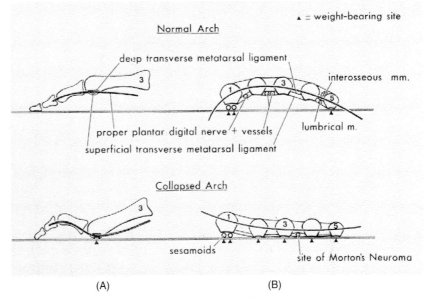

Figure 4.16 Compromise of nerves in the foot with malalignment. Space for the plantar digital nerves is compromised on collapse of the anterior transverse arch (lower 'B') and as they are put under increased tension by the associated 'cock-up' toe deformity (lower 'A'). The lower anterior view 'B' shows how a left lateral shift in weight-bearing (supination) could activate a left Morton's neuroma. (From Schamberger 1987, with permission.)

Discussion here will be limited to some specific orthopaedic entities that can result from or somehow be affected by malalignment.

Iliopectineal bursitis

This bursa lies on the anterior aspect of the hip joint and usually communicates with the joint between the pubococcygeal and iliofemoral ligaments (see Figs 4.2 and 4.3). When inflamed, the bursa may become palpable just distal to the anterior inferior iliac spine and lateral to the pubis; visualization by ultrasound or on magnetic resonance imaging may be necessary to confirm the diagnosis.

Inflammation has been associated with hip joint synovitis and osteoarthritis, as well as with an increase in tension in the overlying iliopsoas or pectineal muscles that may result in these muscles snapping repeatedly across the anterior aspect of the hip joint on hip flexion and extension (see Figs 2.31, 2.40 and 3.38). Iliopectineal bursitis must be considered in the differential diagnosis of anterior hip tenderness and pain in the presence of malalignment, in which tension in the iliopsoas is frequently increased on one or both sides on the basis of:

- an adaptive shortening having occurred on the side of an anterior rotation and which is now limiting hip extension
- an increase in the length-to-tension ratio on the side of a posterior rotation
- reflex contraction in an attempt to stabilize a painful SI joint (see Fig. 2.31B)

- facilitation, frequently triggered by a malrotation of one or more of its proximal origins (the transverse process and lateral aspect of vertebrae T12–L5).

Pain from the axial skeleton

The asymmetry of the spine seen as part of the malalignment syndrome results in increased biomechanical stresses along the length of the axial skeleton (Box 4.5).

Upper extremity pain

Malalignment must be considered in the differential diagnosis of pain affecting the upper extremities, especially if the diagnosis proves elusive and the pain is resistant to standard therapy approaches. The following should be considered.

Asymmetries of ranges of motion

Stress is increased on upper extremity joints by the limitation of movement in specific directions. One most commonly sees, for example:

- at the glenohumeral joints, a limitation of right internal and left external rotation (see Fig. 3.15A), and of left extension (Fig. 3.15B)
- at the elbow, a limitation of left forearm pronation and right supination (see Fig. 3.15C, D).

Box 4.5 Causes of increased biomechanical stress in the axial skeleton

---

1. *Distraction and compression*: structures on the convex side of a curvature of the spine are distracted, whereas those on the concave side are compressed (see Fig. 2.38)
2. *Simultaneous vertebral rotation and side flexion*: the four upper lumbar vertebrae usually rotate into the convexity and side-flex into the concavity (see Figs 2.29, 2.65A, 3.5, 4.6 and 4.22). The pressure distribution is altered, with an asymmetrical loading of the disc. A torsional strain is imposed on the disc and anulus fibrosus, as well as on the muscles and ligaments that attach to each vertebral complex (see Figs 2.23 and 3.63). The facet joints are compressed contralaterally, and distracted ipsilaterally, to the direction of vertebral rotation (see Figs 2.35B, 4.6, 4.26A, 4.27 and 4.28). All of these structures have sensory innervation and can, with time, become a source of localized and/or referred pain
3. *Curve reversal and interruption*: pain and tenderness localize in particular to the junctional (lumbosacral, thoracolumbar and cervicothoracic) areas and any sites of vertebral malrotation (see Figs 2.60, 2.63, 3.12 and 3.13). Thoracolumbar junction involvement can mimic Maigne's 'thoracolumbar syndrome' (discussed below)

Referred symptoms of pain and paraesthesias

Cervical vertebral malrotation can cause referred symptoms in a dermatomal, myotomal or sclerotomal pattern involving the cheek, neck and shoulder region (C2–C5), and from the shoulder to the fingers (C5–T1).

Sclerotomal referral is often not recognized (see Fig. 3.10). C4–C5 and C5–C6 rotational stress can, for example, result in a referral to the C5 and C6 sclerotomal sites along the lateral elbow region, capable of mimicking lateral epicondylitis or 'tennis elbow' (see Fig. 3.10A, B2, 3). An irritation of C8 and T1 can result in symptoms from sclerotomal sites along the medial elbow, capable of mimicking medial epicondylitis or 'golfer's elbow', as well as wrist pain (see Fig. 3.10A). Involvement of the C7 and C8 sclerotomal sites may account for 'unexplained' wrist and finger symptoms (see Fig. 3.10A, B4).

A failure of these sites to respond to standard treatment, and to the injection of local anaesthetic or cortisone, should raise the suspicion that the 'epicondylitis', for example, is occurring on the basis of sclerotomal referral and should prompt a search for vertebral rotation with localizing facet and/or soft tissue tenderness in the immediate region.

Compressive, distractive and torsional stresses

The clavicles are submitted to stresses of this type because they are part of the trunk, which is subjected to rotation and displacement with malalignment (see Figs 2.62 and 2.63B). Pain is likely to localize to the securing ligaments, in particular the sternoclavicular medially and the coracoclavicular laterally (see Figs 2.62 and 4.7).

In comparison to the acromioclavicular joint, the sternoclavicular joint appears less capable of dealing with these stresses. The sternoclavicular joint is more likely to be tender on palpation and to develop a weakness of the anchoring ligaments that eventually allows a frank anterior subluxation of this end of the clavicle relative to the sternum.

Pelvic and lower extremity joint pain and degeneration

LLD, whether anatomical or functional, has been implicated in the acceleration of hip and knee joint degeneration. Dixon & Campbell-Smith (1969) drew attention to 'long leg arthropathy', indicating that degeneration and pain are more likely to involve the hip joint on the long-leg side and the knee joint on the short-leg side. The effect of the functional LLD associated with malalignment is compounded by the asymmetry of lower extremity loading, attributable to the shift in weight-bearing and rotation of the legs in contrary directions (see Figs 3.74 and 3.75).

Sciatica

In its strictest sense, 'sciatica' refers to a pressure neuritis, typically from a disc protrusion. There is irritation of the nerve root fibres or the nerve root sleeve, which gives rise to back pain and muscle spasm, as well as pain or sensory symptoms down the leg in the distribution of the affected root. Nowadays, the term is more commonly used to refer to an entrapment of the sciatic nerve at the level of the sciatic notch, where it exits from the pelvis (Fig. 4.17). Compression at this site can result in intermittent paraesthesias, pain or weakness in the distribution of the tibial and/or peroneal nerve. These arise from the lumbosacral plexus as individual nerves and eventually lie together to form the sciatic nerve proper, the peroneal component lateral to the tibial.

The sciatic nerve leaves the pelvis by way of the greater sciatic foramen. The piriformis muscle divides this foramen into a superior and inferior portion, the other borders of the inferior portion are comprised of the medial edge of the innominate laterally, the sacrotuberous ligament medially, and the upper edge of the

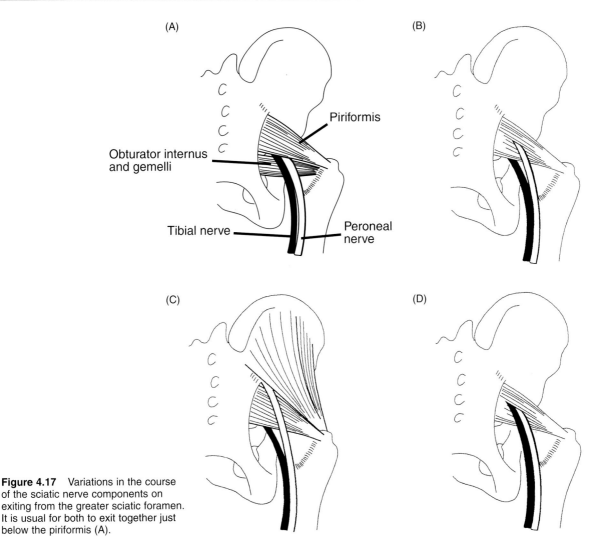

(A)

(B)

C
C
C
C

Piriformis

Obturator internus
and gemelli

Tibial nerve

Peroneal
nerve

(C)

(D)

C
C
C
C

C
C
C
C

Figure 4.17 Variations in the course
of the sciatic nerve components on
exiting from the greater sciatic foramen.
It is usual for both to exit together just
below the piriformis (A).

sacrospinous ligament and ischial spine inferiorly.
Grant (1964) reported that, in 87.3% of 640 dissections,
both the tibial and the peroneal division passed
through this inferior portion, below the piriformis
muscle (Fig. 4.17A). In 12.2%, the peroneal component
actually passed through this muscle (Fig. 4.17B),
whereas in 0.5% it passed above it, exiting between the
superior border of piriformis and the inferior border of
gluteus medius and minimus before joining the tibial
component (Fig. 4.17C). Rarely were both components
found to traverse the muscle mass (Fig. 4.17D).

The lateral position of the peroneal nerve makes it
more vulnerable to compression against the bony
lateral border of the foramen. In the variants in which
the peroneal nerve passes either through or above the
piriformis muscle, this component is at increased risk

of compression by a contraction of the surrounding
muscle. Piriformis functions as an abductor and external rotator of the lower extremity (see Fig. 2.31A).
Sciatic nerve entrapment can therefore occur:

- acutely with an excessively strong piriformis
  contraction
- acutely with a piriformis muscle sprain or strain
  caused by either excessive and/or sudden internal
  rotation and adduction of the leg, especially if this
  occurs while the muscle is in a contracted state
- over a period of time, with repetitive activity that
  incorporates these same mechanisms, for example,
  some of the high kicking actions with simultaneous
  passive internal rotation and adduction that are
  used in martial arts.

The symptoms may be provoked on clinical examination with manoeuvres that combine a passive increase in tension in both the piriformis and the sciatic nerve with simultaneous active piriformis contraction intended to compress the nerve. These effects can typically be achieved by:

1. passive internal rotation, hip flexion and adduction, with simultaneous resisted external rotation, extension and abduction of the hip
2. straight leg raising combined with a resisted contraction of the external rotators.

Irritation of the peroneal or tibial component consistently results in pain in the respective parts of both the lower limb and foot supplied by these nerves (see Fig. 4.12A, B). Those presenting with malalignment frequently use the term 'sciatica' to describe pain felt primarily in the low back and/or buttock region and radiating a variable distance down the back of the leg. In other words, the pain usually stops partway down the thigh or at the knee, although it sometimes goes into the calf and possibly as far as at the ankle.

Symptoms in the foot are rare; when present, dysaesthesias often involve only part of the dorsum or sole and the athlete may be able to state quite definitely that the foot dysaesthesias do not appear to be continuous with the more proximal symptoms. In addition the symptoms may at times be felt only in the leg, at other times only in the foot, and sometimes in both sites simultaneously.

These phenomena are characteristic of referred dysaesthesias, as discussed above (see Figs 3.41, 3.58 and 4.10). On a closer inspection of these athletes, one is likely to find a malalignment-related increase in tension and tenderness of one or more of the structures capable of referring to the posterior thigh, calf, ankle and foot. The piriformis muscle itself and the sacrotuberous ligament are typical of structures that can be activated through malalignment and come to mimic 'sciatica' (see Figs 3.41, 3.58 and 4.10).

Symptoms felt only a variable distance down the back of the leg, or in a patchy pattern as far as the foot, are therefore more likely to be occurring on the basis of referral from structures upset by the malalignment rather than being a true 'sciatica', especially if:

- there is no evidence of a neurological deficit
- root stretch tests and pressure applied over the sciatic notch do not suggest increased irritability of the sciatic nerve or its components and fail to recreate the athlete's dysaesthesias.

Piriformis syndrome

As originally described by Yeoman in 1928, piriformis syndrome consisted of a history of traumatic injury to the sacroiliac and gluteal region combined with the following: pain in the piriformis muscle and the region of the SI joint and greater sciatic notch, causing difficulty in walking; a markedly tender, palpable 'sausage-shaped' mass over the piriformis muscle; a positive straight leg raising test; eventually gluteal muscle atrophy; typical aggravation of the symptoms by prolonged hip flexion, adduction and internal rotation; and an absence of findings in the low back and hip regions.

Pace & Nagle (1976), reporting on a series of 45 patients diagnosed as having piriformis syndrome, noted that only half had a history of trauma, usually minor. Pain and weakness on resisting simultaneous abduction and external rotation of the thigh was one of the most consistent findings on clinical examination.

They also commonly found a trigger point located within the piriformis that was responsible for a distinct tenderness on the lateral pelvic wall, pressure on this trigger point reproducing the original complaint. The point was located fairly high up and felt to correspond to the medial trigger point described by Travell & Simons (1992), the lateral one being located at the junction of the middle and distal third (see Fig. 3.41). The symptoms were abolished with trigger point injections.

A tear of the piriformis muscle results in a circumscribed area that is acutely tender and probably localized most accurately by internal palpation. Nerve conduction and electromyographic studies may be abnormal because:

- injured muscle fibres are still present
- the tear and/or subsequent swelling has resulted in injury to:
  - the nearby tibial or peroneal nerve component
  - the nerve fibres from S1 and S2 that supply piriformis directly.

Many of the athletes who have been labelled as having a 'piriformis syndrome' do not have a history of an acute or repetitive mechanism of injury that might have caused entrapment of the sciatic nerve, and their electrodiagnostic studies are normal. A large number, however, present with an upslip or rotational malalignment and show increased piriformis tension and tenderness, more often on the right (see Ch. 3).

Accompanying symptoms of pain and paraesthesia often led to the diagnosis of a 'piriformis syndrome' with irritation of the sciatic nerve, even though the dysaesthesias actually radiate only a varying distance down the back of the leg, usually not past the knee and very rarely involving the foot. These symptoms are more likely to arise on the basis of referral, originating from the piriformis itself, from trigger points within that muscle, or from nearby ligaments (Fig. 3.41). The medial and lateral trigger points, for example, refer pain to the sacroiliac region primarily, the buttock in general, the hip joint posteriorly and occasionally to the proximal two-thirds of the posterior thigh, but not to the posterior calf nor into the foot (Travell & Simons 1992).

Anterior rotation, particularly when combined with an outflare of the innominate, narrows the space available for the sciatic nerve traversing the inferior foramen. With time, a chronic increase in piriformis tension combined with such a narrowing of the outlet can result in some nerve fibre irritation, in which case one might expect pain and paraesthesias down the leg and into the foot in the distribution of either or both components, in the form of a true 'sciatica'.

> In most athletes, therefore, increased tension and tenderness of piriformis and the referred symptoms are more likely to be just another manifestation of the changes associated with malalignment rather than a *bona fide*, isolated 'piriformis syndrome'.

In keeping with this assumption is the fact that the signs and symptoms usually disappear quite quickly on realignment.

On the other hand, increased tension or spasm following an actual injury of piriformis has been implicated as one cause of the occurrence and recurrence of malalignment. The muscle originates from the anterior sacrum and innominate (greater sciatic notch), crosses both the SI and the hip joints, and inserts into the upper posterior aspect of the greater trochanter (see Figs 2.31A and 3.41). It is therefore in a strategic position to exert rotational forces on all these structures. In addition, the increase in tension in the piriformis muscle typically associated with malalignment puts the athlete at increased risk of suffering a sprain or strain of this muscle and presenting with a *bona fide* acute piriformis syndrome. In this case, treatment of the piriformis injury in isolation, without simultaneous correction of the malalignment, is likely to prolong recovery and increases the risk of the injury recurring.

Thoracolumbar syndrome

As far back as in 1972, Maigne drew attention to the fact that 'low back pain erroneously attributed to lumbar or lumbosacral disease may well be caused by referred pain from the thoracolumbar junction' (1980,

p. 393). In 1980, he reported on a series of 138 patients, all of whom complained of low back pain but whose pain originated from the transitional area of the spine, the dorsolumbar region (see Fig. 3.8). Maigne was referring to the fact that T12 typically had:

1. superior facets that were oriented in the frontal plane, in keeping with the rest of the thoracic spine and allowing primarily for rotation
2. inferior facets that were oriented in the sagittal plane, in keeping with the lumbar part of the spine and allowing primarily for flexion and extension.

The syndrome was attributable to the resultant 'disharmony of movement', usually of T12 relative to L1, but also at times involving the vertebra above or below. The disharmony would eventually result in a painful facet joint on one side, and evidence of the irritation of cutaneous branches originating from the posterior roots of T11, T12 and L1 on the same side. The thoracolumbar level involved could be determined by applying lateral pressure to the spinous processes and applying pressure and friction over the facet joints lying about 1 cm from the midline (Fig. 4.18).

On dissection, the cutaneous branches were shown to descend in the subcutaneous tissue and end in the skin of the lower lumbar area; typical findings on examination included a painful 'crestal point' (where these branches crossed the posterior iliac crest – Fig. 4.19) and acute tenderness on skin-rolling and pinching the subcutaneous tissue supplied by these branches (Fig. 4.20). Subsequently (1986, 1995), Maigne referred to these branches as the 'posterior branch' of spinal nerves T12 and L1, with frequent contributions from T11 and L2 (Fig. 4.21A2, B1), at the same time drawing attention to an 'anterior' and a 'lateral cutaneous perforating' branch that could also be part of the thoracolumbar syndrome.

The *'anterior branch'* (Fig. 4.21A1, B2) is formed by the anterior rami of spinal nerves T12 and L1, and innervates:

- the skin of the lower abdomen, the inner aspect of the upper thighs and the labia majora or scrotum
- the lower part of rectus abdominis and transversus abdominis (see Fig. 2.24A)
- the pubis.

The *'lateral cutaneous perforating branch'* (Fig. 4.21A3, B3) arises from each of the anterior rami of T12 and L1, and innervates the lateral hip, thigh and occasionally also the groin region to a varying extent.

Irritation of these cutaneous branches originating from the thoracolumbar junction area occurred because:

1. the greatest degree of rotation and lateral flexion occurred at the level of this junction

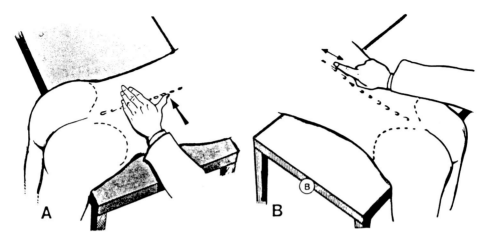

Figure 4.18 Thoracolumbar syndrome: method of determining the thoracolumbar level involved. (A) Lateral pressure over the spinous process at the involved level is usually painful in only one direction – left or right. (B) Seeking the painful posterior articular point (facet joint) by pressure and friction 1 cm from the midline. (From Maigne 1995, with permission.)

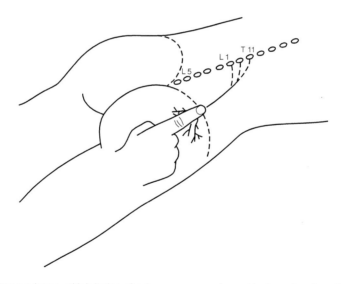

Figure 4.19 Thoracolumbar syndrome, with irritation of cutaneous nerves formed by branches from T11, T12 and L1. The posterior branch, which ends in the skin of the posterior lumbosacral and buttock area, may be found by applying friction and pressure to the posterior iliac crest to seek the 'crestal point'. (After Maigne 1995, with permission.)

2. a rotary twisting movement eventually resulted in a 'minimal vertebral displacement', usually of T12 relative to L1.

Maigne (1980) reported that, in 76% of the subjects, the clinical finding of eliciting pain with pressure applied to the spinous processes and facets joints was limited to the T11–T12 or T12–L1 level. In 1995, his sta- tistics indicated that this particular form of back pain was found in approximately 30% of those presenting with back pain. A lack of pain radiating into the legs, an absence of scoliosis and of an antalgic spine, and a 'usually negative' straight leg raising test should raise the suspicion that the problem is not in the lumbosacral but in the thoracolumbar part of the spine. The clinical presentation could include any or all of the following.

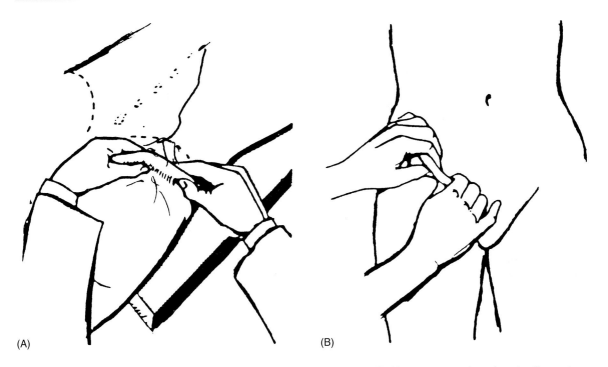

Figure 4.20   Seeking painful subcutaneous tissue by pinching a skin fold supplied by a cutaneous branch and pulling and rolling it. (A) Cellulalgia from the posterior branch. (B) Cellulalgia from the anterior branch. (From Maigne 1995, with permission.)

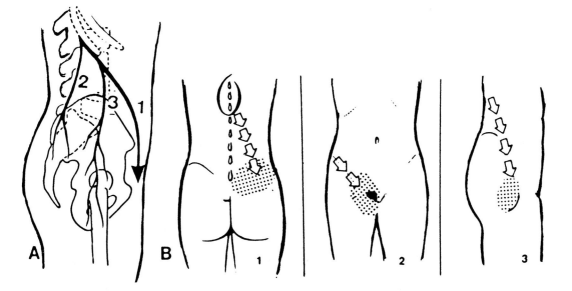

Figure 4.21   Problems relating to the T12 and L1 cutaneous branches. A1, B2: Anterior branch: pseudo-visceral pain. A2, B1: Posterior branch: low back pain. A3, B3: Lateral perforating branch: pseudo-hip pain. (From Maigne 1995, with permission.)

Low back pain of thoracolumbar origin (Fig. 4.21A2, B1; see Fig. 4.19)

The pain is described as being mostly chronic in type, although it can be of acute origin. It is usually unilateral and perceived in the sacroiliac, low back or buttock region, sometimes with referral to the lateral thigh. Patients never complain of symptoms in the thoracolumbar region. Clinical signs include:

- at the posterior iliac crest point, a very tender point, 7–10 cm lateral to the midline where the posterior branch crosses the crest
- *pain on skin-rolling* (see Fig. 4.20A) as irritation of the skin innervated by the posterior branch can result in a limited area of cellulalgia in the upper buttock region; the skin becomes very painful and often feels thickened when rolled between the thumb and index finger
- a relief of the pain on injection or manipulation, the injection of local anaesthetic over selective facet joints in this area, or manipulation, relieving the presenting pain, allowing free movement and resulting in the disappearance of the crestal point and area of cellulalgia.

'Pseudo-visceral pain' (Fig. 4.21A1, B2)

Involvement of the anterior branch can result in pain over the lower abdominal wall, groin or testicle:

It is experienced as a deep, tight pain, perfectly simulating visceral pain; … it is variable and episodic in nature and can occur at the same time as the back pain. (Maigne 1995, p. 88)

If, however, it occurs at separate times, the patient may fail to associate the two pains and end up being seen by a gynaecologist for this part of the pain and an orthopaedic surgeon for the low back pain. Maigne (1995, p. 88) warns that persistence of these pains may lead to:

multiple and sometimes extensive investigations. Minor abnormalities may be found which often lead to inappropriate surgical treatment. This is particularly true in the field of gynaecology.

On clinical examination, the pseudo-visceral problem is characterized by an area of cellulalgia localizing to the lower abdomen and upper inner aspect of the thigh. The pain is unilateral and corresponds to the side of the back pain.

In one out of three cases, involvement of the anterior branch also results in a marked tenderness of the 'hemipubis' on one side, although the patient rarely complains spontaneously of pubic pain. The prevalence of this sign is increased in athletes engaged in sports that involve the abdominal and adductor muscles (e.g. soccer and tennis).

'Pseudo-hip pain' (Fig. 4.21A3, B3)

Involvement of the lateral cutaneous perforating branches can cause pain in the greater trochanter region, sometimes in the groin, and may simulate hip pain. Compression of the overlying area of cellulalgia against the trochanter often leads to the mistaken diagnosis of 'trochanteric bursitis', but local injections (predictably) fail. Tenderness localizes to the point at which the cutaneous fibres cross the lateral iliac crest just above the trochanter, and to the area of cellulalgia that runs vertically between this point and the trochanter.

Mention is made here of the thoracolumbar syndrome because of the large number of athletes who present with malalignment and who have tenderness localizing to the thoracolumbar junction. Of the 96 athletes presenting with malalignment in Schamberger's unpublished 1994 study, 76% had pain when pressure was applied to the spine; in 22% of these, the pain localized to the thoracolumbar junction alone.

> Malalignment will either cause or accentuate an existing lateral curvature of the thoracic and lumbar segments, curvatures that in nearly all athletes reverse at the thoracolumbar junction (see Fig. 3.12B).

If the lumbar segment is straight in the presence of malalignment, a break again usually occurs at the thoracolumbar junction, leading into a right or left thoracic convexity (see Fig. 2.61). The curvature in each segment is formed by the simultaneous side flexion and rotation of the vertebrae in that particular segment. The reversal of a curve therefore means the rotation of adjoining vertebrae in the opposite directions at the point at which these segments meet. That is, T12 would be rotated in the opposite direction to L1 (see Fig. 3.12C).

The commonly seen reversal of the lumbar lordosis to a thoracic kyphosis that occurs at this junction in the sagittal plane can only add further to the stress at this level of the spine (see Fig. 3.12A). In addition, T12 or L1 rank among the vertebrae that most often show malrotation (see Ch. 3).

Given that the thoracolumbar junction is one of the high-stress areas of our spine, particularly in the presence of malalignment, it is really no wonder that bony and soft tissue structures in this area can become tender. The symptoms and signs of a thoracolumbar syndrome could easily develop, even though the athlete may be unable to recall a specific 'rotary twisting movement' that might cause Maigne's traumatic 'minimal vertebral rotation'. Malalignment, for example, increases the stress on the T12–L1 facet joints on one side because the rotation of these vertebrae in opposite directions results in:

1. compression of the facet joint surfaces on one side, with a possible entrapment of the capsule and/or branches of the posterior root fibres innervating the joint
2. distraction of the joint surfaces on the opposite side, which increases the tension on the facet joint capsule and nearby nerve fibres (see Fig. 2.35B)
3. irritation of the nerve fibres, including the cutaneous branches mentioned by Maigne.

The localized increase in tone and tenderness to palpation so commonly seen in the immediately adjacent paravertebral muscles and limited to the thoracolumbar junction area may be no more than a reflex splinting of the muscles overlying a painful facet joint or disc structure. It could also be an indicator of the increased tension that occurs in muscle fibres secondary to the irritation of their nerve supply, in this case the medial branch of the posterior root that innervates the multifidi, rotators and interspinous muscles at each level (see Fig. 2.23).

A number of the athletes also show tenderness of the cutaneous sensory fibres where they cross the posterior and/or lateral pelvic crest, and hypersensitivity of the overlying skin, in keeping with a full-blown thoracolumbar syndrome. Once realignment has been achieved and maintained, muscle tension and tenderness, along with other signs and symptoms localizing to the thoracolumbar, iliac crest, abdominal and hip regions, usually resolve fairly quickly (see Appendix 9).

Another form of 'thoracolumbar syndrome' has been attributed to irritation of either the L1 or L2 root, which contribute to the formation of the LFCN. It can present as anterior abdominal pain – lateralizing on palpation to where the LFCN runs medial to the anterior superior iliac spine – and the symptoms of meralgia paraesthetica: anterolateral hip and thigh dysaesthesias in the distribution of the LFCN (see Fig. 4.13). This problem has been attributed to the hypermobility that can develop with increased stress on the thoracolumbar junction from loss of movement in the low or mid-lumbar segments noted with:

- fusion of these segments (Paris 1990)

- prolonged close-packing of the facets characteristic of an increased tendency to lumbar spine extension, seen with:
  - the 'faulty lordotic posture' typical of those presenting with chronic pelvic pain (Baker 1998)
  - excessive nutation of the sacrum and a secondary increase in lordosis, as occurs with 'bilateral anterior sacrum' (see Ch. 2).

Malalignment and coexisting conditions of the spine

Some common conditions involving the spine do not present any problems for most athletes; they are usually considered to be 'benign', albeit a possible source of trouble. The chance of these conditions becoming symptomatic is, however, increased by the stresses imposed on the spine by malalignment. The key then is for someone to recognize the causal role of the malalignment. Initial treatment should be to correct the malalignment rather than mistakenly to attempt to treat what will often turn out to be a benign underlying condition once it has had a chance to settle down with realignment.

'Scoliosis'

The word 'scoliosis' strikes terror into the hearts of parents and those children old enough to understand its implications: a gradually increasing C-curve or double curve, accelerated degeneration of the spine, deformity, limitation of activity and eventually complications relating to the spinal cord itself or to compromised function of the heart and lungs. The picture described is that of progressive idiopathic scoliosis. The tentative diagnosis is often made at the time of a screening examination, being later confirmed by someone with a special interest in this condition. And yet, how often do those familiar with malalignment see parents presenting with a child or teenager who has already been labelled as having 'scoliosis', but:

- whose X-rays show no congenital malformations, such as hemivertebrae or absent ribs, that might ensure a progressive course
- who by history and on review of the clinical records has no convincing evidence of such a progressive course, or at most only a few degrees change over the years
- and who on examination proves to have no more than the compensatory, albeit perhaps accentuated, curvatures of the spine attributable to the pelvic obliquity caused by an underlying problem of malalignment?

The compensatory curves seen in association with malalignment can easily measure up to 10, 15 or even 20 degrees, large enough perhaps for someone to think that the label 'idiopathic scoliosis' is appropriate (see Figs 3.6A and 3.7). In a large number of these athletes, however, there is no indication of a progressive element, and the curves are either abolished or significantly reduced with realignment. Any residual curvatures then usually amount to no more than the average intrinsic curves of the lumbar and thoracic segments that may be typical for the child's age group.

It would save a lot of grief and worry if some of these children were not labelled 'scoliotic' until the malalignment was first corrected and the residual curvatures measured and followed for a year or two while maintaining realignment and strengthening the trunk and pelvic muscles in particular, in order to see:

1. whether there is indeed a progression of these curves
2. whether the diagnosis of a progressive 'idiopathic scoliosis' is indeed warranted.

> Even if the diagnosis of idiopathic scoliosis is eventually felt to be appropriate, it is still in the child's or adult's best interest to correct any pelvic malalignment and vertebral malrotation on an ongoing basis in order to remove that component of the curvature (and the associated stress) which is strictly attributable to the malalignment (see Fig. 4.6).

In the author's experience, a correction of malalignment of the pelvis has consistently been possible even when it is associated with curves of 30–40 degrees. In addition, although realignment may not have resulted in an appreciable decrease in the measurement of the curves, it has repeatedly brought about a decrease or even resolution of the pain, and an increased ability to pursue work and leisure activities.

A scoliosis often first becomes apparent on examination, when the athlete presents with symptoms. It is, however, this author's contention that:

• most of the athletes who are in their teens and older will present with malalignment and will probably have been out of alignment for some time, given that longitudinal studies already show a prevalence of 75% for malalignment in elementary school children (Klein 1978; Klein & Buckley 1968)
• most would already have shown a scoliosis on routine examination when they were still asymptomatic
• the scoliosis is in the majority of the non-progressive type and represents in part, if not entirely, an attempt to compensate for the pelvic obliquity attributable to:

– a functional LLD seen in all of the approximately 80% who eventually present with malalignment (see Figs 2.47, 2.48, 2.54 and 2.55)
– an anatomical LLD in approximately 10%, in isolation or combined with malalignment (see Fig. 2.42B)
• the malalignment has had a large part to play in the evolution of the pathological stresses that finally resulted in the specific symptoms
• the compensatory component of the scoliosis will in most cases decrease or completely disappear if a correction of the malalignment is carried out early enough (see Fig. 4.6). Persistent scoliosis, however, results in contracture of the myofascial and ligamentous structures (see Fig. 2.38). Therefore, the longer the malalignment has been present, and the older the athlete, the more likely the compensatory component will be to persist or fail to correct completely on realignment.

Realignment combined with a strengthening programme and possibly appropriate supports should initially be the mainstay of treatment and may be all that is needed to relieve the symptoms. The athlete should consider avoiding activities with a rotational component, in order to avoid further stress on the already painful sites and to decrease the chance of a recurrence of the malalignment.

The author recently saw a 3-year-old girl with well-established malalignment and a pelvic obliquity 1.5 cm higher on the right when standing, sitting and lying. Following realignment, the pelvis was level, the leg length equal and the previous scoliotic curves practically non-existent. If malalignment can be seen in children as young as this, and if there is no evidence of abnormality (e.g. hemivertebrae) on examination or X-rays, the question arises as to whether these children can eventually go on to develop a progressive 'idiopathic scoliosis' as a result of not having had treatment for the problem of malalignment earlier in life.

Spondylolisthesis

Spondylolisthesis, even an advanced spondylolisthesis of 25–50%, usually remains asymptomatic. The L5–S1 level is most often involved, a concomitant degeneration of the disc at this level being typical. An anterior displacement of L5 on S1 is most likely to render the L5 root symptomatic by being put under traction, becoming entrapped by a prominent disc bulge or protrusion, spinal stenosis or foraminal narrowing, or a combination of these factors.

Some athletes may experience intermittent back pain with or without transient root symptoms. Exacerbations are more likely with activities that put an extension or torsional strain on the spine, such as gardening, wrestling or playing court sports. Concomitant malalignment with compensatory scoliosis automatically increases the stress on the spondylolisthetic level: L1–L4 inclusive already tend to rotate into the lumbar convexity (see Figs 2.29, 2.65, 4.6, 4.22 and 4.28), and any associated L4 or L5 vertebral malrotation will only increase the stress even further (see Fig. 2.35). In addition, symptoms may relate to an instability of L4 and/or L5 that can eventually develop because of the increased stress on ligaments in this area resulting from the combined effect of the spondylolisthesis and the superimposed recurrent malalignment.

Initial treatment should be aimed at stabilizing the lumbosacral area by combining realignment with a muscle-strengthening programme, the use of a lumbosacral support and possibly the addition of prolotherapy injections to strengthen the ligaments by stimulating collagen formation (see Ch. 7). The athlete should avoid activities with a rotational component to decrease the chance of recurrence of the malalignment. Surgery is not indicated until the effect of the above measures has had a fair trial or unless there is evidence of instability not amenable to prolotherapy, an increasing scoliosis and/or nerve root irritation or compression.

Unilateral lumbarization, sacralization and transverse process pseudoarthrosis

In all three conditions, the vertebra is anchored down on one side (Figs 4.22–4.24). Even simple flexion and extension of the spine results in a rotational strain as the free side of the vertebra rotates forwards and backwards respectively to a varying extent, pivoting around the pseudoarthrosis or unilateral fusion. The effects relating to malalignment are twofold:

1. The torquing of this vertebral segment with spine flexion and extension increases the chance of malalignment occurring or recurring.
2. The pelvic obliquity and sacral torsion associated with coexisting malalignment increase the torquing force constantly exerted on the lumbar vertebrae, especially at the L4–L5 and L5–S1 levels, and the chance of these segments becoming symptomatic.

In some athletes, fusion of the free side may be the logical procedure in order finally to stop any recurrence of the malalignment and permanently to resolve the symptoms. Unfortunately, fusion increases stress on the levels above and below, and accelerates degeneration.

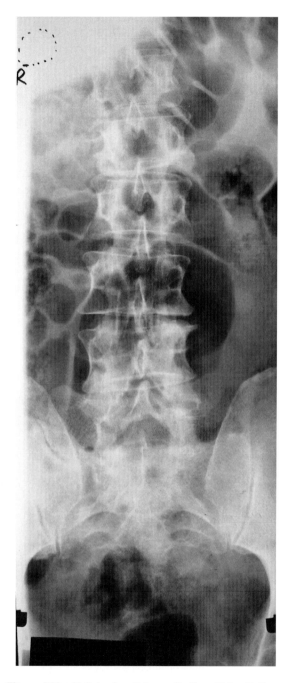

Figure 4.22 Unilateral partial sacralization of L5, with the formation of a pseudoarthrosis between the right transverse process and both the ilium and sacrum. Malalignment is present, with pelvic obliquity, lumbar dextroscoliosis and L1–L4 rotation into the convexity. Asymmetry of the sacroiliac joint articular surfaces relative to the X-ray beam results in different parts of the joint showing on the right compared with the left side. Realignment abolished the right lumbosacral back pain.

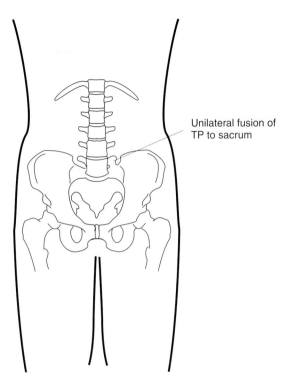

Unilateral fusion of TP to sacrum

Figure 4.23 Complete sacralization of left L5 transverse process (TP) in an athlete who is in alignment and standing.

IMPLICATIONS FOR RADIOLOGY AND MEDICAL IMAGING

> An appreciation of the changes that occur with the development of the SI joint, and with malalignment, is essential in order to allow for the proper interpretation of X-rays and scans of the axial and appendicular skeleton.

Radiographs

The patient with malalignment may have marked difficulty lying on a hard radiology table. The problem in part reflects the difficulty of getting a twisted pelvis, spine and extremities to accommodate to a flat surface, as with the patient who experiences increased pain on attempting to flatten the back doing the 'pelvic tilt' manoeuvre whenever out of alignment (see Fig. 7.2).

Normal changes relating to development and to the asymmetries associated with malalignment could easily result in a misinterpretation of what are essentially normal X-rays. Alternately, the radiologist familiar with the changes attributable to malalignment should be able to comment on the presence of and, on occasions, the actual type of malalignment evident on the films.

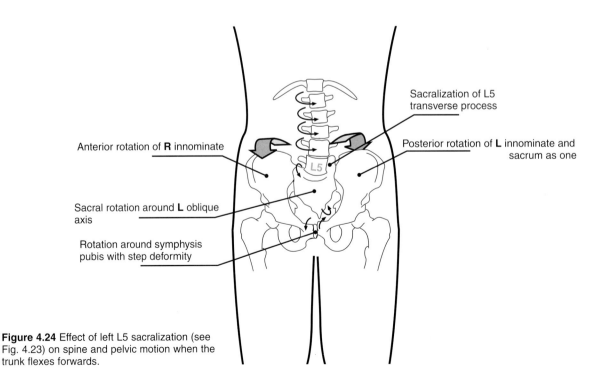

Anterior rotation of **R** innominate

Sacral rotation around **L** oblique axis

Rotation around symphysis pubis with step deformity

Sacralization of L5 transverse process

Posterior rotation of **L** innominate and sacrum as one

Figure 4.24 Effect of left L5 sacralization (see Fig. 4.23) on spine and pelvic motion when the trunk flexes forwards.

Sacroiliac joints

The developmental changes undergone by the SI joint have been described in detail in Chapter 2 and are summarised in Box 4.6.

These physiologically normal intra-articular ridges and depressions may be mistakenly read as 'osteophytes' and misinterpreted as implying advancing SI joint degeneration (Vleeming et al 1990a).

Box 4.6 Development of the sacroiliac joint

- The sacroiliac joint is at birth a planar joint, developing a thick layer of hyaline cartilage over the sacral, and a thin fibrocartilagenous cover over the illiac, surface in the ensuing years (see Fig. 2.5A)
- after puberty, the joint surfaces roughen with:
  - the initial development of a crescent-shaped ridge running the length of the iliac surface and a matching depression on the sacral surface
  - the subsequent development of further irregularities and prominences (Fig. 2.5B), possibly as an adaptation to adolescent weight gain.

Malalignment, especially outflare/inflare (Fig. 4.25) and anterior/posterior rotation (Fig. 4.26; see Fig. 4.28), results in a reorientation of the right versus left SI joint relative to the plane of the film and the X-ray beam being projected. If the reorientation is in contrary directions, as it commonly is, it will compound any difference that already exists in the orientation of the short and long arms of the joint relative to the vertical axis (see Fig. 2.1). Therefore, on reading the film:

1. different parts of the SI joint may appear to be open or closed on the right compared with the left side (Fig. 4.26; see Figs 4.6A, 4.22 and 4.28)
   – the joint may be all 'open' on one side and appear partially or fully 'closed' on most of the other (Fig. 4.26A; see Fig. 4.6)
   – alternatively, some of the joint may be 'open', with the adjacent borders clearly evident but other parts of it hidden by the overlapping of the sacral and iliac surfaces, whereas on the other side, different parts of the joint will be 'open' and 'closed' to the beam (see Figs 4.22 and 4.28)
2. any overlapping of roughened joint surfaces may be misinterpreted as 'sclerosis' and changes indicative of 'osteoarthritis' or other pathological conditions.

On realignment, the same views of the pelvis and spine are, barring any underlying pathology, now likely to show near-symmetry of the SI and facet joints on exposure to the same beam (e.g. Fig. 4.27).

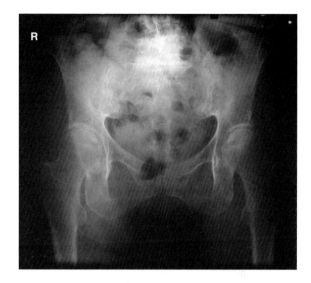

Figure 4.25 X-ray changes with left outflare and right inflare. (A) The femoral heads remain at the same level as the left acetabulum moves outwards and the right inwards in the transverse plane. (B) Innominate width appears to be increased on the left and decreased on the right. (C) The anterior superior iliac spine (ASIS) appears to be increased in overall size and broader on the outflare (left) side, and smaller and narrower on the inflare (right) side. (D) The left femoral neck appears to be further away from, the right closer to, the ipsilateral inferior pubic ramus. (E) The left greater trochanter appears to be smaller with overlapping on external rotation, the right more obvious with internal rotation of the leg (see also Fig. 2.45).

Spine

Rotation of the vertebrae occurs, with the formation of cervical, thoracic and lumbar convexities. Let us consider, for example, the typical rotation of L1–L4 into the lumbar convexity (Fig. 4.28; see Figs 2.29, 2.65, 4.6 and 4.22). Displacement of the spinous processes towards the concavity may also be evident on antero-posterior views of the thoracic and cervical spine (see Fig. 4.26B). As with the clinical examination findings of a spinous process having been displaced relative to the vertebrae above and below, the malrotation of an isolated vertebra will usually be evident on X-rays:

- If the malrotation is also into the convexity, there may be an obvious accentuation of the displacement of its spinous process relative to those above and below (see Fig. 4.26B).
- If the malrotation is in the direction opposite to those above and below, there may be an obvious interruption of the curve traced by the other spinous processes (see Fig. 2.65B).

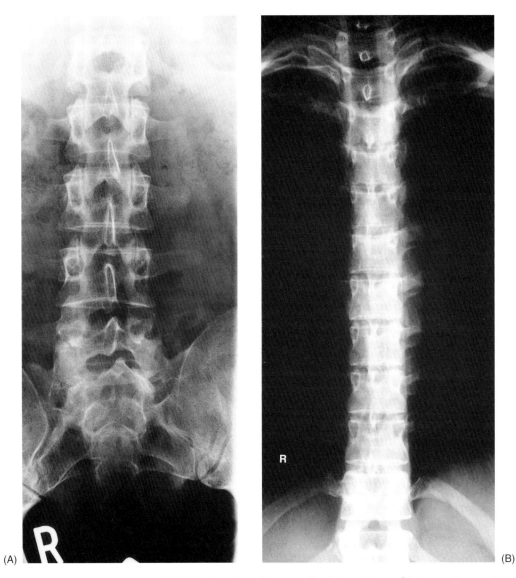

(A)   (B)

Figure 4.26 X-ray changes reflecting a variation in orientation of the sacroiliac joint surfaces and the vertebrae to the beam as a result of right anterior, left posterior rotational malalignment, with the lumbar spine fairly straight and some thoracic levoscoliosis (see also Figs 2.45 and 4.22). (A) Most of the right sacroiliac joint is visualized, whereas the left appears 'closed' except for the lower third. The facet joints appear variably open or closed at the different levels. (B) The mid-thoracic vertebrae (T4–T9 inclusive) have rotated into the left convexity. T5 at the apex appears to be considerably more left rotated than would be expected relative to T4 and T6, suggesting a possible T5 malrotation.

Facet joints

Malalignment also results in a reorientation of the facet joints relative to the beam, so that they will appear open on one side and narrowed or closed on the other. The rotation of L1–L4 into a left convexity, for example, opens the right and closes the left facet joints (Fig. 4.28; see Figs 2.65 and 4.26A). Malrotated individual vertebrae will augment or diminish this effect. The difference will be most evident on oblique films of the lumbar spine (see Fig. 2.44B). The narrowing of the joint space on one side may be wrongly attributed to degeneration of the surface cartilage, widening to laxity of the capsule and the supporting ligaments.

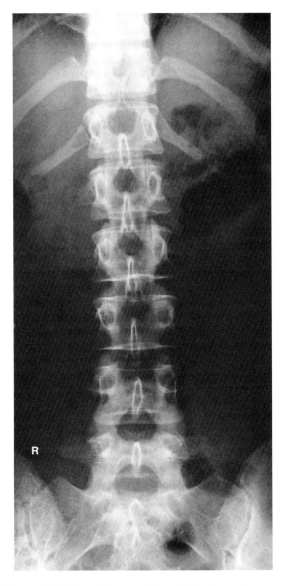

Figure 4.27   On realignment of the athlete shown in Fig. 4.26, the sacroiliac and lumbar facet joints appear to be more symmetrically open and the spine relatively straight.

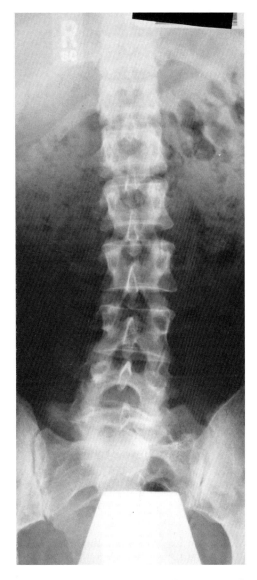

Figure 4.28   X-ray changes with malalignment: the effect on sacroiliac and facet joint orientation to the beam. L1–L4 vertebral rotation into the left convexity opens the left mid-lumbar facet joints and aggravates the closing/compression that results with the simultaneous right side flexion. L5 is sacralized on the left.

Sacrum

A shift of the sacrum may be easily apparent on X-ray. Standing anteroposterior views of the pelvis, for example, may show the following.

In the presence of malalignment, rotation of the sacrum around one of the oblique axes will show that a line through the middle of the sacrum and coccyx runs off centre, the coccyx obviously off to the right or the left of the Y-axis with rotation around the right or the left

oblique axis respectively (Aitken 1986; Fig. 4.29A). The sacrum and coccyx will realign with the Y-axis on correction of the malalignment (Fig. 4.29B).

In the presence of a pelvic obliquity attributable to an anatomical or functional LLD, the sacrum is usually rotated around the frontal plane as part of the pelvis, the sacral base being up on the high side. The sacrum may,

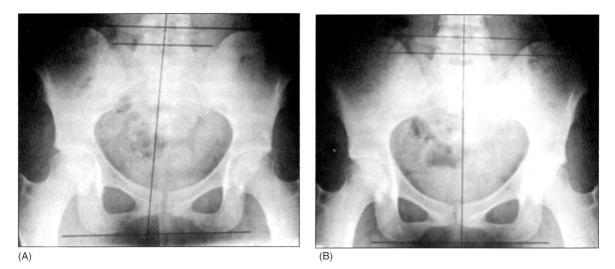

Figure 4.29 Changes in the relationship between the lumbar spine and the pelvis on a standing anteroposterior view. (A) Before manual treatment: left axis deviation is evident. (B) After manual treatment: realigned with vertical axis. (From Aitken 1986, with permission.)

however, eventually adapt to the obliquity in an attempt to decrease the stress on the lumbosacral region and to minimize the compensatory curves of the spine. In this case, the sacral base will be partially or completely level, even though the iliac crests show a persistent obliquity, being high on one side. It is important to know whether or not this sacral adaptation has occurred, especially when contemplating prescribing a lift on the 'short' leg side in the case of an anatomical LLD or the failed correction of a functional LLD (see Fig. 3.83).

Hip joints

Anterior innominate rotation results in an anteroinferior rotation of the superior acetabular rim, with increased overlapping of the femoral head that could be misinterpreted as a narrowing of the hip joint on an anteroposterior X-ray. Posterior innominate rotation has the opposite effect, posterosuperior rotation of the superior rim possibly making the joint appear wider than that on the opposite side (see Fig. 2.45).

There will also be a contrary reorientation of the joints relative to the vertical plane with both outflare/inflare and rotational malalignment (see Figs 2.45 and 4.25).

Other landmarks

Trochanters. The greater and lesser trochanters are rotated into or out of view by the external and internal rotation of the lower extremities (see Figs 2.45 and 4.25).

Symphysis pubis. A step deformity of 2–3 mm or more at the symphysis pubis will reflect changes in the alignment of the superior pubic rami:

● with right anterior, left posterior rotation, the right ramus is displaced downward relative to the left (reflecting anteroinferior and posterosuperior rotation respectively – see Figs 2.7, 2.29 and 2.45)
● with a right upslip, the right is displaced upwards relative to the left.

These findings may be erroneously interpreted as reflecting an instability of the symphysis pubis, but instability should not be presumed until it has been proven radiologically (see Fig. 2.70) and the effect of realignment assessed.

Computed tomography

A computed tomography scan may by helpful for confirming SI joint instability by disclosing a significant displacement of the SI joint surfaces relative to each other, which may correct on realignment (Fig. 4.30). The findings may be enhanced by an injection of contrast material into the joint.

Bone scans

Athletes presenting with pain localizing to the lumbosacral and/or SI joint areas often undergo bone scans to rule out problems such as facet joint osteoarthritis and sacroiliitis. In the presence of malalignment, and

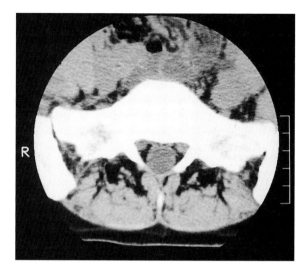

Figure 4.30 An unstable right sacroiliac joint. The computed tomography scan shows 1 cm posterior displacement of the right innominate relative to the sacrum. A block with local anaesthetic resolved the pain.

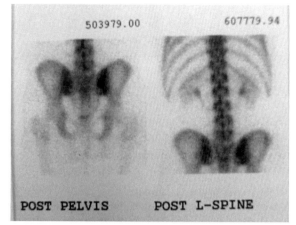

Figure 4.31 Typical changes on a bone scan when malalignment is present: there is a variable tracer concentration, here considerably higher in the right sacroiliac area than in left, as reflected by the asymmetrical SIS ratio (right 1.37 versus left 1.17). The ratio was still, however, within normal limits (less than 1.5), and there was neither any history of remote injury nor any clinical or laboratory indications of spondyloarthropathy.

with no indications of a spondyloarthropathy on clinical examination, these scans:

- are usually normal
- may reveal an underlying problem with increased bone turnover, often indicative of osteoarthritis involving the facet or hip joints.

These scans sometimes do, however, show:

1. asymmetrical, albeit still within normal limits, activity of the SI joint regions
2. one or more small areas of an abnormal increase in activity (Fig. 4.31)
3. an abnormal increase in activity in the symphysis pubis, usually interpreted as representing changes consistent with 'osteitis pubis'.

These changes in activity may be no more than a reflection of an increase in bone turnover that has resulted from the malalignment-related asymmetrical stress on these joints now that the joint surfaces are no longer matching, and there is often a component of instability attributable to a failure of form and/or force closure.

> The presence of malalignment can usually be diagnosed from changes evident on X-rays. Reporting these findings should be part of the regular interpretation of these films to decrease the possibility of their misinterpretation on subsequent reading by those not familiar with malalignment.

Dijkstra (1997) provides an excellent overview of the basic problems relating to SI joint visualization, Jurriaans & Friedman (1997) of the application of computed tomography and magnetic resonance imaging investigation to this area, Fortin et al (1997) of the application of SI joint injection for pain referral mapping and arthrography, and Maigne (1997) of radiology applied to investigating coccydynia. For further information regarding technique and findings related to problems specific to the SI joints and symphysis pubis, the reader is referred to Bernard & Cassidy (1991), Dorman & Ravin (1991) and Mens et al (1997).

IMPLICATIONS FOR RESPIROLOGY

The biomechanical changes and pain associated with malalignment can alter the mechanics of breathing and impair ventilation.

Malalignment typically results in pelvic obliquity and compensatory curves of the spine. Given a thoracic convexity to the left (see Fig. 3.13A):

1. the ribs on the right side move closer together, whereas those on the left separate
2. after costal motion has stopped, there is some further side flexion of the vertebrae to the right (see Fig. 3.13B); this causes the right ribs to rotate anteriorly and the left ribs to move posteriorly

3. the result being:
  – an alteration in the space available for the right compared with the left lung
  – stress on the costochondral junctions, costovertebral and costotransverse joints (see Figs 2.63, 3.13 and 3.14) and pleural irritation with cough
  – increased tension in some soft tissue structures, in particular the thoracic diaphragm and intercostal muscles
  – conceivably, a decrease in the minute lung volume on the right compared with the left side.

The typical finding on clinical examination of the supine-lying athlete is a forwards and downwards displacement of the upper segment of ribs on the left side, usually from the first to the fourth, fifth or sixth inclusive, relative to their right counterparts (see Fig. 2.62B). The reverse finding – the right ribs displacing forwards and down – is seen much less frequently.

Breathing normally involves an elevation of the ribs and a lateral expansion of the chest cage, with a descent of the thoracic diaphragm – so-called 'lateral costal breathing' Fig. 4.32). Joints already placed under stress by pelvic and spine malalignment - sternocostal included – and especially by malrotation of any thoracic vertebrae – costochondral/transverse/vertebral – will be stressed even further by any movement of the rib cage (see Figs 2.62, 2.63, 3.13 and 3.14). Pain from

these joints can impair normal lateral costal breathing and result in one of the following patterns:

1. *Apical breathing*: breathing is carried out mainly using the upper parts of the lungs. The result is a shallow pattern, with a failure to ventilate the major part of the lungs.

2. *Abdominal breathing*: movement of the ribs is limited; instead, the diaphragm descends to allow the lungs to open, but the descent is limited, sometimes as a result of restriction caused by problems with the stomach, liver, spleen or bowel. The result is a shallow breathing pattern that may also impair normal gastric and bowel motility, resulting in a feeling of 'bloating' of the stomach.

The shallow breathing associated with the apical and abdominal patterns results in a compensatory increase in respiratory rate which can result in excessive blowing-off of carbon dioxide, a respiratory alkalosis and earlier fatigue of respiratory muscles. Weakness and early fatigue may eventually become noticeable even on attempts at retraining for lateral costal breathing. A viscious cycle can develop, with pain from the thoracic spine and rib cage limiting retraining efforts and resulting in further weakening.

IMPLICATIONS FOR RHEUMATOLOGY

The malalignment syndrome *per se* is not an arthritic condition, but malalignment can result in irritation and inflammation of the SI joints, symphysis pubis or any other joint put under increased mechanical stress by chronic asymmetrical overloading. The question of whether or not the stresses related to malalignment can actually lead to osteoarthritis, with accelerated joint degeneration, still needs to be answered (see Figs 3.74 and 3.75).

Differentiating between malalignment and arthritis

When attributable to malalignment, any back stiffness and aching experienced on waking are typically temporary. These symptoms tend to resolve on moving around, usually within a few minutes or an hour or two at most, only to manifest themselves again briefly after prolonged sitting or lying down. The stiffness and aching reflect a stretching-out of irritated or inflamed soft tissues, in particular the thoracodorsal fascia and posterior pelvic ligaments, that tend to contract or 'gel' during a rest period. A recurrence of the aching that sometimes occurs when the athlete persists with an activity, such as prolonged walking, probably

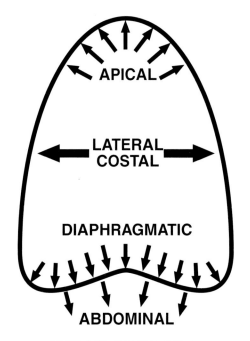

Figure 4.32 Breathing patterns.

reflects the increased stress on the joints and these tender soft tissues as the muscles fatigue.

Back stiffness associated with an inflammatory arthritic condition (e.g. rheumatoid arthritis or spondylotic arthropathy) tends to be much more persistent, often lasting several hours or even throughout the day.

Tests specific for the SI joint area may provoke pain in someone presenting with malalignment, some of the tests discussed in Chapter 2 being appropriate for this purpose. Most of these tests do not, however, differentiate between pain arising from the joint surfaces or the capsule and from the surrounding ligaments.

Radionuclear scans sometimes detect a difference in the degree of activity in one SI joint compared with the other, but the actual amount of activity on both sides is usually still within normal limits (see 'Implications for radiology and medical imaging' above and Fig. 4.31). This relative increase in uptake may just reflect early degeneration that is somewhat worse on one side. It may also, however, simply reflect an asymmetrical increase in bone turnover attributable to the asymmetrical increase in pressure on these joint surfaces and the change in weight-bearing that occurs with the malalignment. Such an increase in pressure could conceivably accelerate the degeneration of the joint cartilage, known to occur at an earlier age on the iliac than the sacral side (Cassidy 1992).

In the case of an inflammatory arthritis affecting the SI joints, bone scans typically delineate a generalized - and symmetrical - involvement of the joints.

'Malalignment syndrome' versus 'chronic pain syndrome'

The malalignment syndrome is frequently confused with some of the chronic pain syndromes thought to arise primarily from muscle, in particular fibromyalgia syndrome and myofascial pain syndrome. These three are, however, distinct entities, even though they may coexist. In addition, the chronicity of the biomechanical stresses and pain associated with malalignment can result in findings consistent with myofascial pain syndrome. There is an ongoing debate over whether malalignment can eventually lead to the development of a coexisting fibromyalgia syndrome.

Myofascial pain syndrome

The key features of this syndrome are as follows:

- It occurs more frequently in females than males (3:1).
- The pain and tenderness usually localize to one quadrant or even just one muscle.

- There is a trigger point – an area of acute tenderness localizing to a taut nodule or band, which is palpable within a muscle in the area of the muscle spindle.
- Transverse snapping of the taut band or the insertion of a needle may elicit a local muscle twitch response that can be seen and recorded.
- Palpation of the trigger point may, in addition to causing localized pain, also elicit pain or altered sensation in a typical referral pattern (see Fig. 3.41).
- The pain from the trigger point can be relieved by stretching or by the injection of a local anaesthetic.

Fibromyalgia syndrome

This syndrome occurs primarily between ages of 30 and 50 years, females being affected 10 times more often than males. The incidence is increased in association with autoimmune diseases such as hypothyroidism, rheumatoid arthritis, systemic lupus erythematosus and Raynaud's disease. Chronic, generalized, muscular aching pain involves in particular the shoulder and hip girdles, neck and lower back.

Tender points occur at specific sites bilaterally: the suboccipital muscle insertion, the anterior aspect of the C5–C6 intertransverse space, the midpoint of the upper border of trapezius, the origin of supraspinatus, the second rib just lateral to the costochondral junction, the lateral epicondyle, the upper outer quadrant of gluteus maximus, the posterior aspect of the greater trochanter and the medial aspect of the knee at the joint line. The diagnosis of fibromyalgia syndrome rests on a history of widespread pain and localized tenderness in at least 11 of these 18 sites.

> The tender points are distinct from trigger points in that there are no palpable nodules or bands, the sites are symmetrical, and their location does not change.

The individual suffers from generalized, chronic stiffness and fatigues easily. There is a non-restorative sleep pattern associated with:

1. a disturbance of the characteristic low-frequency (0.5–2.0 Hz) delta waves of non-rapid eye movement sleep by faster (7.5–11.0 Hz) alpha waves, leaving the person feeling tired rather than refreshed in the morning
2. muscular fatigue, aching and the development of tender points.

Given these distinguishing features of fibromyalgia syndrome and myofascial pain syndrome, it should be easy to differentiate these entities from the malalignment syndrome, which:

- occurs in an approximately equal number of females and males
- may have tender points, less frequently trigger points, associated with it but is more likely to show an increase in tension and tenderness in an asymmetrical pattern in specific muscles as a result of:
  – an increase in the sympathetic response (facilitation)
  – a change in the length-to-tension ratio
  – a reaction to an irritating focus
  – an attempt to stabilize a joint
  – a combination of these factors (see Ch. 3)
- is characterized by musculoskeletal pain from specific structures, mainly in an asymmetrical pattern that can usually be explained on the basis of the factors noted above, and is usually attributable to the biomechanical stresses that typically occur with malalignment
- is not characterized by chronic fatigue, generalized stiffness or a non-restorative sleep pattern.

According to some authors (Barral & Mercier 1988, Selby 1992, Upledger & Vrredevoogd 1983), the chronic increase in pelvic floor tension is considered to be a possible cause for the decrease in vitality, or even the chronic fatigue syndrome, frequently noted in those with the levator ani syndrome (see below).

IMPLICATIONS FOR UROLOGY, GASTROENTEROLOGY, GYNAECOLOGY AND OBSTETRICS

In the peripartum period, acute pain localizing to the symphysis pubis may be wrongfully attributed to a separation of the pubic bones, but a separation is rarely palpable, or even visible on a standing radiological view intended to stress the joint (see Fig. 2.70A, B). The problem is more often the result of the additional stresses being superimposed during this period on a joint that is already under constant stress as the result of a long-standing upslip, rotational malalignment, outflare/inflare or combination of these. The malalignment, and the associated excessive displacement and rotation of the pubic rami relative to each other, may certainly also result from the trauma of delivery or from subsequent muscle spasm.

> Pain originating from the pelvic region as a result of malalignment can mimic gastrointestinal and genitourinary disorders because of its location.

Take, for example, pain originating from the right anterior SI joint ligaments, which are usually located immediately posterior to the appendix. This pain can localize to McBurney's point and mimic the pain of appendicitis. In addition, all of these ligaments and other somatic structures are segmentally related to viscera that have an autonomic supply from the same segment (Barral & Mercier 1988).

Norman (1968) reported on 74 patients who presented with lower abdominal, groin or rectal pain 'which, after extensive investigation … defied the efforts of the examiners to implicate any of the organ systems to explain the protracted pain' (p. 54). Seventy-two of the 74 had no complaint of back pain or sciatic radiation, and none responded to antispasmodic medications. Seventy-one individuals obtained relief from their pain within minutes on the injection of $3 \, cm^3$ 2% procaine into the ipsilateral SI joint; 52 required a second and 32 a third injection, spaced 3 days apart. By 1 month, 58 (81%) were pain-free. The various symptoms reported by some of those who were successfully treated in this way are of particular interest and are given in Box 4.7.

There is no reference to pelvic malalignment in Norman's report, but the types of symptoms listed have all been reported in association with malalignment (see Ch. 3, 'Thoracolumbar syndrome' above and descriptions below). The negative investigations, and the positive response to SI joint injection, suggests that the pain arose from stress on this joint and its ligaments. Norman correctly identified 'sacroiliac disease and its relationship to lower abdominal pain'. The

---

> **Box 4.7** Symptoms encountered in Norman's (1968) study
>
> - An acute onset of right groin pain
> - Right lower quadrant pain with radiation to the groin, treated unsuccessfully by repeated dilatation of the ureter for 'spasm of unknown origin'
> - Severe right lower quadrant pain radiating to the back, with only a partial response using a ptosis corset for bilateral renal ptosis noted on X-ray
> - Left lower quadrant pain in a patient diagnosed as suffering from diverticulitis
> - Symptoms of acute right lower quadrant pain in a patient with a previous appendectomy, felt to indicate 'another attack of appendicitis'
> - Severe pain and muscle spasm in the rectum with radiation down the right leg, which failed to respond to haemorrhoidectomy, improved only temporarily after a paravertebral nerve block and caudal block, and worsened on anaesthetizing the coccyx
> - Severe sciatica, as well as abdominal pain on coughing
> - Pain in the lower left part of the abdomen on taking long steps when walking.

question remains of how many actually had the SI joint problem to begin with because they were out of alignment and would have responded just as dramatically to realignment.

It is not unusual for athletes to experience symptoms involving the gastrointestinal or genitourinary system when they are out of alignment. The acute onset of these symptoms can coincide with the recurrence of malalignment and their abrupt cessation with successful realignment. Typical of these symptoms are:

- an increased need to void (daytime frequency and nocturia), urgency and stress incontinence
- episodic loose stools, or even diarrhoea, lasting 1–3 days and sometimes alternating with the onset of constipation on realignment
- a build-up of gas with abdominal distension
- a marked exacerbation of premenstrual and menstrual pain
- testicular/vaginal wall pain
- sexual dysfunction and pain on intercourse (dyspareunia).

An awareness of the commonly encountered referral patterns involving the gastrointestinal and genitourinary systems is important when questioning athletes as they often fail to report such patterns spontaneously. Male athletes, for example, may not volunteer a history of testicular pain. In the athlete presenting with malalignment who is afebrile and has no evidence of testicular tenderness or swelling, and whose investigations for infection, tumour and hernia are negative, this may well represent pain referred to the testicle from the ipsilateral iliolumbar ligament (see Fig. 3.42). In female athletes, irritation of this ligament may account for dysaesthesias felt in the ipsilateral vaginal wall and/or labia. Irritation of the 'anterior' cutaneous nerve branches of T12 and L1 can also cause dysaesthaesias in the ipsilateral lower abdominal wall, groin, scrotum or labia majora (see Figs 4.21A1, B2).

Effects of malalignment: somatic versus visceral?

The fact that problems involving somatic structures can result in visceral symptoms has long been recognized. In this respect, Hackett (1956) did much to clarify the visceral effects relating to ligaments, Travell & Simons (1983, 1992) documenting those associated with trigger points.

A recognition that visceral problems can result in somatic symptoms is in large part attributable to the translation in 1988 of the landmark *Manipulations viscerales* by Barral & Mercier (1983).

> Barral & Mercier's studies, and the experience of others skilled in 'visceral manipulation', have resulted in an increasing awareness that the problems related to malalignment can, rather than being restricted to the musculoskeletal or somatic system, also affect the autonomic and visceral systems.

In fact, those using visceral manipulation are convinced that it is more often the visceral problem that is the cause of the recurrent malalignment rather than the other way around (Barral & Mercier 1989; J.L. Cole-Morgan, personal communication, 1993; J.S. Gerhardt, personal communications, 1995, 1997, 1999; H.L. Jones, personal communications, 1993, 1995, 1999), and their success in treating these resistant cases would certainly support their contention. They speak of organs or viscera not lying in their proper place as the result of trauma, and not fully functioning because of displacement or a restriction of their mobility, much as one might talk about the malalignment of a vertebra or the pelvis being 'out of place'.

The liver, for example, is suspended in the abdominal cavity by six major ligaments (Fig. 4.33) and normally moves some 200 m a day as it repeatedly ascends and descends in harmony with the movements of the diaphragm on expiration and inspiration respectively. A tightness of any of these ligaments can result from postoperative scar formation or blunt trauma, such as a seat-belt injury, also secondary to inflammation or infection.

Tightness will impair the smooth upwards and downwards movement of the liver and will, by impairing the glide of the fascia that envelops the liver, also interfere with the craniosacral rhythm. These restrictions can eventually interfere with the proper functioning of this organ. Malfunction may initially be experienced as unexplained visceral symptoms attributable to biliary stasis and a decrease in hepatic metabolism. Nervous depression and a decrease in the immune response have been linked to the same mechanism (Barral & Mercier 1989).

> Athletes who present with malalignment that fails to respond to other techniques may finally respond to visceral manipulation, used either alone or in combination with one of the more 'traditional' mobilization techniques.

Ligaments and referral to viscera

Hackett (1958) was probably one of the first to point out that pain originating from somatic structures,

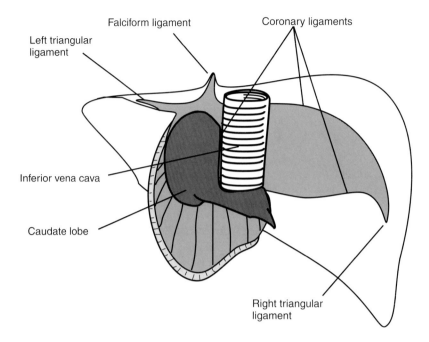

Falciform ligament

Coronary ligaments

Left triangular ligament

Inferior vena cava

Caudate lobe

Right triangular ligament

Figure 4.33 The six ligaments supporting the liver. (After Grant 1980, with permission.)

namely the ligaments, could be referred to the viscera and could therefore result in symptoms involving the gastrointestinal and genitourinary systems. He blamed the problem on a laxity of these ligaments. By injecting hypertonic saline or glucose into specific ligaments, he was able not only to map out the patterns of referred pain into the extremities (see Chs 2 and 3), but also to record consistent responses involving the viscera. Some of his findings warrant repeating here because they have been supported by numerous subsequent publications (e.g. Barral & Mercier 1988, Maigne 1997, Steege et al 1998) and, in this author's experience, have been borne out in clinical practice. Direct quotations regarding the symptoms referred from specific ligaments to the viscera (Box 4.8) are taken from Hackett's monograph (1958).

Hackett writes that:

The pain in the intestine and testicle has been reproduced by needling in the dorsal 12th, lumbar articular and the iliolumbar ligaments, and the tendon attachments to the transverse processes of all the lumbar vertebrae. (pp. 90–91)

Anterior rotation of the coccyx has also been associated with bowel disturbance, possibly by affecting the autonomic supply to the bowel as it exits with the S2, S3 and S4 nerve roots (see Fig. 4.15) in close proximity to the anterior aspect of the sacrococcygeal articulation and the coccyx itself (Barral & Mercier 1988).

Problems relating to the female reproductive system

Female athletes are sometimes reluctant to volunteer information relating to sexual function and menses, in which case specific questions are in order.

Dyspareunia (painful intercourse)

Pain in the ipsilateral vaginal wall or labia may manifest itself as introital dyspareunia. Pain can be referred to these sites from the iliolumbar ligament or result from irritation of the T12/L1 anterior cutaneous branches as part of the thoracolumbar syndrome (see Fig. 4.21A1, B2). The following problems are more likely to result in deep-thrust dyspareunia:

- tension and tenderness involving the pelvic floor muscles themselves
- a painful coccyx, which may reflect:
- a chronic increase in tension in the attached muscles and ligaments (Fig. 4.34B)
- problems involving the sacrococcygeal junction itself, such as rotational or torsional strain, or excessive anterior or posterior displacement (Fig. 4.34C).

These problems are discussed in more detail under 'Coccydynia, pelvic floor disorder and levator ani syndrome' below.

Box 4.8 Viseral symptoms caused by referral from ligaments

Iliolumbar ligament (see Figs. 3.42 and 3.58)
- Ipsilateral testicular discomfort
- Discomfort involving the penis
- Unilateral vaginal or labial pain, with or without dyspareunia
- Unilateral groin pain, known to mimic appendicitis, because its location just above and medial to the inguinal ligament is near McBurney's point
- Nausea

Lumbosacral ligament (see Fig. 3.58):
- Bladder discomfort and a frequent urge to void, which can signal a recurrence of malalignment and may not be relieved by voiding; in addition to an involvement of this ligament, another mechanism to consider is a strictly mechanical one, malalignment having resulted in irritation of the bladder outlet by distorting the bladder and squeezing or twisting the bladder neck (see 'Visceral problems and the pelvic floor' below)
- rectal pain, which can occur with laxity of the lower sacral ligaments.

Sacroiliac ligaments (see Figs 3.58 and 4.10): these may refer pain to the lower abdomen, possibly 'accompanied by tenderness' (Hackett, 1958; p. 91) in that area

Lumbar and lumbosacral spine ligaments (see Fig. 3.63): irritation of these ligaments has been connected to bowel disturbance. Athletes may experience an acute onset of diarrhoea coincident with the recurrence of malalignment that is abolished by realignment. In others, recurrence is associated with episodes of severe constipation, bloating and 'gas'

Dysmenorrhoea

Typical changes in the menstrual cycle include a longer and more painful premenstrual phase, increased back pain, increased abdominal and/or pelvic discomfort, a heavier flow, a longer duration and irregularity, usually with increased frequency, the periods reverting to the habitual pattern with realignment. Possible explanations for these phenomena include:

- increased engorgement of the reproductive organs resulting from torsion of these organs and increased tension in the pelvic floor muscles
- torsion resulting in increased tension in some of the ligaments that suspend the uterus and ovaries
- an actual recurrence of the malalignment, which is more likely to recur around the time of the period, possibly as a result of:
  - an increase in ligamental laxity associated with the transient increase in blood relaxin level known to occur around this time (and also with ovulation)
  - a transient increase in the stress level, which in turn causes an increase in muscle tension; muscles that have previously been tense and tender, whether as a result of malalignment or some other insult, tend to be the first ones to react.

Coccydynia, pelvic floor dystonia and levator ani syndrome

Involvement of the coccygeal region is not uncommon in association with malalignment. In Schamberger's unpublished 1993 and 1994 studies, the author found that 12% of those presenting with malalignment had

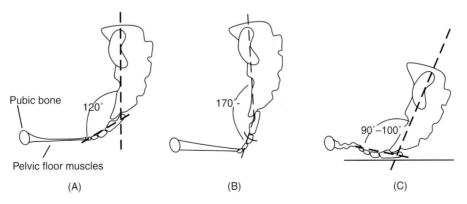

Figure 4.34 Effect of angulation of the coccyx on the inserting ligaments and pelvic floor muscles. (A) A normal angulation of 120 degrees relative to the sacrum, with a 30 degree range of motion; there is normal pelvic floor tone. (B) Excessive extension angulation resulting in hypertonus of the pelvic floor. (C) Excessive flexion angulation resulting in hypotonus of the pelvic floor (e.g. on 'slouched sitting') but which may itself result from a chronic hypertonus.

tenderness over the coccyx. Abnormalities of the sacro-coccygeal joint and the attaching pelvic floor muscles and ligaments are now recognized as a cause of:

1. both acute and chronic pain arising from the 'spine', sometimes hard to differentiate from symptoms that originate from the lumbar region because of the overlap in pain distribution
2. pelvic floor dystonia (both hyper- and hypotonicity)
3. visceral dysfunction
4. levator ani (spasm) syndrome
5. failure to achieve realignment of the pelvis and spine, or to maintain the correction.

The role of coccydynia and pelvic floor dystonia as a cause of ongoing problems, including chronic pelvic pain and visceral symptoms, has been receiving increasing recognition (Maigne 1997, Steege et al 1998). The following is an adaptation of a succinct account of developments in this area by Selby (1992).

The coccyx and sacrococcygeal articulation

Barral & Mercier (1988, p. 260) stressed the importance of the sacrococcygeal articulation in stating that:

it has a physiological role in copulation, defecation and micturition. It plays an integral part in lumbosacral dynamics; problems with the coccyx can contribute to lumbosacral restrictions.

This diarthrosis is normally capable of up to 30 degrees of motion (Fig. 4.34). It is reinforced by the anterior, posterior and lateral sacrococcygeal liga-ments, which help to maintain the position of the coccyx and distribute forces to the coccyx and adjacent structures. In addition, the coccyx serves as a point of attachment for almost all the other soft tissue struc-tures of the pelvis (Barral & Mercier 1988).

Excessive angulation forwards, such as occurs with sacral counternutation or slouching, or as the result of a fall, can result in pelvic floor hypotonus with an even-tual contracture of these muscles and ligaments (Fig. 4.34C). Excessive angulation backwards, as with exces-sive nutation or birth trauma, increases the tension and can eventually stretch out these structures (Fig. 4.34B).

The continuations of the dural tube that exit through the sacral hiatus also blend into the periosteum of the coccyx. Manipulation of the coccyx thus allows those undertaking craniosacral treatment a direct means of acting on the spinal dura.

Anatomy of the pelvic floor

The pelvic floor muscles serve as anchorage for the low back and the hip joints, and as a support for the pelvic organs. The pelvic floor is made up of five layers of muscle and fascia, which attach to the bony ring of the pelvis (see Fig. 2.36).

The anal sphincter forms the *first* (superficial) layer. The urogenital triangle, or *second* layer, consists of the urogenital diaphragm and vaginal and urethral sphinc-ters; it stretches from the ischial tuberosities posteriorly to the pubis anteriorly. The pelvic diaphragm, or *third* layer, is made up of the three levator ani muscles (pub-ococcygeus, iliococcygeus and ischiococcygeus), which blend with the rectal sphincter posteriorly and the superficial perineal muscles anteriorly. Together, these support the base and neck of the bladder.

Herman (1988, p. 87) notes that the levator ani muscles not only:

have the potential to decrease the urethral, vaginal and rectal canals, but they can decrease the anteroposterior relationships of the bony ring; and some authors believe that they can change the angle of the sacrum to the lumbar spine.

In addition, as Heardman pointed out in 1951, there are fascial connections between the levator ani muscles and the piriformis, biceps femoris, semitendinosus and obturator internus muscles, so that tension in any of these muscles can affect the tone of the pelvic floor. The smooth muscle diaphragm and endopelvic diaphragm complete the floor.

The pudendal nerve and vessels that supply these muscles travel within the fascial layers (see Fig. 4.15), which puts them at risk of being irritated or compressed by any abnormal increase in tension and/or contracture of these myofascial tissues. Any compromise of the neu-rovascular supply can result in spasm, trophic changes, vasomotor effects and pain involving the pelvic floor structures (Barral & Mercier 1988, Herman 1988).

Visceral problems and the pelvic floor

Typical visceral problems that have been attributed to pelvic floor dysfunction include:

- incontinence of bowel or bladder attributed to a lax floor
- constipation and incomplete voiding with excessive tension
- dysmenorrhoea, dyspareunia, impotence and sexual dysfunction
- recurrent cystitis and urinary tract infection.

Pelvic malalignment distorts the ring formed by the pelvic bones and therefore disturbs the points of attachment of the pelvic floor muscles. This affects the tone in these muscles. It also puts a twist on structures that exit by traversing the pelvic floor (the urethra and distal rectum/anus) or lie in close proximity to the pelvic floor (the vagina, uterus, bladder and rectum).

Twisting of the bladder and its outlet may be one explanation for the not-infrequent report of urgency and frequency of voiding that disappear immediately on realignment, only to return just as quickly with recurrence of malalignment, a phenomenon that has also been attributed to irritation of the lumbosacral ligaments (Hackett 1958). Distortion of the vagina and uterus may account for problems of dyspareunia and dysmenorrhoea, which can also sometimes disappear just as miraculously with realignment.

Visceral pain can, however, also cause pelvic floor hypertonicity and spasm, which may deform the sacrococcygeal joint and cause back pain. A bladder infection can cause spasm of the levator ani muscles, which can in turn be responsible for the inability to void completely and may also eventually cause back pain.

In other words, sacrococcygeal pain may initiate visceral problems or may itself be the result of an underlying visceral problem.

Therefore, in the absence of a history of trauma to the sacrococcygeal region, a concerted effort must be made to exclude any underlying visceral pathology affecting the bowel, rectum or urogenital system. If preliminary tests (e.g. blood screen, urinalysis and ultrasound scan) are negative, the problem(s) may simply be related to coexisting malalignment. In particular, distortion of the pelvic ring and L5 vertebral and sacrococcygeal rotation should be sought and addressed. Further investigations and treatment (e.g. trigger point injection, pelvic floor exercises and biofeedback) may be in order if the symptoms fail to respond to realignment alone (Costello 1998, Wallace 1994).

Hypotonicity of the pelvic floor muscles has been attributed to anterior movement of the coccyx as a result of trauma or the pressure of faulty sitting. McGivern & Cleveland (1965) were able to show this anterior movement radiologically. They cited radiological studies showing that the coccyx is normally tilted forwards some 120 degrees on the sacrum (Fig. 4.34A). The angle of the sacrococcygeal joint tended to decrease considerably when the patient was placed in a 'slumped position' on the X-ray table, 'indicating substantial flexion of the sacrococcygeal joint' (Fig. 4.34C). Like Thiele (1963), they stressed how a habitual poor sitting posture was common in patients with coccygeal pain, how slumping in a chair caused the sacrum and the coccyx to press against the hard surface and produced increased flexion on the sacrococcygeal joint, and how the coccygeal pain was often relieved simply

by sitting on a firm surface, trunk erect so that its weight was now supported by the ischial tuberosities rather than the coccyx.

Traumatic or habitual anterior rotation of the coccyx moves it closer to the pubic symphysis, bringing the origin and insertion of the pelvic floor muscles, ligaments and fascial sheaths closer together (Fig. 4.34C), muscle strength and pelvic floor tone thereby being decreased. When the bladder and rectum are relaxed in this way, incontinence may result (Barral & Mercier 1988).

Levator ani syndrome

Levator ani syndrome, also called levator spasm syndrome, may result from a persistent increase in pelvic floor tension. Acute trauma to the sacrococcygeal region, such as from a fall, direct blow or unaccustomed and prolonged pressure from a poor sitting posture, can result in reflex hypertonicity of the levator muscles. As Selby (1992, p. 3) has pointed out, this may create further:

irritating deformation of the joint in the same anterior direction as the original traumatic insult … This scenario can go on for years, fuelled by sitting in soft chairs and certain car seats (e.g. bucket seats). However, simple manoeuvres (e.g. direct mobilization of the sacrococcygeal joint) that break into the vicious cycle can often totally alleviate this sort of distress, both acute and chronic, in short order.

A history of trauma to the coccyx is often overlooked or hard to come by in patients who have sustained an injury many years ago. Specific questions may trigger a memory of a tobogganing accident or of a fall from a bike or down a staircase. Athletes are less likely to recall specific incidents if their sport is one in which falls are par for the course. Sexual abuse is another cause to consider.

In female athletes, questions repeatedly bring forth the realization that the symptoms that have now brought them to the doctor's office have, in retrospect, been present since the time of a pregnancy and delivery. Birth trauma and inadequate postpartum strengthening are very likely to result in excessive relaxation of the pelvic floor. This subject is now being studied extensively (Mens et al 1992, Oestgaard 1998).

In Selby's experience (1992, p. 4):

spinal pain due to coccyx strain and hypertonicity of the pelvic floor is commonly felt in the mid to low sacral area referring outward toward the greater trochanter unilaterally or bilaterally (resembling trochanteric bursitis) and not infrequently down the posterior thigh.

He has also documented cases of chronic groin and anterior thigh pain that completely resolved following mobilization of the coccyx. Symptoms are typically provoked by sitting in soft chairs and by prolonged standing and repetitive activities such as stair-climbing that 'demand effort from the pelvic floor muscles to contract in order to stabilize the pelvis and thus are potentially provocative' (Selby 1992, p. 4).

In this respect, Baker (1998) points out that gluteus maximus has tendinous attachments to the sacrococcygeal capsule, and that reproduction of the pelvic floor pain with resisted hip extension (e.g. stair-climbing) 'is indicative of coccyx dysfunction due to that relationship' (p. 225).

Increased pelvic floor tension, in addition to causing localized or referred pain, must be considered as a possible cause of a general decrease in vitality or even a chronic fatigue syndrome that has frequently been noted in these patients (Barral & Mercier 1988, Selby 1992, Upledger & Vredevoogd 1983).

Diagnostic approach

Selby proposes the following approach to assessment:

- First comes an initial evaluation of the gross range of motion of the whole spine, of sacroiliac mobility (using the kinetic rotational or Gillet test – see Figs 2.88 and 2.89) and of the spinal dural system for irritability (using tests such as Maitland's slump test – see Fig. 3.68).
- The coccyx is then palpated through the clothing to note its anterior/posterior angulation, any deviation from the midline, tenderness and thickening or hypertrophy of the soft tissue inserting into it.
- With the patient in standing or side-lying, the edges of the coccyx are then briefly massaged through the clothing, noting its flexibility and end-feel while attempting to release any tension in the soft tissue and gently to mobilize the joint. Alternatively, sustained pressure can be applied 'deeply' on the lateral margins of the coccyx.

- The range of motion of the back and neck is then immediately re-evaluated, as is the slump test (if it was positive).

Selby (1992, p. 5) notes that:

coccydynia and abnormal tonicity of the pelvic floor is almost always associated with loss of lumbosacral extension, unilateral or bilateral side-bending and sometimes loss of flexion.

After rubbing the margins of the coccyx deeply, there is often a marked resolution of these restrictions.

Selby feels that mobilization of the sacrococcygeal joint and the surrounding soft tissues 'frees up sacral extension' so that the sacral base can once again tip anteriorly (which is the physiological movement of the sacrum that occurs with lumbar extension – see 'nutation', Figs 2.8A and 2.15C). He postulates that these effects may come about as a result of influencing inhibitory reflexes mediated by the Golgi tendon organs, proprioceptive changes resulting from mobilization of the sacrococcygeal joint and possibly also a reflex decrease of tension in the iliopsoas and piriformis muscles.

SUMMARY

A recognition of the malalignment syndrome is important in order to allow its differentiation from other specific medical problems. The symptoms arising from malalignment and these other entities may clearly overlap; it is not until realignment has been achieved that the true nature of an underlying problem may become apparent. Malalignment must itself always be considered as a possible unifying cause of the complaints with which the athlete presents, especially when these complaints suggest asymmetry and the examination and investigations fail to reveal one of the 'well-recognized' clinical conditions.

5

Clinical correlations in sports

Malalignment alters body biomechanics and creates stresses that may hinder the athlete's ability to progress and do well in a given sport, predispose the athlete to injury, prolong the recovery time or even prevent full recovery. This chapter takes a closer look at the detrimental effects of malalignment on athletic activities. The first part discusses the clinical correlations relating to specific biomechanical changes, the second looks at the effect of malalignment on specific sports, and the third analyses the biomechanical changes underlying some of the recurrent injuries seen when malalignment is present. The chapter concludes with considerations regarding:

- whether a failure to advance in some sports is primarily a 'natural' process of elimination, or whether it may be determined in large part by the restrictions imposed by the presence of malalignment and may therefore be preventable
- the effect of malalignment on the validity of research in certain areas in sports.

CLINICAL CORRELATIONS: SPECIFIC BIOMECHANICAL CHANGES

Clinical correlations associated with vertebral malrotation and pelvic malalignment relate primarily to stress patterns that result from limitations of ranges of motion, changes in muscle and ligament tension, and alterations of weight-bearing and leg length. The irritation of joint structures and soft tissues, including the peripheral nerves and autonomic nervous system, gives rise to typical pain phenomena.

VERTEBRAL MALROTATION

In the thoracic region, stress is also transmitted through the costovertebral and costotransverse junctions to the ribs, and anteriorly to the sternocostal and costochondral junctions (see Figs 2.63, 3.13 and 3.14). Further rotation into the direction of the malrotation is restricted, affecting the overall movement of the spine and predisposing to injury.

> The term 'vertebral malrotation' refers to an excessive rotation of one or more vertebrae (see Ch. 2), which can result in increased stresses and strains on soft tissue structures, facet joints and discs at the level(s) involved.

Level of malrotation

Vertebral malrotation can affect any vertebra between the occiput and the sacrum, but it does involve certain levels of the spine with increased frequency (see Ch. 3). The general findings on examination at an affected level have been described in Chapter 2.

Malrotation of L4, L5 or both vertebrae (see Figs 2.35 and 2.65)

There are three major problems related to the malrotation of these vertebrae: pain, restriction of range of motion and secondary malalignment of the sacrum and the sacroiliac (SI) joints. Instability of the lumbosacral area may occur with the initial injury or develop subsequently with the stress arising from recurring malalignment.

Pain. Pain may be localized to the low back region, but there may also be radiation to the buttocks or even referral to the lower extremities as a result of:

1. *increased tension* on soft tissue structures, primarily the paravertebral muscles, iliolumbar ligaments and interspinous, supraspinous and other intervertebral ligaments (see Figs 2.2, 2.3, 2.35, 3.57, 3.63 and 7.37)
2. *facet joint compression* on the side contrary to the direction of vertebral rotation and distraction (opening) on the opposite side (e.g. clockwise trunk rotation results in left compression and right distraction – see Fig. 2.35B)
3. *torquing* of the annulus and the disc.

A clockwise rotation of L5, for example, increases tension in the right iliolumbar ligaments as well as the supra- and interspinous ligaments, multifidi and rotatores muscles, primarily from the L3 to the S1 level (see Figs 2.23, 2.35B and 3.63). It compresses the left and separates the right L5–S1 facet surfaces. Distraction or entrapment of the facet joint capsule, ligaments and nerve fibres supplying these joints can account for local-

ized pain and referred symptoms to the ipsilateral buttock and lower extremity as far down as the ankle (McCall et al 1979, Mooney & Robertson 1976, Travell & Simons 1992).

Restriction of range of motion

> Vertebral malrotation is usually multidirectional, consisting not only of rotation in the transverse plane, but also of a combination of either forward flexion (F) or extension (E) with rotation (R) and side flexion (S).

The 'FRS' and 'ERS' patterns result in a restriction of further movement into the directions indicated. L1–L4, for example, would normally rotate into a convexity; therefore, rotation would be counterclockwise into a left convexity (see Figs 2.29, 4.6 and 4.28,) and clockwise into a right convexity (see Figs 2.65A and 4.22). Superimposing a clockwise malrotation of L4 on a preexisting right convexity will accentuate the already existing forwards flexion, rotation and right side flexion, limiting any further movement of L4 into all of these directions; an L4 counterclockwise malrotation will, however, limit further movement into the opposite directions (see Fig. 2.65B).

Malalignment of the SI joints. A clockwise rotation of L4 or L5, for example, exerts a rotational force on the innominates (anterior on the left and posterior on the right) because the simultaneous rotation of the transverse process (backwards on the right, forwards on the left) displaces the iliolumbar ligament origins away from their insertions and increases tension in these ligaments on both sides (see Fig. 2.35). There is also the torsional effect on the sacrum transmitted through the L5–S1 disc indirectly, and through the compressed left facet joint directly (see Fig. 2.35B). Reactive spasm in the adjacent quadratus lumborum and iliopsoas can cause recurrent ipsilateral SI joint upslip (Fig. 2.40). A failure to correct L4 and/or L5 vertebral malrotation, and an instability of L4 and L5, are two common causes for the recurrence of rotational malalignment and upslip.

Thoracolumbar junction: T11, T12 and L1

Degenerative changes at the thoracolumbar junction are common in sports calling for repeated high spinal loading, high-velocity hyperflexion and hyperextension, and rotary motion (d'Hemecourt & Micheli 1997), in particular, gymnastics, ballet, wrestling, diving, waterski-jumping and the bowling action of cricket, gymnastics repeatedly receiving most mention (Kesson & Atkins 1999).

Malrotation of this level involves primarily T12 and L1, less often T11. These vertebrae may be involved in isolation or in combination with the others, for example in 'T12 right and L1 left' rotation. In addition to the discomfort localizing to the thoracolumbar region as a result of the increased stress on facet joints, discs and ligaments, often with reactive muscle spasm, malrotation at these levels may be complicated by:

- the presence of malalignment of the pelvis, with pelvic obliquity and the compensatory scoliosis that creates stress points at the sites of reversal: the lumbosacral, thoracolumbar and cervicothoracic junctions
- thoracolumbar syndrome (see Ch. 4 and Figs 4.18–4.21)
- rotational stresses on the attaching rib(s) and thoracic diaphragm
- facilitation of the left quadratus lumborum muscle with rotation of L1 to the left, also causing increased tension directly on the upper origins of this muscle from the L1 transverse process.

A malrotation of T11 and/or T12 results in increased stress on their costovertebral and costotransverse articulations. The associated torquing increases the stress on the anterior articulation of the 11th rib at the costochondral junction and its continuation as the costal cartilage. Pain can usually be provoked by applying pressure anywhere along the affected rib(s), and localized by direct pressure on the tender anterior and/or posterior articulation(s). Torsion of the lower ribs can also present as discomfort and even spasm of the attaching diaphragm musculature. Any of these structures may become symptomatic, sometimes presenting as 'chest' or 'abdominal' pain and leading to extensive investigations to rule out a cardiac, pulmonary or epigastric problem.

The T4 and T5 level

A malrotation of one or both vertebrae at these levels is a frequent occurrence and may reflect the fact that:

1. reversal of the curvature of the thoracic segment, which helps to ensure that the head ends up in the midline, may start as low as T4 or T5 (see Fig. 2.60B)
2. the forces normally associated with upper extremity activities intersect at this level, unopposed or unequal forces predisposing to malrotation of one or both vertebrae, for example:
   - in throwing events (bowling, curling or athletic events that involve throwing an object)
   - weight-lifting with one arm at a time

- asymmetrical resisted manoeuvres (e.g. canoeing)
- sudden rotational forces on the trunk, especially when the pelvis is fixed (e.g. wrestling or collisions with players and objects).

> The spinous process will deviate from the midline in a direction contrary to the direction of vertebral body rotation. As a result, the otherwise uniform curve formed by the thoracic spinous processes, convex to right or left, will be interrupted at the level of the deviated spinous process (see Figs 2.63A and 2.64).

The associated pain is commonly felt in the interscapular area itself and may be referred to the shoulder girdle on one or both sides. Pain from this site can also be referred directly through the thorax to the anterior chest region, simulating angina (see Ch. 4). The athlete may localize the main discomfort to an area of increased tension and tenderness, or even localized spasm, which may be palpable within the immediately adjacent rhomboid, mid-trapezius and paravertebral musculature (often just on one side). The abnormal tension may reflect simply the increase in distance between the origin and insertion of these muscles: a deviation of the T4 spinous process to the right, away from the left scapula, will, for example, put the attaching left rhomboid and mid-trapezius muscles under increased tension. Pain from T4/T5 can also trigger a reflex contraction of muscles in the vicinity in an attempt to splint this site. One is probably often looking at a combination of factors (see Ch. 3). The area may, however, remain asymptomatic.

On examination, pain may be evoked only with posterior-to-anterior and/or rotatory pressure applied to the spinous process of the vertebrae, and/or pressure on the soft tissues within the immediate vicinity, which, as in tests carried out for thoracolumbar syndrome, may suggest an irritation of specific facet joints (see Fig. 4.18). Trigger points are common in the muscles and ligaments at these levels and the adjacent posterior shoulder girdle regions. In addition, upper extremity ranges of motion may be restricted by pain if they exert a rotational force on the affected segment of the thoracic spine.

The 'T3' or 'T4' syndrome

As described by Maitland (1977), this refers to a symptom complex caused by the malrotation of one or more vertebrae between T2 and T7, T3 or T4 being most commonly involved. The symptoms are vague and widespread, with a report of pain and paraesthesias in the upper limbs and/or head pain (initially described as a dull aching or pressure feeling in an 'all-over' distribution). Symptoms may occur as a result of referral through the autonomic nervous system, originating from the upper thoracic region. In the series of 90 patients with T4 syndrome published by McGuckin (1986), all had an involvement of the upper extremity, either uni- or bilaterally, with a glove-like distribution of paraesthesias up to the wrists, forearm, elbow or even more proximal level (see Fig. 4.9).

Fraser (1993) has described a 'T3 syndrome' following trauma (e.g. a fall onto the shoulder or direct trauma to the anterior rib area). Symptoms may include paraesthesias, pain, vasomotor changes, a loss of sensation, the swelling of an extremity, anterior chest wall or axillary pain, a weakness of grip and/or difficulty breathing. The dramatic results achieved with manipulation to restore joint play at T3, the T3 costotransverse junction and sometimes T2 and T4 has led Fraser to propose that the correction 'affects the vaso-motor system probably via the sympathetic ganglion at T-2' (1993, p. 5). It may also be worth considering injection of local anaesthetic into this ganglion.

Examination and diagnostic techniques

Palpation of the paraspinal muscles in the vicinity of the malrotated vertebra(e) may reveal tenderness and increased tension, or even muscle that has become hard and unyielding with recurrent spasm; chronicity of the problem can result in an increased fibrous content, with the feeling of crepitus. The facet joints are stressed non-specifically on side-bending, back extension alone, and back extension combined with rotation to the right or left, as well as more specifically by applying a translatory rotational force to a spinous process from right or left to compress the contralateral facet joint (see Fig. 4.18).

In the case of vertebral malrotation, a rotational force will also reveal a restriction of any further rotation into the direction of the malrotation – the joint play normally available in this direction may have completely disappeared.

Posterior–anterior movement or 'glide' may be similarly decreased or abolished, making the affected level(s) feel 'stiff' and unyielding. These changes are usually most easily appreciated in the region of T12–L1, where the reversal of the lumbar and thoracic curves itself already results in a restriction of joint play, even in the absence of a superimposed malrotation (Fig. 5.1 and see Fig. 3.12C). The levels adjacent to a site of malrotation sometimes also lack 'give' and feel stiff; hyper-

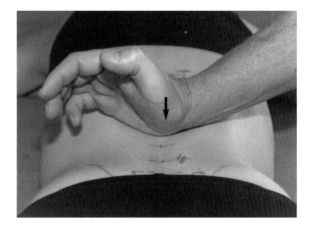

Figure 5.1 Posteroanterior compression of individual spinous processes using the heel of the hand (pisiform bone).

mobility may be evident at sites immediately adjacent or some distance away, where the spine is attempting to compensate for this restriction of movement.

Rib involvement can be assessed by examination for asymmetry and by stressing the anterior and posterior rib attachments, either directly or by selectively springing the individual ribs along their length (see Figs 2.62 and 2.63). Diagnostic nerve root blocks can be helpful if an involvement of posterior root or intercostal nerve fibres is suspected. Selective blocks of the rib articulations – costochondral, costotransverse and costovertebral – may also help to localize the pain (see Figs 3.13 and 3.14).

Correlation to sports

Vertebral malrotation is most likely to become symptomatic with sports that require repeated flexion, extension or rotation of the spine, or movements combining these patterns of motion: in particular, weight-lifting, court sports, sports involving a swinging motion (e.g. golf, baseball and field and ice hockey), rowing sports, canoeing, kayaking, throwing events and martial arts. Whether or not vertebral malrotation actually becomes a problem depends on several factors (Box 5.1)

Sports requiring rotation of the trunk while standing

The orientation of the lumbar facet joints in a near-sagittal direction allows for little rotation of the lumbar vertebrae in the transverse plane. When standing, most of the movement on trunk rotation in sports such as golf, baseball and hockey occurs through the thor-

---

Box 5.1 Factors affecting whether vertebral malrotation becomes a problem

- The level of the spine affected, which in turn determines the restrictions already imposed by the normal orientation of the facet joints (thoracic more flat or horizontal, limiting flexion and extension; lumbar aligned more in the sagittal plane, limiting rotation – see Fig. 3.8)
- The degree of malrotation, which in turn determines the degree of:
  - excessive facet joint compression and distraction
  - stress on the discs and rib joints
  - stress on the soft tissues connecting any of these structures (see Fig. 2.35)
- Whether a particular sport actually results in further stress on the level at which the malrotation has occurred. Malrotation of a lumbar or thoracic vertebra may, for example, be no problem with repetitive, symmetrical flexion/extension activities such as sculling or using a rowing machine. The deciding factor here would be whether the degree of extension required is such that it causes a further increase in the already abnormal facet joint compression on the side on which the surfaces have been brought closer together, to the point of eventually provoking pain.

  Symptoms are also more likely to be precipitated by athlete activities that put an additional rotational stress through the level(s) affected (e.g. court sports or kayaking); this is especially true for the lumbar segment, where the minimal rotation normally available may already have been reduced to a critical point on one side by malrotation

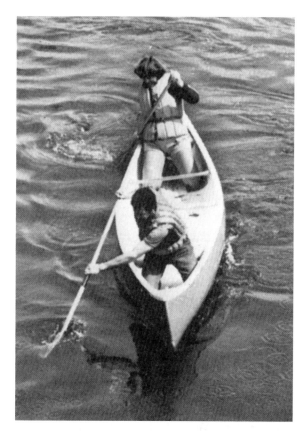

Figure 5.2 Canoeing in the kneeling, half-squatting position: torquing through the trunk, pelvis and even legs to carry out a 'stern pry and bow cross-draw' manoeuvre. (From Harrison 1981, with permission.)

acic segment. There is some simultaneous rotation of the lower extremities possible, the pelvis and lumbar segment rotating more or less as one unit. Rotation of the trunk results in stress, particularly through the thoracolumbar junction. Stress through the lumbosacral junction is maximal once all the rotation of the thoracic segment, pelvis and lower extremities has occurred and the few degrees of rotation possible in the lumbar spine segment above L5 have been exhausted.

Sports requiring rotation of the trunk while sitting

The pelvis is now fixed, rotation again occurring primarily in the thoracic segment and at the thoracolumbar junction. Once rotation available through these levels has been exhausted, the lumbar spine will start to rotate as one segment. Rotation of this segment is limited and quickly results in increased stress on the lumbosacral junction. An athlete may, therefore, develop symptoms from the mid- (thoracolumbar) and low back (lumbosacral) regions with activities such as

kayaking, yet have no problem with asymmetrical paddling such as when canoeing in the kneeling position, when the rotational stress can be distributed along the length of the spine, the pelvic region and even partly through the lower extremities (Fig. 5.2).

SACROILIAC JOINT UPSLIP, ROTATIONAL MALALIGNMENT AND OUTFLARE/INFLARE

The changes associated with these three types of malalignment may result in limitations of sports performance by:

- interfering with the desired or required range of motion
  - limitation of range in a direction specifically needed for a particular sport (e.g. reaching outwards and back to catch a ball, or trunk rotation in kayaking)

- a limitation of combined trunk, pelvic and limb ranges of motion, which could create problems particularly in those sports which require all parts of the body to be able to move through a full range of motion at any time, sometimes at high speed (e.g. court sports)
- provoking discomfort or pain
- causing problems with muscle weakness and fatigue
- changing weight-bearing, balance and controlled progression
- disturbing symmetry and style.

Appendix 10 notes the key changes that can occur and some of the sports affected as a result.

CLINICAL CORRELATIONS: SPECIFIC SPORTS

Specific sports create specific demands, and malalignment can affect the ability to meet these demands, often in a predictable manner. We are sometimes too quick to blame hand and foot preference, muscle tightness or weakness in an attempt to explain why one athlete is unable to change his or her style and repeatedly carries out a manoeuvre in the same way, or why another athlete has suffered a specific injury. A knowledge of the limitations imposed by malalignment may allow for a rational explanation based on the biomechanical changes that occur as a result of malalignment. Appendix 11 details the clinical correlations related to some specific sports and Appendix 5 those specific to running.

CLIMBING

Climbing can demand the utmost in agility and strength, as dictated by the terrain. Any weakness or restriction of range of motion puts the climber at increased risk. Slopes augment any shift in weight-bearing and therefore predispose to inversion or eversion sprains, especially when climbing in other than supportive hightops or boots (see Fig. 3.27). The climber should get into the habit of being on the look-out for any recurrence of malalignment during the climb, or at least checking on return to base camp or home, in order to carry out corrections as soon as possible.

COURT, RACQUET AND STICK SPORTS

A specific sport may appear to have been singled out as carrying an increased risk for a particular injury, but the injuries outlined below are common to a number of

these sports, and the mechanisms of injury often similar. Malalignment may well be the unifying factor.

Excessive rotation into a pelvic or thoracic restriction

Typical here is the rotation of the trunk required in tennis or golf (see below). Take the example of a right-handed tennis player with right anterior, left posterior innominate rotation and a lumbar segment convex to left (see Fig. 2.29). When he or she attempts a backhand with both feet fixed to the ground (Fig. 5.3), the initial left rotation is restricted:

- through the lumbar segment, by the fact that the vertebrae have already rotated partly to the left, into the convexity (see Fig. 2.29)

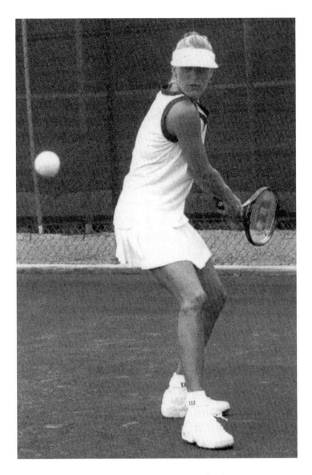

Figure 5.3   A right backhand in tennis: the feet are relatively fixed to the ground and the trunk is rotated counterclockwise in preparation for hitting the oncoming ball. (From Schwartz & Dazet 1998, with permission.)

- through the pelvis in the transverse plane, because of the left posterior rotation (see Fig. 3.4C)
- through the legs, particularly by a limitation of further internal rotation of the left leg, which is already partially rotated in that direction.

The combined effect is to restrict rotation through the lumbar spine and below. The rotational component has to occur in large part through the thoracolumbar junction and thoracic spine. Reaching backwards in preparation for the backhand further increases the possibility of causing an injury to any one of these regions. This manoeuvre, which requires a counterclockwise rotation, again occurs primarily through the trunk when the feet are fixed. The player may be able to compensate by increasing rotation through the knees, but is at increased risk of suffering an acute knee injury and acceleration of wear and tear because the counterclockwise rotation augments the tendency towards:

1. right pronation, with internal rotation of the tibia relative to the femur, increased stress on the medial knee structures (e.g. the medial collateral ligament) and increased pressure within the lateral joint compartment (see Figs 3.33 and 3.74B) ˙
2. left supination, with external rotation of the tibia relative to the femur, increased stress on the lateral knee structures (e.g. the lateral collateral ligament) and increased pressure within the medial joint compartment (see Figs 3.33 and 3.74B).

Actually hitting the ball involves a clockwise thoracic rotation which is suddenly slowed, arrested, or even forced counterclockwise as the racquet contacts the ball. If clockwise rotation of the pelvis and lower extremities continues, there results a torsional stress, maximal through the already compromised thoracolumbar junction.

A lay-up in basketball requires a maximum range of trunk and pelvic rotation. Limitations associated with malalignment may make it more difficult to approach the basket from one direction and may in fact be responsible for a preference to execute a lay-up from right or left, clockwise or counterclockwise. The risk of injury is increased should circumstances such as the proximity of other players or a blocking of the preferred approach force the player into choosing a different angle or rotating into the restricted direction in order to complete a lay-up.

Excessive movement into a restricted hip range of motion

Right anterior innominate rotation results in a limitation of right hip flexion and internal rotation, and left hip

extension and external rotation (3.64–3.72). There is therefore an increased risk that a quick forwards or backwards movement of one or other leg may exceed the available hip flexion or extension range of motion respectively. Similarly, rotation of the body to right or left over a fixed foot may exceed the available external or internal rotation of that extremity respectively, 'engaging' the anatomical barrier to the point of causing injury.

Thoraco-abdominal injuries

Injuries involving the rectus abdominis, transversus abdominis and external and internal abdominal oblique muscles have been noted to occur more often in tennis players than in those playing handball and racquetball. Lehmann (1988) may well be right in attributing these injuries to the increased need for overhead activity in tennis. Malalignment can, however, also increase the chance of suffering a sprain or strain of these muscles with the sudden rotational, reaching and extension movements characteristic of some of these sports.

> Injury is especially likely if such movement occurs at a time when that muscle is already shortened by contraction and/or tension increased, for example, because of facilitation or reactive spasm triggered by malalignment.

Athletes with malalignment sometimes complain of pain in the lateral flank and abdominal region on one or both sides. Problems relating to transversus abdominis or the external or internal obliques can, given the overlapping of these muscles, cause pain in these generalized areas. Tenderness may localize to their origins from the ribs, the main muscle bulk or insertions onto the innominates (see Fig. 2.24A, B, C).

External abdominal obliques

Most frequently injured, unilaterally or bilaterally, are the external abdominal obliques (Fig. 2.24B). The right external oblique originates from the posterolateral aspect of the lower eight ribs and runs forwards and downwards to attach to the right iliac crest and, along with the inferior segment of transversus abdominis and lateral rectus abdominis, into the iliohypogastric and ilioinguinal region and onto the lateral aspect of the superior pubic ramus (see Fig. 2.24B). Tension in the external muscle is increased directly by right anterior innominate rotation, and by clockwise trunk and counterclockwise pelvic rotation in the transverse plane. Tension increases simultaneously in other abdominal muscles, such as transversus abdominis and rectus abdominis, which are interlinked with the external obliques.

Internal oblique

In the example given (right anterior rotation), tension is especially likely to increase in the contralateral (left) internal oblique (see Fig. 2.24C) if there is the usual compensatory posterior rotation of the (left) innominate. This muscle originates from the thoracodorsal fascia and anterior iliac crest, inserting into ribs 9–12, through the aponeurosis into the linea alba and to the superior pubic ramus and pectineal line.

Transversus abdominis

Tension will increase in the ipsilateral transversus abdominis (see Fig. 2.24A). This muscle originates from the lateral inguinal ligament, iliac crest, thoracodorsal fascia and cartilages of the lower ribs, inserting into the linea alba and the superior pubic ramus and the pectineal line.

Rectus abdominis

Anterior innominate rotation increases tension in the ipsilateral half of rectus abdominis (see Fig. 2.24A) by separating its origin and insertion. As indicated above, the transversus abdominis and external and internal obliques blend with rectus abdominis and are therefore also affected indirectly by changes in tension in this muscle.

Tension in all four muscle groups is further increased by reaching and extension movements (e.g. serving in tennis, going up for a spike in volleyball and bowling in cricket). Injury is more likely when rotation, reaching and extension movements occur at a time when these muscles and their tendons are already under increased tension because of pre-existing malalignment.

Low back pain

Marks et al (1988) state that the four strokes used in racquet sports – forehand and backhand ground-strokes, the overhead serve and the volley – all put the back at risk. The overhead serve in tennis, for example, is a combined action of rotation and hyperextension of the back. Rotation occurs through the lower extremities, pelvis and primarily thoracic segment of the spine. Any malalignment-related restriction of movement increases the stress on sites that are already attempting to compensate.

Field hockey deserves special mention here because of the prevalence of low back pain in its participants. Part of the problem stems from the constant need to flex the trunk while handling what, for many of the players, amounts to a relatively short stick. In addition, the trunk is repeatedly rotated clockwise and counterclockwise when attempting to hit the ball from the left or right respectively. If this manoeuvre is carried out while moving forwards, the ability of the pelvis to rotate into the side of the leading leg is restricted, further increasing the rotational stress on the thoracic spine in particular.

Players may already be aware of a mechanical restriction on wind-up or follow-through. The pelvic restriction is more likely to be to the left, in keeping with the more common left posterior innominate rotation and associated restriction of pelvic rotation in the transverse plane to that side (see Fig. 3.4C); left inflare will have a similar effect.

Pelvic restriction can only increase the stress on the thoracic spine, whose ability to rotate to one or other side – usually the left – may be further decreased by the malrotation of individual thoracic vertebrae (see Fig. 3.45B). It should be remembered that thoracolumbar dysfunction, rather than causing mid-back pain, may be felt as low back pain (see 'Thoracolumbar syndrome', Ch. 4).

Shoulder injuries

> Partly as a result of the compensatory scoliosis, causing the glenoid socket to face either more upwards or more downwards and an increased tendency to shoulder protraction on one side and retraction on the other, malalignment impairs both shoulder stability and range of motion (see Fig. 3.15).

When a player is serving overhead or hitting an overhead volley, the shoulder is initially in a position of maximum external rotation, and the anterior capsule and internal rotators maximally stretched. Malalignment will increase these stresses by restricting external rotation on the serving side, which it usually does on the left side of those with the 'alternate' presentations or upslips (see Fig. 3.15A). To avoid an irritation of tight structures, the player can try to compensate by increasing the extension and/or rotation of the spine, at the risk of precipitating or aggravating back pain.

Groin strain

Balduini (1988) has described two mechanisms that can result in groin strain in tennis players, both resulting from an attempt by the player to stop lateral progression. One tends to occur on clay surfaces and involves the leading foot sliding outwards. A loss of traction can result in the slide ending up a split, in which case the adductors, and less often the iliopsoas, can be strained or the lesser trochanter avulsed. The other mechanism occurs by 'posting' the leading foot outwards on a surface where the footing is secure, such as a synthetic court. In other words, lateral movement is abruptly stopped. Here 'the efforts of the adductors and hip flexors are opposed by lateral momentum, and contraction results in muscle tearing rather than the anticipated deceleration' (Balduini 1988, p. 352). Malalignment results, in the vast majority, in a restriction of both left hip adduction and abduction range. Tension is typically increased in:

- the left hip abductors and tensor fascia lata/iliotibial band (TFL/ITB) complex, through facilitation (see Figs 3.37 and 3.40A)
- the iliacus component of iliopsoas (see Figs 2.31B, C, 2.37, 3.38, 4.13 and 4.14), especially when posterior innominate rotation is present (which it more often is on the left side)
- iliopsoas as a unit, in an attempt to stabilize an SI joint
- psoas, as a result of facilitation caused by T12, L1 or L2 vertebral malrotation.

The combined effect of these restrictions predisposes to injury of the hip adductors, as well as the individual components of iliopsoas, and pectineus (see Figs 3.46, 4.2 and 4.14), with either a lateral 'slide' or 'posting'. Forced adduction can cause pain by compressing these same structures, while putting a tight TFL/ITB complex at risk of sprain or strain (see Figs 3.40A and 5.15).

Reference should also be made at this point to the occurrence of a painful hemipubic bone in court sports as a result of irritation of the anterior cutaneous branches in association with T12/L1 malrotation and the thoracolumbar syndrome (see Fig. 4.21A1, B2; Appendix 9). These branches are particularly vulnerable in tennis – and soccer – players (Maigne 1995). Certainly, repeated trunk hyperextension and reaching manoeuvres (e.g. serving), as well as excessive or repetitive hip extension, will put these branches under stretch while simultaneously narrowing the intervertebral foraminal outlets as the player leans backwards.

Knee injury

Typical alterations of knee biomechanics relating to malalignment, and predisposing to acute injury or the

acceleration of wear and tear, have been discussed above under 'Excessive rotation into a pelvic or thoracic restriction'.

Ankle sprains

The 'alternate' presentations and upslips predispose to various types of ankle sprain (Box 5.2) (see Ch. 3).

Collision with a fixture or opponent

As a result of a collision, parts of the body may be involuntarily rotated into one of the malalignment-imposed restrictions of range of motion, to the point of exceeding the anatomical barrier and causing injury.

Recurrence or aggravation of malalignment

> These torsional sports are among the worst that athletes with malalignment could engage in while symptomatic and undergoing treatment.

The activities are asymmetrical, with rotational components, and involve repeatedly jumping from one leg to the other. Because of the competitive element of the game, movements are often almost reflex in nature, with little or no time for thought as the athlete throws all caution to the wind, something which can only add to the risk of sustaining an injury or causing the recurrence or aggravation of an existing malalignment.

CYCLING

The legs should move symmetrically in the sagittal plane, knees equidistant from the crossbar, in order to

---

Box 5.2 Ankle sprains predisposed to by 'alternate' presentations and upslips

- *Left ankle inversion sprains*: caused by the tendency to supination and lateral weight-bearing, weakness of the peroneal muscles and pre-positioning by internal rotation of the left lower extremity
- *Right ankle inversion sprains*: probably attributable to a momentary instability as the increase in varus angulation noted in the non-weight-bearing state causes the lateral aspect of the right foot to hit the ground at a more acute angle
- *Right ankle eversion sprains*: caused by the tendency to pronation and medial weight-bearing, weakness of the ankle invertors, and pre-positioning by external rotation of the right lower extremity

generate an equal amount of force. The cyclist who presents with malalignment may, however, be aware of an asymmetry of form and strength in that:

- leg strength feels different, the leg on one side tending to feel weak in terms of the amount of power it can generate and in having a tendency to fatigue more rapidly
- the legs appear to move differently, movement generally feeling less smooth on the weak side.

Several laboratory studies have attributed these problems to a malalignment-related leg length difference (LLD). On the side of the 'short' leg, Dunn & Glymph (1999) have shown:

1. an up to 5% decrease in the power generated
2. a loss of pedal stroke efficiency, the round and smooth 'electronic motor' type effect being replaced by a piston-like action.

Studies were carried out using a standard bicycle mounted on a CompuTrainer, which allowed for a measurement of torque applied to each crank arm at every 15 degrees of rotation, as well as of the power split percentage between the right and left legs. These studies have documented that, on realignment, the cyclist:

- regained a smoother, more rounded stroke on the previous short side, more in keeping with that on the other side
- could ride for longer at his or her maximum output
- showed a continuing improvement on repeat studies over time, which was thought to be indicative of the body's continuing adaptation to the newly aligned position.

The right leg is more likely than the left to feel weak. Given the large percentage of those presenting with right anterior rotation and right upslip (around 80%), the right leg is more often the shorter leg in the sitting position (see 'Sitting–lying test' in Ch. 2).

Foran (1999) points out that an LLD of more than 3 mm is a sign of 'spastic contracture' (perhaps caused by facilitation) originating at an upper motor neuron level, and that:

The spastic musculature responsible for the functional leg insufficiency remains hypertonic, even while wearing orthotics and heel lifts. This means a torqued pelvis and microtrauma on one side while seated. (p. 12)

Only realignment will improve matters.

In addition to the above observations regarding form and strength, the following may become obvious to the cyclist or trainer.

The knees end up a variable distance away from the crossbar

With right anterior innominate rotation, the right knee comes closer to midline than the left as the foot reaches the lowest point on pushing down on the pedal (Fig. 5.4A). This inward movement reflects the tendency to external rotation of the right leg, with a tendency to foot pronation and knee valgus angulation on this side. As the right pedal moves upwards, the right knee flexes and very obviously moves away from the crossbar, a movement again reflecting the fact that the right leg is in exaggerated external rotation (Fig. 5.4B).

Seen from the front, the right knee appears to be moving in a circle in the frontal plane, alternately moving to and from the crossbar. In contrast, the left knee moves more straight up and down in the sagittal plane, maintaining a more consistently even distance from the bar. The overall movement of the left leg also appears to be smoother in comparison to that of the right.

The cyclist can improve matters by adding toe clips in the hope of stabilizing the feet in order to counteract the tendency towards pronation. The right toe clip can be adjusted by rotating it counterclockwise so that the right foot, rather than pointing outwards as the malalignment would dictate, now ends up pointing more or less straight ahead or even slightly inwards. Fixing the foot in this position might be expected to counteract the tendency to external rotation of this leg, improving the mechanical advantage of the right leg and its ability to generate a force by:

- orienting the leg muscles more in the sagittal plane, so that they are working more in the line of progression
- increasing right ankle stability by decreasing the tendency to pronation.

Unfortunately, the right leg has really had to be forced into this 'straight' position because, as long as malalignment is present, there will be a force to rotate this leg outwards. If the toe clip now counteracts this tendency to external rotation as the foot forces the pedal down, the rider may start to experience pain on either:

1. the medial aspect of the knee, as a result of arrested foot pronation, decreased tibial internal rotation and straining medially on forced femoral external rotation.

2. the lateral knee, owing to the increased tension in TFL/ITB and stress on the lateral compartment that results with augmentation of these external rotational forces.

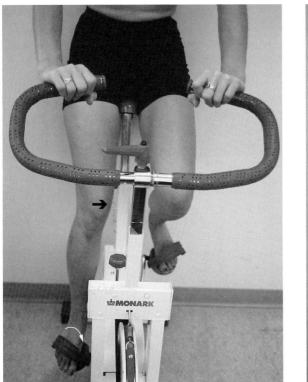
(A)

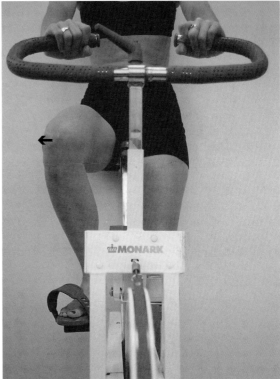
(B)

Figure 5.4   Relationship of the knees to the midline (crossbar) in a cyclist with an upslip or 'alternate' rotational malalignment and typical rotation of legs (right external, left internal). (A) The right knee is moving towards midline on knee extension, with foot pronation and a tendency towards genu valgum; the left knee is relatively neutral, travelling more in the sagittal plane. (B) The right knee is moving away from the midline with external rotation of the leg as the knee flexes. The left knee maintains a relatively neutral position.

One solution is to angle the toe clip outwards as far as is needed so that the external rotation of the leg can actually be accommodated, in that way perhaps providing some increased stability for the foot while resolving the problems at the knee level. The addition of an orthotic modified to counteract pronation may also be helpful, but the only long-term solution is realignment.

Cycling precipitates back pain

In some cyclists, riding with the trunk in a forward-flexed position (Fig. 5.5A) precipitates or worsens mal-alignment-related back or pelvic pain by:

- increasing the stress on the cervicothoracic junction as the cyclist keeps the head and neck in compensatory extension throughout the ride in order to see the road ahead

- increasing the tension in already tense and tender paravertebral muscles or posterior pelvic ligaments (particularly the iliolumbar, sacrotuberous and interspinous ligaments)
- putting direct pressure on tender sites such as the sacrotuberous insertions, hamstring origins and coccyx.

> One alternative is temporarily to use a stationary bicycle, sitting with trunk straight upright and the arms relaxed at the sides. This minimizes tension on the muscles and ligaments of the back, sacral and coccygeal regions. Weight-bearing is more effectively shifted onto the ischial tuberosities and may in fact spare the coccyx.

An even better option may be to use a recumbent bicycle, which effectively relaxes the back muscles and ligaments by providing support, helping to maintain

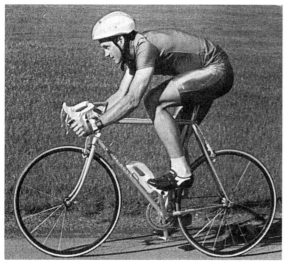

(A)

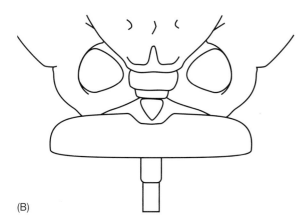

(B)

Figure 5.5 Seating in cycling. (A) The supposedly 'good' position, with the back flat and the head up, may still cause problems when malalignment is present by stressing tense/tender structures (e.g. the paravertebral muscles and posterior pelvic ligaments). (From Matheny 1989, with permission.) (B) A bicycle seat with a central depression relieves pressure on the coccyx and concentrates weight-bearing on the ischial tuberosities (see also Fig. 7.40).

the lumbar lordosis and thereby decreasing the tension in these structures. It may also avoid putting pressure directly on tender sites, although this is not always guaranteed.

When out on the road, trunk flexion can be minimized by raising the handle bars as high as possible. Mountain bikes, ridden on smooth surfaces, are preferable; shock absorption can be further increased by using a visco-elastic gel seat or similar cover. Seats

with a groove that accommodates the coccyx are also available (Fig. 5.5B).

Seating may be impaired

In addition to the problem of sitting on painful structures, discussed above, impaired seating can also relate to the uneven weight-bearing characteristic of malalignment. With right anterior rotation or upslip, for example, the right ischial tuberosity may be raised by as much as 1 cm relative to the left (see Figs 2.41F, 2.46D, 3.69A, 3.79C and 6.5). The cyclist may be aware that he or she is bearing more weight on the left side and that the pelvis is shifting to accommodate; alternatively, he or she may try to compensate by filling the gap between the right buttock and seat with a thin pillow, or by material stuffed inside the training pants.

Toe cleats, orthotics, cleat shims and adjustments to the saddle, peddle and crankshaft to accommodate for the short leg may result in some improvement, but realignment remains the only definitive treatment. If cycling repeatedly stirs up coccygeal symptoms or other musculoskeletal pains, this activity is best avoided until the problem has responded to treatment. Finally, those who are cycling and still going out of alignment must make sure that they are not doing so when getting on and off the bicycle. If that is the case, a bicycle without a crossbar is preferable, and making use of a stool or the curb also cuts down the amount of asymmetrical rotation through the hip girdle and pelvis that will otherwise occur.

DANCING

Today's dancers start training at an earlier age and often train longer and harder than those in previous decades in order to excel. Chronic or overuse-type injuries are more common than acute ones, and the lower extremities are injured more often than other areas in most forms of dance. The biomechanical limitations imposed by malalignment probably play a key role in causing these injuries.

Take, for example, the turnout of the legs. As Adrian & Cooper (1986, p. 409) indicate:

the amount of turnout is influenced by bony, ligamentous, and musculotendinous factors [and] optimum turnout … will result if the dancer has adequate strength in the deep external rotators and adductor muscles of the hip joint and uses appropriate muscle activation patterns.

This may be true for the dancers who are in alignment, but those who present with malalignment are fighting needlessly imposed restrictions on ranges of motion and, in addition, limitations relating to altered strength and activation patterns. The following discussion will refer to the more common upslips and 'alternate' presentations of rotational malalignment.

The five basic positions of classic dance

Dance is a flow of movements based on fundamental patterns of alignment of the head, arms, trunk, pelvis and legs. These movements repeatedly strain the available ranges of motion of these various parts of the body to their limit. The five basic positions in classical ballet, for example, involve a progressively increasing degree of difficulty in terms of their effect on the orientation of the lower extremities in relation to the rest of the body (Fig. 5.6). In all five positions:

- the pelvis remains facing forwards; that is, it is aligned in the frontal plane
- the trunk is usually aligned in the frontal plane, but it can rotate on the pelvis with some manoeuvres (e.g. *ports de bras*)
- the lower extremities are externally rotated (*en dehors*).

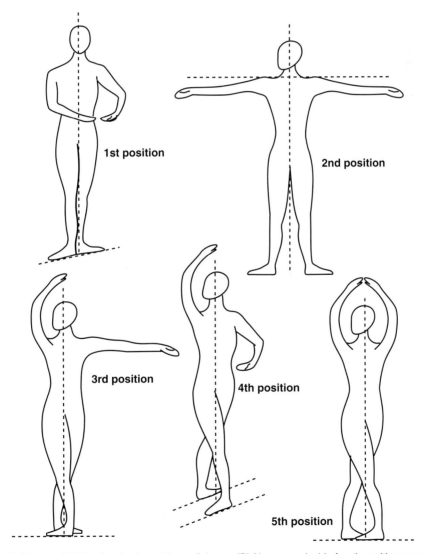

(A)

Figure 5.6   Classical dance. (A) The five basic positions of dance. (B) Narrow and wide fourth position preparations for a *pirouette en dehors*. (From Laws 1984, with permission.)

Fig. 5.6 (B), see overleaf

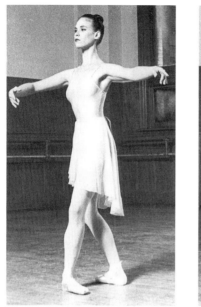 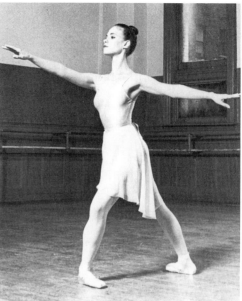

(B)

Figure 5.6 *Continued*

In the *first position*, the lower extremities are externally rotated so that the feet are aligned at an angle of 45 degrees or less relative to the frontal plane, with the heels touching (Fig. 5.6A, 1st). The *second position* resembles the first except that the lower extremities are abducted to an equal extent in the frontal plane and are externally rotated to 90 degrees (Fig. 5.6A, 2nd). In the *third*, *fourth* and *fifth positions*, the lower extremities are adducted so that the legs are crossed and placed either together (Fig. 5.6A, 3rd and 5th), or with one foot in front of the other (Figs 5.6A, 4th and 5.6B), with the overall orientation of the feet in line with the frontal plane. The stress created in the lower extremities, pelvis and trunk by these five positions is further augmented by progressing from the *à plat* (flat) to *sur la demi-pointe* to *sur la pointe* (up on the toes) placements of the foot, combined with the various possible positions of the head and arms, and whether the dancer is supported on one or two legs.

Problems related to the basic positions

The ranges of motion particularly taxed by these positions are external rotation and adduction of the lower extremities, and to a lesser extent pelvic and trunk rotation in the transverse plane. Nixon (1983, p. 465) has bluntly stated that:

The position of the leg en dehors (turned out) is contrary to nature. The position necessitates constant training from a very early age and laborious exercise to force it. There is little wonder … that musculoskeletal strain becomes manifest.

Micheli (1983), on discussing the causative factors of back pain in dancers, indicates that the increased lordosis noted in a large number of dancers is usually acquired; the accompanying extension of the pelvis actually allows increased external rotation of the lower extremities and would therefore facilitate turnout. He also identifies the following as risk factors for overuse injuries in dancers: 'anatomic malalignment of the lower extremity, including differences in leg length; abnormality or rotation of the hips; position of the kneecap; and bow legs, knock-knees, or flat feet' (p. 474). Sammarco (1983) makes the point that 'children who begin classical ballet training during their juvenile years … have the benefit of developing turnout while at the same time developing the femoral neck angle', whereas:

after the age of 11 the shape of the femoral neck can no longer be altered through the moulding process of continual pressure, such as lying on the floor with the hips abducted and externally rotated … turnout is achieved by stretching the hip capsule. (p. 487)

He points out the common complications that occur around the hip region (Box 5.3).

Box 5.3 Hip region complications in dancers

- Prolonged forced hip abduction stretches the capsule, whereas strain at turnout puts the medial internal capsule under stretch and compresses the superolateral aspect of the acetabulum; there is eventual capsule scarring and calcification, with osteophyte formation on the acetabular rim and the femoral neck (see Fig. 4.3)
- Hamstring origin pulls
- Hamstring tears, in particular of the short head of biceps femoris
- Strain of the adductor origins or muscle belly
- Iliacus tendonitis and myositis, often seen bilaterally and in association with the *developpé* manoeuvre, in which: the hip and leg are brought from the first dance position outward and upward in external rotation [at which point the flexed knee is extended] and the lower extremity returned to the first position again. (Sammarco 1983; p. 493)
- Greater trochanteric bursitis
- A snapping sensation as the tendon of tensor fascia lata moves across the greater trochanter, this being most likely to be visible when the dancer lands from a leap
- Snapping in the groin region, probably of iliopsoas, when the hip is still 45 degrees flexed 'as the leg is brought from a flexed, abducted, externally rotated position with the knee extended back to the first position' (Sammarco 1983; p. 495) in the second half of a *developpé*
- Traumatic sciatic neuritis from striking the buttocks against the floor when doing the splits

---

In addition to these, there are the problems related to the Achilles tendon, knee and great toe. Howse (1983) stresses the importance of this toe in allowing the dancer to 'maintain the correct line through the foot', thereby avoiding 'the secondary production of injuries elsewhere in the lower limbs', which could result from 'the difficulty or inability to maintain correct line and weight distribution from the foot up the leg and through the trunk' (p. 499). He notes the following problems in particular:

1. metatarsus primus varus, resulting in secondary hallux valgus
2. a short first ray, forcing the dancer into attempts to try to maintain stability by weight-bearing over the second and third toes (commonly known as Morton's toes – see Fig. 3.35A)
3. hallux rigidus, with pain and a progressive loss of dorsiflexion
4. injury to the capsule and ligaments of the first metatarsophalangeal joint, aggravated by a rotational twist of the toe itself.

Effect of malalignment

The above are among the more common injuries seen in dance. Some of them can be related to repetitive movements that place an abnormal stress on a specific structure.

On looking at the structures commonly involved, however, it becomes obvious that these are also in large part the structures that can be put under abnormal stress merely by the occurrence of malalignment, even before superimposing the additional stresses incurred in dancing.

> The stresses arising from dance manoeuvres and malalignment must be regarded as being capable of augmenting each other and increasing the risk of the dancer becoming symptomatic.

The following is a consideration of how some dance manoeuvres can be affected by the specific stresses associated with malalignment in a dancer afflicted with one of the 'alternate' presentations.

Turnout

The malalignment-related limitations that will interfere with the ability to achieve maximum, symmetrical turnout include:

- a restriction of left lower extremity external rotation and abduction as a result of asymmetrical orientation of the hip socket
- the asymmetrical increase in muscle tension around the hip joint, in particular the right hamstrings and left iliopsoas
- tightness of left hip abductors and TFL/ITB complex.

The dancer may try to force the feet past the amount of left turnout that is readily available. Adrian & Cooper (1986, p. 409) point out how the dancer may be able to:

assume the perfect turned-out position while the lower legs are flexed, and then straighten the legs and attempt to adjust alignment from the floor ... by pronating the feet excessively, by 'screwing (twisting) the knees' and/or by hyperextension of the back – all of which may cause a myriad of dance injuries if continued over time

When one of the 'alternate' presentations or upslips is present, attempts at such faulty adjustments would be further compromised by:

1. an inability to pronate the left foot as much as the right or, at worst, not at all because of a tendency towards frank left supination

2. an inability to 'twist' through the left knee as easily as the right, with a limitation of the amount of internal rotation of the left tibia relative to the femur, compared with the right (see Fig. 3.74)

3. any decrease in lumbar lordosis, and with it decreased flexibility of the lumbar spine segment and ability to extend, that can result with compensatory lateral curvature, the addition of vertebral malrotation, excessive posterior rotation of the sacral base (counternutation), coccygeal involvement and pain from stress on the junctional regions (lumbosacral and thoracolumbar) with a reactive increase in tension in the adjacent paravertebral muscles.

Pattern of weight-bearing

The typical dance shoe offers little, if any, support. The feet are therefore at liberty to pronate and supinate on movement and to collapse into positions of medial and lateral weight-bearing respectively. The left foot tends to supinate and becomes more rigid, increasing the chance of developing metatarsalgia, plantar fasciitis, stress fractures and other complications related to an impaired ability to absorb shock.

A relative increase in right pronation under high load, especially with the impact on landing, results in excessive or repeated traction on the abductor hallucis longus and plantar fascia, as well as the origins of tibialis posterior, predisposing to longitudinal arch pain and medial 'shin splints' respectively. Medial shin pain may also occur from a sustained contraction of tibialis posterior as the dancer attempts to prevent excessive pronation (Kravitz 1987).

Excessive internal rotation of the right tibia and increased right knee valgus angulation predispose to an excessive stress on medial knee structures and patellofemoral compartment syndrome or 'dancer's knee' (see Figs 3.33 and 3.74). The risk of ankle sprains is increased, given the shift in weight-bearing and the weakness of specific ankle muscles. Increased right pronation results in increased stress on the medial aspect of the first metatarsophalangeal joint and rotation of the great toe, increasing the chance of hallux vulgus formation and progressive degeneration. These and other asymmetries affecting the lower extremities may be responsible for a dancer's disconcerting sensation of instability of one or the other ankle or extremity when pushing off or landing, more usually involving the right leg (see Ch. 3).

Asymmetry of strength, tension and range of motion

Muscular imbalance, relating to differences of strength, endurance and flexibility in opposing muscle groups, is frequently cited as a cause of pain in dancers if left uncorrected (Adrian & Cooper 1986, Fitt 1987). The imbalance is attributed to structural factors and to 'consistent patterns of misuse or overuse' (Adrian & Cooper 1986, p. 412). Although these factors may indeed be operative in dancers, there is also the possibility that the dancer prefers to carry out these manoeuvres in a particular way for the simple reason that it feels better or is easier to do that way, or that there just is no choice if the manoeuvre is to be executed at all.

> If malalignment is present, it probably plays a big role in determining the easiest way to carry out a particular manoeuvre.

Most of the imbalances cited above can in fact be more easily explained by the asymmetries associated with malalignment rather than inherent structural changes or limitations resulting from faulty repetition. It is more likely to be that the malalignment has played a major part in determining the evolution of these structural changes and faulty patterns.

Failure to progress

Dancing, especially ballet, is one of the disciplines that calls for a stepwise progression to more and more demanding routines in terms of physical skill, balance and grace. The dancer is at risk of dropping out at the point at which the restrictions imposed by the malalignment make it increasingly difficult, if not impossible, to advance to the next stage of the progression.

DIVING

The asymmetries associated with malalignment will affect those dives which have a sagittal or vertical component by preventing perfect symmetry and increasing the splash at entry. Examples include dives incorporating vertical take-off followed by a somersault back layout or a somersault pike.

The restrictions imposed by malalignment are, however, even more likely to affect those dives incorporating a twist produced by simultaneous rotation around two or three axes. A dive starting with a vertical take-off with an angular component, followed by 1.5 reverse somersaults and 1.5 twists, will incorporate rotation around all three axes (Fig. 5.7). If the diver leans into the twist too soon, it may be difficult to initiate the somersault. A problem of a similar nature could conceivably result because malalignment pre-sets the body in a 'twisted' position from top to bottom.

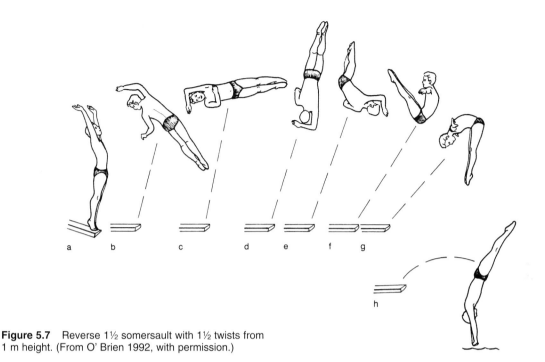

Figure 5.7 Reverse 1½ somersault with 1½ twists from 1 m height. (From O' Brien 1992, with permission.)

Another problem common to diving, particularly with dives that incorporate a twist, is the recurrence of malalignment. The recurrence can occur either while performing the twist or on entry into the water, especially if the entry is not perfectly symmetrical and/or there is still a spinning component at the time the body hits the water. Some teams actually make sure that someone skilled in the assessment of malalignment examines the diver following each dive and, if necessary, carries out immediate realignment in an attempt to ensure the quality of a subsequent dive and to decrease the risk of injury.

Dives from a springboard may be affected by asymmetry in the ability of the ankles to dorsiflex as the board is depressed, and to plantarflex maximally on pushing off (see Figs 3.68 and 3.77). The ability to gain lift will be affected by the asymmetry in the strength of the hip and knee extensors, and by the weakness attributable to the tendency towards excessive right pronation and knee valgus angulation. The diver may actually complain of one leg, usually the right, feeling weaker.

The coccyx is particularly vulnerable in somersaults, 'lead-ups' and other reverse dives and training drills in which the feet enter the water first and the body leans back. On back dives from the 5 or 10 m board, for example, the body tends to overlean backwards as the feet enter the water, the coccygeal area ending up

taking the brunt of the blow. The amount of buttock cushioning may play a protective role here and with some dry-land drills, such as somersaults carried out at floor level or off a low box where the diver actually lands on the mat sitting on his or her buttocks, with the legs in front. Always suspect the possibility that pelvic floor dysfunction may have developed and is complicating recovery when coccygeal pain fails to respond to rest, repeated realignment and the modification of dives and dry-land drills (see Ch. 3).

FENCING

Classical fencing is a 'unidirectional' sport requiring speed, balance, strength and timing as the body repeatedly lunges forward and retreats. The feet are placed at a right angle to each other; a right-handed fencer will have the right foot pointing straight at the opponent (Fig. 5.8A). This stance provides stability in both the frontal and sagittal directions. Stability also comes from a proper positioning of the knees: 'the knees should be above the feet to reduce the moments of force and stress at the knee joints' (Adrian & Cooper 1986, p. 623). Stability is decreased by any deviation of the knees to either side from this ideal position directly over the feet (Fig. 5.8B).

The lunge is initiated by kicking the front foot towards the opponent and rapidly extending the knee

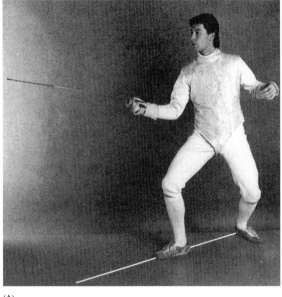

(A)

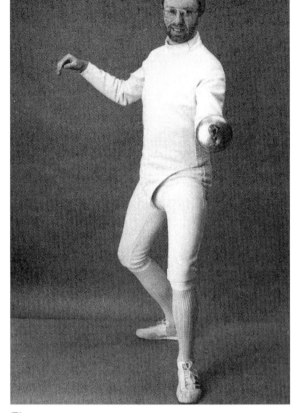

(B)

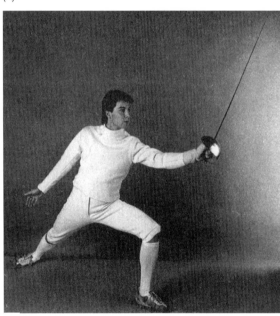

(C)

Figure 5.8 Classical fencing: positioning for speed, strength, balance and timing. (A) Side view of a right-handed fencer in the 'on guard' position: the right foot is pointing at the opponent, the left foot is at a right angle and the trunk is turned one-half to three-quarters to the front. (B) Front view of a left-handed fencer (in the 'on guard' position: the left knee is balanced directly over the foot. (C) The sabre lunge: note how the left knee is balanced over the left foot, and the feet are at a right angle. (From Pitman 1988, with permission.)

of the back leg so that the body moves forwards in as straight a line as possible (Fig. 5.8C). There is a simultaneous extension of the back arm and hand from their initial position: held overhead, with the shoulder, elbow and wrist bent to 90 degrees. The knee of the front leg stays flexed and, in order to increase the force of the lunge, is flexed even further after the lead foot has been planted securely. This knee flexion is con-

trolled by eccentric quadriceps contraction. Forward motion and flexion of the front leg are eventually arrested by a concentric contraction of the quadriceps, hamstrings and gluteus maximus. The motion is then reversed by the combination of the front leg extending, the back leg pulling the weight of the torso backwards, and the back arm resuming the bent position overhead.

The lunge requires, of necessity, some pelvic rotation in the transverse plane; bringing the hip forwards augments the distance by which the foot can advance (as in the swing phase in walking – see Fig. 2.9). In the fencer leading with the right leg, pelvic rotation will be counterclockwise. Throughout the encounter, the trunk is turned one-half to three-quarters to the front in order to minimize the chest surface area exposed to the opponent (Pitman 1988).

> Needless to say, fencing is a precision sport. Malalignment can ruin that precision, with the result that the fencer may miss the target, becomes more vulnerable and is at increased risk of injury.

The possible impact is illustrated here using the example of a fencer who leads with the right leg and presents with one of the 'alternate' patterns of rotational malalignment, that of right innominate anterior rotation.

As indicated, stability is greatest when the feet are at right angles, which requires that both lower extremities are in a position of relative external rotation. The malalignment will limit external rotation of the left leg while increasing it on the right. If left external rotation is less than 45 degrees, the left foot may end up angled at less than 90 degrees to the sagittal plane, diminishing stability in the frontal and perhaps even sagittal planes. Compensation may be achieved by active clockwise rotation of the pelvis, to ensure the right foot points at the oponent and simultaneously increase the amount of external rotation of the left leg. This clockwise rotation of the pelvis may help improve stability in both planes, albeit at the cost of:

- resulting in passive clockwise rotation of the trunk, increased exposure of the vulnerable chest area and more compensatory manoeuvres to ensure the right arm moves in the sagital plane if the trunk is actively counter-rotated
- placing the right acetabulum further backward so that it takes more time to advance from and retreat to this position with a lunge.

Forced external rotation on the left side puts the hip joint ligaments and the TFL/ITB complex under even more tension and risks precipitating pain from the left hip, greater trochanter and thigh area (see Fig. 3.37). Other internal rotators of the left lower extremity (e.g. gluteus medius) will also be wound up passively and put at risk.

Any compensatory posterior rotation of the left innominate bone will restrict the counterclockwise rotation of the pelvis in the transverse plane, decreasing the ability to use pelvic rotation to help to advance

the right leg (see Fig. 3.4C). In addition, the decrease in left hip abduction range may further decrease the length and force of the right forward lunge that would otherwise be possible.

If the above limitations make it impossible to have the right foot point directly towards the opponent, and move forwards and backwards in a straight line, balance will be impaired. For maximum stability, the knees should be positioned directly over the feet at all times. The right arm is said to deviate by 2 degrees for every degree that the leading right knee deviates medially or laterally from that ideal position, increasing the chance of missing the target (M. Conyd, personal communication, 1993). The right knee may deviate because of:

1. *a tendency of the right lower extremity towards external rotation*: because of the tendency for external rotation of the right leg, the foot may end up pointing out from midline (see Figs 3.3B, 3.16B and 3.17). As the knee flexes to go into the lunge, the foot tends to pronate. The associated valgus angulation of the knee predisposes to an inward deviation of the knee relative to the foot, decreasing stability, increasing tension in the medial knee structures (e.g. the medial collateral ligament) and compressing the lateral compartment (see Figs 3.33 and 3.74). The movement pattern, and the stresses, will be reversed on extending the knee to recover from the lunge

2. *compensatory internal rotation of the right foot*: the fencer may try to increase the stability of the lunge by actively rotating the leg inwards to bring the outwardly-rotated right foot back to midline and the knee more into the sagittal plane. As with the cyclist using toe clips, however, the femur will still want to rotate externally on the fixed foot. On a right forward lunge, the knee may actually drift outwards into varus, decreasing stability, increasing stress on the lateral knee structures (e.g. the lateral collateral ligament) and compressing the medial compartment

3. *weakness of the quadriceps*: the functional weakness of the right rectus femoris, possibly coupled with an actual wasting of the right vastus medialis, will make the eccentric contraction of the quadriceps mechanism less effective in stopping the lunge. The knee is more likely to collapse inwards (valgus strain) and the patella to track outwards, increasing the tension across and compression within the patellofemoral compartment. Weakness may also affect the subsequent concentric contraction needed to extend the knee and reverse the lunge.

The knee is the most common site of injury in fencing (M. Conyd, personal communication, 1998).

Increased valgus angulation at a time when the right knee is under load, coupled with a wasting of the right vastus medialis, increases the risk of developing knee injury (Box 5.4).

The fencer can try to overcome the restriction of stride length that results with malalignment by lifting the right leg higher, but this unfortunately means coming down harder on the heel, increasing the chance of sustaining a heel bruise. It also increases the amount of shock transmitted upwards to the knee joint, where it can accelerate the degeneration of the menisci and cartilaginous surfaces. Perhaps more importantly, it also raises the centre of gravity and decreases stability even further at a moment when the fencer is already in a precarious position.

The left foot is more likely to supinate, which may increase the tendency towards:

- the knee collapsing towards varus angulation at times when the fencer is in a more upright position
- the foot and ankle collapsing towards inversion at push-off, increasing the risk of an inversion sprain at a time when the trailing leg is helping to accelerate the body forwards in a lunge.

The fencer with the left anterior and locked presentation (see Figs 3.3A and 3.18B) who leads with the right foot will have:

1. *a limitation of right external rotation*: it will be more difficult to rotate the right leg externally in order to point the right foot directly at the opponent. A clockwise rotation of the pelvis can compensate for this limitation. Simultaneous clockwise rotation of the trunk may be inevitable and will make the chest more vulnerable; compensatory active trunk rotation counterclockwise will result in increased rotational stresses and increased energy output

2. *problems related to supination*: the tendency is for right foot supination and right knee varus angulation, which increases the risk of an inversion sprain. The increased rigidity of the right foot predisposes to injury of the heel and knee at foot plant

3. *impaired left leg stability and push-off strength*: these will result if the left foot collapses into pronation and the knee buckles into valgus at the time of the lunge.

Malalignment affects the classical fencing form in particular, decreasing versatility by limiting the repertoire of actions. It is less likely to affect the modern form, which consists in large part of a 'flash' combining a running motion, jump action and quick recovery. It has, however, adverse effects on both types, particularly in terms of increasing susceptibility to injury by limiting certain ranges of motion and decreasing stability.

GOLF

For the right-handed golfer, the initial action is one of winding up the spine by twisting the trunk clockwise and then unwinding to strike the ball and continuing into swing-through, effectively winding up counterclockwise. Adrian & Cooper (1986) have described the golf swing as a combination of the arms moving across the body primarily in the frontal plane while the trunk rotates in the transverse plane. The shift of weight onto the right foot on the backswing, and the left on the forward swing, increases the range of hip rotation. According to their analysis, at the height of the backswing 'pelvic action is seen to have rotated the pelvis almost 90 degrees and spinal rotation to have turned the upper torso more' (Adrian & Cooper, 1986, p. 558).

In the right-handed golfer presenting with malalignment, problems relate to the following.

Asymmetrical limitation of upper extremity rotation

Asymmetrical limitation of rotation may become a factor as the right arm rotates externally and the left internally on the backswing, the reverse occurring on swing-through (see Fig. 3.15A).

Box 5.4 Knee injuries in fencing

- *Patellofemoral compartment syndrome and chondromalacia patellae*: if retropatellar pain is already a problem, the fencer can sometimes avoid the pain by forcing the knee into varus angulation. The improved patellar tracking might avoid putting pressure on tender patellar facets or femoral condyles, but it comes at the cost of decreasing stability
- *Injury to the medial or lateral meniscus and compartments*: varus or valgus angulation under load increases the pressure in the medial or lateral compartment respectively and predisposes to premature degeneration of the joint. Anything that counteracts the increased tendency towards external rotation of the right leg associated with upslips and 'alternate' presentations increases the pressure on the medial compartment. Medial meniscal entrapment is more likely when:
  - the foot is fixed and does not allow the tibia to rotate externally when the knee extends
  - the knee quickly moves from a position of flexion and valgus angulation with the tibia in internal rotation to a position of extension and neutral (or even varus) alignment with associated external rotation of the tibia

Limitation of rotation through the thorax

Trunk rotation to one side is typically decreased (see Fig. 3.45). This results from a combination of factors including the direction of the thoracic convexity, an asymmetrical increase in paravertebral muscle tension, the presence of any vertebral malrotation and rib rotation (Lee 1993).

Limitation of pelvic rotation in the transverse plane

Left posterior innominate rotation and left inflare both limit pelvic rotation to the left and will affect the right-to-left swing-through (see Fig. 3.4). With a right posterior rotation or right inflare, the limitation is to the right and will affect the right backswing. To avoid compromising the backswing or swing-through, the reduced pelvic rotation may be compensated for by increasing rotation primarily through the thoracic segment of the spine and the lower extremities, albeit at the cost of increasing the stress on these structures.

Asymmetrical limitation of lower extremity rotation

The golfer with the left anterior and locked presentation has a limitation of right external and left internal leg rotation, both of which could affect the right-to-left swing-through. On the other hand, the golfer with one of the more common 'alternate' presentations or an upslip has a restriction of right internal and left external rotation, which could create problems with the left-to-right backswing. Problems are more likely to occur if the feet move inadequately or, worse still, remain planted on the ground.

Interference with thoracic rotation

When the golfer driving from right to left takes a divot the wrong way or hits a covered root or rock in the rough, thoracic rotation to the left can be suddenly slowed or even completely stopped, whereas the rotation of the pelvis continues. This twisting of the pelvis on a fixed trunk can cause an aggravation of problems relating to malalignment (e.g. if there is already a limitation of pelvic rotation counterclockwise) or actually a recurrence of the malalignment.

The author is reminded of the golfer who goes out of alignment each and every time he 'takes a divot'. He has solved this problem by lying down on the links in order to carry out an immediate correction using a muscle energy technique. This allows him to get on with the game until he takes the next divot. The suggestion of having someone assess his style in the hope

of cutting down on the number of times he took a divot was not well received.

The use of graphite clubs should also be considered, particularly on the driving range where there is a risk of repeatedly hitting the mat. Unlike traditional steel clubs, these will yield a bit on impact and absorb some of the shock.

Increased stress on the thoracolumbar junction

> Restrictions imposed by limitations of pelvic and lower extremity rotation require a compensatory increase in rotation more proximally, the resulting stress being maximal at the thoracolumbar junction or mid-back region.

A typical history is that of the golfer who presents fit and unaware of any problems at the start but develops back pain over the first half of the course. The pain typically increases as the game progresses, sometimes forcing him or her to abandon play before reaching the 18th hole. The pain is often limited to the mid-back region or may be maximal in this area. Other parts of the back may eventually become a problem as impaired rotation and pain result in protective muscle spasm and a faulty technique. An irritation of the T12 and L1 cutaneous fibres can trigger a full-blown thoracolumbar syndrome.

Posterior pelvic ligament stress

Malalignment results in increased stress on these ligaments so that some or all of them are often already tender or outright painful (see Fig. 2.3). They are more likely to become a problem with golf, particularly when working out on the driving range. To drive the ball, the trunk is slightly flexed on the pelvis, further increasing the tension in these ligaments. Maintaining this stance while repeatedly adding a twisting insult can eventually precipitate or worsen pain from these ligaments.

The results of treatment can be most gratifying, with repeated reports that realignment finally allowed a completion of the 18 holes without pain being 'par for the course'. The biggest problem in most cases is one of convincing the golfer not to play for a while to ensure that treatment attempts will be successful. Unfortunately, few are willing to stop for the 3–4 months sometimes required to get to the point of maintaining the realignment and tolerating the rotational stresses inherent to playing golf without triggering a recurrence of the malalignment.

GYMNASTICS

Gymnastics may be divided into floor exercises and those carried out on apparatus. Some problems, including back and knee pain, are common to both.

Back pain

Tsai & Wredmark (1993) have postulated that the increased incidence of back pain in gymnasts relates to the commonly noted hyperlordosis aggravated by repeated hyperextension manoeuvres, an increased trunk length and a low sacral inclination. Micheli (1985) has identified four entities responsible for back pain in gymnasts.

Pars interarticularis fracture or spondylolysis

These presentations can sometimes be attributed to trauma or to a single episode of hyperextension. It is, however, more often felt to be related to the increased lordosis and/or repeated and extreme degrees of hyperextension required for some routines.

Stinson (1993) cites studies also implicating heredity and the combination of lordotic stress on a neural arch weakened because of an inherited defect in the modelling of the cartilage. He notes, however, that the high prevalence in certain athletic disciplines (gymnastics, diving, football, weight-lifting and wrestling) makes 'spondylolysis in the athlete in some respects a unique entity' (p. 519). It may occur unilaterally or bilaterally. The history is usually one of an insidious onset of low back pain with or without radiation to one or both buttocks, 'often first noted when the gymnast does a back flip or back-walkover' (p. 86).

Vertebral body fracture

Micheli (1985) cites fracture of the vertebral end plates as another cause of back pain in young athletes. Fractures are noted particularly at the anterior margins and 'appear to be usually the result of repetitive micro-trauma – most probably repeated flexion ... and can result in frank vertebral wedging' (p. 89). He goes on to say that 'in the gymnast, these fractures usually occur at the thoracolumbar junction and may involve three or more vertebral bodies, although one or two levels of involvement are more common' (p. 89). The athletes may be mistakenly labelled as having Scheuermann's disease.

Discogenic back pain

Micheli (1979) has reported an increasing incidence of this condition in the athletically active adolescent pop-

ulation. Back pain may actually be overshadowed by unilateral or bilateral hamstring tightening or the development of a 'sciatic scoliosis'.

Spondylogenic back pain

This is often a presumptive diagnosis based on the exclusion of the above three categories and ruling out a tumour or infectious process.

Malalignment augments the stress on both the discs and the pars interarticularis, and conceivably increases the chance of the gymnast developing any of the above complications. In the gymnast presenting with malalignment, manoeuvres that call for a maximum movement of the vertebrae in all three planes are superimposed on a spine that is already moving abnormally. Malrotation of the L5 vertebra to the right, for example, compresses the left L5–S1 facet joint and will automatically increase the stress placed on the left pars whenever a movement involving extension, left side flexion or clockwise rotation of the trunk is superimposed (see Fig. 2.35B). As stated by Ciullo & Jackson (1985, p. 97), the pars can fail 'when subjected to unusual repetitive forces of hyperextension, tension, torque and compression'.

Malalignment can cause or augment all of these stresses. The compensatory lumbar convexity to right or left, for example, entails a rotation of L1–L4 into the convexity, bringing the facet joint surfaces on the concave side closer together and reducing the overall flexibility of the lumbar segment (see Figs 2.29, 2.65, 4.6, 4.22 and 4.28). The problem will be even worse with the addition of a malrotation of one or more individual vertebrae (see above and Fig. 2.65B). Any malalignment-related increase in sacral nutation would accentuate the lumbar lordosis and further increase the pressure on these facet joint surfaces, as would any side-flexion from reflex contraction of psoas, quadratus lumborum or the paravertebral muscles on one side.

A mention by Micheli (1985) that vertebral body fractures in gymnasts usually involve the anterior aspect of only one or two vertebrae in the thoracolumbar junction area could be explained by the change from a lordosis to a kyphosis at this site, with a change from extension to flexion stresses respectively. If, however, these fractures are indeed related to increased or repetitive flexion stresses, the flexion stress caused by the kyphosis would be expected to be least at the thoracolumbar junction and maximal at the apex of the thoracic kyphosis. In addition, because of the orientation of the facet joint surfaces, most flexion and extension movement occurs in the lumbar segment, to lesser extent at the thoraco-lumbar junction and least in the thoracic segment (see Fig. 3.8).

Malalignment can offer a more probable explanation for finding vertebral fractures at the thoracolumbar junction. There is the torsional and lateral flexion strain on the discs attributable to the reversal of the lumbar and thoracic convexities, L1 being rotated one way and T12 in the opposite direction (see Fig. 3.12C). In addition, vertebral malrotation involving T12 or L1 is very common, typically occurring in conjunction with a rotational malalignment of the pelvis. All these changes result in a loss of the normal joint play or 'glide' so that there is, typically, increased resistance or stiffness at the level of the junction, the stiffness diminishing the ability of this area to yield to stresses of any type (see Fig. 5.1).

Superimposing a flexion stress more readily increases the load on the anterior disc and adjoining vertebral margins, predisposing to fracture. The fact that pain elicited by posterior–anterior and transverse pressure on the spinous processes often localizes to the thoracolumbar and lumbosacral junction areas is indicative of the increased stress on these sites attributable to the malalignment (see Figs 3.12 and 4.18). Even though tenderness can often be elicited from either site on examination of the asymptomatic athlete, that athlete may, however, have no actual complaint until something, such as a tear of the annulus fibrosus or an end plate fracture, finally occurs and brings these areas to his or her attention.

Knee pain

A review published by Andrish (1985) indicates that knee pain in gymnasts relates primarily to patello-femoral compartment problems, ligament sprains, meniscal tears, contusions and Osgood–Schlatter's disease. The stresses on the patellofemoral region that result with malalignment must always be borne in mind (see Ch. 3). If there is no history of direct trauma, or if the complaint is unilateral, there should be particular concern that malalignment may be playing a role (see Figs 3.33, 3.74, 3.75 and 4.5).

Let us now look at the effect of malalignment on the demands of the individual gymnastic disciplines.

Apparatus

Malalignment will primarily affect the dismount, those routines which are asymmetrical and those requiring rotation around the vertical axis and in the transverse plane. Problems relate to the following changes that occur with malalignment.

Limitations of thoracic spine and pelvic rotation. These affect the ability to do somersaults and twists as part of routines carried out on the rings, parallel bars, the side-horse and the balance beam or in the course of vaulting.

A limitation of rotation of the pelvis in the transverse plane into the side of the posterior innominate rotation or inflare may become a problem, particularly when the gymnast is holding on to the apparatus with both hands, for example, with manoeuvres on the pommel horse (Fig. 5.9B, C) or the rings (Fig. 5.9D). Holding on this way automatically decreases the ability to rotate through the thoracic region and therefore increases the rotational stresses through the thoracolumbar, lumbosacral and pelvic regions, including the SI and hip joints.

> The ability to rotate through the lower extremities is restricted in some routines by holding the legs closely applied to each other, as when doing double-leg circles on the pommel horse or horizontal bars (Fig. 5.9A, B) as opposed to a scissor-action (Fig. 5.9C).

The restriction increases the rotational stresses through more proximal structures. If the pelvis and spine cannot accommodate because of a malalignment-related limitation of rotation in specific directions, the result can be awkwardness, a decreased ability – or even inability – of the gymnast to carry out these routines, and injury.

The ultimate test of any limitation of the hip, pelvic or thoracic range of motion must occur while carrying out high double-leg circles on the pommel horse (Fig. 5.9B). This requires rotating the closely applied legs in one direction across the top of the horse while the rest of the body, supported alternately by each arm holding on to one of the handles, rotates in the opposite direction.

The ability to rotate the upper trunk to either right or left while in the cross-hang (iron cross) position on the rings will be compromised in particular by limitations of the thoracic spine and/or pelvis to rotate or twist into one direction (Fig. 5.9D).

Asymmetry of lower extremity muscle strength, a feeling of weakness in one leg and a problem with balance. These may present difficulties particularly on dismount and with routines carried out on the balance beam, especially those incorporating a twist of the trunk relative to the pelvis or around the long axis of the body. Dismount stability is further compromised by the various asymmetries affecting the lower extremities, the right one being more likely to be a problem (see Ch. 3).

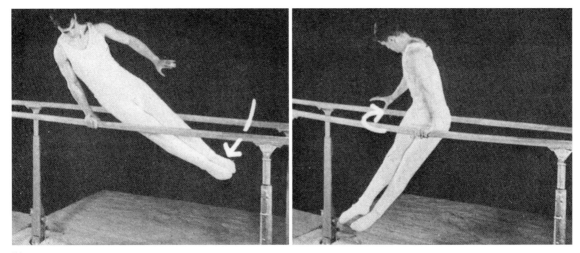

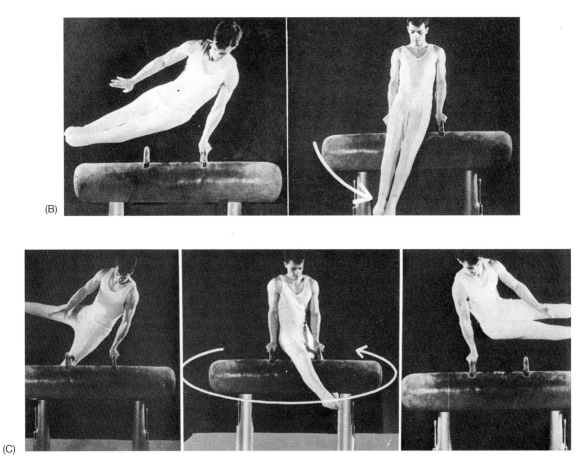

Figure 5.9 Gymnastic manoeuvres. (A) Front support turn on the parallel bars. (B) Double-leg circle on the pommel horse. (C) Single-leg circle with scissor-action. (D) Straight-body cross-hang (iron cross) position on the rings. (From Loken & Willoughby 1977, with permission.)

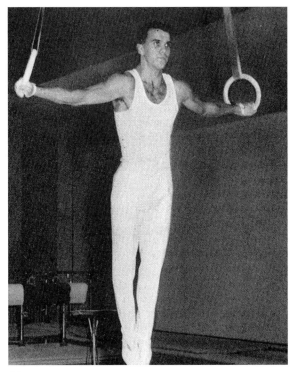

(D)

Figure 5.9 *Continued.*

Floor exercises

Floor exercises require the ultimate in flexibility and balance as the gymnast carries out tumbles, springs and double and triple twists in quick succession, landing on either one or both feet or in the split position. As the difficulty of the routines increases, so does the chance that the asymmetries associated with malalignment will become a limiting factor or a cause of injury.

The athlete may appreciate asymmetries in push-off strength, stiffness or limitations of movement, as well as a feeling of insecurity or imbalance on trying to come to a controlled stop at the end of a routine. Athletes probably tailor their routines, consciously or subconsciously, in order to avoid these problems, for example, by repeatedly landing on the more stable leg, putting more weight on that leg when landing on both or repeatedly carrying out a manoeuvre in the direction that avoids a restriction of range.

> This repetition predisposes to overuse problems, whereas an inadvertent deviation from these routines puts the gymnast at risk of injury.

INTERCEPTIONS IN TEAM SPORTS

Interceptions result in an unexpected turn-over of the ball or puck to the opposition; they are mentioned here because they are an important part of a number of athletic activities. The opposition player usually cannot plan for the event, that is, prepare the body for any associated impact, excessive rotation or loss of stability. The athlete can easily end up at increased risk of:

- exceeding a restriction of range of motion
- losing equilibrium
- having to twist the pelvis and spine, sometimes in opposite directions and sometimes with the addition of acute trunk flexion or extension.

Interceptions are therefore more likely to result in injury, especially in the athlete already presenting with malalignment. They must also be considered as a possible cause of an initial malalignment or of recurrence.

JUMPING SPORTS

Limitations relating to malalignment affect primarily the following aspects:

1. *Rotation*: most jumps have a rotational component, for example, after the take-off in a high jump using the Fosbury flop (Fig. 5.10), or on ascending and when reaching the top in the pole vault.

2. *Hip extension and flexion*: right anterior, left posterior rotation restricts right hip flexion and left hip extension, the reverse occurring with the left anterior, right posterior presentation (see Figs 2.72 and 3.65). These changes will affect the stride length required for clearance (hurdles and steeplechase), the extent of reach (the long and triple jumps) and push-off (pole vault and high jump). The final upward thrust in the vault and high jump, for example, comes from simultaneously kicking one leg up in the air (hip flexion) and extending the opposite hip and knee after initial flexion. Stride length can also be affected by an asymmetry of pelvic rotation in the transverse plane, for example, by a limitation into the side of a posteriorly rotated innominate or an inflare (see Fig. 3.4).

The jumper may be able to change style to adapt to the limitations imposed by malalignment. Leading off with the left leg in steeplechase and hurdle events might, for example, get round any restriction of right hip flexion caused by right anterior rotation, right outflare or increased tension in the right hamstrings (see Figs 3.64–3.66). For the same reason, the pole vaulter might fare better swinging up the left leg and pushing off with the right, provided that functional weakness affecting the right hip extensors is not a major problem. The way in which an athlete finally executes a particular manoeuvre is probably arrived at by trial and error, largely influenced by the limitations imposed by malalignment. Take, for example, the high-jumper with one of the 'alternate' presentations and right anterior, left posterior rotation who intends to execute a Fosbury flop by approaching the bar in one of the following ways.

From the right side (Fig. 5.10)

The jumper will run towards the bar in a curved approach (1). After planting the left foot, lift-off is combined with simultaneous counterclockwise rotation of the pelvis and trunk, forcing the left leg into external rotation (2). Lift-off comes through initially flexing the left leg and then simultaneously fully extending that leg while kicking the right leg (closest to the bar) up in the air (2). Once airborne (3), the thorax and pelvis continue to twist, hopefully to allow clearance of the bar with the buttocks while sailing backwards with the extended back 'draped' across the bar (4).

In other words, acceleration is converted into a vertical force by the kicking action of the right leg with simultaneous left leg extension, initiating a counterclockwise rotation of the trunk and then pelvis, and final back extension (Paish 1976, Worth 1990). The malalignment may affect the factors listed in Box 5.5.

Box 5.5 Factors affected by malalignment in a right-side Fosbury flop approach

- The ability to drive the right thigh upwards (hip flexion) may be limited by:
  - the mechanical restriction of the femur that occurs with anteroinferior rotation of the superior rim of the acetabulum (see Figs 3.64–3.66).
  - tightening of the hamstring/sacrotuberous complex by a change in the length-to-tension ratio and complicating facilitation of the hamstrings (see Figs 3.38 and 3.39)
- A decreased ability to externally rotate the weight-bearing left leg, external rotation being restricted on this side
- An increased risk of a left ankle inversion sprain, given the weakness in the left peroneus longus and a tendency to supination on this side (see Figs I.1, 3.18A and 3.49B)
- A torsional stress on the spine, especially thoracolumbar junction, if there is a restriction of counterclockwise rotation of the thorax (see Fig. 3.45)
- Stress on the already 'ill-fitting' thoracolumbar junction – especially the facet joints – by hyperextension of the back (see Fig. 3.12)

From the left side

Acceleration is converted into a vertical force by simultaneous extension of the flexed right leg and kicking up the left leg, which is followed by clockwise rotation of

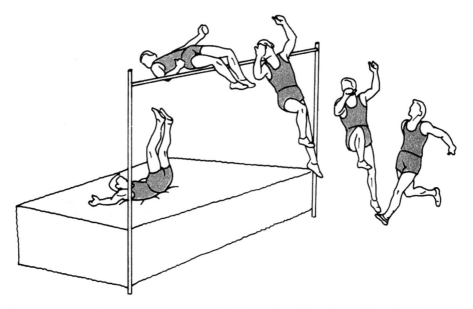

Figure 5.10 Fosbury flop: approaching the bar from the right. (After Worth 1990, with permission.)

the trunk and then the pelvis. The malalignment may lead to the following:

- stability of the push-off foot and strength of the right leg is decreased, given the asymmetrical functional weakness that typically affects the right hip flexors and extensors, tibialis anterior and posterior, extensor hallucis longus and other toe extensors, so that the right leg may feel weak compared with the left (see Figs 3.49–3.53)
- a decreased ability to plantarflex the right foot (see Fig. 3.77)
- torsional strain on the spine and thoracolumbar junction (see Figs 3.12 and 3.45).

Depending on the type of malalignment present, and which pattern of restriction is dominant, the jumper may find that it 'feels easier' to approach the bar from one side than the other, with better results. In that respect, the malalignment may be thought of as providing a 'biomechanical' advantage to the athlete. If malalignment does indeed appear to result in improved performance in an 'established' jumper, there may be no point in attempting realignment, provided that the athlete is asymptomatic.

MARTIAL ARTS: KARATE

Karate involves fighting with the hands and feet, punching and kicking being the two most common forms of attack. The intent is to deliver as forceful a blow with as small a surface area as quickly as possible, while at the same time maintaining balance. When advancing to deliver a punch or kick the athlete – or karateka – moves forward in a straight line in order to minimize the displacement of the centre of gravity and to shorten the time required to reach the opponent. Increased mobility occurs at the expense of stability: the 'one-and-a-half-footed' cat stance (Fig. 5.11A), for example, provides mobility but is less stable than the wide-based 'two-footed' horse stance (Fig. 5.11B) or back stance (Fig. 5.11C). Increasing the distance through which an extremity moves increases the amount of force generated, but this again comes at the expense of stability.

The karateka with one of the 'alternate' presentations and right anterior innominate rotation has limitations that may decrease effectiveness and increase the risk of injury, as described below.

First, stride length is decreased as a result of a restriction of:

- counterclockwise rotation of the pelvis
- right hip flexion and left hip extension.

This karateka is at increased risk of a sprain or strain of the tight right hip extensors and left hip flexors when advancing the right foot in front stance or lunging, especially with the 'lunge punch', a particularly deep lunge required to deliver a low blow (Fig. 5.11D). The karateka can compensate for a decreased stride length by moving closer to the opponent in order to 'connect', at the increased risk of being hit and injured.

Second, the reach of the right leg is usually decreased and the high kicking action hampered, making this leg a less formidable striking weapon. Reach could be increased by plantar flexing the right foot, but this motion is already restricted on this side (see Fig. 3.77B).

The restrictions affecting counterclockwise rotation of the pelvis, and internal rotation of the right and external rotation of the left leg, may become a limiting factor for any rotational manoeuvre of the trunk carried out while supported on one or both feet. These restrictions could, for example, impair those manoeuvres in which the body quickly rotates through 180 degrees to face alternately to right and left while both feet remain on the ground. These restrictions could also interfere with assuming a specific stance, such as:

- the horse stance, in which both feet point forwards or out and the knees are flexed, externally rotating both legs (Fig. 5.11B)
- the back stance, the feet being placed at a right angle to each other (Fig. 5.11C)
- the straddle stance, in which the feet are rotated outwards at the start, simultaneous knee flexion then accentuating this external rotation.

The force that can be generated with either leg may be decreased because of decreased strength and/or the decreased range through which the leg can now be moved, with a decrease in the length of the resulting lever arm:

1. The weakness of the right hip flexors and the decrease in right hip flexion can result in a decreased strength and range of kicks with a flexion component (e.g. the high right forward kick – Fig. 5.12A).

2. The weakness of left hip abductors and the decrease in left hip extension can result in a decreased strength and range of kicks with an abduction and extension component (e.g. the left backward roundhouse kick – Fig. 5.12B).

The ability to abduct the lower extremity is usually less on the left than the right. This could decrease the effectiveness of a left forward roundhouse kick because the kick might end up being delivered low. The karateka can compensate by side-bending to the right to

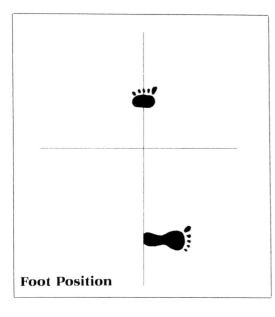

Foot Position

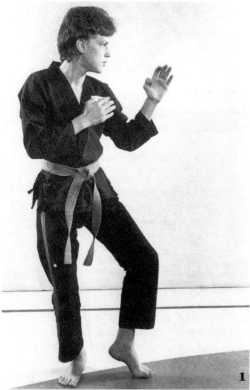

(A)

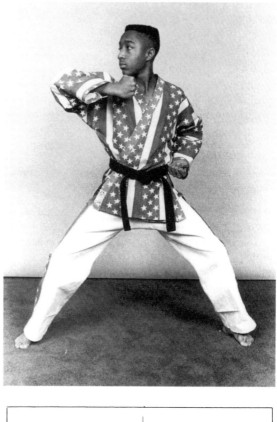

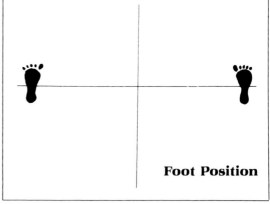

Foot Position

(B)

Figure 5.11 Karate: typical positions and movements. (A) Cat stance. (B) Horse stance. (C) Back stance. (D) The 'lunge punch' from the front stance position. (From Queen 1993, with permission.)

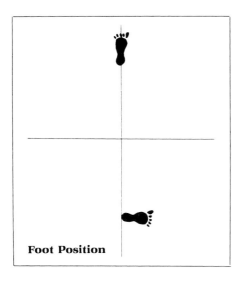

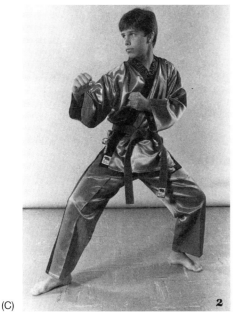

Foot Position

(C)

2

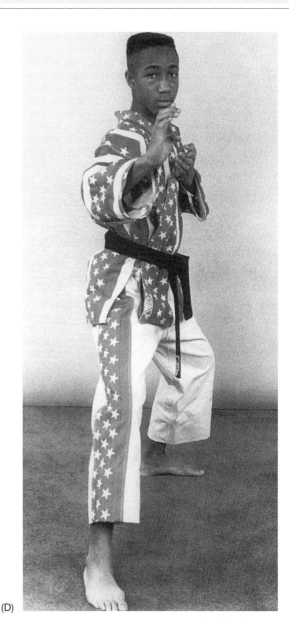

(D)

Figure 5.11 *Continued.*

elevate the left thigh further, but this will be at the expense of stability as the centre of gravity is displaced to the right of the midline (Fig. 5.12C).

An impaired ability to externally rotate the left lower extremity may interfere with the ability to 'close the gap' properly in the roundhouse kick, which requires that the left foot rotate outwards 90 degrees from its starting position (Hobusch & McClellan 1990).

Limitations of ranges of motion can decrease the effectiveness of the impact of a kick:

• In *side-kicking*, there may be difficulty striking the opponent with a small surface area, such as the lateral edge of the foot, because of a limitation of internal or external rotation of the leg and variations in the varus/valgus angulation of the non-weight-bearing foot (see Fig. 3.22). The blow is more likely to be delivered with the sole of the foot, which is less effective because the force is dissipated over a larger area. There is also an increased risk of fracturing the toes.

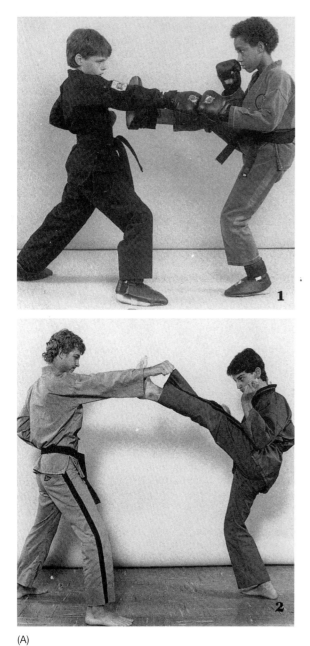

(A)

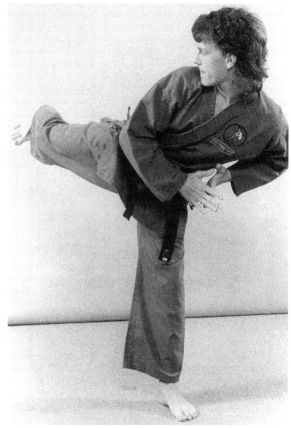

(B)

Figure 5.12 Typical karate kicks. (A) Right (1) and left-sided (2) 'crescent' kick incorporating hip flexion (limited on the right side). (B) Right 'spinning back' or 'roundhouse' kick. (C) Left forward roundhouse kick. (From Queen 1993, with permission.)

- A *direct kick* to the body should impact at the ball of the foot; that is, the foot is in maximal active dorsiflexion and may be passively pushed into further dorsiflexion on contact. With the roundhouse kick, impact with the dorsum of the foot requires maximum active plantar flexion, and the foot is forced into further plantar flexion passively on contact. The malalignment-related limitation of plantar flexion on one side, and dorsiflexion on the other, may decrease the effectiveness

of these kicks and increase the risk of injury by passively forcing the foot past a physiological or even anatomical barrier (see Figs 3.77 and 3.78).

Instability when standing on one leg alone may be more noticeable on kicking, particularly when using a forward or reverse roundhouse kick, in which the kicking action is combined with rotation to increase the force of the blow. The right single-leg stance is more

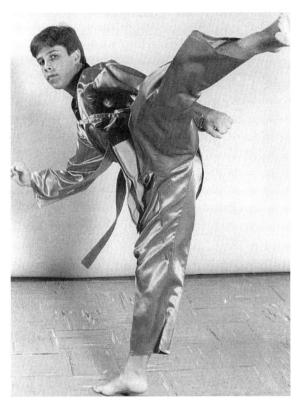

(C)

Figure 5.12 *Continued.*

often a problem, which may become evident with the kinetic rotational (Gillet) test (see Figs 2.88 and 2.89).

The karateka requires a stable base when advancing and when delivering punches. As in fencing, advancing rapidly requires a quick forwards movement of the foot and flexion of the knee on one side, combined with extension of the other hip and knee (see Fig. 5.8C). Maximum stability in the sagittal plane is achieved by having the right and left knees end up directly over their respective feet (see Figs 5.8 and 5.11D). Instability results with deviation of the knee to either side because of the inward or outward rotation of the leg, and valgus or varus angulation of the knee with a tendency towards pronation or supination respectively. Instability attributable to these factors is even more likely with leaping movements, both forwards and backwards, along the sagittal plane.

MARTIAL ARTS: JUDO

The intent is to throw the opponent off balance without losing one's own. Adrian & Cooper (1986) have pointed out that 'the weight is often maintained over the leading foot so that the rear foot can be quickly used for sweeping and for other attacks' (p. 629). In the presence of malalignment, the stability of the lead leg will be decreased by the same factors discussed above for fencing and karate. Impaired balance is a factor to consider when weight is borne on one leg only.

In addition, the ability to use the sweeping leg effectively may be decreased by limitations of rotation. Right anterior innominate rotation, for example, limits the ability of the right leg to sweep behind the opponent from right to left by:

1. decreasing the ability to internally rotate the right leg
2. limiting the ability of the pelvis to rotate counterclockwise in the transverse plane, which would normally allow the right hip and leg to swing forward to gain extra length for the sweep (see Fig. 3.4C).

The torquing forces used to throw the opponent in judo increase the chance of injury by inadvertently forcing the thorax, pelvis or legs into the direction of a restriction.

ROWING, SCULLING, KAYAKING AND CANOEING

These sports differ primarily in the amount and symmetry of trunk rotation, flexion and extension that occur from the 'catch' through the 'drive' and eventual recovery phase (Dal Monte & Komor 1989).

Sculling

The rowing action for single, double and quadruple sculls is symmetrical, a similar action occurring when the athlete uses a rowing ergometer. The force generated by the extending legs and trunk is transferred to the arms and finally the oar. At the 'catch', the scapulothoracic muscles, in particular serratus anterior, are maximally contracted, which helps to stabilize the scapula against the thorax. The 'drive' phase involves extension of the lower extremities, extension of the trunk and flexion of the upper extremities. Style is determined primarily by the timing and the degree of initial trunk flexion and final extension.

Malalignment will increase the possibility of developing back pain and restricting ranges of motion by:

- increasing tension in tense, and often tender, thoracic (and sometimes lumbar) paravertebral muscles and posterior pelvic ligaments, thus restricting forward flexion
- increasing the amount of stress on the now asymmetrical facet joints, sacrum and SI joints, restricting extension and flexion.

There are other complicating factors relating to malalignment:

1. There is a functional inequality of leg length and strength.

2. Forward flexion can provoke pain by further increasing tension in other tender and/or tight muscles (e.g. the right hamstrings, which very often already show an increase in tension – see Figs 3.38 and 3.39).

3. Tender structures subjected to direct pressure will limit sitting time. Seat comfort varies with body proportions and seat design. Appropriate cut-outs on the seat help to avoid direct pressure on the ischial tuberosities and coccyx but may not spare a tender piriformis, gluteus maximus muscle or sacrotuberous ligament. The peroneal and tibial components of the sciatic nerve are also vulnerable to pressure on the posterior thigh region.

4. Asymmetry of the ribs and of the associated rib rotation increases the chances that the bellows-type effect on the chest cage will result in irritation of the costochondral, costotransverse, costovertebral and clavicular joints (see Figs 2.62–2.64).

Sweep-rowing

> The significant asymmetry involved in sweep-rowing results in specific injury patterns not seen in sculling as there is considerable forwards flexion combined with repetitive rotation to the side of the boat.

Complications with malalignment relate in particular to limitations of range in these directions because of tender or asymmetrically tight soft tissue structures and an impaired rotational ability of the pelvis and the various segments of the spine, with or without complicating vertebral malrotation. The compensatory curves and changes in muscle tension resulting from malalignment can, for example, easily limit trunk rotation into either the port or starboard side by 5–15 degrees (see Fig. 3.45B).

Sweep-rowing also results in unbalanced muscle development and strength, particularly involving latissimus dorsi and quadriceps on the side of the rigger frame; this asymmetrical development could well predispose to a recurrence of malalignment.

Kayaking

In the typical recreational kayak, the double-bladed paddle allows for stroking on alternate sides in a cyclical fashion. The legs and pelvis are essentially fixed because of the low seating position and the fact that each foot may be stabilized on a foot pedal for rudder control, and the knees braced against the sides of the boat. In a flat-water kayak used for competition on lakes, there is no rudder and the knees are not braced when racing, so that the trunk is subjected to more intrinsic forces, whereas in whitewater kayaking – racing down a canyon or other natural challenge – the body is subjected to more extrinsic forces.

The cyclical paddling action in all events is primarily one of forward flexion, combined with alternate side flexion, and clockwise or counterclockwise rotation of the trunk in the transverse plane. Most of this rotation occurs through the thoracic segment, which, in the presence of malalignment, usually shows restriction into one side (see Fig. 3.45B). The maximum stress will be through the transitional region for facet orientation: the thoracolumbar region (see Figs 3.8 and 3.12). Back pain is therefore more likely to develop in the mid-back region. Low back pain also occurs because there is some rotation of the lumbar segment as a whole once thoracic rotation reaches its limit, compounding the stress already imposed on the lumbosacral junction by the malalignment.

The increased demands for trunk rotation associated with whitewater kayaking might be expected to precipitate back symptoms more readily than flat-water kayaking, but the repetitive nature of the action, and the generally increased duration of ocean and river kayaking, may make these outings just as devastating. Factors that prove complicating in any situations include:

- the pressure exerted on tender sites (e.g. coccyx and ischial tuberosities, the site of sacrotuberous insertion and hamstring origin)
- increased tension forces on structures that are already tender (e.g. the posterior pelvic ligaments and muscles such as piriformis and quadratus lumborum), exerted by prolonged or repetitive forward flexion and/or the repetitive rotation.

Canoeing

A stroke on the left side is initiated by reaching forwards and out to the left with the paddle, that is, by simultaneous forward flexion and left side flexion. There follows a counterclockwise rotation of the trunk and pelvis, and progressive trunk and hip extension as the blade is driven backwards.

The positioning and combination of movements makes the stroke the most asymmetrical of the ones described and therefore probably more vulnerable to the effects of malalignment. Left posterior innominate rotation, for example, limits both left hip extension and left pelvic rotation in the transverse plane. There is often also a complicating increase in tension in the left hip flexors, reflecting a change in the length-to-tension ratio and sometimes facilitation, which further restricts left hip extension (see Fig. 3.64A). These changes could create problems for the canoeist who drives the blade backwards on the left while kneeling on the left knee, left hip in neutral or slight extension, and weight-bearing on the right foot with the right hip and knee flexed to 90 degrees (see Fig. 5.2). Problems include:

- *when driving the left blade backwards*: increased rotational stress on the thoracic segment because of a limitation of left pelvic rotation; increased stress on tight left hip flexors as the trunk and left hip extend
- *in the right semi-squat position (right hip and knee flexed)*: increased stress on the right sacrotuberous ligament and the gluteus maximus and hamstrings, augmented whenever the pelvis rotates counter-clockwise.

Even though sculling and kayaking may be symmetrical, these activities, along with sweep-rowing and canoeing, are all associated with an increased risk of having the athlete go out of alignment when:

1. getting in and out of the boat
2. getting the boat into and out of the water or on and off a transport vehicle.

The risk of losing alignment on these occasions can be decreased by having the athlete try to preserve symmetry as much as possible (Box 5.6).

If malalignment recurs as a result of being unable to heed these precautions, or even when activity is limited to symmetrical sculling or recreational kayaking, the athlete should avoid these activities until realignment is being maintained.

RUNNING

Problems relating to running have been discussed throughout the previous chapters, particularly with regard to problems resulting from:

- an asymmetry of weight-bearing, pronation and supination (see Figs 3.18, 3.33, 3.74 and 7.1)
- contrary rotation of the legs (e.g. a whipping action of either heel, or 'clipping' of the opposite side – see Fig. 3.17)
- functional leg weakness, fatiguing and instability
- a tendency of the pelvis to rotate towards the side of an outflare, with a limitation of stride length in the opposite direction.

Box 5.6 Techniques to try to preserve symmetry

- *Slide in and out of the boat*: use the dock or side of the boat to sit on, or hang on to both sides of the boat at the same time for support while stepping in or out (Fig. 5.13A)
- *When getting up from or down onto the seat*: have someone steady the boat and hang on to both sides (Fig. 5.13B)
- *When getting in or out of the boat*: if at all possible, avoid leading with one leg (which usually requires excessive hip abduction, flexion or extension, rotation or a combination of these), but try instead to move the legs together while sitting on the dock or side of the boat
- *When alone and carrying the boat to and from the water*: with the boat lying parallel to the water's edge, face the boat and pick it up with both hands as symmetrically as possible (Fig. 5.14A); preferable would be a two-person low carry (Fig. 5.14B)
- *When having to lift the boat*: try to get someone to help by simultaneously lifting the boat up on the other side or end in order to avoid as much torsional strain as possible (Fig. 5.14B, C)

Appendix 5 lists some of the typical problems encountered by runners with one of the 'alternate' presentations.

SKATING

The skater has to defy gravity while at the same time trying to balance the weight of the body over a thin blade. In the presence of malalignment, these challenges may become highly problematic.

Edges

There are basically four edges – inside and outside, forward and backward – and the skater has to be able to switch from one to another quickly. The more the lean of the body, the 'deeper' the edge and the less support available from the blade.

Edging is affected by any tendency to pronation or supination, the tendency to go either way being in turn augmented by the lack of a supporting base, any angulation and/or off-setting of the way in which the blade is fixed to the boot, and the fact that the foot is elevated by the boot.

These factors can make for a very insecure foot in terms of weight-bearing support and push-off stability.

Falling inwards or 'losing the edge' on the side of the pronating foot appears to be a more common complaint

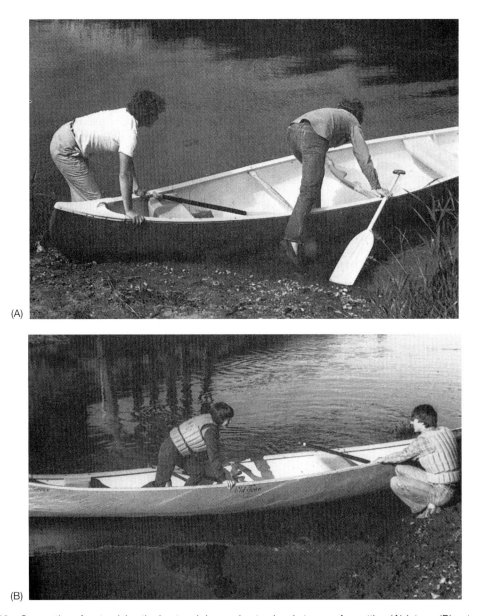

(A)

(B)

Figure 5.13 Suggestions for steadying the boat and decreasing torsional stresses for getting (A) into or (B) out of the boat. (From Harrison 1981, with permission.)

than toppling outwards probably because the supinating foot is a more rigid foot, better suited for supporting the skater, for push-off and for 'holding the edge'. Any medial or lateral deviation of the knee from a position directly over the foot will further decrease stability (as for judo and karate; see above and Figs 5.8B, C and 5.11D).

The combination of custom-made skates with medial or lateral reinforcement, and possibly longitudinal arch supports with or without posting, may increase the sta-

bility at the ankle and minimize such deviations of the knee. If, however, the tendency towards excessive and asymmetrical pronation or supination is attributable to malalignment, only realignment can be expected to resolve the problem completely, by:

- putting the feet into a more secure and symmetrical position for weight-bearing
- removing any resistance to controlled shifting on to the inner or outer edge.

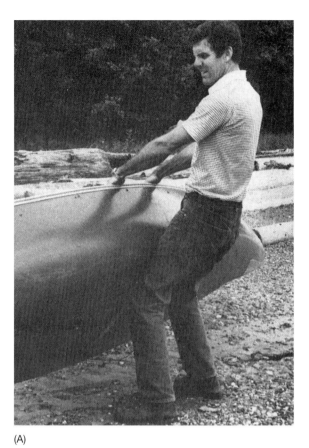

(A)

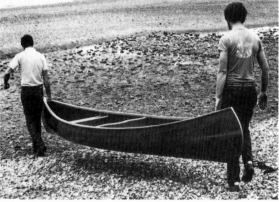

(Bi)

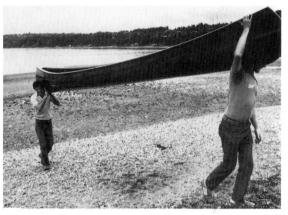

(Bii)

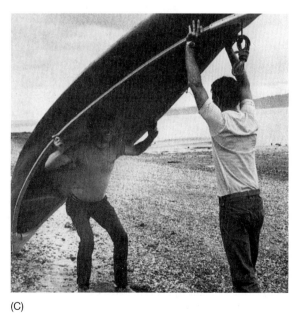

(C)

Figure 5.14 Safe carrying and lifting techniques. (A) One-person carry over a short distance (minimal torquing).
(B) Two-person (i) low and (ii) high carry (minimal torquing).
(C) One-person assisted lift (no torquing). (D) One-person unassisted lift (with considerable torquing). (From Harrison 1981, with permission.)

Figure 5.14 (D), see overleaf

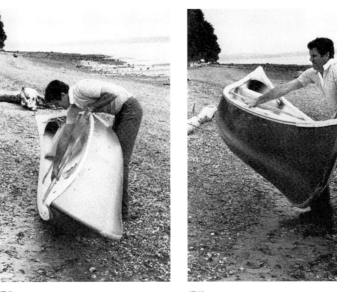

(Di)

(Dii)

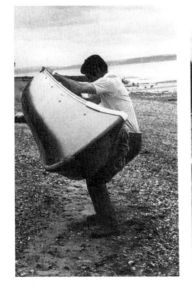

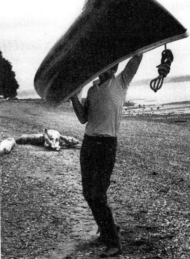

(Diii)

(Div)

Figure 5.14 *Continued.*

Executing turns

Turning is accomplished by shifting the weight on to the appropriate inner or outer edge (see Fig. 5.16A, B). To make a left turn, for example, the skater can simply lean on to the left outer and/or right inner edge. Malalignment, by affecting the ease with which the skater can shift on to a particular edge, will make it easier to make a turn in one direction. Whether this is

to right or left may be predictable from the presentation of the malalignment.

'Alternate' presentations and upslips

The tendency to supinate on the left and pronate on the right facilitates turning to the left; the skater is already predisposed to leaning on to the left outer and right inner edge. By the same token, the same skater may find it harder to execute a turn to the right because of the increased difficulty of shifting weight on to the left inner and right outer edges. Biomechanically, making a left turn is like 'going with the flow', whereas on attempting a turn to the right, the skater is 'going against the current'.

The right foot and ankle may, however, tend to feel 'sloppy', collapse inwards and fatigue more easily than the left because of the weakness of tibialis anterior and posterior, and the collapse of the medial longitudinal arch, so that the skater may prefer to put more weight on the more stable left foot and ankle.

If the same skater attempts to skate circles of a small diameter, such as figure-skating or compulsory figures, the following might occur.

It might again be easier to go counterclockwise. Counterclockwise circling requires alternately transferring the weight on to the left outer and right inner edges and back. The transfer from left to right is achieved by adducting the right leg to cross it in front of the left. This manoeuvre again requires getting on to the skater's preferred edges. It also calls for adduction with the right leg, which happens to have a greater passive adduction range than the left in nearly 100% of those presenting with malalignment (see Figs 3.40 and 3.70). The 'alternate' presentations will also favour the speed-skater going counterclockwise around the track, especially when the right leg has to adduct to cross in front of the left leg while leaning to the left into a curve (Fig. 5.15).

It will be relatively more difficult to go clockwise. Attempts to transfer weight to the right outer and left inner edge run counter to the tendencies usually imposed by malalignment. In addition, there is the restriction of left hip adduction relative to the right. The skater may try facilitating getting onto the left inner, right outer edge by leaning towards the ice more on the right side, but this comes at increased risk of falling.

An exception to the above is an attempt to go counterclockwise supported only on the right outer edge. This is required, for example, on the 'back or backward outside eight' part of a figure-of-eight or as part of another configuration (Fig. 5.16B). Here, the skater with an 'alternate' presentation or upslip is at risk of 'losing the edge'; that is, attempts to stay on the right outer edge may eventually fail as the foot falls inwards. An astute 'pro' may notice that the right knee also falls inwards the moment that the edge is lost. If both edges on the right skate end up contacting the ice, this constitutes a 'flat', which, in competition, results in loss of points.

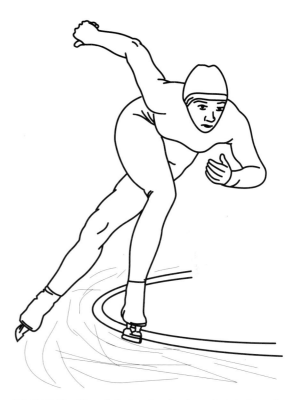

Figure 5.15   Speed-skating: leaning inwards to help push off from the right inner and left outer edge while adducting the right and left leg simultaneously.

Left anterior and locked presentation

This skater tends to pronate on the left and supinate on the right and may therefore find it easier to execute circles clockwise rather than counterclockwise. The speed-skater with this presentation would be at a disadvantage when racing in the usual counterclockwise direction.

Balance and recovery

The skater with an 'alternate' presentation or upslip may feel insecure when landing on the right leg, for example, on completion of an Axel-Paulsen loop jump (Fig. 5.16A). The skater in the illustration takes off from the left outer edge, does a full rotation counterclockwise and lands on the right outer edge. On landing, there may be extraneous movements of the arms, trunk and left leg in an attempt to maintain balance because stability is decreased by the combination of:

- losing the outer edge as the right foot tends to pronate
- the right knee collapsing inwards into valgus, away from its more stable position directly over the foot.

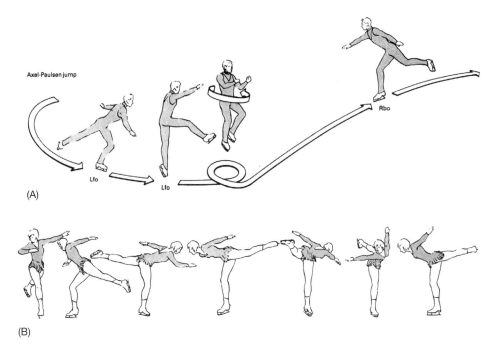

Figure 5.16 Edging and weighting during typical ice-dancing routines. (A) Axel-Paulsen jump; note the weighting of specific edges (Lfo, left forward outside; Rbo, right backward outside) and the landing on the right leg after the jump. (B) A 'camel spin' (which incorporates the 'spiral') carried out weight-bearing on the right leg. (From Worth 1990, with permission.)

The biomechanical limitations imposed by malalignment can become blatantly obvious with some of the routines. The 'spiral', for example, calls for flexion of the trunk to horizontal, arms out to the side, gliding along supported on only one skate with the other leg extended in a horizontal position, in line with the trunk (Fig. 5.16B). The skater with right anterior, left posterior innominate rotation doing the spiral:

1. will be able to raise the right leg further up in the air while supported on the left leg than he or she could raise the left leg while supported on the right. This is consistent with the increased amount of hip extension possible on the side of the anterior rotation. When attempting the spiral supported on the right leg, the left posterior innominate rotation may interfere with the ability to bring the left leg to horizontal or higher by:

– creating a mechanical block to extension (see Figs. 3.64 and 3.65)

– tightening up the left iliacus and rectus femoris by separating their origin and insertion even further (see Fig. 3.38)

– limiting compensatory counterclockwise rotation of the pelvis in the transverse plane (see Fig. 3.4C).

2. Will find it easier to flex the trunk to a horizontal position when supported on the left leg than on the right. The right anterior rotation tightens the right gluteus maximus, the hamstrings and the sacrotuberous ligament, thereby limiting right hip flexion.

Balance is also more likely to be a problem with right single-leg support. Balance becomes progressively more precarious with routines that combine single-leg support, trunk flexion and cutting a circle. For example, the addition of a turn to the spiral (Fig. 5.16B), known as a camel spin, calls for staying on a specific edge. For a 'back inner edge', for example, the skater in the spiral position supported on the left leg would place the weight on the left inner edge.

Because of the tendency towards supination on the left, those with one of the 'alternate' presentations may lose that inner edge more easily and end up with a flat or even move on to the outer edge of the left skate.

This results in a simultaneous increase in varus stress on the knee. If the knee ends up no longer positioned directly over the foot, the stability of the left lower extremity will be decreased.

Malalignment can only compound the difficulty of mastering the progressively more demanding routines, such as the triple axle or quadruple toe loop, or combinations like the triple axle–triple toe loop. It will also increase the chance of a mishap occurring when attempting these routines, particularly given that most require a high-speed landing on one blade – in most cases the right – as the body continues to rotate. Malalignment, by affecting balance and edging, interferes with recovery and increases the margin of error.

Propulsion and speed

Because of the low coefficient of friction between the ice and the blade, propulsion in ice-skating is not possible by pushing the blade straight backward. As van Ingen Schenau et al (1989) point out:

- the blade has to be positioned at right angles to the gliding direction of the skate; this requires some external rotation of the lower extremity on the side pushing off
- the smaller the angle between the push-off leg and the ice, the more effective the push-off; the angle is decreased by increasing the amount of abduction of that extremity.

The skater with an 'alternate' presentation or upslip, in particular the speed-skater going around the track counterclockwise, may derive some benefit from the malalignment. The tendency toward pronation, coupled with the increased ability to externally rotate and abduct the right lower extremity, should make it easier to position the right blade properly and to move on to the inner edge for push-off from this extremity. However:

1. *on the right side*: the combination of pronation, weakness of the ankle invertors (especially tibialis posterior) and increased fatiguability of the right lower extremity in general may result in a feeling of weakness and instability that could affect right push-off unfavourably
2. *on the left side*: the limitation of left hip external rotation, and usually also of abduction, plus an exaggeration of the tendency towards supination and the weakness of peroneus longus, all combine to make it more difficult to get on to – and stay on – the inside of the left blade, diminishing the ability to push off from that side. In the skater with posterior rotation of the left innominate, the left push-off may be further compromised by the restriction of left hip extension and the limitation of left counterclockwise rotation of the pelvis.

Increased velocity is associated with an increased forward inclination of the trunk, as seen in the tendency of speed-skaters to hold the trunk in a near-horizontal position. This is partly to counterbalance push-off, but mainly to lower the centre of gravity and to reduce drag. van Ingen Schenau (1982) has shown that the drag force increases by more than 20% with a vertical deviation of the trunk of only 20 degrees from the horizontal position. In the presence of malalignment, the ability to achieve the maximum forward inclination possible may be limited by:

- right or left anterior innominate rotation, resulting in an ipsilateral restriction of hip flexion
- an inability to tolerate a further sustained increase in tension in structures that have become tender because of the malalignment (e.g. the trunk extensors, posterior pelvic ligaments and piriformis muscles).

Stopping

A stop is usually accomplished by digging in the opposite edges perpendicularly to the line of progression. The skater with one of the 'alternate' presentations or upslip is already oriented to bear weight more easily on the right inside and left outside edges, which should make it easier to make a sudden stop with a quick turn to the left. Stopping by turning to the right may prove both awkward and ineffective in comparison. Excessive right pronation and the right ankle feeling 'sloppy' or insecure may, however, prevent the skater getting onto the right inside edge, a problem that is sometimes solved with an orthotic that provides increased support for the collapsing medial arch.

The ice hockey goalie

Goalies frequently use their legs to stop the puck. Injuries are often blamed on lack of flexibility or on having had to elongate a muscle that has not yet had time to relax completely after having been activated for some other manoeuvre immediately preceding the one that caused the injury. Malalignment, by restricting some ranges of motion and increasing the tension in certain muscles and ligaments, is another cause to consider, especially if the goalie is subject to recurrent injuries. In that respect, structures particularly vulnerable include the following:

Hip adductors

A quick abduction of one or both legs (e.g. doing the splits) can protect a large area of the goal crease and may block a sliding or low-flying puck, but these manoeuvres risk tearing the adductors, pectineus and/or iliopsoas, and may even avulse the lesser trochanter (see Fig. 3.46). Left hip abduction is decreased in the majority of those with malalignment, increasing the risk of injury on that side.

Iliopsoas

- Posterior innominate rotation increases the tension in iliacus, anterior rotation that in psoas major and minor, through a separation of their origin and insertion (see Fig. 3.38).
- The tension in iliopsoas may be *per se* increased in an attempt by part or all of that muscle to stabilize the SI joint (see Fig. 2.31B), through facilitation triggered by rotation of any of the origins (T12–L3 vertebrae – see Fig. 2.40) or passively with internal rotation of the lower extremity.

Piriformis

Tension in the right and left piriformis (Fig. 2.31A) is increased in a large number of those with malalignment. A tense piriformis is at risk of being sprained or strained if:

- the muscle contracts further to externally rotate the leg but that movement is suddenly blocked
- the muscle is subjected to an increase in tension by a manoeuvre that results in internal rotation, adduction or flexion of the leg or a combination of these; in a goalie with right anterior rotation, the ranges of right internal rotation and flexion are already limited, making the right piriformis more vulnerable when the leg is forced into those directions (see Figs 3.64 and 3.71B)

Hip flexors and extensors, and sacrotuberous ligaments

Increased tension in the gluteus maximus, hamstrings and sacrotuberous ligaments on the side of the anterior innominate rotation puts these structures at risk in attempts to block a puck by kicking the leg straight out, hyperflexing the hip on this side. The increased tension in iliacus and rectus femoris on the side of the posterior rotation puts these structures at risk when kicking the left leg straight back, thus hyperextending the hip. A sagittal split would jeopardize these structures on opposite sides simultaneously, and the ability to perform these movements would also be affected by facilitation causing increased tension in any of these muscles.

Pelvis, trunk, shoulders and neck

A goalie has to be extremely agile in order to move quickly from one side of the goal to another, or to

---

> **Box 5.7** Areas of the ice-hockey goalie's body particularly vulnerable to injury
>
> 1. *The trunk*, especially on collision with the goal posts or other players, and even more so when the pelvis is fixed by sitting on the ice and trunk rotation is attempted (or forced) into the restricted side (see Fig. 3.45C)
> 2. *The shoulders*, especially on reaching attempts that require rotation into a restricted range or being passively forced into one of these directions, for example, in a goalie with an 'alternate' presentation or upslip, having the left arm forced into extension or external rotation, or the right arm into internal rotation (see Fig. 3.15A)
> 3. *The neck and back*, pain often being triggered by having to assume an awkward stance for longer periods of times. This may be seen if the trunk is flexed and the head and neck extended, resulting in a prolonged increase in tension on structures that are often already tender because of the malalignment: the paravertebral muscles (some of which run from the cervical region to attachments as far down as the T4 or T5 level), the posterior pelvic ligaments, sites of curve reversal and vertebral malrotation

rotate to the right or left when standing or sitting in the goal crease. Any malalignment-related limitation of range of motion can interfere with this agility and increase the risk of injury. The areas listed in Box 5.7 are particularly vulnerable.

Hockey players are particularly at risk of having their trunk, pelvis or extremities moved passively into directions of restriction and past anatomical barriers on collision with other players, the boards and goal posts.

> Ice-skaters and goalies are particulary prone to suffering the complications of coccydynia and pelvic floor dysfunction from repeated falls onto the coccyx.

A single incident of shear injury, or repetitive microtrauma, from a single or repeated falls onto one buttock can result in SI joint instability. Given the increased potential for collisions and/or falls, skaters are also at increased risk of going out of alignment in the first place and encountering problems when trying to maintain correction.

SKIING: ALPINE OR DOWNHILL

Alpine skiing is one of the athletic activities that maximally stresses the ability of all body parts to move through the full available ranges of motion. As so aptly described by Luttgens et al (1992, p. 572):

The movement problems encountered by the alpine skier revolve around changing directions and maintaining balance at high speeds while undergoing a variety of horizontal and vertical disturbances.

Executing a normal turn

Turns are initiated primarily by a rotation of body parts, unweighting and transferring the weight to the appropriate edges. Almost any body part can be used to initiate a turn, but the feet and arms tend to be the least effective because they are the farthest away from the centre of gravity. In addition, as indicated by Adrian & Cooper (1986, p. 672):

Arm and trunk rotations, initiated by movements at the shoulder, hip and spinal column will cause the skis to turn if the action is forceful enough. This necessity for force, acceleration, and large motions is a source of 'overturning' and loss of control.

Rotation of the pelvis in the transverse plane thus proves most effective for initiating a turn, given the proximity of the pelvis to the centre of gravity and the need for only a minimal displacement of this part of the body (see Fig. 3.85).

An intermediate skier travelling to the right and perpendicular to the fall line is gliding on the inner edge of the downhill (left) and outer edge of the uphill (right) ski while putting more load on the downhill than the uphill ski (Fig. 5.17). The edging is facilitated by leaning with the hips and knees into the mountain while the trunk is maintained in a vertical position or leans downhill, creating a varus stress (outer soft tissues and medial compartment) on the right knee, and valgus stress (inner soft tissues and lateral compartment) on the left one (see Figs 3.33 and 3.74). In order to execute a left (downhill) turn, the skier:

1. transfers weight to the inner edge of the uphill (right) and outer edge of the downhill (left) ski; this transfer is aided by leaning the body downhill, the combined effect being to:
   – unload the downhill ski while at the same time loading the uphill one
   – create a force towards valgus angulation of the uphill (right) and varus angulation of the downhill (left) knee
2. rotates the pelvis counterclockwise in the transverse plane, which helps to initiate the turn by advancing the uphill leg and increasing the ability to weight the inside edge of that ski
3. progressively pivots through the turn, the uphill (right) leg pivoting from external to internal rotation, the downhill (left) leg pivoting in the opposite direction.

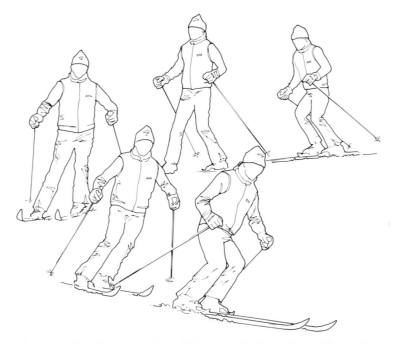

Figure 5.17 The basic 'stem turn' in skiing: proceeding initially perpendicularly to the fall line and then down the fall line and on around the turn. (From Parker 1988, with permission.)

When the first half, or 90 degrees, of the turn has been completed, the skier will be facing downhill with the legs and trunk in alignment and the weight equally distributed on both skis. If the skier decided at this point to head straight down the mountain, the pelvis would rotate clockwise back to neutral, facing the fall line. In order to continue the turn to a full 180 degrees, the skier has to:

- maintain the forward rotation of the right side of the pelvis
- help weight the inside of the right (now downhill) and outside of the left (now uphill) ski.

This weight transfer is aided by leaning the knees and hips into, and the body away from, the hill, thereby accentuating the left varus, right valgus angulation strain on the knees.

Effect of malalignment on executing a turn

Adrian & Cooper (1986) rightly observe that 'human beings tend to be asymmetric, that is, they perform a turn more successfully in one direction than in the other'. They go on to state that 'leg dominance with respect to balance usually determines the preferred turning direction' (p. 674). While 'leg dominance with respect to balance' may be involved, the chief determining factors in this author's experience relate to the presence of malalignment that affects:

- *rotation in the transverse plane* with limitation into the side of a posterior rotation or an inflare
- *edging*
  - limiting the ability to get onto the right outer and left inner edge with upslips or one of the 'alternate' presentations
  - the reverse when the left anterior and locked pattern is present.

Those presenting with a left posterior rotation will generally find it easier to execute a turn to the right; those with a right posterior rotation, a turn to the left. The tendency to right or left pronation and supination does not appear to be as influential as the limitation imposed by the side of posterior rotation.

Let us look at the difficulties that four different presentations of malalignment create for skiers attempting a turn.

Right anterior, left posterior presentation

When attempting a left turn, there should be no problem unweighting the left (downhill) and weighting the right

(uphill) ski, unless the skier is one of those athletes who has difficulty balancing on one leg (something that might become apparent on single-leg stance doing the kinetic rotational or Gillet test – see Figs 2.88–2.90).

The weight is transferred more easily to the outside of the left and inside of the right ski, which should favour making a left turn. However, some athletes with an 'alternate' presentation report how the right foot feels 'sloppy', how it is difficult to 'get an inner edge' on the right side and how the addition of a right medial longitudinal arch support increases the stability of that foot and ankle and allows them to dig in that edge more convincingly. A weakness of the right ankle invertors, combined with external rotation of the right leg and a tendency to right pronation, may account for this feeling of right foot and ankle instability.

Pelvic rotation in the transverse plane is restricted to the left. The side-to-side difference can be appreciable: 10–25 degrees is not unusual (see Fig. 3.4). In addition, the restriction of left pelvic rotation increases as the degree of left posterior innominate rotation increases, and can actually progress to the point at which it becomes ineffective for initiating the turn. The skier may then accomplish the turn by:

- transferring all the weight on to the left ski and literally 'hiking up' the right hip, in order to clear the right ski and allow the skier to rotate the right leg and attached ski internally by muscle action, in combination with
- increasing left trunk rotation to compensate for the loss of left pelvic rotation.

All the above is occurring at a time when the skier is supposed to be unweighting the left ski and weighting the right. Needless to say, having to unweight the right ski to effect a left turn completely forfeits the benefits that would usually derive from transferring on to its inner edge.

Trunk rotation in the transverse plane is typically restricted to the left, although restriction to the right can also occur (see Fig. 3.45). Left limitation will decrease the ability to use trunk rotation to the left to help to initiate or carry through a left turn, even though this would be considered poor technique.

To compensate, the skier may resort to using the arms to help to initiate and control turning; this unfortunately proves to be an even poorer technique in that it results in a greater displacement of the centre of gravity and a further decrease in stability.

Left anterior, right posterior innominate rotation; right sacroiliac joint locked

The main problem with this 'alternate' presentation is the restriction of clockwise rotation of the pelvis, which is likely to make it harder to use the pelvis to initiate a turn to the right and easier to initiate a turn to the left.

Left anterior and locked

The tendency for the left foot to pronate, and the right to supinate, should be of help in digging in the appropriate edges to initiate a right turn. However, the associated limitations of lower extremity rotation – with a limitation of left internal and right external rotation – and the decrease of clockwise rotation of the pelvis in the transverse plane all become a hindrance to initiating and carrying out a right turn.

Right outflare, left inflare

The pelvis tends to rotate clockwise and the left swing/right stance stride is increased, facilitating a turn to the right. The reverse will occur with left outflare, right inflare.

Turning problems related to degree of malalignment

As indicated, the difficulty with turning into the side of the posterior innominate rotation appears to be directly related to the degree of posterior rotation. The ability to turn in one direction can certainly worsen from one day to another, or may even deteriorate as the day progresses, perhaps because the amount of posterior rotation has increased. Aggravating factors include the following.

Tightness in the muscles attaching to the innominate, which can exert a pull. This can occur:

- in a posterior direction (e.g. from the gluteus maximus, hamstrings and external abdominal oblique – see Figs 2.24B and 2.37), which increases the tendency towards posterior rotation of the ipsilateral innominate
- in an anterior direction on one side (e.g. from the rectus femoris, iliacus, TFL, quadratus lumborum and internal oblique) which could worsen an anterior rotation and thereby aggravate a compensatory posterior rotation of the contralateral innominate (see Figs 2.24C, 2.31 and 2.37).

Unskilled turns initiated by excessive trunk rotation. Excessive trunk rotation at a time when the lower extremities are fixed can exert a rotational effect on the innominates:

1. *directly*: by way of the attachments of muscles (e.g. quadratus lumborum, latissimus dorsi and the abdominal obliques) and ligaments (e.g. the iliolumbar – see Fig. 2.35A)
2. *indirectly*: by exerting a rotational force down through the lumbar spine, straining the lumbosacral junction and compressing the facet joint on one side to cause torsion of the sacrum (see Fig. 2.35B).

Impact to the innominate bone. The direction of rotation that results from a direct blow to the innominate as a result of a fall or collision depends on whether the impact has come from an anterior or posterior direction, and whether the force was applied above or below the transverse axis of rotation (see Figs. 2.33 and 2.34).

Leverage effect on the innominate. A fall or collision can easily turn the lower extremities into levers capable of effecting innominate rotation: anterior with inadvertent hyperextension of the hip, posterior with forced hip flexion (see Fig. 2.32).

Simultaneous inflare on the side of the posterior rotation. The skier with marked left posterior rotation will often note that turns to the right can be carried out with increased ease and speed, and at a more acute angle, if necessary. In contrast, turns to the left are harder to execute, tend to take more time and are less acute. At worst, the skier literally lifts the right leg and twists the body into the direction of the turn.

Whenever these limitations become apparent, he or she should carry out one of the self-treatment techniques intended to correct innominate rotation (see Chs 7 and 8) in the hope of being immediately able to return to unhindered skiing. Alternatively, a trip to the therapist at the foot of the slope might prove worthwhile. Correction will certainly make for a better day of skiing in that it should again allow turns to be carried out with equal ease, speed and angulation to either side, as well as decrease the risk of injury.

Problems: 'getting a good edge'

> Skiers are acutely aware of side-to-side differences in the ability to fit comfortably into a boot and to dig in the inner or outer edge, and they often make modifications on their own through trial and error.

The following comments apply also to Nordic and cross-country skiing and telemarking.

One common complaint is that of feeling a weakness of the ankle, with an inward collapse of the foot. Skiers may use terms such as 'pronation', this condition being countered using either a medial arch support or a build-up under the binding. Skiers who supinate bilaterally may feel an improved ability to get onto the inner edge by adding a lateral raise under the binding. For those with one of the 'alternate' presentations or an upslip, the tendency towards supination is likely to be accentuated on the left, so that they may end up with a left lateral raise only, or one on the left that is higher than the one on the right side.

The binding on one side is often rotated outwards in an attempt to accommodate for an increased tendency towards external rotation of that leg, typically on the right side in those with an 'alternate' presentation or upslip (Fig. 5.18A). Provided that the amount by which the binding is rotated outwards exactly matches the external rotation of the leg:

- it will help to minimize stresses at the ankle and knee that would otherwise result from a mismatch

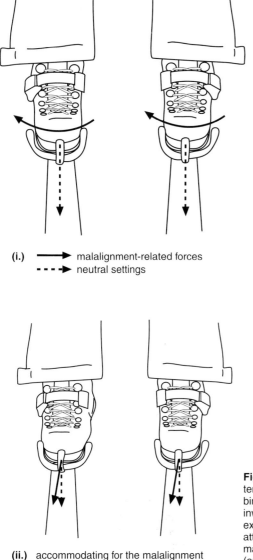

(i.) ⟶ malalignment-related forces
- - -► neutral settings

(ii.) accommodating for the malalignment
⟶ new settings

(A)

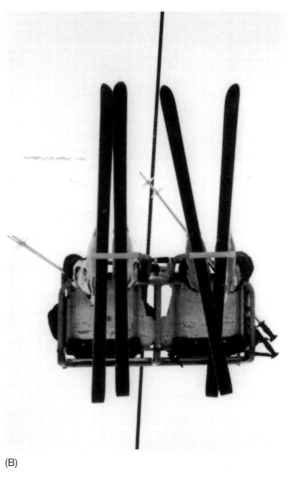

(B)

Figure 5.18 Typical manifestations of a malalignment-related tendency to right external, left internal rotation in skiing. (A) The ski bindings have been offset outwards from the midline on the right and inwards on the left in (ii) to accommodate for the increased stress exerted on the right lateral and left medial foot in (i) as the legs attempt to rotate within the boot. (B) When riding the lift: malalignment is probably present in the skier sitting in the left seat (appearance from below), where right ski (leg) is turned outwards relative to the left. The skier in the right seat is probably in alignment, with both skis pointing in the same direction.

- the foot, ankle and knee may feel more stable, and there may be a relief of the discomfort previously felt on the lateral aspect of the foot and knee; this is not unlike the case of the cyclist who has rotated the toe clip outwards for increased comfort, stability and ability to generate power with that leg (see 'Cycling' above)
- it will do little else to counter the stresses relating to the malalignment (e.g. on the pelvis and spine).

If the binding is maintained in a neutral position (sagittal plane), so that the boot points straight forwards (Fig. 5.18Ai), or if the amount by which the binding is offset outwards fails exactly to match the external rotation of the leg, and given that the foot is fixed in the boot, the persistent tendency for the leg to rotate outwards will:

1. accentuate the tendency to external rotation of the femur relative to the 'fixed' tibia, increasing stress on the medial structures (e.g. MCL), pressure on the lateral joint compartment and tension in TFL/ITB (see Figs 3.33 and 3.74)

2. probably result in a pressure feeling along the lateral aspect of the foot, particularly the forefoot, as it tries to rotate outwards but is restrained by the boot

 – this pressure sensation may be aggravated by the addition of an orthotic made to counteract the tendency towards pronation: by raising the medial longitudinal arch, the orthotic shifts weight-bearing laterally and encourages a further external rotation of that leg, thereby increasing the pressure exerted by the boot against the lateral edge of the foot

 – an orthotic with a lateral raise of the forefoot may relieve the pressure on the outside of the foot but will accentuate the forces tending towards pronation, knee valgus and lateral tracking of the patella.

The initial temptation is often to offset both bindings outwards, usually to the same degree. In someone with one of the 'alternate' presentations or an upslip, whose left leg has actually rotated inwards (sometimes to the point at which the foot now points straight ahead or may even have crossed the midline – see Fig. 3.16B), offsetting the binding outwards on the left side will create a counter-rotational force:

- There will now be increased pressure against the medial aspect of the left forefoot as the leg tries to turn inwards. This pressure may be alleviated with an orthotic to 'counter pronation'. An orthotic that shifts weight-bearing laterally would, however, further increase the rigidity of a foot that is often already in a neutral to supinated position.

- There will be a residual varus stress on the knee as the femur attempts to rotate inwards relative to the 'fixed' tibia. The skier may complain of symptoms related to stress on lateral soft tissues and the medial compartment.

> The ongoing need for any modifications that have been made to skis, orthotics, bindings or boots must be reassessed following the correction of the malalignment.

Weight-bearing and lower limb orientation may change dramatically with realignment, so the biomechanical effect of these previous modifications may, if they are left in place, now be completely inappropriate. In fact, these modifications could now actually cause malalignment to recur.

Problems relating to 'getting' a good inner or outer edge are also influenced by the inherent weight-bearing pattern (neutral, excessive pronation or supination) and the alignment of the lower extremities (neutral, genu valgum with compensatory pronation, genu varum with a tendency towards supination, or external or internal rotation of a lower extremity). Following realignment, these factors have to be reassessed and accommodated for as indicated (see Fig. 3.29).

Knowing whether or not the skier is in alignment may be helped by observing the orientation of the skies on the next ride up on the lift: are both pointing forwards or outwards by the same amount, or is one rotated outwards (usually the right) relative to the other (Fig. 5.18B)? If malalignment is suspected, the next step is to confirm this and establish the type of presentation occurring before proceeding with any realignment procedures.

Difficulty weight-bearing on one lower extremity

> The skier may describe a feeling of weakness and/or insecurity when weight-bearing on one leg alone, usually the right.

Alpine, cross-country and telemark skiers often end up unexpectedly having to place most or all of their weight on one ski for short distances. How they fare when that happens to be the insecure leg depends in part on their level of skill, the speed at which they are travelling and the difficulty of the terrain. The problem may be attributable to malalignment, in which case it can be corrected by realignment.

Preference for attempting a sudden stop

A sudden stop, which Parker (1988) appropriately refers to as a 'hockey stop', entails 'a rapid two-footed twisting and resultant two-footed skid' (p. 52), the skis ending up parallel to the fall line but the skier still looking down the hill (Fig. 5.19). In other words, the pelvis rotates with the skis, whereas the trunk continues to face the fall line to a varying degree. This rotation occurs in the transverse plane, with trunk rotation primarily through the thoracic segment and in a direction opposite to pelvic rotation.

For most skiers, the combination of impaired rotation of the pelvic and thoracic segment to one or other side, difficulty getting an edge and perceived weakness on one side makes it consistently easier to accomplish such a quick stop by turning to either the right or left. The

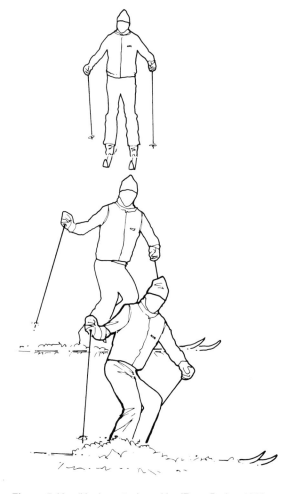

Figure 5.19 'Hockey-stop' on skis. (From Parker 1988, with permission.)

Box 5.8 Factors affecting the ability to undertake a 'hockey stop'

1. The ability of the pelvis to rotate in the transverse plane is limited into the direction of the posterior innominate rotation or inflare (see Fig. 3.4C)
2. In some, the ability to dig in the more 'secure' edges may be a more important factor. The more common pattern of right pronation, left supination should make it easier to dig in the right inner and left outer edges; this pattern, especially when combined with a left anterior rotation, may make it easier to complete a left turn. If, however, the pronating right ankle feels weak and insecure, the skier may prefer to get onto a more secure right outer edge and turn to the right instead; right innominate anterior rotation or outflare will facilitate a turn in this direction

---

main determining factors appear to be those listed in Box 5.8.

The skier is at increased risk of injury at times when the terrain or fellow skiers prevent the quicker, and usually more stable, turn into the preferred direction for stopping. For those in competitive ski events, the combination of problems relating to turning preference and the asymmetry of turning, getting an edge and lower extremity strength and balance, assumes more significance as a potential cause of poorer performances and injuries.

The ability to crouch in order to reduce drag may be hampered, especially by:

- an inability to tolerate a sustained increase in tension on tender posterior pelvic ligaments and muscles
- restrictions imposed by anterior innominate rotation, especially a restriction of right hip flexion (see Figs 3.64A and 3.69B).

SKIING: NORDIC OR CROSS-COUNTRY, AND TELEMARK

Differences between the various styles relate primarily to the method of achieving propulsion and making turns.

Traditional Nordic and track skiing

Propulsion is usually achieved using an alternating stride pattern, the most common being the diagonal stride, in which pole action is coupled with a backward thrust of the opposite, trailing ski. This thrust is produced by rapid hip extension with terminal plantar flexion of the foot, and results in the forward gliding action of the lead ski. Speed is determined, in part, by the following.

The strength of the backward thrust

With upslips and right anterior rotation, the strength of push-off could be decreased on either side as a result of:

- any ankle weakness and instability, associated in particular with an increased tendency towards right pronation and external rotation
- a limitation of left ankle dorsiflexion (see Fig. 3.77A), which has been associated with a decrease in plantar flexor peak torque (Mueller et al 1995)
- functional weakness and increased fatiguability of the muscles acting on the ankles, in particular the left peroneal muscles, and the right extensor hallucis longus and tibialis anterior and posterior.

Stride length

Stride length will be influenced by the asymmetry of hip and ankle ranges of motion and the limitations imposed by the innominates. Left hip extension is, for example, decreased with left posterior rotation (see Figs 3.64 and 3.65). The problem is compounded by the limitation of left ankle dorsiflexion noted in those with the 'alternate' presentations and upslips (see Fig. 3.77A). As weight is transferred to the left forefoot in preparation for push-off, further stretching of the already tight calf muscles and plantar fascia engages the 'windlass' mechanism prematurely and results in earlier, accelerated plantarflexion of the ankle.

In an attempt to compensate for the limitation of left hip extension, the skier may try actively to exaggerate left plantarflexion in order to increase the leg length on push-off. Active counterclockwise rotation of the pelvis in the transverse plane will also increase left leg length to help to even out the stride length, but this action is limited in those with left posterior innominate rotation or inflare. Either way of dealing with the asymmetry means more work and an increase in energy expenditure.

Problems on turning are primarily related to difficulties in getting an inside or outside edge, and restrictions of rotation of the pelvis and trunk, similar to those discussed above for downhill skiing.

Ski-skating: marathon and V-skate stride

These are presently the two main types of skating stride used in cross-country skiing. The marathon skate stride is accomplished with the thrust coming from only one lower extremity while the other glides in a track (Fig. 5.20A), whereas with the V-skate the thrust comes alter-natively from one and then the other leg (Fig. 5.20B). In both methods, the rear or thrust ski is angled at approximately 30 degrees to the direction of the glide (Watanabe 1987).

The skier with an upslip or one of the 'alternate' presentations, for example, is affected by the limitation of left hip abduction and external rotation, as well as the tendency to left supination, all of which make it more difficult to angle the left ski outwards to 30 degrees and get onto the left inner edge. As a result, the left push-off thrust may be decreased compared with the right.

With the left anterior and locked presentation, the tendency towards inward collapse of the left foot and ankle, and an increased ability to rotate that extremity outwards, may make it easier to get onto the left inner edge, while making these same manoeuvres more difficult on the right side.

Telemarking

A turn to the right can be initiated from the 'half-wedge' position, where the right (inside) ski points straight and the left is wedged, or pointed inwards, by a slight internal rotation of the left leg (Parker 1988 – Fig. 5.21). Although most of the weight remains on the straight-running right ski, 'the pressure that develops on the wedged ski initiates a slight direction change' (p. 34).

To make a telemark turn to the right, the left ski leads and assumes the half-wedge position, pressure being applied to the left inner edge. The right leg is 'tucked under', the hip extended and the knee flexed, and the foot moves back, with an application of pressure to the right outer edge. The left half-wedged ski continues to advance so that the right hip extends and the right knee flexes even further to allow the skier to sink into the telemark stance: the left foot forwards and the right slightly back. The weight is primarily on the leading (left) leg at the beginning of the turn. As the turn progresses, the skier rocks back, putting increasingly more weight on the trailing (right) leg (C. Adamson, personal communication, 1993).

Turns therefore require a partial squat, dorsiflexion of the foot and ankle, and partial flexion of the hip and knee on the leading half-wedged leg (which will end up being downhill at the completion of the turn), while trailing the eventual uphill leg with the hip extended, the knee flexed and the ankle plantarflexed.

Turns will be affected by limitations of ranges of motion:

- dorsiflexion and plantarflexion (see Figs 3.68A and 3.77)

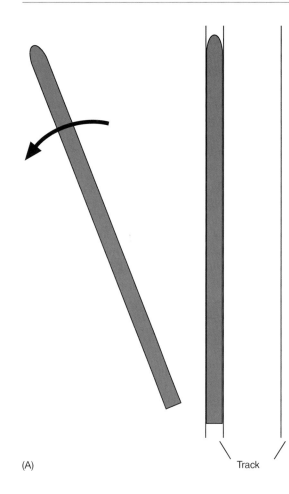

(A)

Track

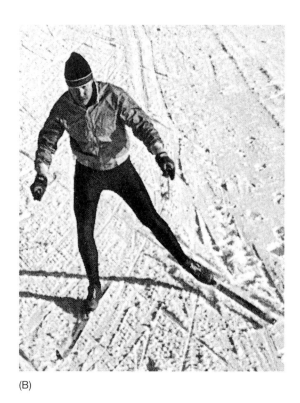

(B)

Figure 5.20 Ski-skating: (A) Marathon skate stride; (B) V-skate stride. (From Matheny 1989, with permission.)

• hip extension and pelvic rotation on the side of the posterior rotation (or an inflare); hip flexion on the side of the anterior rotation (see Figs 3.4, 3.64, 3.65 and 3.69).

> A restriction of pelvic rotation will be even more of a problem than in downhill or nordic skiing, given that the telemark skier is squatting to a variable degree, and the turns are much tighter. The tendency will be to compensate by rotating more through the trunk on executing a turn into the restricted side.

SNOWBOARDING

Snowboarders have their feet placed on the board pointing towards one edge of the board or rotated to a varying degree towards the front relative to a line dissecting the board (the so-called stance angle – Fig. 5.22A). The left foot leads in a 'regular', the right

in a 'goofy-foot' boarder (Fig. 5.22B). Steering is accomplished largely with the rear foot when the board is on the ground, as well as with rotation of the hips and pelvis; the trunk is angled at about 45 degrees to the fall line. In a 'regular' snowboarder, whose feet face the right edge of the board and who uses his or her right (rear) foot for steering, the effects of malalignment with right anterior rotation are as follows.

The more the feet face forwards the greater the stance angle and the more the bindings are actually fixed in a way that runs counter to the abnormal tendency towards right external, left internal rotation of the lower extremities.

> The snowboarder may eventually feel more comfortable with adjustments, perhaps even with the bindings mounted so that the stance angle is zero degrees (Fig. 5.22A).

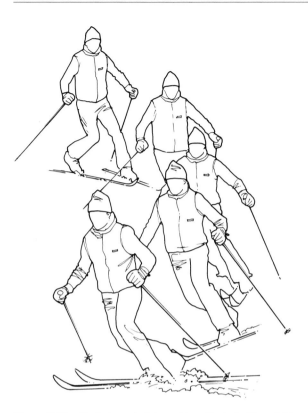

Figure 5.21 Basic turns in telemarking. Illustrated is a right 'half-wedge turn', initiated by 'wedging' what will become the leg on the outside of the turn, by rotating the left leg and ski inwards. Most of the weight remains on the straight-running right 'inside' ski; while the pressure on the inside edge of the wedged 'outside' ski is gradually increased as the turn progresses. For progression to a right 'telegarland' or telemark turn: as the 'outside' left ski is 'wedged', the left leg is simultaneously internally rotated and slid forward, the skier sinking into the 'telemark' stance by flexing the right knee further and extending the hip on that side. (From Parker 1988, with permission.)

The feet will then be in better alignment relative to the tendency to right external and left internal rotation, and there may be more comfort and ease of control; this is similar to the adjustments made by a cyclist or skier (see above).

The limitation of counterclockwise rotation of the pelvis in the transverse plane may interfere with the ability to rotate the pelvis to the left; this is likely to create more of a problem with 'zero stance angle' when trying to manoeuvre the board on the ground (see Fig. 3.4C).

Limitations of ranges of motion become a problem particularly at the time of a fall or collision, not only when riding the board, but also when performing vertical 'tricks'. When 'riding the half-pipe', for example,

a number of torsional stresses initiated in the air continue once the rider has contacted the ground, so that trunk and pelvis are repeatedly subjected to rotation into extreme ranges of motion while the feet are 'fixed'; alternatively, the board may already be rotating in the opposite direction as this part of the rider twists to prepare for the next trick.

The less the rider can get onto an edge because of malalignment-related limitations of pronation or supination, the more he or she depends on rotating the trunk and arms or on leaning the body towards the ground in order to carve a turn.

SWIMMING

Detrimental effects relate primarily to asymmetrical propulsion, increased resistance and the increased energy required to correct for any torquing of the pelvis, trunk or lower extremities.

Head and neck

The frequently noted limitation of head and neck rotation to the right and of side flexion to the left (see Fig. 3.9) may interfere with the ease with which breathing can be carried out on the right side when attempting alternate breathing on doing the crawl or freestyle swimming. The increase in tension noted in the right upper trapezius in particular, compounded by repeatedly straining to rotate the head and neck into the direction of the limitation, may precipitate or exacerbate neck and upper back pain. The swimmer may compensate for any limitation by increasing the clockwise rotation of the trunk, but this could prove costly in terms of efficiency of style and energy expenditure.

Upper extremities

Decreased right internal and left external rotation (see Fig. 3.15A). Asymmetry of upper extremity internal and external rotation will affect arm entry and pull-through where these are dependent on utilizing maximum range in the direction of the restrictions. The end result is:

- increased strain at the end of the restricted range of motion
- an asymmetrical contribution of the arms to propulsion and lift.

Decreased left arm extension (Fig. 3.15B). The butterfly swimmer who has less left than right arm extension should conceivably be able to compensate by:

- pulling with more force on the left side than the right

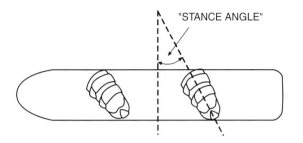

i. increased stance angle with feet facing toward tip

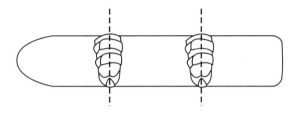

(A)   **ii.** zero "stance angle"

Figure 5.22 Snowboarding. (A) A 'regular' foot placement relative to a line dissecting the board: (i) increased stance angle, with the feet facing towards the tip; (ii) zero stance angle. (After Bennett & Downey 1994, with permission.) (B) A 'regular' snowboarder (left foot leading) and a 'goofy-foot' (right foot leading). (From Bennett & Downey 1994, with permission.)

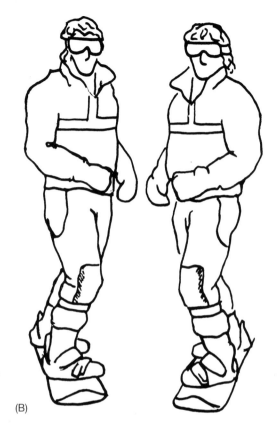

(B)

- torquing the body counterclockwise, to the point at which the left and right arms clear the water to an equal extent.

These manoeuvres may assure symmetry of stroke strength. Any torquing could, however, introduce a 'wobble' that would increase energy expenditure by decreasing efficiency and increasing overall resistance.

Lower extremities

Propulsion using extension and external/internal rotation. The kick used for the breaststroke requires initial hip and knee flexion followed by forceful extension. Richardson (1986) describes how 'maximal valgus force is applied to the knee and the foot is maximally dorsiflexed and everted' during the flexion phase, so that 'abduction of the hips is minimized during the pushing phase' (p. 110). As a result, the lower extremities go from an initial position of internal rotation and extension, to one of external rotation and flexion, finally again assuming an adducted and fully extended position by the end of the kick.

> In other words, the propulsion phase consists of simultaneous hip and knee extension, internal leg rotation, ankle plantarflexion and foot inversion.

The propulsive force is created in large part in reaction to the water displaced by the inner aspect of the shin and the bottom of the foot.

Any asymmetry of movement will result in an asymmetrical contribution to the propulsion force. With upslips and the 'alternate' presentations of malalignment, for example, there is more external rotation possible on the right than the left side. The sole of the right foot is, unfortunately, set in increased varus angulation compared with the left when non-weight-bearing (see Fig. 3.22), decreasing the surface area that can generate a propulsion force on extension. This balance of factors may result in asymmetrical propulsive forces being generated by the right and left sides.

Lower extremity orientation, joint range of motion and strength. The efficiency of propeling the body is also affected by lower extremity side-to-side diferences of orientation and asymmetries of joint ranges of motion and strength. Upslips and 'alternate' presentations, for example, limit right internal rotation and plantarflexion, left external rotation and dorsiflexion. These asymmetries may help to explain the predicament of swimmers who are slow to move forwards, or worse, fail to move forwards or even move backwards when using the flutter kick hanging on to a board but procede forward without problem once in alignment.

It helps to think of the lower extremities as acting like two propellers. Because of the malalignment, each of these propellers is set at a different angle. In addition, there are side-to-side asymmetries in strength. Significant here is the common finding of a relative decrease in right hip flexor and extensor strength, whereas these same muscles are usually of full strength on the left side. These muscles are crucial for doing the flutter kick. In comparison, weakness on the left side affects primarily the hip abductors, hamstrings and ankle evertors, none of which plays much of a part. The combined effect of these asymmetries appears to be that, in some swimmers, the 'propellers' actually work against each other, so that the propulsion effect is reduced, cancelled or even reversed. Correction of the malalignment serves to realign the propellers and promote forward propulsion.

Swimming is, with exceptions such as the sidestroke, a mainly symmetrical activity. However, asymmetrical stresses imposed by malalignment increase the likelihood of a particular injury occurring on one side. Frequently seen knee injuries, for example, include medial collateral ligament stress syndrome, patellofemoral compartment syndrome, medial synovitis and medial synovial plica syndrome. These are more likely to occur on the right side with upslips and 'alternate' presentations, and on the left with the left anterior and locked pattern. Ankle and foot extensor tendonitis commonly associated with the flutter and dolphin kick are more likely to occur on the side on which the extensors are tight and plantarflexion is decreased.

In addition, symmetrical strokes will result in increased stress on structures that are now asymmetrical; in the butterfly, for example, back extension further compresses facet joints that are already approximated on one side by vertebral rotation, especially in the thoracolumbar junction, where this problem is compounded by the curve reversal (see Fig. 3.12). Box 5.9 summarizes the overall effects of these asymmetries.

In a sport in which races are sometimes won by one-hundredth of a second, these effects can prove costly indeed.

Box 5.9 Effects of asymmetry on swimming

- Speed is reduced by any decrease or asymmetry in propulsion and the lift forces generated
- Energy is wasted by the need for corrective action in order to 'keep an even keel' and counterbalance any asymmetry in propulsive forces generated by the right versus the left side
- Asymmetry and corrective torquing further increase energy requirements by increasing drag
- Injuries, particularly involving the back, hips and knees, are more likely to occur

---

SYNCHRONIZED SWIMMING

Problems with malalignment relating particularly to an asymmetry of lower extremity ranges of motion may be more easily evident in routines in which the body is submerged with the legs protruding from the water. In an athlete who is not blessed with a general degree of increased mobility, malalignment may well result in difficulties.

Limitations of hip flexion and extension will affect those positions in which one leg flexes to 90 degrees and one leg remains vertical, either completely (e.g. the 'crane' – Fig. 5.23A) or partially (e.g. the 'knight' – Fig. 5.23C3). Restrictions of flexion or extension may also cause a problem with a 'split' in the sagittal plane (Fig. 5.23C4), which the athlete may be able to correct by 'opening' the pelvis, rotating the pelvis in the transverse plane – forwards on the side of restricted flexion and backwards on the side of restricted extension (see Fig. 2.9). In those with left posterior rotation, however, the limitation of pelvic rotation in the transverse plane to the left side may make this manoeuvre less effective to compensate for the restriction of right flexion and left extension (see Fig. 3.4C).

Extension can also be increased by accentuating the lumbar lordosis, at the risk of precipitating back pain.

For the split in the frontal plane, both legs should abduct 90 degrees to become horizontal with the water (Fig. 5.23B), but malalignment may result in an obvious limitation to one side. Symmetry may be preserved by actively limiting abduction on the more mobile side to match that on the restricted side, but then both will fall short of horizontal. The asymmetry of plantar flexion may result in an obvious inability to point the foot on one side as much as on the other (see Fig. 3.77B).

As in swimming, asymmetries related to malalignment may also play a role in the causation and

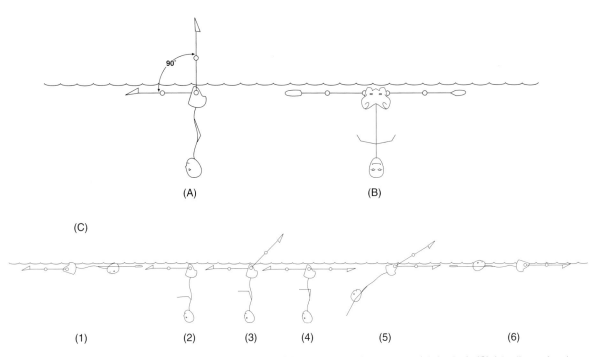

Figure 5.23 Synchronized swimming positions. (A) 'Crane'. (B) A 'split' in the frontal plane (abduction). (C) A 'walkover front' sequence: (1) initial position and (6) finale; (2) back pike; (3) 'knight' or 'castle'; (4) 'split' in the sagittal plane (extension/flexion).

localization of injuries seen with synchronized swimming. Weinberg (1986) has noted the following common problems.

Back pain

Back pain has been attributed to an increased lumbar lordosis and to the hyperextension required to carry out manoeuvres such as the split in the sagittal plane, the knight position and the walkover sequence (Fig. 5.23C); for example, going from the back pike (2) into the knight position (3), with one leg extended and the other vertical, into a sagittal split (4), and finally bringing the trunk into horizontal alignment with the legs.

Needless to say, back pain is more likely to develop when an increased lordosis or repeated hyperextension is superimposed on the asymmetry of pelvis and spine, and the rotational stress, particularly on the thoracolumbar and lumbosacral junction, that results with malalignment.

Knee injuries

Cited as one of the common overuse injuries is chondromalacia patellae, possibly related to 'the constant emphasis on forceful extension of the knee' (p. 161), and to a repeated use of the eggbeater kick, as well as exaggerated Q-angles, which increase the tendency to lateral tracking of the patella on knee extension (see Figs 3.33, 3.74 and 4.5). These knee problems are more likely to occur on the right side in those with an upslip or 'alternate' presentations, for reasons previously noted to predispose to patellofemoral compartment syndrome (see Ch. 3).

Shoulder injuries

Aside from rotator cuff impingement syndrome, shoulder pain can be produced by extensive support sculling. The shoulder is 'slightly abducted and maximally rotated [externally] on the outward phase, and adducted and internally rotated on the inward phase. The major stress … is a stretching of the anterior capsule at the point of maximal external rotation' (p. 162), which predisposes to developing laxity, subluxation or even dislocation. A malalignment-related limitation of external rotation on one side and internal rotation on the other, combined with asymmetrical strength, may reduce the overall effectiveness of the sculling manoeuvre. Stress on the anterior capsule will be increased on the side on which external rotation is relatively reduced (see Figs 3.15A and 4.7).

THROWING SPORTS

In most sports, the execution of a throw involves the whole body rather than consisting of an isolated arm action. Most throws basically require some rotation of the pelvis, thorax and extremities in order to generate maximum velocity. The following two throws serve to illustrate these points.

Javelin

At the end of the run up, the right-handed athlete transfers weight from the right to the left foot in preparation for release. Just prior to this transfer, the athlete 'winds up' for the throw by rotating the trunk clockwise, simultaneously extending the spine, side-flexing to the right and rotating the right arm externally (Fig. 5.24). The transfer to the left foot is accompanied by a counterclockwise rotation of the pelvis to advance the right hip and thereby add to the length of the step. The trunk then flexes and unwinds counterclockwise as the right arm rotates internally. 'The final force, added to the forward movement of the body, is derived from pelvic and spinal rotation, [and] medial rotation ... of the humerus' (Adrian & Cooper 1986, p. 526), with simultaneous passive internal rotation of the weight-bearing left leg.

Pitching

The movement of the throwing arm and the trunk is much the same as the sequence after the run-up described for throwing the javelin. Looking at a right-handed pitcher throwing overhand, the initial 'wind-up' phase calls for balancing on the right leg while accentuating the passive internal rotation of that leg as the body winds up (Fig. 5.25A). Simultaneous pelvic rotation to the right during this phase 'can be more than 90 degrees from the intended direction of flight of the projectile' (Adrian & Cooper 1986, p. 498). The trunk rotates along with the pelvis until it also is at a right angle to the intended direction of the throw. As the 'wind-up' proceeds, the left leg rises upwards in the air, partly to counterbalance simultaneous right side flexion of the trunk and partly in preparation for stepping forwards on to the left foot. During the 'forward force' phase or actual 'cocking' phase, the hands separate (the right hand moving backwards), the throwing arm moves into extreme external rotation, and weight is transferred onto the left foot (Fig. 5.25B).

'Acceleration' sees an increased weight-shift forwards onto the left foot, and a simultaneous 'unwinding', consisting of a counterclockwise rotation of the pelvis that subjects the now-supporting left leg to passive internal rotation (Fig. 5.25C). Further rotation of the pelvis, unwinding, and forward flexion of the spine, combined with internal rotation and extension of the upper extremity, constitute the 'deceleration' phase and all aid the force of the release (Fig. 5.25D). Control of the throw is perfected by going through the 'follow-up' phase, which also involves passive internal rotation of the left leg (Fig. 5.25E).

Some of the restrictions imposed by malalignment are capable of affecting the 'four axes of motion' felt to be crucial for the execution of any of these throws. Limitations of joint ranges of motion, combined with asymmetries of strength and problems with balancing on one leg, distract from speed and accuracy and can result in a suboptimal throw. Take the example of the pitcher. In the 'wind-up' phase, any limitation of right arm external rotation results in:

- a compensatory increase in elbow flexion, which will increase tension on the ulnar nerve and increase the chance of precipitating or aggravating nerve subluxation, irritation and inflammation

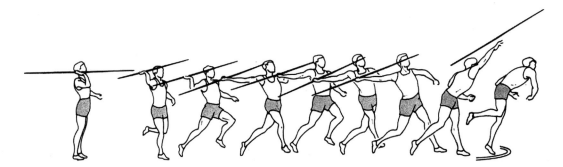

Figure 5.24   Javelin throw: the wind-up phase leading to weight transfer onto the left leg, with passive internal rotation of that leg just prior to release. (From Worth 1990, with permission).

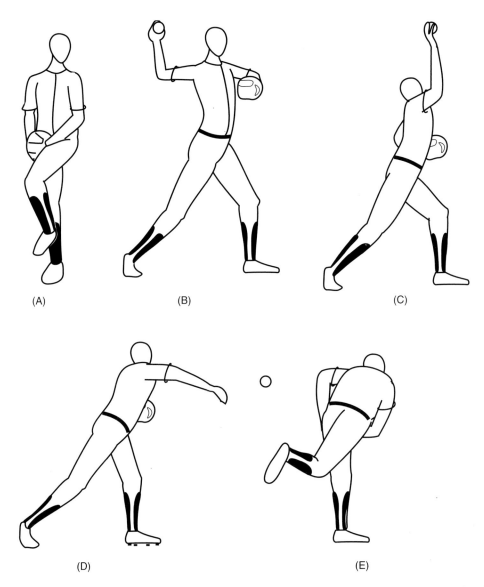

Figure 5.25 Phases of ball throw: right-handed pitcher (see Fig. 3.47). (A) Wind-up (including 'cocking' of the left leg). (B) True 'cocking' phase. (C) Acceleration. (D) Deceleration. (E) Follow-through.

- increased valgus stress (medial elbow stress syndrome and injuries to the medial elbow ligaments and capsule)
- increased lateral elbow joint compression (e.g. radiohumeral joint).

As the arm rotates internally in preparation for the release, any limitation of internal rotation will increase:

1. the traction forces on the lateral ligaments and capsule

2. the medial elbow joint compression forces (e.g. medial humero-ulnar joint).

In the absence of any other shoulder pathology, the actual total number of degrees of internal plus external rotation will be the same on the right and left sides. The limitation of either internal or external rotation will, however, alter the rotation around the axis of the arm and may decrease its contribution to the throw.

In the pitcher with an upslip or one of the 'alternate' presentations, internal rotation of the right lower extremity is restricted compared with that of the left.

> Once the limit of internal rotation has been reached, any further movement into the right required for the wind-up either cannot occur at all or has to take place through increased right side flexion and/or increased clockwise rotation of the pelvis, trunk or both.

In the presence of right posterior innominate rotation or inflare, the limitation of clockwise rotation of the pelvis will increase the stress on the trunk.

The right-handed pitcher with left posterior rotation or inflare will have a restriction of counterclockwise rotation of the pelvis in the transverse plane. This may limit the ability to rotate the pelvis to the left through the throw, especially when both feet are fixed to the ground.

Any restriction of pelvic rotation to the right or left increases the torquing force through the thoracic segment – in particular through the thoracolumbar junction – in either the wind-up or acceleration/deceleration phases.

Restrictions of thoracic spine side flexion and rotation, as a result of a compensatory curvature of this segment and an asymmetry of paravertebral muscle tension, could limit its contribution to these phases and decrease its ability to cope with any increase in rotational stress that occurs because of restrictions of pelvic and lower extremity movement.

Balance may also be a problem, whether because of a functional weakness, an alteration of proprioceptive input or both. This is more likely to occur during the single-support phase on the right leg in conjunction with one of the 'alternate' presentations.

WATERSKIING

The waterskier's success depends in large part on maintaining balance while trying to execute turns and other manoeuvres by getting onto an inner or outer edge of the ski(s).

Two skis

The ability to turn to the right or left is determined largely by the ease with which the skier can simultaneously get onto the inside edge of one and the outside edge of the other ski. The skier can seemingly accomplish this simply by leaning the body to one or other side. The ease with which this shift can occur will, however, also be influenced by the facilitating or restricting effect imposed by any coexisting malalignment. It will, for example, conceivably be easier to execute a turn to the left with an upslip or any of the 'alternate' presentations that would make it easier to get on the right inside and left outside edge.

Slalom

Malalignment will have a more pronounced effect on the ability to execute turns in this event. Most slalom skiers have the left foot mounted forwards on the ski, the rear right foot steering by selectively weighting the inner or outer edge. In those with an upslip or one of the 'alternate' presentations, the associated tendency to right pronation and left supination:

- increases the ease with which they can weight the left edge
- may make it easier to turn and to fall to the left
- allows a more acute lean of the body to the left before triggering a fear of falling
- may allow them to raise a higher wall of water more easily when executing a left turn.

The insecurity experienced by some on a right turn may relate in large part to the difficulty they have with shifting onto the right edge and with an increased need to lean towards the water in order to do so.

The skier who has the right foot mounted forwards is known as a 'goofy foot' (Fig. 5.26). This may again be an expression of malalignment. Certainly the left anterior and locked presentation increases the ease with which weight can be shifted to the inside of the left foot and the outside of the right, which will make it easier to steer with the left foot trailing and to get onto the right edge to execute a right turn.

WEIGHT-LIFTING

Some power lift competitions, such as the squat exercise or deep knee bend, are judged partly on style. A spotter on each side looks to see whether each buttock has dropped below the level of the ipsilateral bent knee when the athlete is in the full-squat position. Points may also be deducted if the height of the buttock and knee on one side does not match that on the other side.

With right anterior innominate rotation, the right buttock (ischial tuberosity) and iliac crest are usually noticeably elevated relative to the left (see Figs 2.46B, D, 3.69A and 3.79A). The right thigh may be noticeably higher or lower than the left (Fig. 3.69B), with counterclockwise pelvic rotation in the frontal plane causing elevation, whereas tight hamstrings, anteriorly rotated

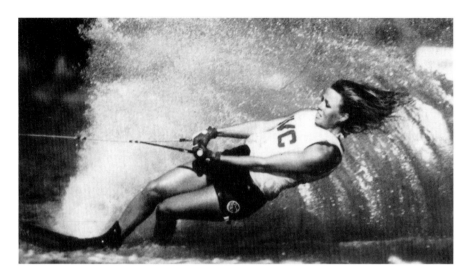

Figure 5.26 'Goofy-foot' slalom water skier: the right foot leads, the left steers. (From West 1989, with permission.)

superior acetabular rim, or painful iliopsoas and ligaments all counter hip flexion. The full squat may also be limited on one or both sides by pain provoked from tender muscles or posterior pelvic ligaments put under increased tension by this manoeuvre. Pain from these structures may also create problems with the full squat required part way through:

1. the snatch lift, when the weight-lifter is in the 'catch' or 'receiving' position (Fig. 5.27A3)

2. the clean-and-jerk lift, when the weight-lifter is in the catch or receiving position for the clean (Fig. 5.27B3).

The clean-and-jerk lift proceeds to the catch or receiving position for the 'split' jerk, which is an asymmetrical position with one leg fully extended behind the body and the other flexed to approximately 90 degrees at the hip and knee. At the same time, the fully extended arms balance the weight directly above the head (Fig. 5.27B5).

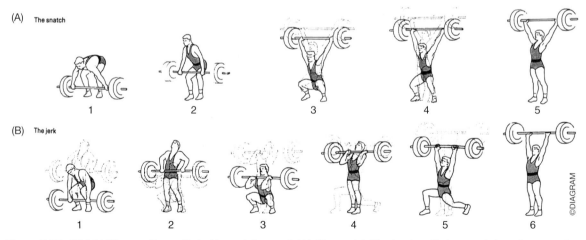

Figure 5.27 Weight-lifting positions affected by malalignment. (A) *The snatch.* The bar is pulled upwards from the ground (1, 2) to the full extent of both arms being vertical above the head (3), 'splitting' or bending the knees to a deep squat in the process (3), before proceeding to the full standing position (4, 5). (B) *The clean-and-jerk lift.* For the 'clean', the bar is brought in a single motion to the shoulders (1, 2, 3), simultaneously 'splitting' or bending the legs (squatting) into the catch or receiving position for the 'clean', which is then achieved by going on to stand (4). The arms are next brought vertically above the head, the legs at the same time being split by flexing one hip and extending the other. This manoueuvre results in the catch or receiving position for the 'jerk' (5) which is then achieved by standing up while maintaining the arms vertical (6). (From Worth 1990, with permission.)

The weight-lifter who presents with right anterior, left posterior rotation or a right outflare, left inflare may experience a problem with this part of the lift if he or she is supported by the flexed right hip and knee with the left leg in extension, because of the associated limitation of right hip flexion and left hip extension. The tight right gluteus maximus, hamstrings and sacrotuberous ligament, and left iliacus and rectus femoris, are at particular risk of injury, given the rapidity of this movement and the superimposed weight.

Weight-lifters with an 'alternate' presentation have also reported:

- the legs in the squatting, split or bend positions not being oriented in the same direction, often with the right knee and foot pointing more outwards relative to the left (in keeping with external rotation of the right leg)
- the right leg not feeling as strong as the left, something that disappears on correction of the malalignment, or that they can correct for in part by actively rotating the right leg inwards so that the foot now points forwards.

Any exercises with weights, whether resting on or held above the shoulders (Fig. 5.28), increase the risk of going out of alignment. This risk may relate to:

1. weights that are excessive and therefore more likely to result in even a momentary aggravation of any asymmetries of balance and muscle contraction
2. asymmetries in the weights being handled, either individually in each hand or attached to the ends of a bar
3. torsional movements carried out with the trunk while supporting a weight in this manner.

> Interestingly, the weight-lifter's belt is applied in exactly the same location as the sacroiliac belt and has been shown on magnetic resonance imaging studies to run across the short upper arm of the L-shaped SI joint.

This finding led Snijders et al (1992) to speculate that the benefit derived by a weight-lifter from wearing a belt when in a stooped position may relate more to its ability to stabilize the SI joint than to improving back strength by increasing the intra-abdominal pressure.

WINDSURFING

A windsurfer needs to be able to control the board and sail it from either side, yet many will have a side pref-

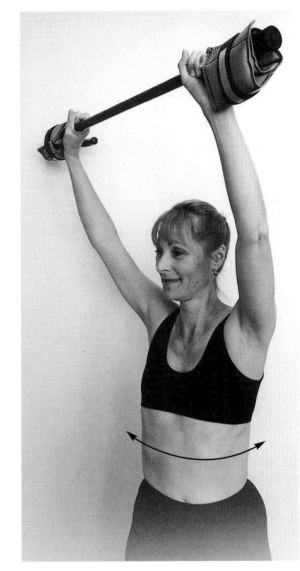

Figure 5.28 Weight-lifting: torquing the trunk with a bar and weights supported above the shoulders, while the feet (and pelvis) are relatively fixed.

erence. This sport requires, in addition to agility, flexibility and the ability to rotate the limbs and trunk through the maximum available ranges of motion. Whereas the preference for one side may be determined in part by laterality and habit, a restriction of motion in directions frequently called upon as part of manoeuvring the board and sail probably also play a role. A problem in shifting weight on to the medial or lateral edge of a foot could affect the ability to maintain a stable position and to steer the board. Asymmetry in the pectoral muscles, increased on one side by malalignment-related shoulder retraction and/or facilitation, might help to account for the observed increase in pectoral muscle ruptures (Woo 1997).

WRESTLING

Wresting has been referred to repeatedly in discussion relating to excessive torsion of one part of the body, particularly when another part is 'fixed' and unable to move. Typical examples are given in Box 5.10.

Box 5.10 Effects of torsion in wrestling

1. *torsion of the trunk* into the limitation at a time when the pelvis is 'fixed'
   – a contestant forming a bridge to prevent a fall (Fig. 5.29A)
   – an opponent somehow preventing the pelvis from moving while forcing rotation of the trunk (Fig. 5.29B)
2. *torsion of the pelvis and legs* into the direction of limitation. Consider one contestant with a right anterior, left posterior rotation, now lying supine with the hips and knees flexed; the opponent, while pinning down the trunk, somehow forces the flexed lower extremities to the left (Fig. 5.30A, B), into the combined limitations of left pelvic rotation (see Fig. 3.4C) and right internal, left external leg rotation (see Figs 3.71 and 3.72 respectively).

FORETHOUGHT TO CHAPTER 6: HORSEBACK RIDING AND PLAYING POLO

The interplay of malalignment and horseback riding is covered in detail in Chapter 6, the comments here being limited but intended to precede in part the material in 'A "natural" process of elimination?', below.

Failure to advance in riding

Riding may well be one of those sports in which malalignment makes the difference between whether the athlete progresses as expected, gives up riding altogether or settles for less challenging equestrian pursuits. Wanless (1989) more or less said as much in her lesson on 'The positioning of the body and an introduction to asymmetry'. She cites the case of Jan who:

had reached a stage in her riding where she was continuously depressed about her apparent inability, whilst simultaneously becoming desperate in her attempts to 'get it right'. Finally … she decided to take up long-distance riding in the hope that

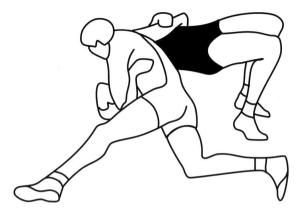

(A)

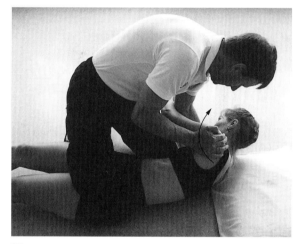

(B)

Figure 5.29 Wrestling action in which the trunk may be forcefully rotated (actively or passively) relative to a 'fixed' pelvis. (A) Forming a bridge (black shorts) to prevent a fall, with the pelvis 'fixed' by keeping both feet anchored to the ground. (B) The opponent (white top) is rotating the trunk clockwise while pinning the pelvis down on the floor.

'letting herself off the hook', combined with long hours in the saddle, might somehow give her the seat and the abilities for which she longed. She is not the first person I have met who had made this transition; however, she is also not the first to have admitted that although long-distance is great fun, it is for her a substitute – and if she felt competent enough she would really prefer to do dressage. (p. 78)

Wanless describes how a rider may feel that he or she is sitting symmetrically in the saddle when in fact the right thigh is turned outwards (external rotation) and the left inwards (internal rotation), and how placing the rider symmetrically in the saddle makes him or her feel rotated to the left (Fig. 5.31). The description is in

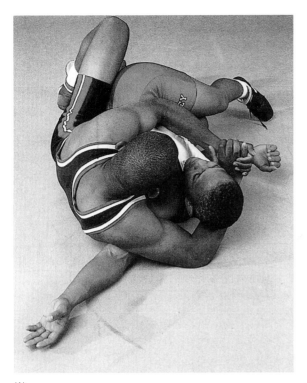

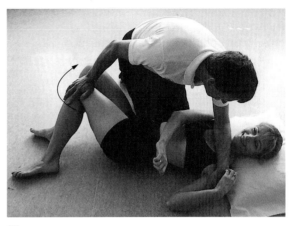

(B)

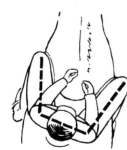

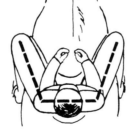

(A)

Figure 5.30 Wrestling action in which the pelvis may be forcefully rotated (actively or passively) relative to a 'fixed' trunk. (A) A clockwise rotational force on the pelvis of the red-white [lower] opponent, whose shoulders (= trunk) are pinned to the mat. (From Savage 1996, with permission.) (B) The flexed hips and knees are forced to the right, rotating the pelvis clockwise relative to the 'fixed' trunk.

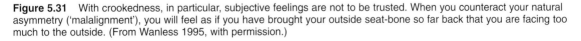

CROOKED RIDER TO THE RIGHT IS ACTUALLY PLACED LIKE THIS

BUT SHE FEELS SYMMETRICAL

WHEN SHE IS ACTUALLY WELL PLACED SHE FEELS LIKE THIS

Figure 5.31 With crookedness, in particular, subjective feelings are not to be trusted. When you counteract your natural asymmetry ('malalignment'), you will feel as if you have brought your outside seat-bone so far back that you are facing too much to the outside. (From Wanless 1995, with permission.)

keeping with a rider who most probably has an upslip or one of the 'alternate' presentations of malalignment, with rotation of the lower extremities: the right externally and the left internally (see Figs 3.3B, 3.16B, 3.71B and 3.72A, B). These changes would make it more difficult to maintain a proper seat. Loss of contact with the right thigh probably also interferes with being able to communicate properly with the horse (see Ch. 6).

Wanless then gives Jan's presentation, which is really typical of someone with an upslip or 'alternate' presentation of rotational malalignment. She goes on to describe, complete with illustrations, how the right leg was turned outwards and concludes with the advice to Jan that she should start the recovery process by making a conscious effort to turn the right leg inwards when both riding and walking. This conscious change did indeed improve Jan's posture, and indeed the horse 'responded beautifully with this change in her carriage ... Jan could feel a distinct difference in the way she was moving' (Wanless 1989, p. 86). However, Wanless goes on to point out that:

This initial change can happen in a very small amount of time, but it can take years for it to become so ingrained that it feels natural and effortless. *With every lapse of concentration, the rider tends to fall straight back into her old pattern* – but at least she knows how to redeem herself. (p. 87)

The temporary nature of these treatment attempts is really not very surprising given that the problem identified is probably attributable to an underlying malalignment.

> Unfortunately, malalignment can be corrected only in part by voluntary effort and will recur as soon as that conscious effect ceases even momentarily.

Realignment of the rider, and often also of the horse, may offer the only long-term solution. Maintaining the alignment of the horse and rider may become as simple as checking regularly to detect – and reverse – recurrence early, using mounting blocks, and getting into the habit of mounting from alternate sides (see Ch. 6 and Wagner-Chazalon 2000).

Playing polo

Polo deserves special mention here because of the extreme demands on the ability to:

- side-flex the trunk to reach the ball
- twist backwards in preparation for reaching the ball
- rotate the trunk on the pelvis for hitting the ball and for follow-through.

Whenever the player is sitting, the pelvis is relatively 'fixed', increasing any rotational stress through the thorax, especially the thoracolumbar region. Added to all this is the momentum of the action and the possibilities for close contact or collision with an opponent. The stage is set particularly for injury related to the limitations of trunk and shoulder ranges of motion typically seen with malalignment.

In conclusion, Appendix 10 notes clinic correlations typical for some specific sports other than running, and Appendix 11 provides some non-specific correlations that apply to a number of sports. It is obviously not possible to mention every individual athletic activity in this book. It is, however, to be hoped that the discussion of the basic biomechanical changes in the preceding chapters, and the application of this information to the sports above, has given those working with athletes the insight needed to make use of this material when trying to analyse problems and injuries encountered in their particular sport.

RECURRENT INJURIES

The following are the most common recurrent problems seen in association with right anterior, left posterior innominate rotation.

- left hip abductor and ITB sprain
- left trochanteric bursitis
- left ankle inversion sprain
- right patellofemoral compartment syndrome
- back 'sprain' or 'strain', typically localizing to the right and/or left of the lumbosacral junction, or one or both SI joints
- 'shin splints': medial, lateral and anterior

Factors contributing to the first five conditions have been discussed throughout the text, and are noted again in Appendix 12, but shin splints deserve further mention at this point.

'SHIN SPLINTS'

> Whether athletes presenting with malalignment develop medial, lateral or anterior shin splints will be determined in part by factors such as their inherent weight-bearing pattern, tibial torsion, genu valgum or varum and patterns of referral.

Medial shin splints

These are usually activity related and result from excessive traction on the medial periosteal origins of tibialis posterior. With 'alternate' presentations, they may be present just on the right side, or worse on the right than the left, because of the increased tendency towards pronation and medial weight-bearing on that side, aggravated by the functional weakness of tibialis posterior and the increased ease of fatiguability of this muscle.

Lateral shin splints

These are usually the result of excessive traction on the lateral compartment muscles, peroneus longus and brevis. With upslips and 'alternate' presentations, lateral shin splints may occur just on the left, or be worse on the left than the right, because of the increased tendency towards supination and lateral weight-bearing on that side, compounded by the functional weakness and ease of fatiguability of these muscles. Like medial shin splints, they are usually activity related.

Pain may also be referred to the lateral shin region from the upper posterior SI joint ligaments (see Fig. 3.58A,B), and to the anterolateral shin region from the anterior hip (flexor origin) ligaments (Hackett 1958; see Fig. 3.62).

Other sources of 'lateral shin pain' include:

- a tender ITB, vastus lateralis or biceps femoris insertion
- a painful, displaced proximal tibiofibular joint.

Prolonged discomfort following the cessation of activity is more in keeping with a lateral compartment syndrome or stress fracture.

Anterior shin splints

In the presence of malalignment, and with stress fracture having been ruled out, anterior shin splints usually reflect referred pain. Hackett (1958) has shown how irritation of the sciatic nerve associated with SI joint instability 'resulting from relaxation of posterior sacroiliac, sacrospinus and sacrotuberus ligaments' (p. 30) can result in a pain that localizes 'to either side' of the upper anterior tibia (Fig. 5.32).

In the presence of malalignment, therefore, one must always suspect that shin splints tending to localize medially, laterally or anteriorly may be occurring on the basis of referred pain, especially if:

- the shin splints are not necessarily activity related, at times coming on even at rest
- there is no localized soft tissue or bone tenderness to suggest a possible stress fracture, and the bone scan is negative
- the shin splints are relieved by realignment or by injecting a local anaesthetic into the ligaments from which they are felt to originate.

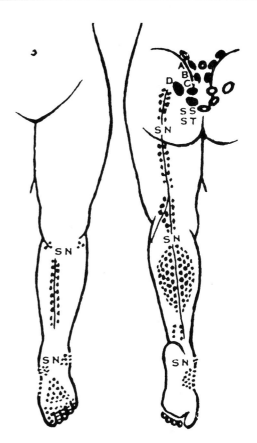

Figure 5.32 Pattern of 'sciatica' caused by sciatic nerve (SN) irritation that can occur with sacroiliac joint instability from 'relaxation' of the posterior sacroiliac (A, B, C, D), sacrospinous (SS) and sacrotuberous (ST) ligaments. (From Hackett 1958, with permission.)

WORK AND HOBBIES

Many athletes work either part or full time, and a number have physically demanding hobbies. If they are adhering to recommendations in respect to curtailing their athletic activities, yet have ongoing symptoms and the malalignment keeps recurring, their work or hobbies may be the culprit. Of particular concern are those activities requiring:

1. asymmetrical movement, such as repeatedly having to lift, reach and twist (e.g. putting things onto high or low shelves, or into filing cabinets; getting on and off a bike or horse; or getting down to and up from a rowing machine, or other piece of exercise equipment, that sits low on the floor)

2. repeatedly getting in and out of bed or vehicle with one leg leading, thereby exerting a torsional force through the pelvic region

3. dealing with periodic or constant stress (e.g. competitive, emotional or financial)

4. repeated squatting, especially when this is combined with rotation of the trunk and reaching with the arms (e.g. gardening).

The problem may be as simple as that of the runner who had stopped running while undergoing mobilization treatments but who continued to go out of alignment. At the author's recommendation, he had discontinued running in favour of the 'symmetrical' activity of cycling. The recurrence of malalignment was attributable to the torquing of the pelvis required to swing one leg over the seat and crossbar on getting on and off the bicycle. The problem was solved by using a step-up stool or the curb to decrease the amount of torquing.

A 'NATURAL' PROCESS OF ELIMINATION?

> Malalignment is a ubiquitous condition, yet not everyone who is out of alignment develops problems.

In a recent study of 136 cardiac patients being seen at an intake clinic for admission to a cardiac rehabilitation programme, 80% were out of alignment (W. Schamberger, unpublished data, 1998). Thirty-seven per cent of these were asymptomatic other than for their cardiac problems and on examination had no musculoskeletal findings (e.g. tenderness of specific muscles or ligaments, or pain with pressure over the spine or on stressing the hip or SI joints) that could be related to the malalignment. The other 63% had either complaints or findings on examination that could be attributed to, or aggravated by, the malalignment. These patients were admittedly in an older age group (60–80 years) and had been relatively inactive, most of them for many years. There are, however, definitely athletes who have been known to be out of alignment for some time but who have become symptomatic only recently. There are several precipitating causes to consider (Box 5.11).

Nonetheless, a large number of those athletes who do make it to the top are also out of alignment. There are several possible reasons why they have been able to succeed despite the malalignment:

1. They have somehow been able to compensate, surmounting the limitation imposed by the malalign-

---

> **Box 5.11** Factors precipitating symptoms in malalignment
>
> - Problems relating to malalignment may in fact begin when another insult – such as a fall or collision – is imposed on a system already subjected to the stresses inherent to malalignment. Athletes are, depending on their sport, obviously at increased risk of such a mishap occurring
> - Another mechanism, one that also applies to athletes in particular, is the sheer increase in demand placed on the musculoskeletal system. Aggravating factors include starting up or accelerating an exercise programme too quickly, or subjecting specific parts of the system to increased forces by changing equipment or terrain (e.g. adding up and downhill runs to a previous all-flat terrain). This 'overuse' increases the chances that one of the structures already under excessive stress from the malalignment will eventually fail and become overtly painful
> - A third mechanism sees the athlete progress to a level of difficulty at which the malalignment finally interferes with performance, to the point at which it prevents the athlete advancing in that sport. A typical scenario is the previously cited example of the skater with one of the 'alternate' presentations who considered dropping out of the training programme because the malalignment-related right leg instability and inability to hold the right edge prevented her from advancing to more difficult routines. It is for reasons like these that athletes who have problems related to malalignment may get 'eliminated' from their sport along the way.

ment. Compensation may have been achieved through selective stretching and strengthening or the use of devices such as a lift, orthotics, ankle supports or weight-belts.

2. They may be able to use the malalignment to their advantage. A high-jumper may, for example, adopt a certain style and side of approach in order to incorporate the best ranges of motion available and to avoid any of the restrictions imposed by the malalignment (see Fig. 5.10).

3. They are naturally hypermobile, or they have increased their mobility with stretching to the point at which they have been able to overcome any restrictions attributable to the malalignment.

4. The restrictions do not matter because of the way in which they deal with the demands of their sport, their particular 'style', so to speak. Alternatively, the very nature of the sport may never require them to go past the point at which a limitation of range or a functional weakness will become a problem. For example, an oarsman in a four or an eight:

– is less likely to be affected by lower extremity asymmetries

– may be able to compensate for any limitation of pelvic or trunk range of motion by always rowing on the same side

– may not have to flex or extend the trunk to the point at which these actions might pull on posterior ligaments and/or muscles which have been put under increased tension by the malalignment, or compress facet joints to the point of provoking pain, respectively.

EFFECT OF MALALIGNMENT ON THE VALIDITY OF RESEARCH IN SPORTS

> Malalignment affects a number of parameters that in turn alter the biomechanics of the athlete's body. The results of any research that involves biomechanics should therefore be suspect if the investigator has failed to take into account whether or not malalignment is present.

This includes in particular research looking at or influenced by range of motion, muscle strength, muscle tension, leg length and weight-bearing patterns.

Numerous studies have, for example, looked at the effect of orthotics on weight-bearing and oxygen consumption. Most make no mention of whether the athlete was in alignment or not; some (e.g. Delacerda & McCrory 1981) make mention of 'leg length differences'.

Let us assume that the athlete presents with right anterior, left posterior innominate rotation, the right leg rotated externally, and with obvious pronation on this side, the left leg rotated internally, with the left foot and ankle appearing to be in neutral or to supinate slightly on weight-bearing. Because we are generally more attuned to detecting pronation, and because the pronation on the right side is often so easily discernible when this presentation of malalignment is present, the fact that the left foot really remains in neutral or actually supinates slightly may be easily overlooked unless those carrying out the research are familiar with malalignment and specifically looking for an asymmetry of weight-bearing. The athlete, therefore, stands a good chance of being labelled as a 'pronator'.

Initial force plate studies will probably show some difference between the right and left side. This difference may well end up being attributed to the 'leg length difference' that may have been evident on examination. One iliac crest may have been noted to be higher than the other in standing, or one leg longer than the other in long-sitting or supine-lying, but it is unlikely that the length was checked in two positions, and even more unlikely that the sitting–lying test was performed to note the change or even reversal in length that typically occurs with rotational malalignment. Any measurement of leg length, other than by standing X-ray (see Figs 2.44A and 2.45) would have been erroneous, having been based on an assessment using asymmetrically displaced landmarks.

Following initial oxygen uptake studies, the athlete is made to run without orthotics, with orthotics that are in neutral, and with pairs of orthotics that are built-up or 'posted' to varying amounts on the medial aspect to counteract the supposed 'bilateral pronation'. The right and left orthotics of each pair will probably have been posted by the same amount, for example 2 degrees medial posting, hindfoot and forefoot, bilaterally. Repeat testing is noted to show a continued side-to-side difference on force plate studies, with no significant change in oxygen consumption for the same workload while wearing the different types of orthotic.

The results should hardly be surprising. What has really happened with the addition of the orthotics? On the right side, the medial posting may have decreased pronation and provided some feeling of stability; on the left, the orthotic will have increased the tendency towards supination (Fig. 5.33). The end result is persistent side-to-side differences on repeat force plate studies, differences that are unlikely to decrease the workload of walking or running. The workload may actually have been increased by:

- an accentuation of the side-to-side differences, and compensatory changes involving the limbs, pelvis and trunk
- a loss of shock absorption that results from throwing both feet, especially the left, towards increased lateral weight-bearing and thereby making them more rigid.

By looking at combined results for several athletes, one also runs the risk of diluting or cancelling out data if different presentations of malalignment (e.g. upslip, left anterior and locked, and 'alternate') are unknowingly included in the sample.

The correct procedure would be to look for malalignment initially, correct it if present and then reassess weight-bearing. In a number of the athletes, any previously noted pronation may be less obvious, or the pattern may now actually be one of bilateral supination (see Fig. 3.29). The posted orthotics that are then provided should be appropriate for the weight-bearing pattern now evident: medial for pronation, lateral for supination. In about 90% of cases, the leg length will be equal following realignment. An appropriate lift for the other 10% will ensure that the pelvis is level in all the subjects.

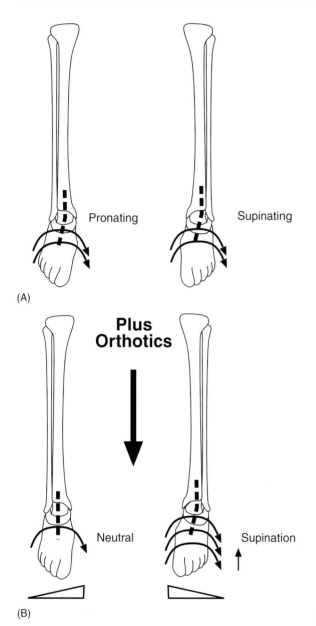

(A)

Plus Orthotics

(B)

Figure 5.33 An athlete with right anterior, left posterior innominate rotation. (A) Tendency towards right pronation and left supination. (B) The effect of provision bilaterally with orthotics that have a medial raise: a decrease of right pronation and an accentuation of left supination.

The only factor being studied will now be whether oxygen consumption is affected by providing a pair of orthotics, neutral or appropriately posted to correct for any residual tendency towards pronation or supination. In addition, the weight-bearing pattern is now more likely to be symmetrical, something that will become evident from the initial and repeat force plate studies.

In summary, researchers frequently appear to assume, usually incorrectly, that we are built more or less symmetrically or that 'minor' asymmetries do not matter, but malalignment can in fact result in asymmetries that may significantly affect the impact of an intervention. To ascribe side-to-side differences to discrepancies in leg length may be in part true, especially when malalignment is present; to suggest, however, a functional LLD without identifying the cause, or to imply that it is the result of an anatomical LLD, ignores the fact that 80–90% of athletes are out of alignment, and that approximately 90% of these will have an equal leg length on realignment. Restrictions in range of motion are easily attributed to a tightness of capsules, ligaments or muscles when these are in fact rarely true restrictions but merely the asymmetries typically seen in association with malalignment. Asymmetries of weight-bearing, muscle bulk and strength may be just as misleading.

Much of the research on biomechanics published today has completely ignored the entity of the malalignment syndrome and may, therefore, be based on erroneous assumptions. Side-to-side differences may be attributable to malalignment rather than to the effect of an intervention. Alternatively, the malalignment may have a 'cancellation' effect on some interventions if these act differently on the asymmetries on one side compared with the other. The malalignment should, therefore, be corrected before carrying out research likely to be influenced by these asymmetries.

Research involving biomechanics that can be influenced by malalignment, but that fails to acknowledge the presence or absence of an underlying malalignment syndrome, should be suspect.

6

Horses, saddles and riders

THE EQUESTRIAN TEAM

Equestrian sports – be they dressage, hunter-jumper, eventing or endurance – are team sports of horse and rider; the two must be in balance before optimum training and performance can occur. Problems with imbalance of the spine and pelvis can mar the interaction of this team. Injuries to either horse or rider are the most common reason for abnormalities of movement and balance.

No injury is trivial, even though it may seem so at the time. Following an injury, many riders seem to be unable to follow advice to curtail their riding and frequently fail to seek early treatment. The end result is that postural changes occur, and an untreated injury becomes chronic. Alterations in bony structures and soft tissues make these chronic injuries much more difficult to treat. The rider may unfortunately be unaware of malalignment until pain occurs. The physiotherapist is far too often called to evaluate the horse for malalignment as a possible cause of poor performance, whereas the problem lies really with the rider.

> To determine the cause of the problem, the conformation of both the horse and the rider must be evaluated, individually and as a working team.

ASSESSMENT OF THE HORSE: CONFORMATION AND GAIT

The therapist should begin with an examination of the horse. A key component of the evaluation is that of conformation, important because it is the position of the horse's head and neck, and the length of the back, that determine its centre of gravity. Gait evaluation must look at the horse performing various movement patterns, from a walk to a trot, canter or gallop.

Conformation

The back

The function of the back of the horse is to carry the weight of the rider. There are bands that run from the poll at the top of the head to the sacral vertebrae. The thoracic, lumbar and sacral vertebrae have dorsal 'fins' (spinous processes) that, up to and including the 15th thoracic vertebra, slant backwards towards the sacrum, whereas the 16th stands vertically, and the remaining two thoracic dorsal (and the lumbar) fins slant forwards toward the head (Fig. 6.1). It is this construction of the thoracic spine that maximizes the ability of the horse to carry loads.

Head and neck

> The carriage of the head and neck and the contents of the intestines determine the position of the centre of gravity.

At the halt, when the horse stands with its front and hind legs in line, it is said to be 'standing square'. In this position, the centre of gravity is approximately at the height of the sternum under the centre of the trunk, closer to the front legs or 'forehand' (Fig. 6.2).

The forelegs

The forelegs carry 10% more weight than the hind legs, both at the halt and in motion; they function to support and brake the horse's weight. An imbalance between the fore- and hind legs can shift the centre of gravity, and a large part of the training works at shifting the centre of gravity back so more weight than normal is carried by the hind legs.

The hind legs

The hind legs are an angled lever mechanism. They create a thrust and are capable of producing a strong propulsive force, which is transmitted forwards through the spine and is received in the forelegs. Because the hind legs are directly connected to the pelvis and spine, a malalignment of the pelvis or at the lumbosacral junction will interfere with this propulsive force. An imbalance, with one hind leg stronger

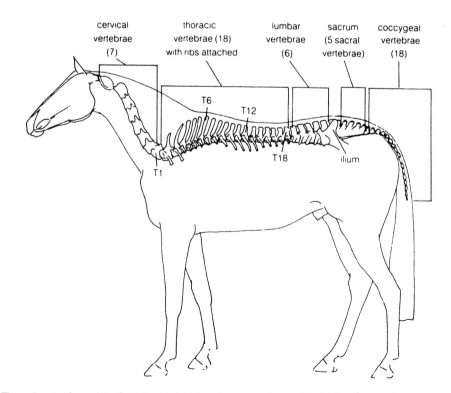

Figure 6.1 The spine: conformation of the dorsal 'fins' or spinous processes. (From Hayes, as revised by Rossdale 1987, with permission.)

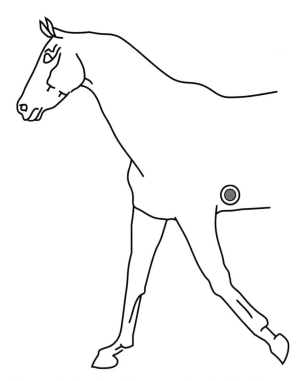

Figure 6.2 Location of the centre of gravity. (After Strasser 1998, with permission.)

than the other, will lead to rider compensation and ultimately malalignment of the rider's pelvis and back.

Gait

Walk

At the walk, the horse takes separate steps with each leg, one after the other. From the halt, the first step will be with a hind leg. This is followed by the front leg on the same side – that is, left hind, left front – and then by the right hind and right front leg (Fig. 6.3). The steps are generally even. At the walk, there is no moment of suspension with all four feet off the ground.

Trot

At the trot, the horse springs from one diagonal pair of legs to the other, the left hind and the right front coming to the ground together. When the horse springs off that pair of legs, there is a moment of suspension before the right hind and left front legs are placed on the ground together (Fig. 6.3). The movement is continuous and should be rhythmic, with a two-time beat. An imbalance in the gait will bring the foreleg down to strike the ground with more weight.

Canter and gallop

An imbalance can also occur at the canter or the gallop, a three-time pace: e.g. left hind to left diagonal, onto right hind and left foreleg, then to right foreleg, followed by a period of suspension with all four legs off the ground (Fig. 6.3). Problems occur more commonly in a young horse or a horse that is not fit, and the rider will ultimately overcompensate to counterbalance. As a result, the rider can develop an increased rotation in the thorax with a shift of the pelvis, so that the opposite ischium bears more weight.

CONFORMATION OF THE RIDER

One of the most common problems that arises in training is that the horse shows signs of stiffness or a lack of willingness to flex the neck and body to right or left and to perform evenly (Fig. 6.4B). The assumption is all too frequently made that this lack of willingness to perform comes from the temperament of the horse. Changes in equipment are made, or stronger aids (the signals by which the rider communicates with the horse, for example, rein aids, leg or hand signals, and the weight and seat position of the rider) are used to make the horse comply. In some cases, temperament may be the problem, but an increase in force and change of equipment frequently does not result in the ability of the horse to flex and to perform equally to both sides. There is a sign of an imbalance, but whether the problem originates with the horse or the rider needs to be determined. In most chronic cases, both the horse and the rider are affected, and both will require treatment.

When trying to decide whether the problem is originating from the horse or the rider, ask the rider the following questions:

1. When riding, is there any pain or aching between the shoulder blades (scapulae) or on one side of the neck or shoulder?
2. Has the trainer commented that, when sitting square in the saddle, the rider has:
   – one shoulder higher than the other? (Figs 6.5 and 6.6A)
   – the pelvic crest elevated on one side? (Figs 6.5 and 6.6A)?
3. Is there low back pain during or after riding?
4. Does the rider have trouble sitting deep in the saddle?

If the answer to any of these questions is 'yes', the rider's weight is not distributed evenly through the

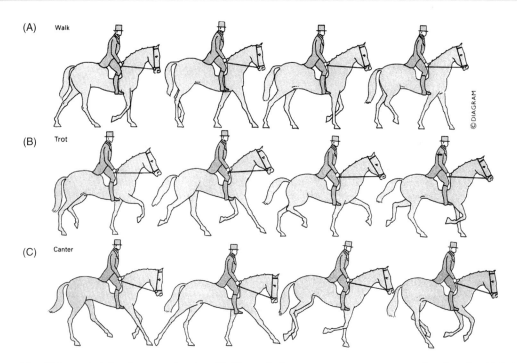

Figure 6.3 Riding gait: thé walk, trot and canter. (A) *The walk*: there are separate steps, one after the other (right hind, right front, then left hind and left front). There is no moment of suspension. (B) *The trot*: the horse jumps from one diagonal to another (right hind and left front, then left hind and right front). There is a moment of suspension with all four legs in the air. (C) *The canter*: a three-time pace. In the right canter, the sequence is left hind leg, left diagonal (right hind and left foreleg) and right foreleg, followed by a period of suspension. (From Worth 1990, with permission.)

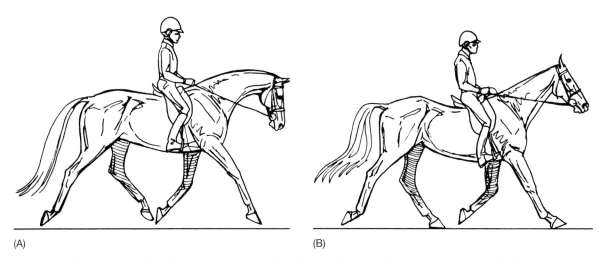

(A)   (B)

Figure 6.4 The horse's back and neck as an indicator of problems. (A) *Correct*: The horse moves 'round' with the back raised. Proper movement can occur with a round, swinging back and not too much tension in the back, neck and hind legs. (B) *Incorrect*: The horse moves 'hollow' with the back dropped. A tense, hollow back may be caused by problems relating to the horse, the rider or an ill-fitting saddle; it results in a high head and a stiff, uncomfortable gait that prevents the horse engaging the hind legs well, responding correctly to seat aids and 'working on the bit'. (C) When the horse 'overbends', the rider's trunk tends to tip onto the 'fork', the body tilts forwards and the thigh moves too much towards the vertical, the foot tending towards plantarflexion. (A, B from Harris 1996, and C from Wanless 1995, with permission.)

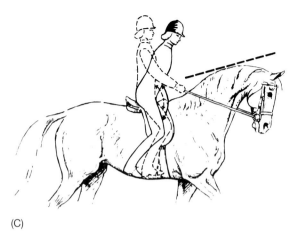

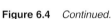

(C)

Figure 6.4 *Continued.*

saddle, producing an incorrect seat. 'In balance' in the saddle means that the pelvic (iliac) crests are even (Fig. 6.7; see Fig. 2.41B), each ischium sits deeply in the saddle. There is no rotation noted in the spine (lumbar to cervical). When the horse is working 'in balance', there is a rhythmic upward thrust to the pattern of movement conveyed to the rider through the horse's back.

When a rider is not in alignment, or is significantly rotated around the pelvis, problems occur with regard to the ability to control and give aids to the horse. Problems usually arise with injuries that lead to asymmetry. Even though chronic pain may not yet be in evidence, the rider often exhibits a limited range of motion that, combined with decreased flexibility, can prevent the rider reaching peak performance.

The rider's seat is the key to identifying rider-based malalignment. The pelvis must be level and symmetrical in the transverse and sagittal plane to allow the horse to be balanced and free to move (Fig. 6.7; see Fig. 6.4A). The rider with an uneven pelvis compromises this balance and ability to move. Someone with an anterior rotation of the left innominate will, for example, have the left side high when sitting (Fig. 6.5) and will have the hip and knee on that side raised and forwards (the reverse of the situation illustrated in Fig. 6.6). These changes can be enough to block the horse from flexing and moving easily to the left.

TEAM ASSESSMENT

It is very important to examine the horse and rider as a working team. An error frequently made by trainers is to have another individual ride the horse, but the

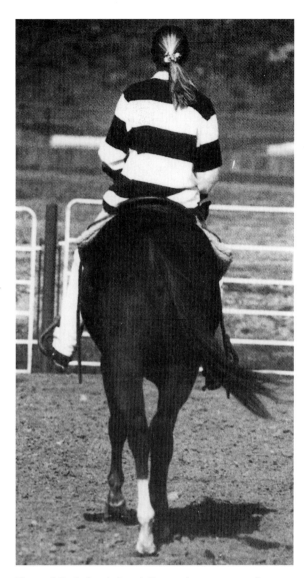

Figure 6.5 Left anterior rotation can be one cause of an abnormal sitting position or 'crookedness'. The left ischial tuberosity is raised off the saddle, losing contact and resulting in a shift of position, with the left pelvis and shoulder in forward rotation. (From Hill 1992, with permission.)

team is just that, the horse and the rider together. It is the team that must be worked and evaluated in order to solve a problem.

Another rider, except possibly an instructor who is trained to notice these types of difficulties, may complicate the situation by bringing a new set of skills and often new problems to the scene.

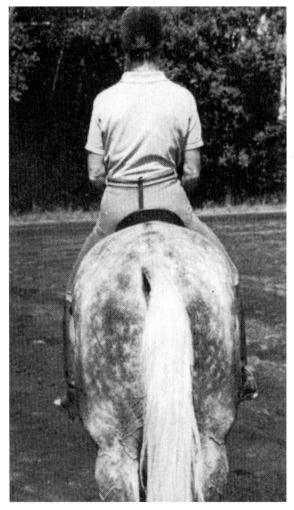

(A)

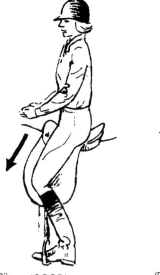
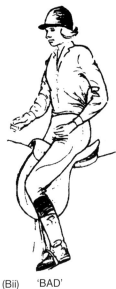

(Bi)　'GOOD'　　　　(Bii)　'BAD'

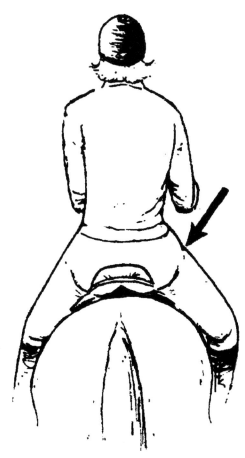

Figure 6.6 A rider sitting 'off centre'. (A) The right shoulder and pelvic (iliac) crest are obviously higher than the left, the pelvis being rotated to the left (forwards on the right). (B) 'The rider's 'good' (i) and 'bad' (ii) sides. As the rider collapses (i.e. goes out of alignment, with right anterior rotation), more of her chest shows, and the twist carries through to her thigh, so that it hangs away from the saddle: she clings on with just part of it. (C) The 'collapse', seen from the back. The rider's inside leg–body angle closes, whereas the outer angle opens. (A from Swift 1985, and B, C from Wanless 1995, with permission.)

(C)

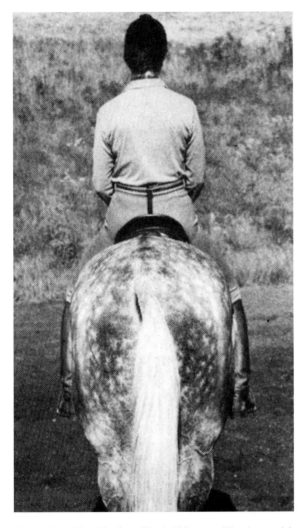

Figure 6.7 The rider from Fig. 6.6A is now sitting 'squarely' in the saddle: the pelvic crests and shoulders are even and the spine straight. (From Swift 1985, with permission.)

The first basic assessment is whether the horse and rider are suited to one another. Is the horse too big or too small for the rider and vice versa? If the 'fit' is correct, one must evaluate their age and skill. In many experienced riders, for example, the spine and back are mobile but controlled. The spine moves laterally from a convex to a concave position with ease, and the low back moves primarily forwards and backwards with the sway of the horse (Fig. 6.8B; see Fig. 6.4A). The rider can apply an aid to the horse with the action of the spine to urge the horse forwards. This mobility and control are, however, often not seen in the novice or the older rider.

When the horse and rider veer off to the left as they start moving, the assessor needs to decide whether incorrect guidance from the rider throws the horse off balance. In this instance, the rider may have a malalignment of the pelvis with a right anterior innominate rotation. The right ischium will be found to be high (see Figs 2.46, 3.69 and 6.6A). The rider's right shoulder and hip are too far ahead of the action, so that the rider appears to be perching in the saddle (see Fig. 6.6B). The right hip ends up in extension, and the right leg goes too far behind the girth of the saddle. The sitting position of the rider is incorrect, and guidance from rider to horse is impaired (see Figs 5.31 and 6.6C).

Next, the horse should have a smooth rhythmic gait. A disturbed rhythm, or a head that is held high or is bobbing (see Fig. 6.4B), may also be a sign of an ill-fitting saddle. All of these problems result in unwanted stresses that affect both horse and rider.

In many cases, the rider presents complaining of muscle spasm and in some cases stiffness when mounting and dismounting. Muscle spasm can be evoked in the vicinity of an injury or lesion, as a protective reflex reaction to prevent any movement of the affected area. This protective reflex is also operative if the pain originates from a joint. The muscles are not necessarily in constant spasm around the injured joint, but movement beyond a critical point can trigger specific groups to contract. The observed pattern of spasm can then be interpreted to determine the type of malalignment present in the horse and/or rider. Spasm in the left quadratus lumborum, the left paraspinal muscle at L2 and L3, and/or the left latissimus dorsi can, for example, indicate pelvic malalignment with thoracic and shoulder involvement.

Malalignment in the horse

> Malalignment in the horse can cause malalignment to develop in the rider and vice versa.

Malalignment in the horse results in secondary muscle spasm, stiffness and pain at predictable sites. The rider can run into grief as he or she unwittingly compensates for alterations of the gait pattern stemming from problems affecting the horse's back and sacroiliac (SI) joint(s).

The back

A horse with back problems manifests a reluctance to move out when the rider is seated. Muscle spasm along

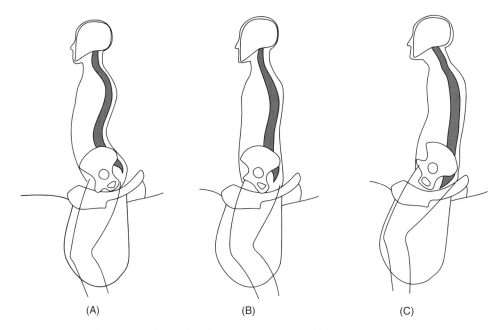

Figure 6.8   The balance of the rider relative to the alignment of the horse. (A) The pelvis is rolled forwards (anterior rotation; an attempt to balance in the saddle when the horse's head is held high), causing an increased lumbar lordosis and rounded shoulders. (B) The pelvis is correctly balanced, resulting in the normal slight curves of the spine and a straight, strong back. (C) The pelvis is rolled backwards (posterior rotation), causing a rounded back and shoulders, a collapsed chest and a protruding head. (After Swift 1985, with permission.)

the paravertebral muscles produces a stiff back, and the horse has a tendency to hold its head high. Persistence of this problem can bring the rider's trunk forwards in an attempt to balance in the saddle, and to bring the trunk back to vertical, the rider compensates by increasing the lumbar lordosis (Fig. 6.8A; see Fig. 6.4B).

A false positive for a back problem in the horse is created by an imbalance on the diagonal gait, that is, the trot (see Fig. 6.3). Here the propulsion from the hindquarters falls heavily through the forelegs. With uneven propulsion, weight falls more heavily through the opposite forequarter. If, for example, the right hind is stronger than the left, weight falls more heavily through the left shoulder and foreleg. The diagonal imbalance can result in spinal rotation in the rider as he or she attempts to compensate.

At the walk or trot, the forelegs pivot around the upper part of the shoulder blades, whereas the hind legs pivot around the hip joints. At the gallop, the lumbosacral junction becomes the pivot point for the hind legs. The length of the back determines where the intermittent stresses from the G-forces will impact: the longer the back, the more forward the impact. The propulsion forces travel through the gluteal muscles and then angle forwards and terminate at the fourth or sixth cervical

vertebrae. There are two impact energies, one from the left and the other from the right hind, which cross in the lumbosacral and thoracolumbar areas. With fast speeds and jumping, the stresses maximize at the point of the lumbosacral junction (see Fig. 6.1). Diagnosis is made by looking for muscle spasm specific to this junction. In cases of acute lumbosacral pain, the horse will frequently get down in the stall and try to roll immediately after being unsaddled.

The horse's sacroiliac joint

In the rider, a small amount of rotation occurs between the sacrum and the ilium. This movement at the SI joints is elicited at the extremes of flexion and extension of the back and the pelvis. It allows an increase in the normal range of movement in these directions and relieves part of the flexion strain at the lumbar spine. The belief is that no true movement occurs between the SI joint surfaces in the horse, but the author is unaware of any studies to definitively prove or disprove whether movement occurs. The joint is, however, an articulating joint with ligamentous support. Furthermore, it has been documented that injury to the sacral ligaments produces an instability, movement in the hind limb being affected by such instability. The horse may give the appearance of having a stiff limb, and the canter gait will be stiff to the side of the instability.

Malalignment in the rider

Malalignment in the rider can affect the harmony that should exist between rider and horse. This harmony is, in large part, determined by the ability or inability of the rider to maintain a proper seating position, one that meets the specific demands of a particular style of riding.

The balance and seating positions of the rider

To apply effectively aids or communications that guide the movement of the horse, the basic pre-requisite is a 'correct seat', which means that the rider follows the movement, the centre of gravity of the rider being in harmony with that of the horse. Malalignment affects the seating and disturbs this harmony. The rider can influence the horse by changing the position of his or her back and seat, but the use of the rider's weight and back as a driving or impulsion-producing force remains controversial and complex.

There are three main seating positions in equitation (Fig. 6.9):

- the dressage seat (also called the basic seat)
- the light seat
- the forward (or jumping) seat

The dressage seat

> The dressage seat is considered to be the basic seat for training a horse and rider in flat work (Fig. 6.9A).

To achieve this seat, the following posture must be assumed by the rider.

The upper body should normally be positioned vertically above the pelvis and sacrum. The trunk should be erect and the pelvis and sacrum level and in balance. The paraspinal muscles contract and relax to enable the back and spine to move in harmony with the movement of the horse. The shoulders of the rider exhibiting a correct dressage seat are slightly retracted and depressed at the scapulae. This posture allows a vertical line to fall from shoulder to heel.

The upper arms should be relaxed and move freely in a flexion–extension motion from the shoulder joint. The elbow is flexed, and the forearm is in a mid-position with the wrists straight, the fingers flexed and the thumbs uppermost. Relaxed shoulders, elbows and wrists ensure that the body movements of the rider are not transmitted to the hands. The head is carried erect, the rider looking ahead in the direction of movement. The chin must stay in line and not push forward.

The ischia and symphysis pubis form the triangle of the seat. The thighs lie flat against the saddle, and sufficient internal rotation must occur at the hip to

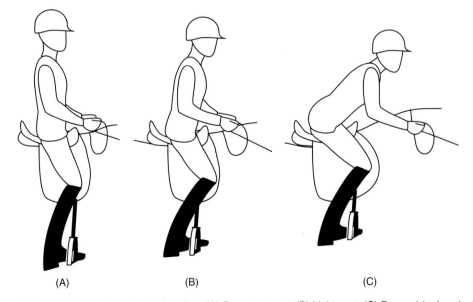

(A)   (B)   (C)

Figure 6.9 The three main seating positions in riding. (A) Dressage seat. (B) Light seat. (C) Forward (or jumping) seat. (After Harris 1996, with permission.)

allow the medial surface of the knee to be in full contact with the saddle. The line of the rider's thigh should be as vertical as possible without taking the weight off the ischium (see Figs. 6.4A, 6.6Bi and 6.8A). Having a long line to the thigh is to ensure a deep knee position, which then enables the rider to apply the lower leg to the barrel of the horse.

The rider's legs below the knee should usually slope backwards and downwards. Depending on the length of the leg, the knees are flexed to approximately 30 degrees. The medial surface of the calf keeps a light contact with the side of the horse. The toes and forefoot are dorsiflexed and everted, the toes always pointing forwards and slightly outward. The stirrup is positioned under the metatarsophalangeal joints and the weight of the rider normally transfers backwards from the metatarsophalangeal joints to the heel. At the ankle, the joint needs to be able to flex freely with the horse's movements.

Given an imbalance to the foot and ankle with supination of the forefoot, the foot will plantarflex, and the heel can end up higher than the forefoot. In this position, the imbalance prevents any distribution of the weight backwards through the heel. This imbalance can also change the position of the rider's upper body as the muscles must strongly contract to fight gravity. The end result is that the rider leans forward, the hands dropping to prevent the rider falling forwards. The head moves forwards as well, into a 'poking chin' posture (see Fig. 6.8C).

An imbalance in the rider's seat, such as sacral torsion and/or locking of one of the SI joints, can prevent the rider maintaining a correct position. With an anterior rotation of the pelvis on one side, for example, the pelvis will be rotated forwards and elevated on that side (see Figs 6.5 and 6.6). When this rider attempts to achieve the vertical position of the thigh, the knee on the side of the anterior rotation will do one of two things:

1. The knee will turn out because of external rotation of the leg (see Figs 5.31 and 6.6B). This 'turning out' automatically makes the seat insecure.
2. The knee will be pressed against the saddle by internally rotating the femur.

The rider actively rotates the femur internally in order to achieve the vertical thigh position. This brings the thigh closer into the saddle but causes the lower part of the leg to move away from the barrel of the horse. The rider may no longer be able to feel the horse adequately with the medial side of the calf or heel to give effective leg aids (see Fig. 6.6Bii, C).

The light seat

> The light seat (Fig. 6.9B) is useful for flat work with showjumpers and when there are frequent changes between flat work and jumping.

The purpose of the light seat is to lighten the burden of the rider's weight on the horse's back. The stirrups are shortened two holes to increase flexion at the knee and make the rider lean the upper body and trunk forwards. This position releases some of the weight through the ischium and puts more weight through the upper leg. It also brings the hip flexors and adductors into play.

Pelvic malalignment results in an asymmetry of strength in hip girdle and leg muscle strength (see Appendix 4). This imbalance of strength, in addition to the malposition of the legs and innominates, contributes to an uneven weight distribution in the saddle. If the rider is to achieve a true light seat, there can be no malalignment of the pelvis and spine.

The forward (jumping) seat

> The purpose of the forward seat is to give freedom to the horse's back, and enables the rider quickly to follow all the balance and movement changes of the horse.

Only when the rider has acquired a safe, balanced dressage and light seat can the forward seat be developed (Fig. 6.9C).

This seat must be mastered before attempting jumping or galloping, and the rider must be able to change between the light and the forward seat between jumps. An inability on the part of the rider to do this, and to be in balance, can throw the horse off stride.

In the forward jumping gait, the stirrups are again shortened, causing increased knee flexion and ankle dorsiflexion. The stirrup placement is mid-metatarsal rather than at the metatarsophalangeal joints. The ankle joint can be immobilized:

- when the stirrup is incorrectly positioned
- when the forefoot plantarflexes rather than dorsiflexes.

Presentations of the malaligned rider

Box 6.1 outlines two common presentations of malalignment in the rider; in both, the left hip is lowered and the right ilium elevated.

Presentation A: there is rotation of the lumbar vertebrae to the right into a right convexity of the lumbar spine, usually from L1 to L4 (see Fig. 2.65), the maximum rotation generally being found at L2. A mild compensatory rotation to the left occurs throughout the thoracic spine. The scapulae are uneven and the left shoulder is elevated and rotated forwards. The rider complains of pain in the low back and between the scapulae.

Presentation B: there is no rotation of the lumbar spine, but rotation occurs throughout the thoracic spine, beginning to the right at T10 and being maximal at T3–T5. There is also a compression and narrowing of the space between the right transverse processes of T1 and C7. Stress on the cervical spine is increased. The rider exhibits a bobbing head and reports pain between the scapulae and often numbness and tingling radiating into the right shoulder and arm

Complaints of the rider

Malalignment is most likely to result in complaints involving the SI, facet and hip joints, and the scapular region. Pain can result from these sites being put under stress either directly or by a malalignment-related impairment of pelvic, spine or limb function having adversely affected the riding style and in turn indirectly increased stress at these sites.

Sacroiliac joint pain. A decrease in mobility at the SI joint can alter the ability of the rider to achieve a deep seat in the saddle. When the range of movement is lost at the hip joint, back and SI joint movement must increase to compensate. Pain from the SI joint, when it occurs, usually radiates into the buttock, into the groin and/or down the leg of the affected side. On examination, the pelvis is no longer balanced, the right ilium probably being elevated, if the left hip is lowered (see Fig. 6.6). Tests intended to stress specific structures, such as the anterior and posterior sacroiliac ligaments, for pain originating from the SI joint, may be positive (see Ch. 2). In addition to realignment, the preferred treatment for sacroiliac and lumbosacral pain includes:

- an SI joint support in the form of a lumbosacral support (see Ch. 7), to be worn while riding and working with the horse
- electrotherapy, for example with the Interferential Current with Vacomed attachment or the HeNe Scan Laser with infrared beam component (2–4 J/cm^2; area 10×15 cm), which have been found to be particularly helpful.

Facet joint pain. Facet joint injury can result from:

1. *prolonged or excessive compression* (see Fig. 2.35): for example, when the right innominate is rotated anteriorly and the pelvis elevated on the right, there is usually a lumbar curve, convex to left, and the vertebrae compensate by rotating into the convexity of the curve (see Fig. 2.29). The facet joint surfaces on the right are compressed, whereas those on the left are separated. The pain that can result with prolonged or excessive compression is often felt as a 'deep in the bone' ache, which is commonly referred from the low back to the buttock, and can also be referred down the thigh to the knee

2. *an acute sprain or strain*: with an acute right lumbar facet sprain or strain, spasm of the surrounding muscles (e.g. paravertebrals and quadratus lumborum) elevates the right pelvis, narrows the lumbar disc spaces on the right side and prevents rotation through the lumbar spine. Pain is commonly referred forwards or around the iliac crest and into the pubic area.

Alteration of weight-bearing and ranges of motion
Leg orientation and foot posture patterns. The therapist should look at the legs with the feet in the stirrups when the horse and rider are stationary and when they are moving towards and away from him or her.

With 'alternate' presentations and right anterior rotation (see Figs 5.31 and 6.6B, C), the right leg may be obviously externally rotated, with the knee falling outwards to the point at which the right foot ends up on tiptoe, the heel up in the air (plantarflexed). The left leg may, however, be internally rotated, the left knee hugging the side of the horse and the foot collapsed inwards and dorsiflexed (pronated). The opposite pattern may be seen with, for example, the left anterior and locked presentation.

Hip ranges of motion. These are tested to determine the effect of the malalignment on the ability of the rider to have the correct leg position needed to control the horse's movement and pace using pressure signals from the calf, knee and thigh. The major problem is that there is now an asymmetry of hip ranges of motion. With the right pelvis elevated and rotated forwards in the sagittal plane, for example:

- external rotation of the right leg is increased, as is adduction and abduction, whereas right internal rotation is limited (see Figs 3.40, 3.71, 3.72 and 6.6C)
- right hip flexion is decreased, whereas extension is increased (see Figs 3.64, 3.65 and 3.69B).

Hip joint pain. Pain from the hip is referred forward to the groin and then down the front of the thigh to the knee (see Fig. 3.62). This pain can continue to radiate down the anterior aspect of the lower leg but stops proximal to the ankle joint. Hip joint pain can be assessed by determining the hip ranges of motion and passive and resisted movement (see Chs 2 and 3). Any weakness, whether pain occurs on passive and/or active movement and whether the pain is experienced at a particular point of the available range should be noted.

Scapular pain. With an imbalance of the scapulae, the rider complains of pain in the paraspinal muscles between the shoulder blades. This imbalance also decreases the range of scapular abduction and retraction on the side on which the shoulder is elevated and can lead to an inconsistency with the rein aids. It is important to maintain a correct balance with the rein aids so that the hands do not become too strong, preventing the horse bending or flexing correctly.

Begin the examination with the rider standing and then sitting on a stool with no back support. Note the level of the scapulae, bearing in mind that alterations of the level can indicate weakness in the trapezius muscles, serratus anterior or latissimus dorsi. Ask the rider to shrug his or her shoulders; this simple movement can demonstrate abnormal mobility of the scapulae against the thorax. Riders occasionally develop numbness in the hands when riding, this being more common with riders who engage in hunter-jumper, 2–3 day eventing and endurance activities. If thoracic outlet syndrome is suspected, one test is to have the rider elevate the scapulae and shrug the shoulders, holding this position for approximately 1 minute. Adson's manoeuvre and the military position should also be tried. Pain into the arms or tingling may indicate thoracic outlet syndrome, other tests and appropriate investigations being needed to confirm or negate this often elusive diagnosis.

EQUIPMENT

The final focus of this chapter will be on the effect of poor equipment, particularly the saddle, on malalignment-related problems of the horse and rider.

The saddle

The horse's saddle all too frequently does not fit. The horse first tries body manoeuvres, such as raising its head or dropping and swaying its back, to avoid the pain caused by the rider's weight being added to an ill-fitting saddle (see Fig. 6.4B). The rider may try to remedy the problem by using blankets or pads, which can unfortunately have the effect of narrowing the saddle base

and result in compression of the thoracic spine. The horse's attempt to manoeuvre away from the saddle can produce an increased thoracic lordosis, or sway back. In addition to hollowing of the thoracic spine, there can be actual bruising of the spinous processes.

The tree, or 'spine' of the saddle, must be evaluated to determine whether there is any rotation or narrowing that could result in weight not being evenly distributed along the horse's spine, so the paraspinal muscles become bruised and go into spasm. The muscles can swell and become inflamed, or, as a protective mechanism, the connective tissue may thicken and leaves an area of callus and scar tissue. A wide gutter on a full tree saddle:

- ensures that the weight of the rider is well distributed lateral to the horse's spine
- protects the spinous processes
- allows the horse's spine to function as a spring, so that the shock of the rider weighting and unweighting is absorbed by the saddle and paravertebral muscles.

> Both the rider's weight and the weight of the saddle should be evenly distributed over the thoracic spine of the horse.

When the saddle is a proper fit, imbalance can occur for two main reasons:

1. *Malalignment of the pelvis and spine of the rider*: when one ischium is more heavily weighted than the other, for example, there results a maldistribution of weight and a shifting or rotation of the saddle. Right anterior rotation and right upslip both result in unweighting on the right side, the right ischial tuberosity moving upwards; increased weight now has to be borne by the left ischial tuberosity, which can easily come to lie a good centimetre lower than the right (see Figs 2.46D, 3.39 and 3.79C).

2. *Malalignment in the lumbosacral region of the horse*: the propulsive G-force is uneven, and the centre of gravity changes (see Fig. 6.1). This can cause a torsion in the movement of the horse's thoracic spine, which can eventually result in a breakdown in the front part of the saddle where the rider's knee grips. This breakdown can cause pain in the shoulder of the horse, and the rider may experience a drop of the thigh and pelvis on the side of the breakdown.

> The saddle should be checked for fit every 4–6 months.

It should be remembered that the horse moving in balance causes an even pattern of upward thrusts to be experienced by the rider through the pelvis, SI joints and back.

Malalignment and the coordination of the aids

As indicated above, an aid is a form of communication between the horse and rider, this being achieved by the use of hands, legs and seat position. Weight transferred from the spine and pelvis, together with a deep seat and relaxed legs, stimulate impulsion and the movement of the horse's back. The rider creates and maintains the horse in a forward movement. In doing so ,the rider seems to 'sit the horse on the bit', that is, to convey a message via the reins and bit. Contact with the bit via the reins to the rider's hands permits communication between the team. The horse must be supple and in balance with the rider in order to take the rein aids willingly. The horse rebalances itself by movement of its head and neck. The following influences on the giving of aids should be considered.

The rider's seat: giving the weight aids

Only a relaxed rider sitting correctly can apply the weight aids efficiently. An effective but soft seat is dependent on the correct position of the rider's pelvis and spine, malalignment reducing the stability of the rider in the saddle by altering the 'correct' position and hence the distribution of the weight.

Shoulder girdle and upper extremity: giving the rein aids

The intensity of the rein aid depends on whether it is made by slight pressure from the ring finger, by a rounding of the wrists or by using the whole arm. This rein aid is sustained while increasing forward drive aids to the horse. When the horse submits, the hand relaxes and light control is maintained. The imbalance and asymmetry of the scapulae associated with pelvic malalignment will interfere with any application of the rein aids.

SUMMARY

Harmony in riding can only be achieved when the horse and the rider are both in alignment and the saddle fits properly. The following are some of the problems that result from malalignment.

Malalignment of the rider

Let us consider the rider presenting with right anterior, left posterior rotation.

The right hip and knee end up elevated and positioned forwards to the point of possibly blocking the horse from flexing and moving easily to the right (see Fig. 6.6Bii). The right shoulder and hip similarly end up too far ahead, so that the rider appears to be 'perching' in the saddle on this side (see Fig. 6.6Bii).

The right hip ends up excessively flexed, and with time there is contracture of the iliolumbar ligament. This contracture can eventually result in a compensatory increase in the lumbar lordosis in an attempt to lengthen the leg and may create difficulties when attempting realignment.

The right leg ends up moving too far behind the girth of the saddle and may be obviously externally rotated (see Fig. 5.31); in this case, the foot tends to go into a plantarflexed position so that the heel is higher than the forefoot, preventing proper distribution of the weight backwards through the heel, and the stirrup may require lengthening on this side compared with the left. Active internal rotation of the legs normally helps the knees to act as anchor points for the pelvis, stopping the rider falling back into the 'armchair seat' with the pelvis rotated backwards and the back being rounded (see Fig. 6.8C).

The outward rotation of the right knee with external rotation results in an insecure seat because the right thigh and the medial aspect of the knee no longer lie in full contact with the saddle (see Figs 5.31 and 6.6C). The rider can actively rotate the right leg internally in an attempt to achieve a vertical position, at the cost of losing contact between the medial calf and the barrel of the horse.

The iliac crests are no longer even, the right probably being higher than the left, and weight distribution is also uneven – heavier on the left buttock and stirrup (see Fig. 6.6A). The compensatory curves of the spine result in an imbalance of scapular position and range of motion (decreased abduction and retraction on the side of the elevated shoulder) and interscapular pain, often with referral to the shoulder or arm.

Insecurity of the seat with right external rotation, imbalance of leg strength and uneven weight distribution in the saddle will also stop the rider achieving a true 'light seat' (Fig. 6.9B). The rider may notice difficulty with control and giving aids, recurrent spasm, and stiffness when mounting and dismounting, if not outright back and SI joint pain.

Malalignment of the horse

Malalignment results in muscle spasm, stiffness and pain in predictable sites and leads to a reluctance to move out; lumbosacral spasm may cause the horse to roll in the stall. Neither the saddle nor the rider will now fit properly:

- The saddle causes compression of the thoracic spinous processes, and the horse tries to manoeuvre away: the end result is often a thoracic lordosis or sway back, possible bruising and a tendency to hold the head high (see Fig. 6.4B)
- The rider may end up shifting or rotating, with a maldistribution of his or her weight.

Malalignment involving the lumbosacral region results in an uneven centre of gravity and torsion of the horse's torso.

The horse may sometimes be felt to display 'antisocial behaviour' when in fact malalignment is limiting some ranges of motion and makes it hard for the horse to comply with certain commands; the horse that will lead on the left side but not the right may, for example, already have a back problem that is triggered or worsened by attempts to turn to the right.

The rider may develop problems secondary to malalignment of the horse on attempting to compensate for alterations in the gait pattern and adjusting to postural changes, for example an increased lordosis in an attempt to counteract the tendency to fall forwards when the horse's head is held high (see Figs. 6.4B and 6.8A).

These ongoing efforts may ultimately result in malalignment in the rider as well. A lack of willingness to lead, to flex or to perform to one side, and signs of stiffness may be attributable to the horse or the rider, but in chronic situations usually involve both.

Disturbance of seating

Problems with the saddle will disturb the harmony of movement between the rider and the horse and can be responsible for malalignment occurring in one or both. The wear and tear of the saddle can serve as an indicator that malalignment is actually present in one or other party.

This chapter has not tried to cover all the problems relating to malalignment of horse and rider. Instead, key areas of difficulty have been discussed and suggestions regarding assessment techniques given. Following an evaluation of horse, saddle and rider, the therapist should list the problems and plan the treatment and the protocols to be followed to correct any malalignment.

One of the principles of a treatment programme is to facilitate healing after an injury. This is achieved by regaining a full range of movement and muscle strength as soon as possible. In addition, the rider must be taught to recognize when he or she is in balance. Whenever movement balance is lost, uneven and unequal stresses are created, which can produce malalignment, albeit minimal at first. Failure to correct the situation can result in serious worsening of the malalignment–related problems of both horse and rider.

7

A comprehensive treatment approach

Seventy-five per cent of athletes in elementary school are out of alignment, 80–85% by the time they graduate from high school (Klein 1973, Klein & Buckley 1968). Treatment is indicated if the history and examination suggest that there is an associated malalignment syndrome that:

- may be putting the athlete at increased risk of injury
- may be precipating the athlete's symptoms or injury
- may be perpetuating and/or aggravating the symptoms
- may be slowing down or preventing recovery from an injury
- may be preventing the athlete advancing in a chosen sport.

This chapter looks first at the shortcomings of using standard treatment approaches for back pain caused by malalignment. It then outlines a logical and proven treatment programme. Participation of the athlete in the treatment programme is emphasized, thus increasing the chances of achieving the best results quickly and helping to maintain improvements. The chapter concludes with a differential diagnosis of other conditions to consider, appropriate investigations and alternate treatment options should this treatment approach fail to achieve lasting realignment and improvement.

FAILURE TO RESPOND TO STANDARD TREATMENT

The judicious use of anti-inflammatory medication and electrical modalities, combined with a graduated stretching, strengthening and range of motion programme, may well bring an injured athlete back into play.

> If the symptoms are in any way related to, or influenced by, the malalignment, however, all these measures may amount to no more than sticking plaster (band-aid) therapy as long as the malalignment itself is never considered and corrected.

MALALIGNMENT AND THE STANDARD TREATMENT OF LOW BACK PAIN

Low back pain is one of the most common musculoskeletal complaints in our society. The aetiology is varied yet the treatment approach often singularly unvaried: the repeated application of heat or cold and electrical modalities (e.g. ultrasound, laser or interferential current), advice regarding posture and proper lifting techniques, strengthening of the back and abdominal muscles, stretching of the hip extensors and flexors, arching the back while lying prone, traction and, thrown in for good measure, the pelvic tilt. Some of the 'standard' exercises are more likely to trigger or aggravate pain in someone who is out of alignment.

The posterior pelvic tilt

The posterior tilt consists of actively rotating the pelvis posteriorly in order temporarily to decrease or eliminate the lumbar lordosis (Fig. 7.2B). In someone who presents in alignment but suffers from mechanical back pain, the tilt may be helpful in that it decreases pressure on the lumbar facet joints and may decrease the pressure within the disc and any tendency of the disc to bulge posteriorly.

Case history

A runner presented with a history of gradually increased left lateral thigh and knee pain, coming on consistently during the last 10 miles of running a marathon. The pain would settle completely with time and standard treatment measures, only to recur again with the next marathon.

Examination 1 week after the last marathon revealed rotational malalignment with anterior rotation of the right innominate. There was increased tone and tenderness to palpation in the left hip abductor muscle mass and the length of the iliotibial band down to its insertion; on Ober's test, passive left hip adduction was significantly restricted compared with that on the right (see Fig. 3.40). Gait examination showed that the runner pronated on the right and supinated on the left side. A pair of running shoes used in training for 6 months showed changes consistent with this weight-bearing pattern: the heel cup collapsed inwards on the right and outwards on the left (Fig. 7.1A).

Correction of the malalignment quickly resulted in a resolution of symptoms and signs, and allowed for an immediate return to a full training schedule. Symptoms did not recur during the next marathon competed 6 months later, and, on reassessment shortly after, alignment had been maintained, and the left hip abductors and iliotibial band were relaxed and non-tender. The heel cups of a new pair of running shoes of the same make still maintained a vertical, symmetrical position after a comparable 6 months in use (Fig. 7.1B).

> In someone presenting with malalignment, however, the posterior pelvic tilt may cause more pain.

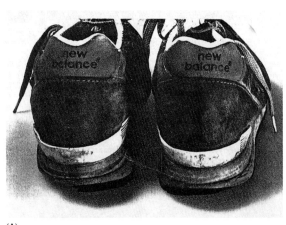

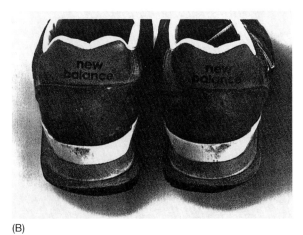

(A) (B)

Figure 7.1 Marathon runner's training shoes. (A) A pair used for 6 months prior to the correction of malalignment. Note the heel cup collapse (inwards on the right, outwards on the left) and excessive left lateral heel wear with supination. (B) A pair used for 6 months while maintaining realignment. The heel wear is even, and both heel cups are in neutral.

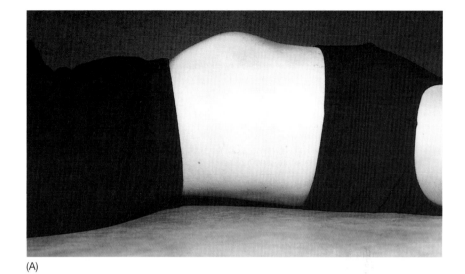

(A)

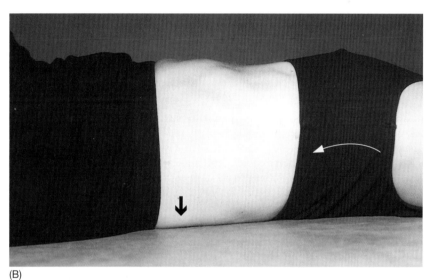

Figure 7.2 Pelvic tilt. (A) The normal resting position showing a hollow (lumbar lordosis). (B) Active posterior rotation of the pelvis flattens the spine.

(B)

As we have seen, rotational malalignment is usually associated with sacral torsion, locking of one or other of the sacroiliac (SI) joints and a lateral lumbar curve that reverses at the thoracolumbar junction to give rise to a thoracic curve going in the opposite direction (see Fig. 3.12). Spinal tenderness localizes primarily to the sites of increased stress: the lumbosacral and thoracolumbar junctions.

The posterior tilt aims to flatten the lumbar segment in one plane – the sagittal – in order to decrease the lordosis. This completely ignores the fact that, when malalignment is present, there will also be an accentuated convexity of the lumbar segment to the right or left. In order to create that lateral lumbar curve, the vertebrae must have undergone simultaneous axial rotation into the convexity and side flexion into the concavity, in other words, simultaneous movement in the frontal and transverse planes respectively. A left lumbar convexity, for example, results from L1–L4 inclusive side-bending to the right and rotating to the left, this being maximal at the apex (see Figs 2.29, 4.6 and 4.28). There will usually also be an element of extension, in keeping with a lumbar lordosis of varying degree (see Fig. 3.12A). As a result, facet joint surfaces have been moved closer together on the right and separated on the left side (see Fig. 2.35).

In someone presenting with malalignment, this pelvic tilt may therefore be painful (Box 7.1).

Box 7.1 Factors causing the posterior tilt to be painful

- Trying to flatten a curve in one plane (sagittal), ignoring the fact that the curve exists in two planes (sagittal and frontal) and that the individual vertebrae are rotated in three planes (sagittal, frontal and transverse)
- Further increasing stress on the high-stress sites of curve reversal (thoracolumbar junction) and the twisted lumbosacral junction
- Increasing the tension on already tender posterior soft tissue structures (e.g. the supra- and interspinous ligaments, and thoracolumbar myofascia)
- Stretching the tender posterior pelvic ligaments
- Aggravating the facet joint irritation that results with vertebral rotation:
  - by increasing the joint separation already present on the convex side, further stretching capsules, ligaments and nerve supply
  - by increasing the joint compression already occurring on the concave side, with a risk of entrapment of these soft tissues and nerve fibres

Doing the posterior pelvic tilt lying supine on a hard surface also risks putting direct pressure on structures that just may not bear to be pressed against a hard surface in the process of attempting the tilt:

- tender posterior pelvic ligaments (especially those crossing the posterior SI joint, and the sacrotuberous origins)
- the sometimes protuberant and very stiff and unyielding coccyx and spinous processes of malrotated vertebrae, particularly the vertebrae around the thoracolumbar junction (see Chs 4 and 5 and Fig. 5.1).

Traction

Traction is unlikely to straighten the curvatures of the spine if these are caused by:

1. the compensatory segmental vertebral rotation (lumbar, thoracic and cervical) associated with malalignment
2. the malrotation of one or more isolated vertebral complexes.

The malrotated spine, pelvis and attaching myofascia have to be regarded as a spiral structure that one may not be able to unwind just by pulling on both ends at the same time. Samorodin aptly explains this using the analogy of the wound-up telephone cord (see Ch. 8). Traction alone may precipitate or augment pain by:

- increasing stress on sites of curve reversal and vertebral malrotation

- further increasing the tension in myofascial and ligamentous structures already under tension because of the malalignment.

Gentle repetitive traction, aimed at relaxing in particular the paravertebral muscles, may, however, be a useful adjunct to help to achieve and maintain the correction of vertebral malrotation. Gentle traction can certainly help subsequent efforts at mobilization, probably temporarily decreasing the tension in these attaching muscles by:

1. achieving some relaxation through the 'contract–relax' mechanism (see below)
2. opening up the spaces between the vertebrae and facet joints to relieve compression and reactive muscle tightening
3. minimizing or abolishing strain in muscles that have been facilitated.

Extension exercises and back extensor strengthening

Extension of the back while lying prone, maximal in the 'cobra' position (Fig. 7.3), further increases the pressure on facet joints that are already compressed on one side by vertebral rotation in the presence of malalignment. Back extension also causes further stress on the sites of curve reversal (see Fig. 3.12B, C).

This is not to say, however, that one cannot have the athlete do exercises for the back extensor muscles. Given the frequent involvement of these muscles (e.g. reflex spasm, tenderness, disuse weakness), a stretching and strengthening programme should be part of rehabilitation - provided a core strengthening programme is well under way (see Figs. 7.24–7.28) and alignment is starting to be maintained. Arching of the

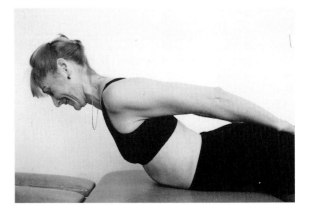

Figure 7.3 Hyperextension of the back: the 'cobra' position.

back should continue to be limited to the pain-free zone to avoid triggering reflex muscle spasm. A contraction of these muscles that avoids excessive back extension can be initiated in the prone position simply by:

1. extending initially only the head and neck (Fig. 7.4A), progressing eventually to lifting also the shoulders, but no more than 2–3 cm off the surface at the same time (Fig. 7.4B)
2. raising the *straight* right and left leg alternately 1–2 cm off the surface (Fig. 7.4C) and eventually both legs simultaneously: initially just clearing the bed and then progressing to 10–15 cm as the pain decreases and the strength increases (Fig. 7.4D).

The emphasis is on frequent repetition. Contractions should initially be brief: holding to a slow count of 1 is adequate.

This is to avoid decreasing or cutting off the entry of blood and the exit of waste for too long, something that will only compound the problem in those muscles along the spine which have already been subjected to the detrimental effects of a chronic increase in tension.

Each contraction should be followed by complete relaxation to allow for a maximum inflow of blood and clearance of waste (Fig. 7.4E).

Once the athlete can do three sets of 10, the duration of each contraction is prolonged to a slow count of 2 for the first set of 10. This is preferable to increasing the degree of extension. As strength increases, the prolongation of the count is carried over into the second and eventually the third set of 10, at which point the workload is again raised by increasing either the count or, eventually, the degree of extension, first for one set, then two and so on. Extension should not be increased unless the athlete is in alignment. This simple progressive approach can be used for strengthening any other muscles.

Sit-ups

There seems to be some obsession in our society with doing vertical sit-ups, the ultimate perfection of the 'abdominal crunch' being the ability to touch the nose or the right and left elbow alternately to the opposite knee (Fig. 7.5). Most athletes presenting with back pain, whether it be on the basis of malalignment or some other cause, are likely to run into grief with these manoeuvres. Pain often increases as they start from the sitting position to try to lie down again. At this point, the paravertebral muscles contract maximally to splint the back, effectively increasing the pressure on both the disc and the facet joints. In someone with malalignment, the addition of twisting the trunk alternately to right and left has to be viewed as another factor capable of causing:

1. pain
   - from attempted rotation into a restriction and from a further compression of the facet joints on one side
   - by increasing the tension on the posterior pelvic ligaments and the thoracolumbar muscles and fascia
2. a recurrence of malalignment following successful correction, because of the torsional element.

The intent is to strengthen the abdominal muscles. In someone with severe back pain, a good contraction primarily of rectus abdominis can be initiated simply by raising the head and neck while lying supine (Fig. 7.6A), progressing eventually to raising the shoulders just 2–3 cm off the surface (Fig. 7.6B). Similar to attempts at strengthening the back extensors, the contractions should initially be of short duration, the muscles being completely relaxed between these contractions. Instructions are for an initial set of 10 contractions daily, increasing to two and then three sets as strength and endurance improve. At that point, either the duration of the contraction and/or the degree of trunk flexion can gradually be increased, following the progression outlines above for the back extensors.

It cannot be stressed enough that strengthening of the above muscles must be preceded by efforts at realignment and graduated core strengthening which are both an intricate part of the overall treatment programme for the malalignment syndrome and will be discussed in that context later (see Figs 2.22–2.27 and 7.24–7.28).

Always consider the possibility of an underlying problem of malalignment when:

1. the standard treatment measures discussed above fail to resolve, or actually worsen, the pain
2. there is no suggestion of a disc, facet or other underlying problem on examination
3. investigations have proved negative.

MANIPULATION, MOBILIZATION AND MUSCLE ENERGY TECHNIQUES

The key to recovery from the malalignment syndrome is to relieve the stresses and strains on the skeleton and attaching soft tissues attributable to the malalignment.

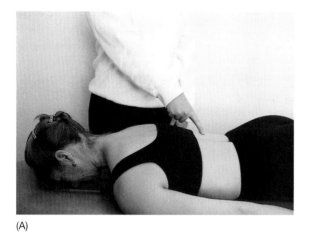

(A)

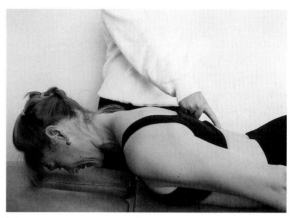

(B)

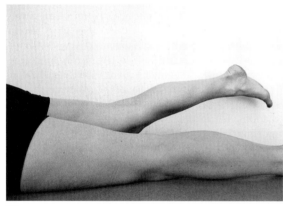

(C)

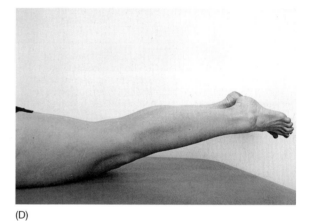

(D)

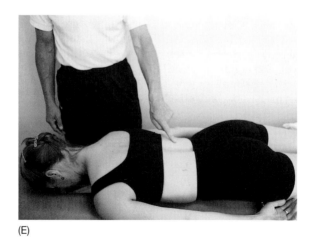

(E)

Figure 7.4 Strengthening of the back extensor muscles in prone-lying. (A) Extending only the head and neck to a limited degree. (B) Clearing the shoulders off the plinth 2.5–5 cm in addition to extending the head and neck minimally. (C) Alternately raising the right and left straight leg 5–15 cm off the plinth. (D) Simultaneously raising both legs 5–15 cm straight off the plinth. (E) All the muscles are completely relaxed between contractions (the head and legs resting on the plinth).

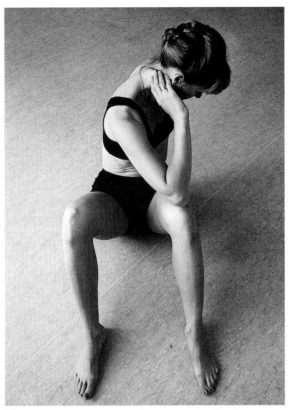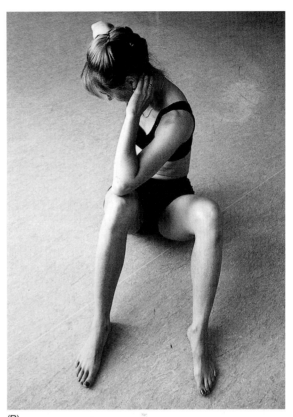

(A)   (B)

Figure 7.5   Risking a recurrence of malalignment doing the abdominal 'crunch' with the addition of a torsional component by alternately touching (A) the left elbow to the right knee, and (B) the right elbow to the left knee.

Realignment using an appropriate manual therapy technique should therefore be the first treatment measure and remains the mainstay of treatment.

In approximately 85–90% of athletes presenting with malalignment, correction can be achieved quite easily. In a small number of these, probably less than 5%, realignment is maintained after only one or two treatments, something that is more likely to occur in younger athletes. In the majority, correction can be achieved but the malalignment keeps on recurring. Realignment is maintained for longer and longer periods following each correction. Within 3–4 months, most of these athletes will finally maintain alignment and require no further correction. That is not, however, to say that they may not go out of alignment again at some point in the future and require further treatment, especially if they again become symptomatic.

In approximately 5–10%, correction cannot be achieved or is quickly lost following each correction. The majority of these athletes prove to have laxity involving one or both SI joints and/or one or more

lumbar vertebrae (especially L4 or L5), a generalized joint hypermobility or both. In others, recurrence may be the result of some as yet undiagnosed problem, such as a missed central disc protrusion (see 'Asymmetries that fail to respond' below).

There are numerous manual therapy techniques that find application in the treatment of malalignment; these are discussed at length in Chapter 8. They range from the high-velocity, low-amplitude (HVLA) manipulations traditionally associated with chiropractic, the long-lever, low-velocity (LLLV) osteopathic techniques to re-establish joint play and the seemingly more gentle methods (e.g. cranio-sacral release, zero-balancing, NUCCA) which are now being embraced by many chiropractors, osteopaths, physicians and physiotherapists alike because they may be more successful in achieving long-term correction.

As suggested by Richard (1986), the success of these more gentle techniques possibly results from the fact that they address not just the issue of the bones being out of alignment, but also any persistent asymmetries

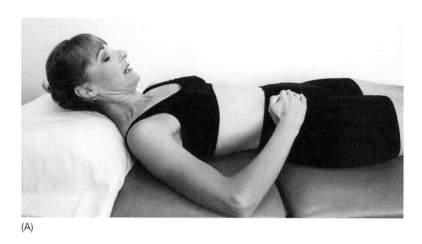

(A)

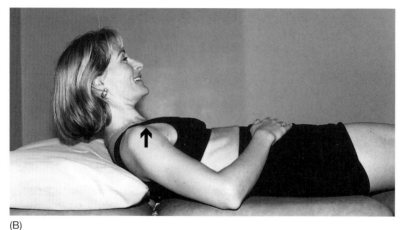

(B)

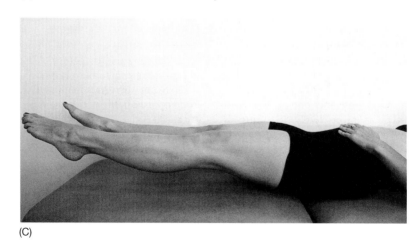

(C)

Figure 7.6   Graduated abdominal muscle strengthening. Simultaneously drawing the umbilicus towards the plinth and tightening up the muscles around the rectum will ensure a strengthening of not only rectus abdominis, but also transversus abdominis and the pelvic floor muscles (see Figs 2.24A and 2.36). (A) Initially only the head is lifted off the plinth. (B) The shoulders clear plinth, along with the head. (C) Both heels are just clearing plinth (with the knees straight).

of flexibility, muscle tone and strength. A failure to treat all of these aspects relating to malalignment can result in subsequent recurrence or even an inability to achieve initial correction. An HVLA manipulation may well, for example, put a rotated vertebrae or pelvic bone back into alignment, but the malalignment may keep on recurring as long as residual asymmetrical tension in the attaching muscles or ligaments continues to exert a rotational stress on these bones. Simultaneously treating the malalignment and any asymmetry in tension is more likely to achieve long-lasting realignment and resolution of the symptoms.

In practice, simply achieving relaxation of the tight myofascial tissue may result in a spontaneous realignment of the bones. In other words, **the problem with malalignment is often more one of asymmetrical tension or tightness in the soft tissues attaching to the bones rather than the fact that the bones are not properly aligned**. For example:

1. the myofascial tissue on the concave side of a curve in the spine is put in a relaxed position and will shorten with time (see Fig. 2.38). When the curve is

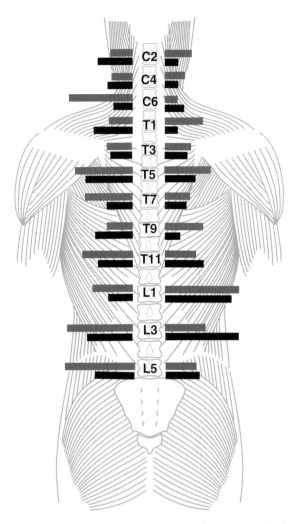

Figure 7.7 A surface electromyograph of the paravertebral muscles to detect the tension level (see the case history). The light horizontal bars indicate the findings after injury; note the asymmetry and the large number of levels showing an increased activity. The dark horizontal bars denote the findings after 3 months of treatment, including manual therapy; the asymmetry has significantly decreased, and there are now fewer levels showing increased tension. (After D.J. McCallum, unpublished data 1999, with permission.)

Case history

This 37-year-old female runner presented, following a fall downstairs, with symptoms of cervicogenic brachalgia, a left C6 and C7 dermatome referral pattern and frequent headaches. On examination in August 1998, the cervical spine range of motion was reduced in all planes of movement, the deltoid muscle weak (a score of 4/5) but the neurological screen otherwise unremarkable. In addition to a postural scoliosis, there was evidence of anterior rotation of the left innominate and rotation at the C2/3, C6/7 and T11/12 levels. Surface electromyography (SEMG) showed increased paravertebral muscle activity readings throughout the spine, worse on the left than the right and worse at the levels noted to have rotated (the light bars in Fig. 7.7). SEMG findings were consistent with postural compensation and a reactive increase in paravertebral muscle tension throughout the back.

Therapy was aimed at mobilizing the pelvis and spine, and relaxing the paravertebral muscles. On repeat examination in November 1998, the frequency of headaches had significantly decreased and the athlete was otherwise asymptomatic, the neurological screen now being negative. Repeat SEMG (the black bars in Fig. 7.7) still showed some higher readings, now localizing to the left C2–C4, left T7 and right L3 levels, probably indicative of a compensation for the changing postural pattern. The muscle tension overall was, however, significantly reduced and much more symmetrical than that recorded the previous August.

decreased or eliminated with realignment, these shortened structures, unless stretched out at the same time, will exert an asymmetrical force on the vertebrae that can result in a recurrence of the malalignment

2. the persistence of a trigger point in the right quadratus lumborum after realignment may gradually result in a general increase in tension in that muscle and cause the recurrence of a right upslip (see Fig. 2.40)

3. mobilization may effectively correct the malalignment of the pelvis initially caused by an L1 rotation that resulted in the facilitation of the iliopsoas muscle on one side and an inhibition on the other. The pelvic malalignment is, however, sure to recur if the L1 rotation, and any persistent asymmetry of tension in right compared with left iliopsoas, is not also attended to.

TECHNIQUES FOR CORRECTION OF ROTATIONAL MALALIGNMENT

Some easily learned manual therapy techniques are particularly useful for treatment of rotational malalignment in a clinic or home setting. It must be stressed at this point that none of these techniques should be painful.

> A technique may be successful in achieving alignment, but the correction is often quickly lost if the procedure has provoked pain and with it a reflex increase in asymmetrical muscle tension.

In most cases, pain can be avoided by a minor modification of the technique.

Sometimes, however, the athlete has such generalized discomfort and soft tissue ténderness that one just cannot use these techniques during the initial stages of treatment. In that case, one of the more gentle and less 'invasive' methods may be more appropriate (e.g. craniosacral release or the NUCCA technique – see Ch. 8). One can then try reintroducing these techniques at a later date once the athlete's condition has started to improve.

Muscle energy technique

> Muscle energy technique (MET) is one mobilization method particularly useful for correcting rotational malalignment, harnessing the athlete's own muscles to generate a rotational force on a specific structure.

Take the example of an athlete presenting with an anterior rotation of the right and a compensatory posterior rotation of the left innominate.

A resisted voluntary contraction of the right gluteus maximus can be harnessed to create a posterior rotational force on the right innominate in order to correct the **anterior rotation** (Fig. 7.8B). Essentially, gluteus maximus originates from the ilium behind the posterior gluteal line and inserts primarily into the greater tuberosity of the femur; if the thigh is free to move, its primary action is to extend the hip joint (Fig. 7.8A). By resisting right hip extension, however, one effectively reverses the origin and insertion (Fig. 7.8C). Gluteus maximus will now exert a posterior rotational force on the right innominate, which is still free to move. The athlete attempts to extend the hip, but this movement is prevented by having the athlete:

- hold on to the thigh or shin, with the knee flexed (Figs 7.8C and 7.9A)
- push against another person who provides the resistance needed (Fig. 7.9B).

Following each contraction, the muscle usually relaxes and lengthens a bit; one can take up the slack by letting the thigh drop towards the chest and, if tolerated, even towards the opposite shoulder (given that gluteus maximus is somewhat diagonally oriented across the buttock) before attempting the next contraction (Fig. 7.9C). For those who have knee pain with flexion, the procedure can be modified by supporting the lower leg (calf) on a chair or the helper's shoulder to decrease the knee flexion angle (Fig. 7.9D). The repeated contraction and relaxation of gluteus maximus in this manner will successfully correct an anterior rotation in 80–90% of the athletes.

Two different sets of muscles can be harnessed in order to correct a **posterior rotation** of the left innominate.

Iliacus

Iliacus originates primarily from anterior iliac crest and upper iliac fossa, inserting into the tendon of psoas major and directly into the lesser trochanter (Fig. 7.10A; see Figs 2.31B, 2.37, 2.40, 4.2 and 4.13). If the thigh is free to move, its primary action is to flex the hip joint (Fig. 7.10C). By resisting hip flexion, one effectively reverses the origin and insertion, and creates a force that will rotate the left innominate anteriorly (see Fig. 7.10C). The athlete attempts to flex the hip, but movement is prevented by:

- having the athlete provide resistance, overlapping the hands resting against the upper part of the left thigh, the elbows preferably locked (Fig. 7.11A)
- having another person provide resistance as the athlete tries to flex the left hip by pulling the thigh towards the chest (Fig. 7.11B).

Rectus femoris

Rectus femoris originates from the anterior inferior iliac spine and anterior rim of the acetabulum; it inserts indirectly into the tibial tubercle by way of the patellar tendon (Fig. 7.12A; see Figs 2.37 and 3.38). It is the only

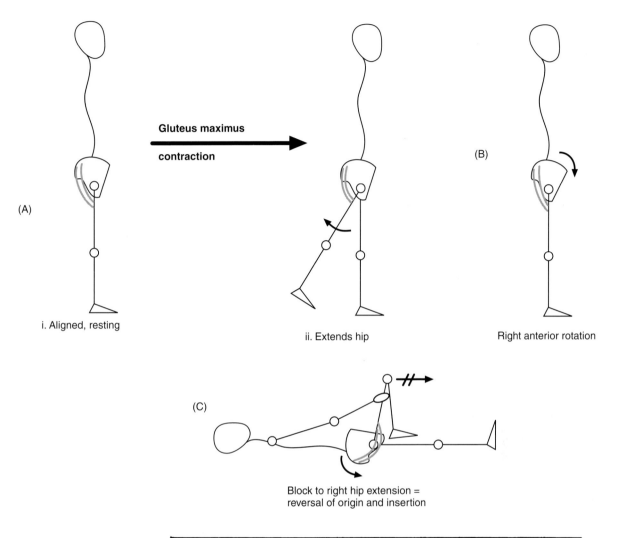

(A)

i. Aligned, resting

Gluteus maximus

contraction

ii. Extends hip

(B)

Right anterior rotation

(C)

Block to right hip extension =
reversal of origin and insertion

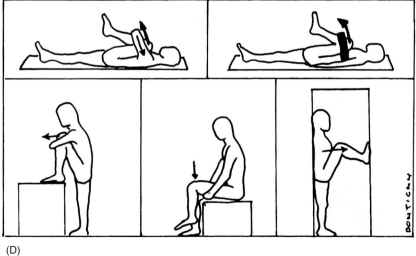

Figure 7.8 Muscle energy technique: the biomechanics of using gluteus maximus to correct a right innominate anterior rotation (B). (A) The muscle acts as a hip extensor when the leg is free to move. (C) Blocking right hip extension reverses the muscle origin and insertion, creating a posterior rotational force. (D) Muscle energy for anterior rotation initiated in a variety of positions. (From DonTigny 1997, with permission.)

(D)

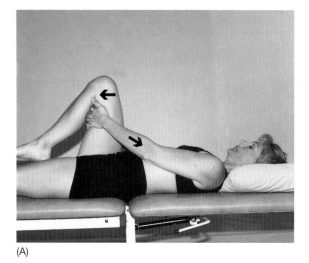

(A)

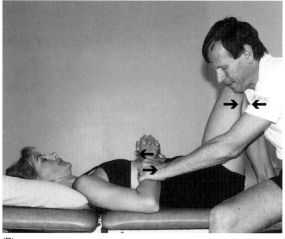

(B)

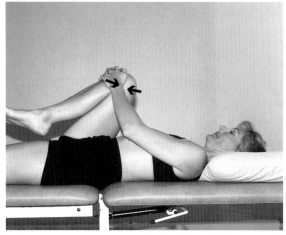

(Ci)

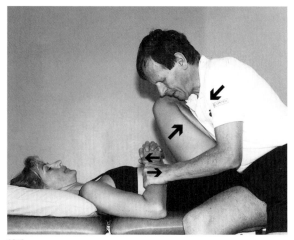

(Cii)

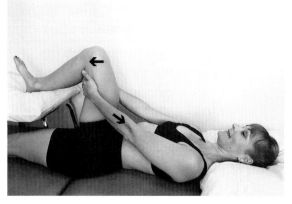

(Di)

Figure 7.9 Muscle energy technique for the correction of right innominate anterior rotation using gluteus maximus: blocking an attempted right hip extension. (A) One-person technique. (B) Two-person technique. (C) To take up any slack in the relaxing hip extensors, gradually increase the hip flexion angle (provided that this is pain-free): (i) one-person technique; (ii) two-person technique. (D) To modify the technique for painful knee (e.g. osteoarthritis or patellofemoral compartment syndrome), decrease the knee flexion angle: (i) one-person technique; (ii) two-person technique. (E) Incorrect technique: the effectiveness of hip extensor contraction is decreased by simultaneous quadriceps contraction, which is here holding the knee in 90 degrees flexion and the lower leg up in mid-air while the rectus femoris is exerting an anterior rotational force on the innominate bone (see Figs 2.31C, 2.37 and 7.12).

Fig. 7.9 (Dii) & (E), see opposite

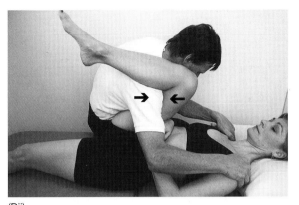

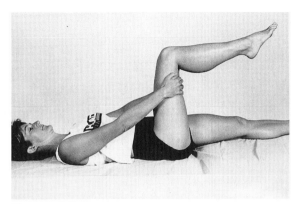

(Dii)

(E)

Figure 7.9 *Continued.*

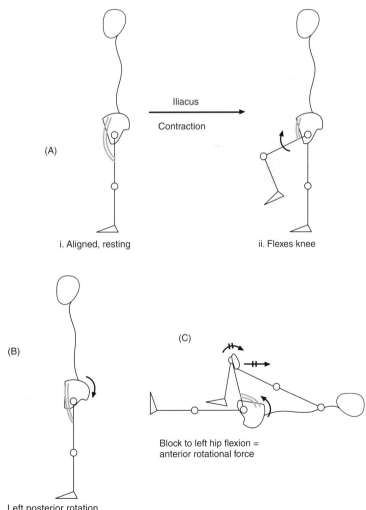

Iliacus

Contraction

(A)

i. Aligned, resting

ii. Flexes knee

(B)

(C)

Block to left hip flexion =
anterior rotational force

Figure 7.10 Muscle energy technique:
the biomechanics of using left iliacus to
correct an innominate posterior rotation
(B). The muscle acts as a hip flexor when
the thigh is free to move (A). Blocking hip
flexion reverses the muscle origin and
insertion, creating an anterior rotational
force (C).

Left posterior rotation

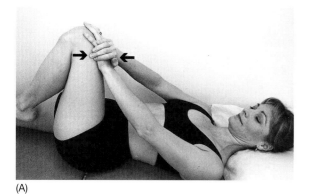

(A)

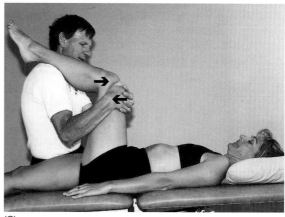

(C)

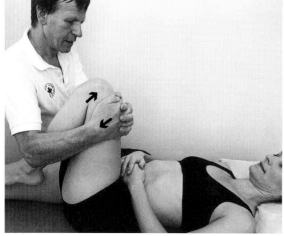

(B)

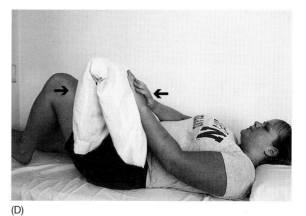

(D)

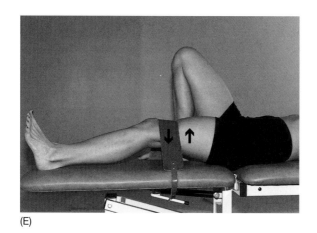

(E)

Figure 7.11　Muscle energy technique for correcting left innominate posterior rotation using iliacus: blocking attempted hip flexion. NB. The hip is maintained at 90 degrees flexion (or less, should this prove difficult or painful, for example, during pregnancy or postpartum). (A) One-person technique. (B) Two-person technique. (C) Modification for a painful left knee. (D) Modification for short arms and/or an inability to flex the hip: using a pillow to fill the gap. (E) Modified one-person technique: the fixed belt provides resistance when hip flexion is limited or proves painful at greater angles.

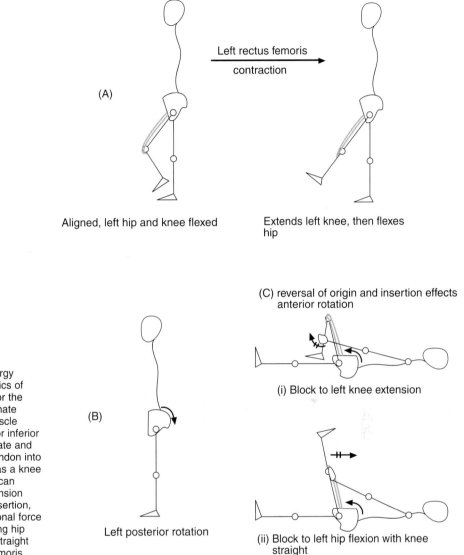

(A)

Left rectus femoris
contraction

Aligned, left hip and knee flexed

Extends left knee, then flexes
hip

(C) reversal of origin and insertion effects
anterior rotation

(i) Block to left knee extension

(B)

Left posterior rotation

(ii) Block to left hip flexion with knee
straight

Figure 7.12 Muscle energy technique: the biomechanics of using left rectus femoris for the correction of a left innominate posterior rotation. The muscle originates from the anterior inferior iliac spine on the innominate and inserts with the patellar tendon into the proximal tibia. It acts as a knee extensor when extension can occur. Blocking knee extension reverses the origin and insertion, creating an anterior rotational force on the innominate. Blocking hip flexion when the knee is straight will also engage rectus femoris.

muscle of the quadriceps complex that crosses both the hip and the knee joint so that, in addition to extending the knee, it can also flex the hip joint when the knee is in full extension (Fig. 7.12A). This muscle can therefore be effectively used to create an anterior rotational force on the posteriorly rotated left innominate (Fig. 7.12B) by:

1. blocking attempted extension of the left knee when that knee is flexed (Fig. 7.12Ci)
2. blocking attempted left hip flexion when that knee is straight (Fig. 7.12Cii).

As illustrated, a one- or two-person technique can again be used. The hip is best kept at 90 degrees flexion;

bringing it any closer increases the chance of using the femur on that side like a lever and accidentally causing a recurrence of the posterior innominate rotation (see Fig. 2.32A). The following recommendations therefore apply.

The athlete lies supine, with the hip flexed to no more than 90 degrees. When the athlete is carrying this manoeuvre out alone, he or she should hang onto a towel or wide belt placed around the shin at the level of the ankle, in order to resist the repeated attempts at knee extension (Fig. 7.13A); a sling looped around the flexed knee and secured at the other end (Fig. 7.13B) not only offers resistance to knee extension, but also

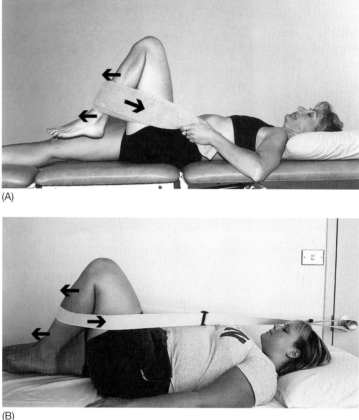

(A)

(B)

Figure 7.13 Muscle energy technique for correcting left innominate posterior rotation using rectus femoris: blocking attempted extension of the flexed left knee. (A) One-person technique (here using a towel for an extension of the arm, to avoid any posterior rotational force that could result with greater than 90 degrees hip flexion). (B) One-person technique using a sling: as an extension of the arms, to provide resistance to knee extension at a reduced left hip flexion angle, and/or as a substitute for the arms, to allow sore neck, upper back and shoulder girdle muscles to relax while doing this muscle energy technique.

allows for a relaxation of any sore neck, upper back and shoulder girdle muscles, a point to consider especially when an athlete has, for example, sustained 'whiplash' injuries.

When you are helping an athlete with this manoeuvre, you can offer resistance to knee extension:

• with your hand around the ankle (Fig. 7.13C): unfortunately, the strength in your arm is probably less than that of the quadriceps in most athletes and will therefore allow for only a suboptimal quadriceps contraction. In addition, your pelvis is fixed by sitting, so that your trunk is subjected to a unilateral rotational force that puts you at risk of going out of alignment

• with the distal part of the leg/ankle region pushing up under your armpit (Fig. 7.13D): this set-up allows you to use your body weight to counteract the quadriceps contraction more effectively, the torsional forces on your body being minimized.

The application of the technique to the wrong side will obviously only make matters worse. Two simple rules are of help here (Box 7.2).

The correction of an anterior or posterior innominate rotation will usually simultaneously resolve a coexisting SI joint movement dysfunction, such as a relative decrease of movement or actual locking (see Fig. 2.90). It may also correct a coexisting vertebral malrotation, for example the rotation of L1 typically seen in association with rotational malalignment. MET can also be used to correct the malrotation of specific vertebrae (see below).

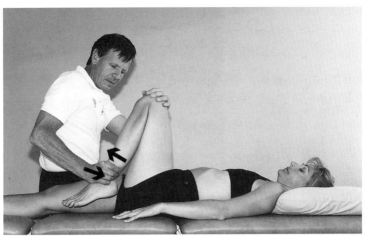

(C)

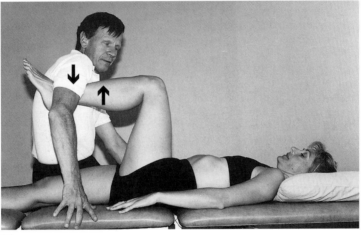

(D)

Figure 7.13 (C) Two-person technique: the twisted position of assistant's trunk increases the risk of putting himself out of alignment. (D) Improved two-person technique: the assistant can offer more resistance using his body weight to advantage, at decreased risk to himself.

Box 7.2 Rules to determine the side of muscle energy technique application

- The anterior rotation is on the side on which the leg lengthens on going from the long-sitting to supine-lying position; asymmetry of all the pelvic landmarks verifies the presentation. These examination findings and conditions that can result in a false test have been discussed in Chapters 2 and 3.
- If the anterior rotation recurs, it will probably do so on the same side. This is a safe assumption in the majority of athletes. In approximately 5–10%, the anterior rotation may be on the right side at one time and the left on another. Those who switch sides are mainly athletes who:
  - Have generalized joint hypermobility, either congenital or postpartum
  - Have suffered some recent asymmetrical stress, such as from a fall onto one side, or when carrying a heavy weight either unilaterally or awkwardly across the body, with rotation in the opposite direction from usual (e.g. going down a staircase carrying a heavy suitcase on one side)
  - Have laxity of one or both sacroiliac joints, or instability of L4 or L5 allowing rotation to either right or left

If the athlete reports pain, the MET may have to be modified as follows:

For right anterior rotation

The athlete lies supine. If the initial attempt to flex the right hip to 90 degrees proves painful, or if the initial effort to extend the right hip in the sagittal plane causes pain, try the same manoeuvre with the thigh adducted or abducted 5–10 degrees. If this makes no difference, try starting with the right hip flexion angle decreased to 60 degrees or even less, resistance being provided by a helper (Fig. 7.14A) or by lengthening the reach using a towel or wide belt (Fig. 7.14B). The manoeuvre can even be performed with the right leg lying almost straight and hip extension attempted against the forearm of the helper, whose hand is secured on the athlete's opposite (left) thigh (Fig. 7.14C).

The mechanical advantage of gluteus maximus decreases as the right hip flexion angle is decreased, but most athletes will still derive benefit with repeated contractions. In these situations in particular (e.g. postpartum), the emphasis is on *repetitions* rather than on the strength of the contractions.

If pain does not occur until some point after the right hip has already been flexed to more than 90 degrees with progressive stretching and relaxation of the gluteus maximus, simply bring the thigh back to the previous position that did not provoke pain. After repeating the manoeuvre a few times in that position, try it once more at an increased hip flexion angle to see whether that still provokes pain. If it does, go back to the previous pain-free position and stay there from then on. It may be that progressive right hip flexion is provoking pain by:

- Putting tender posterior pelvic ligaments and buttock muscles under increasing tension
- Compressing a tense and tender right iliopsoas muscle, which is particularly vulnerable within its narrow space when hip flexion is combined with adduction.

Left posterior rotation

The athlete lies supine, the left hip flexed to 90 degrees and repeatedly resisting either left hip flexion or left knee extension, for a set of 6–10 times each (see Figs 7.10–7.13). If either manoeuvre proves painful, the athlete may have to try changing the angle of the thigh, decrease the strength of the contractions or abandon one or both manoeuvres for the time being. Concentrating on the correction of the right anterior rotation (see Figs 7.8 and 7.9) will often actually result

in simultaneous correction of what amounted to a compensatory contralateral (left) posterior rotation.

> Always remind the athlete to relax all the muscles other than those needed for a particular MET manoeuvre.

The most common mistake is to tense up the muscles in the neck and upper back region while hanging on to the towel or belt to provide the required resistance. Worse still is actually to raise the head and/or shoulders off the plinth. Tensing these muscles inevitably results in a domino-like involvement of the abdominal, erector spinae and other trunk muscles, all the way down to their attachments to the superior pubic rami, iliac crests and the thoracodorsal fascia. A contraction of these muscles can easily interfere with achieving rotation of the innominates in the desired direction.

Contract–relax

The contract–relax method is one way of achieving both progressive relaxation and realignment.

> The relaxation of a muscle following an isometric contraction is usually more profound than can be achieved voluntarily.

Sometimes just relaxing any tense attaching muscles allows the bones to rotate back into proper alignment. This is the same principle as the hold–relax method used to treat localized muscle spasm. The decrease in tension following each contraction allows for the further passive movement of a body part into the direction of the restriction.

The contract–relax manoeuvre can be useful for the correction of innominate rotation, in particular the rotation and displacement that occurs anteriorly at the symphysis pubis. Realignment of the pubic bones, for example, may be achieved by alternate bilateral hip abduction and adduction against resistance while sitting or lying supine (Fig. 7.15). The symmetrical activation of these muscles exerts an equal pull on pelvic structures that are in an asymmetrical position to begin with, thereby allowing them to come back to the midline or to a 'neutral' position. The technique is covered in some detail below under 'Self-help techniques to correct malalignment' (pp. 346–348).

When malalignment is present, there is often increased tone in the left hip abductors and right piriformis, which exert opposite rotational forces on the lower extremities. Asymmetrical tension in the piriformis also creates a sacral torsion strain by way of its

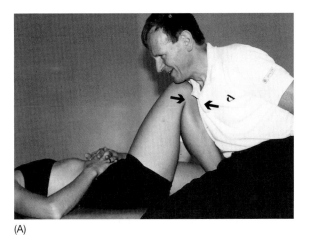

(A)

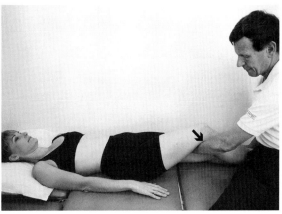

(Ci)

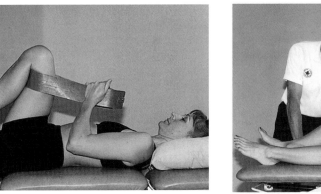

(Bi)

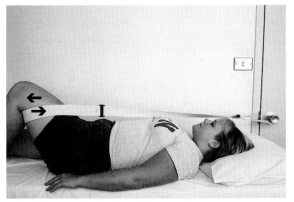

(Cii)

(Bii)

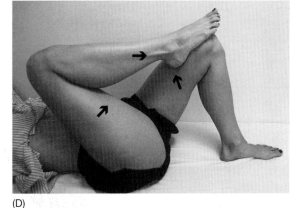

(D)

Figure 7.14 Modifications of the muscle energy technique using resisted hip extensor contraction for the correction of anterior innominate rotation. (A) Decreasing the hip flexion angle to avoid pain. (B) Using a towel or wide belt: (i) to serve as an extension for short arms; (ii) to allow for a decrease in the hip flexion angle and/or a relaxation of the neck/upper back muscles during the manoeuvre. (C) When the hip flexion angle needs to be markedly reduced because of obstruction (e.g. during maternity) or pain (e.g. postpartum or after surgery). The assistant's forearm: (i) can provide resistance; (ii) can be steadied by securing the hand on top of the opposite thigh. (D) Simultaneous resisted right hip extension (versus right anterior rotation) and left hip flexion (versus posterior rotation).

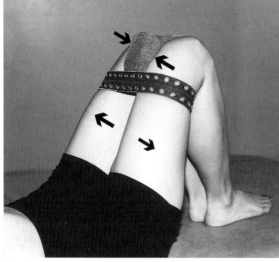

(A)

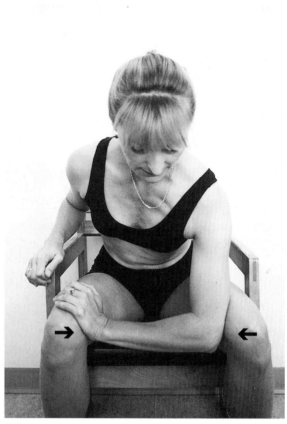

(Bii)

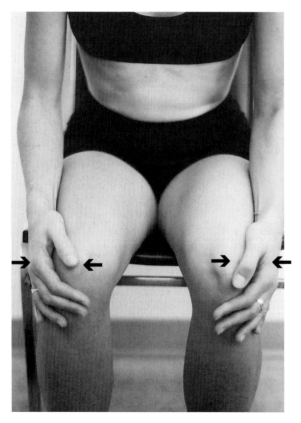

(Bi)

Figure 7.15 Contract–relax method for the correction of innominate rotation: alternating simultaneous right and left resisted hip abduction and adduction. (A) One-person technique lying supine: a belt acts to resist abduction, with a cushion between the knees to prevent bruising on adduction. (B) One-person technique sitting: (i) the hands (or chair arms) resist abduction; (ii) the forearm resists adduction. (C) Two-person technique lying supine: (i) resisted abduction (ii) resisted adduction.

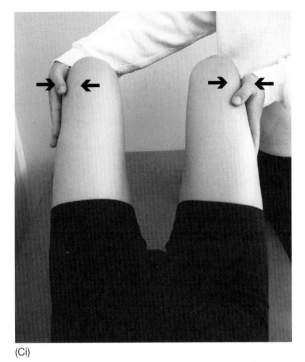

(Ci)

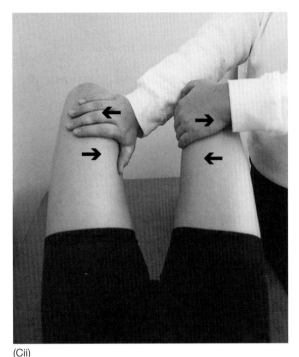

(Cii)

Figure 7.15 *Continued.*

origins from the anterosuperior aspect of the sacrum (see Fig. 2.31A). The hip abductors and the external rotators of the thigh can be activated by resisting bilateral hip abduction while lying supine or sitting, maintaining the hips in a flexed position, the knees some 20–40 cm apart and the feet together (Fig. 7.15). The repeated simultaneous isometric contraction of these muscles may correct a sacral torsion or rotation of the lower extremities, and cause relaxation to the point of re-establishing symmetry of muscle tension.

Simultaneous hip adduction against resistance with the knees held 20–30 cm apart reverses the adductor origin and insertion, resulting in a symmetrical traction force on the inferior pubic rami (Fig. 7.15). These forces can sometimes re-establish symmetry at the symphysis pubis. It may do so by temporarily separating the symphysis and then allowing the adjoining pubic bones to fall back into the normal, aligned position as the adductors relax. It is this separation that is felt to be responsible for the frequently reported sensation of something having 'moved' in the region of the symphysis, often accompanied by an audible popping sound, much like 'popping' a knuckle.

Reassessment may show the partial or complete reduction of a previously noted step deformity at the symphysis and even the correction of rotational

malalignment, suggesting that the manoeuvre can also exert a rotational force on the innominates through the previously asymmetrical pubic bones, to bring them all back to the neutral point.

Pain experienced with this technique is primarily attributable to contracting the muscles too forcefully, too often or both.

> Athletes easily get caught up in thinking that 'more is better' and can end up with an 'overuse' type pain.

The hip adductors and abductors seem particularly vulnerable, perhaps because they are not likely to be very strong muscles in comparison with the hamstrings and quadriceps, except in goalies and others who repeatedly adduct and abduct the legs as part of their sport. Discomfort from overuse may not be felt for some hours after an overzealous attempt at this manoeuvre. Therefore, the following guidelines seem appropriate:

- Limit the strength of the contraction to 50% of maximum to start with
- Do only five repeats to a slow count of 3 initially; add one more contraction each week until you are up to a total of 10

- Once 10 repeats at 50% strength are easy, progressively increase either the length or the strength of the contractions.

Leverage to effect counter-rotation

The femur can act like a lever to effect rotation of the ipsilateral innominate. Progressive hip flexion, for example, eventually puts the posterior soft tissues under maximum tension and causes the femur to impinge on the anterosuperior rim of the acetabulum (see Fig. 2.32A). At that point, further passive hip flexion creates a mechanical force capable of rotating the innominate posteriorly. Progressive hip extension will eventually have the opposite effect: anterior rotation of the innominate (see Fig. 2.32B). This leverage effect can sometimes be used to correct a rotational malalignment. Passive right hip flexion carried out with the athlete lying supine may, for example, correct for an anterior rotation on that side (Fig. 7.16A). Passive left hip extension with the athlete lying prone may correct for a posterior rotation (Fig. 7.16B). Leverage forces for the correction of a right anterior, left posterior rotation can also be achieved by:

1. pushing the right thigh onto the athlete's chest while applying a gentle downward pressure on the left thigh (or letting it hang freely over the edge of the bed - see Fig. 7.16C), to force the left hip into extension

- *Combined trunk and hip flexion* (Fig. 7.17):
  - the athlete's right foot is securely placed on a fairly high support
  - the athlete then lets the trunk bend forwards as far as comfortably possible, the head and arms hanging down in a relaxed position, to help to exaggerate right hip flexion and create a right posterior rotational force
- *A modified lunge* (Fig. 7.18):
  - the athlete puts the right foot up on a chair or other high support, with the knee flexed
  - the left foot is on the floor behind, the knee being in full extension
  - leaning forwards with the trunk, and allowing the pelvis to gradually sink downwards, the athlete turns the right and left femurs into levers capable of exerting a posterior and anterior rotational force on their respective innominates.

Leverage manoeuvres may cause pain from stressing a degenerating hip joint or an inflamed or malaligned SI joint. More often, pain arises from putting tense and tender structures under even more tension. For example, passive hip flexion on the side of the anterior rotation, especially with the knee straight, typically precipitates pain from the involved piriformis and hamstring muscles, and posterior pelvic ligaments, passive hip extension on the side of the posterior rotation, pain from a tender iliacus, rectus femoris, tensor fascia lata (TFL) or anterior SI joint ligament. The vigour with which counter-rotation manoeuvres can be carried out should be guided by the attempt to avoid, if at all possible, precipitating any pain and triggering reflex muscle spasm.

TECHNIQUES FOR CORRECTION OF A SACROILIAC JOINT UPSLIP

Gradual relaxation of the hip girdle muscles achieved with traction may allow the SI joint on that side to 'come down' and resume its intended position. This manoeuvre lends itself to a one- or two-person approach. Repeatedly having someone apply a steady downward traction force 10–12 times to the leg on the side of the upslip may be adequate to resolve the problem with time (Fig. 7.19A). When alone, the athlete can try standing with a weight attached to the foot and the leg freely suspended on the side of the upslip (Fig. 7.19B). This approach is described in more detail under 'Self-help techniques to correct malalignment', below (pp. 346–348).

Manipulation is particularly helpful for correcting some types of malalignment. An SI joint upslip, for example, can usually be corrected with quick downward traction on the leg. The exact position of the innominate needs, however, to be determined in order to establish how the manoeuvre should be carried out. The reader is referred to Lee (1999), Lee & Walsh (1996) and Vleeming et al (1997) for further reading on this topic, and should have supervised hands-on training before applying these techniques to athletes.

Basically, the athlete is asked to lie in either the supine or the prone position. The therapist gets a firm hold of the ankle on the side of the upslip, moves the leg into position – with the hip flexed, extended or in neutral depending on the examination findings – and then gently moves it about in order to ensure complete relaxation of the hip girdle muscles. The athlete is distracted by keeping up a conversation, and a traction force is exerted by pulling downwards on the extremity. Another technique is to have the athlete concentrate on breathing in and out. Sudden traction is applied during the exhalation phase on the second or third cycle.

Successful reduction is usually indicated by the sensation of a joint having moved, similar to the feeling associated with 'popping' a knuckle.

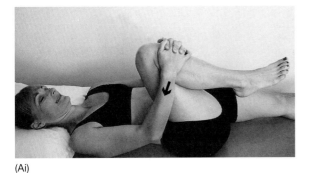

(Ai)

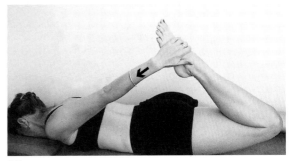

(Bi)

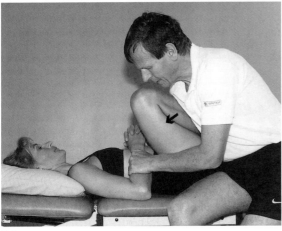

(Aii)

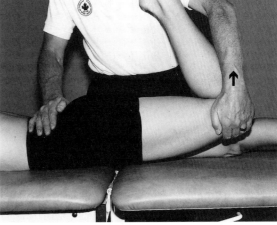

(Bii)

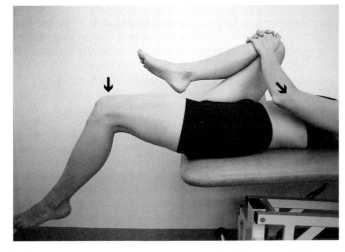

(C)

Figure 7.16 Using a leverage effect to correct rotational malalignment. (A) Passive hip flexion to counteract right anterior rotation: (i) one-person technique; (ii) two-person technique. (B) Passive hip extension to counteract left posterior rotation: (i) one-person technique; (ii) two-person technique. (C) Simultaneous correction of right anterior and left posterior rotation by passive right hip flexion and left hip extension respectively.

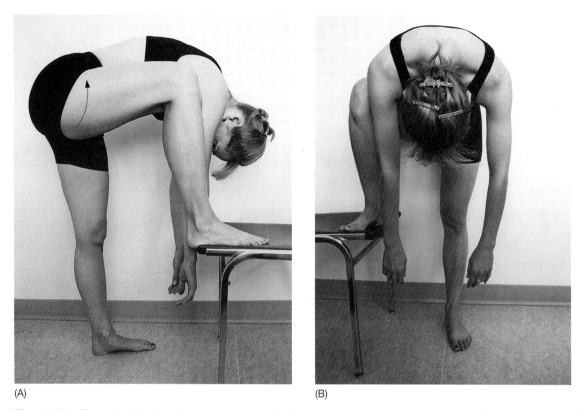

(A)

(B)

Figure 7.17 To correct right innominate anterior rotation, a right posterior leverage effect can be created by resting the right foot on a high support and then letting the trunk hang down in forward flexion as far as feels comfortable.

This sensation can be felt by the therapist as it is transmitted through the femur and tibia down to his or her hands around the ankle. There is sometimes also an audible sound. The athlete may spontaneously report the feeling of one bone having slotted into proper alignment with another. It just 'feels right again', and the discomfort is often immediately decreased or abolished. If the athlete's anatomical leg length is equal, successful reduction is confirmed by finding that leg length once again matches on the long-sitting to supine-lying test, and the pelvis is level in both sitting and standing (see Figs 2.50 and 2.51A). The bony landmarks and hip ranges of motion will be symmetrical.

Several attempts may be required to achieve correction. Even when the manoeuvre appears to have failed to achieve complete correction, one will usually afterwards note a change for the better. Leg length difference (LLD), for example, may have been reduced, and the hip ranges of motion become less asymmetrical. The stretch imparted by repeated downward traction has probably relaxed whichever hip girdle muscle or muscles (e.g. iliopsoas and quadratus lumborum) that

have been exerting an upward pull on the innominate and displacing it relative to the sacrum (see Fig. 2.40). It is for this reason that it may still be worthwhile carrying out the traction and/or manipulation on a repeated basis in the hope that this will relax the muscle(s) enough eventually to allow these bones to slot back into normal alignment.

TECHNIQUE FOR CORRECTION OF OUTFLARE AND INFLARE

Outflare and inflare occur normally with pelvic movement (see Figs 2.10 and 2.14). Excessive outflare or inflare can occur in isolation, but the most common presentation is with outflare on one side and inflare on the other (see Figs 2.10 and 4.25). When associated with rotational malalignment, inflare is often seen with an anterior and outflare with a posterior rotation, but the reverse findings are not uncommon. Correction of the outflare using MET:

- often resolves a contralateral inflare

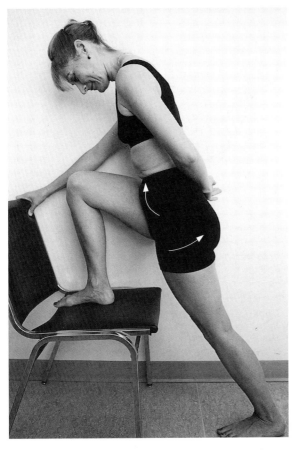

Figure 7.18 When there is a right anterior, left posterior rotation, this modified lunge position (right foot forwards and up on a support, left leg in extension with the foot on the floor) simultaneously creates a right posterior and left anterior rotational force.

- may be necessary before a coexisting rotational malalignment will respond to attempts at correction
- may simultaneously correct a coexisting rotational malalignment or upslip, regardless of whether these are on the same side as the outflare.

If an outflare co-exists with an upslip and/or rotational malalignment, it seems appropriate initially to attempt correction of the outflare, given that it will usually correct the other conditions simultaneously. A right outflare may correct with an MET that uses the resisted contraction of what are primarily the following muscles (Fig. 7.20):

1. posteriorly: primarily the external rotators and abductors of the hip, whose posteromedial origins from the innominate allows them to pull this part of

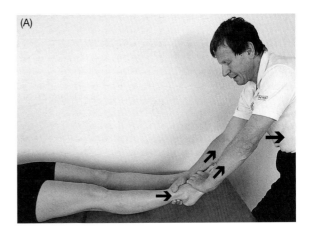

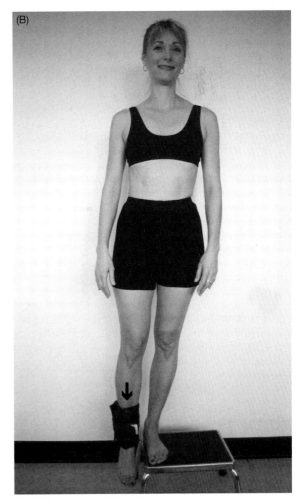

Figure 7.19 Correction of a right upslip with traction on the leg. (A) Two-person approach: repetitively pulling down on the leg. (B) One-person approach: using a weight suspended from the foot.

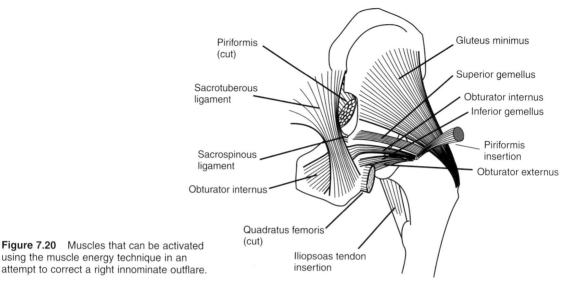

Figure 7.20 Muscles that can be activated using the muscle energy technique in an attempt to correct a right innominate outflare.

the innominate laterally on reversal of their origin and insertion

- obturator internus and externus (from the ischiopubic ramus)
- superorior gemellus (from the outer surface of the ischial spine)
- inferior gemellus (from the ischial tuberosity)
- quadratus femoris (from the ischial tuberosity)
- to some extent, the inferomedial part of the origins of gluteus maximus and minimus (from the posterior ilium)
- piriformis (through its origins from the greater sciatic notch area)

2. anteriorly: primarily iliacus which, through its superolateral origins from the innominate, can pull it medially.

A simultaneous left inflare can be corrected using primarily adductor longus and magnus which originate from the inferior pubic ramus and outer inferior ischial tuberosity and are, therefore, capable of rotating the innominate outward on reversal of origin and insertion.

For a right outflare, the supine-lying athlete would undergo the sequence shown in Box 7.3.

In other words:

- with a right *outflare*, the right leg is in external rotation so that the right knee drops *outwards*, and resistance is applied to the *outer aspect* of the right knee as the athlete attempted to push it *outwards*
- with a left *inflare*, the left leg is also positioned in external rotation, but resistance is applied to the *inner* aspect of the knee as the athlete attempts to push it *inwards*.

Box 7.3 Technique to correct right outflare

- Flex the left hip and knee, leaving the left foot on the plinth
- Flex the right hip and externally rotate the thigh in order to place the lateral aspect of the right ankle against the anterior aspect of the left thigh (the so-called 'figure-4' position)
- Carry out a set of four or five contractions against a resistance supplied by either the athlete (Fig. 7.21A) or a helper (Fig. 7.21D) against the outer aspect of the right knee; with these contractions, the athlete is attempting simultaneously to externally rotate, abduct and extend the right thigh
- Carry out three further sets of four resisted contractions
- After each set of four contractions, progressively increase passive left hip flexion, which results in:
  - the left foot rising gradually further off the plinth (Fig. 7.21B)
  - a progressive increase in passive right hip flexion (and external rotation), which will increase the tension in most of the muscles activated – particularly piriformis – by taking up any slack after each contraction, in order to make the next contraction more effective
- The correction of right outflare is then followed by a correction of left inflare, if this has not already occurred:
  - the left leg is held in external rotation, the left foot being anchored by the flexed right thigh
  - pressure is applied to the medial aspect of the left knee, to resist attempted internal rotation of that leg (Fig. 7.21C)
- Reassessment and a repeat of the manoeuvres if the outflare is still present
- Once the outflare is no longer evident, the correction of any residual rotational malalignment (or upslip)

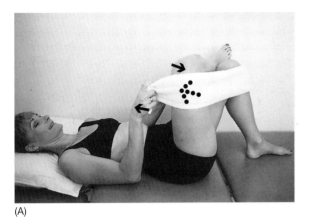

(A)

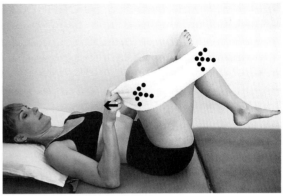

(B)

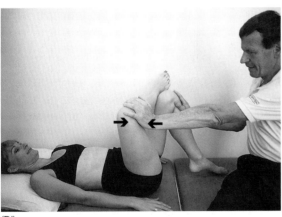

(Ci)

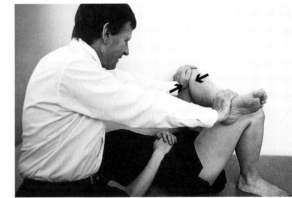

(Cii)

(Di)

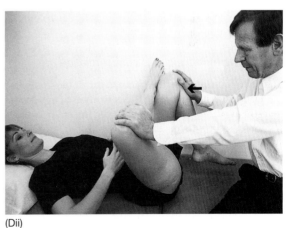

(Dii)

Figure 7.21 Muscle energy technique: to correct a right outflare. Note the starting position for resisting right external rotation, with the right foot anchored on the left thigh and the left foot resting on the plinth (A). (A) A towel against the right anterolateral knee provides resistance (dotted arrow) against active right external rotation. (B) A towel against the right and left shin helps passively (dotted arrows) to increase bilateral hip flexion after every set of four resisted contractions (as in Fig. 7.21A). (C) The reverse manoeuvre to counteract left inflare: resisting left internal rotation: (i) one-person technique; (ii) two-person technique. (D) Two-person technique for resisted external rotation: (i) starting position; (ii) progressing by passively increasing left hip flexion with pressure against the left shin after every set of four resisted contractions.

SELF HELP TECHNIQUES TO CORRECT MALALIGNMENT

> It cannot be stressed enough that a lasting correction of the malalignment will be achieved more quickly if the athlete can supplement this formal treatment with a regular home exercise programme.

Visits to a therapist usually occur once, twice or even three times a week initially and are subsequently tapered to increasing intervals as the athlete starts to respond. However, it serves little purpose to have the therapist correct the malalignment only to have the athlete lose that correction within hours or days and then wait, out of alignment, until the next formal treatment session. Any recurrence of malalignment between treatments is a step backwards because it keeps subjecting the pelvis, spine, limbs and attaching soft tissues to ongoing stresses and strains. Recurrences also interfere with the gradual adaptation that myofascial tissue has to undergo in order eventually to readjust to the aligned position.

If recurrence during these intervals between formal treatment sessions can be minimized or prevented altogether, the whole treatment process can be expected to take less time to complete and to be much more effective in returning the athlete to full activity.

Correction of rotational malalignment

If recurrent rotational malalignment is one of the problems, a home programme with the following components is recommended.

Muscle energy technique to correct rotation

The technique, as described above, can achieve several things. First, it may result in the correction of any recurrence(s) of malalignment between the formal treatment sessions. Second, even though it may fail to achieve 100% correction, it can usually decrease the extent of the rotation and will, in doing so, often decrease discomfort.

It can also play an important part in helping to maintain correction because it results in a strengthening specifically of those muscles which help to counteract anterior rotation on one side (e.g. gluteus maximus) and posterior rotation on other (e.g. rectus femoris and iliacus).

> Finally, a home muscle energy technique programme allows the athlete to carry out a self-reduction manoeuvre whenever and wherever malalignment recurs. This is particularly important when formal help is not immediately available.

A typical example is that of the skier who has taken a fall and afterwards notes difficulty executing turns to the left because the recurrence of a left posterior innominate rotation is restricting left pelvic rotation in the transverse plane (see Fig. 3.4C). Successful self-correction of the rotational malalignment right there on the slope, using the MET outlined above, will allow for immediate return to unhindered skiing. It will also prevent, or at least help to minimize, any recurrence of symptoms that are the result of the increased stress on skeletal and soft tissue structures associated with malalignment, a phenomenon that is definitely time-contingent: the longer any one recurrence of the malalignment is allowed to persist, the more likely it is that these same structures will again become symptomatic.

The athlete is instructed to:

1. start by resisting hip extension 6–10 times on the side of the anterior rotation (see Figs 7.8 and 7.9), taking up any slack in the gluteus maximus following each contraction (by letting the knee drop towards the chest)

2. follow this with resisting hip flexion (see Figs 7.10 and 7.11) and knee extension (see Figs 7.12 and 7.13) 6–10 times each on the side of the posterior rotation

3. repeat the manoeuvre of resisted hip extension on the side of the anterior rotation 6–10 times more, after which it is time to

4. recheck to see whether realignment has been achieved; if not, the above sequence can be repeated and another check made.

If there is any pain on attempting correction of the anterior rotation, the athlete can often avoid this by trying resisted hip extension with the thigh moved further away in order to decrease the hip flexion angle. The thigh may, however, end up so far away that it is out of reach. In this case, the athlete can usually compensate by using a towel or wide belt, either around the back of the thigh or over the upper part of the shin (see Figs 7.13 and 7.14B).

Contract–relax of hip abductors and adductors

The athlete can do this manoeuvre alone in a number of ways.

Lying supine, the hips and knees flexed to 90 degrees (see Fig. 7.15A)

● *Abduction phase*: resistance to abduction is best achieved using a broad belt. The loop is slipped directly around the upper part of the thighs or over the flexed knees and should encircle the thighs just below the popliteal space or 5–10 cm below the patellae respectively (see Fig. 7.15A). The knees should be able to separate by about 20–30 cm on attempted abduction

- *Adduction phase*: a cushion or ball placed between the knees protects the inside of the knees from bruising on adduction.

Sitting

- *Abduction phase* (Fig. 7.15Bi): the athlete can push with the hands against the outside of the knees to resist repeated attempts at abducting both thighs simultaneously. Alternatively, the arm rests of a chair or a narrow doorway or other arrangement can serve to stop abduction
- *Adduction phase* (Fig. 7.15Bii): adduction can easily be resisted by wedging a forearm between the knees, the elbow flexed to 90 degree. The inside of the knee on one side ends up pushing against the arm just above the olecranon, the other against the heel of the hand, with the wrist in extension.

Leverage manoeuvres

The leverage principle can also be incorporated into some effective self-help manoeuvres that attempt to correct both an anterior and posterior rotation simultaneously:

1. The athlete sits over the edge of the bed or plinth, then lies back supine and starts gradually to pull the thigh on the side of the anterior rotation onto the chest. At the same time, the thigh on the side of the posterior rotation passively extends as it hangs over the edge (see Fig. 7.16C).
2. The foot on the side of the anterior rotation is put on a fairly high support (see Fig. 7.17A). The trunk is then allowed to hang forwards and down so that the right thigh ends up alongside the chest (see Fig. 7.17B). This manoeuvre, which results in acute flexion of the thigh, is often described by the athletes as being probably more effective than techniques (1) and (3).
3. The athlete can put the foot on the side of the anterior rotation up on a chair or other type of raised support (see Fig. 7.18). The other foot remains on the ground, the hip and knee on that side fully extended. The body is then allowed to lean forwards into the 'sprint start' or 'lunge' position in order slowly to hyperflex the hip on the side of the anterior rotation while at the same time hyperextending the hip on the side of the posterior rotation. The athlete should be warned to avoid bouncing but instead to sink down gradually and hold that position for 30–60 seconds, like a stretch. The manoeuvre should be repeated four or five times in succession.

These simple manoeuvres have an advantage in that the athlete does not have to lie down, so they can easily be carried out anywhere: in the home or office, by the playing field or while travelling. They can afford many athletes at the very least some temporary relief.

Sacroiliac joint upslip

If the problem is one of an upslip that fails to correct or that keeps recurring, the athlete should be instructed in a daily home traction programme. For the athlete with a recurrent right upslip the following can be tried.

One approach has the athlete lying either supine or prone while someone exerts a steady downward pull on the right leg for 30–60 seconds, followed by complete relaxation (Fig. 7.19A). A check should be done after 10–12 traction–relaxation cycles to decide whether further treatment is needed.

The athlete can also stand with the left leg up on a stool, chair or staircase and initially hang the affected right leg down over the side with a weight attached (see Fig. 7.19B). The progressive addition of wrap-on ankle weights may suffice. Alternatively, the athlete can start with a hiking or ski boot, which serves as a basic weight of approximately 2–3 kg as well as helping to protect the skin and allow for the gradual addition of further weight in 1 kg increments every 3 or 4 days as tolerated. This progressive increase in weight can be achieved simply by hanging a small bucket containing an increasing amount of water or sand from the boot, or a bag gradually filled with hand-weights, cans of food and so on. Most athletes can eventually hold 7–9 kg.

Traction is applied for 15–30 minutes once or twice a day. While the weight is attached, the athlete is encouraged to move the right leg gently through a limited range of motion at the hip joint (e.g. circumduction through no more than 15–20 degrees). This movement, combined with the traction, gradually helps to relax the muscles and stretch out any tight structures in the hip girdle and pelvic region in order to allow for a reduction of the upslip.

Recurrences of the upslip may be decreased in frequency, or altogether prevented, by carrying out traction manoeuvres on a regular basis, both before and immediately after any activity likely to precipitate a recurrence.

Correction of outflare and inflare

The MET manoeuvres described above for the correction of these presentations can be carried out with the athlete providing the required resistance (Fig. 7.21A above). In the case of a right outflare, this is done by having a towel or sheet cross the right anterolateral knee region and the left upper shin. This support can be used to provide the force required to prevent the right knee moving. It can also be used to bring the left thigh gradually closer to the trunk after each set of four contractions, simply by pulling on both ends to increase the overall tension in the set-up (Fig. 7.21B above).

INSTRUCTION IN SELF-ASSESSMENT AND MOBILIZATION

Athletes presenting with the malalignment syndrome who will benefit from carrying out mobilization exercises at home are given a handout describing how to carry out the self-assessment to determine whether or not they are out of alignment in the first place and, if so, whether there is an upslip, a rotational malalignment, outflare and/or inflare or a combination of these. The handout instructs them how to carry out the appropriate MET, traction or other manoeuvre, either on their own or with someone's help. Athletes receive the handout after having been taught how to do the exercises by their therapist as part of the treatment sessions and by the author at the time of initial assessment or reassessment.

They are also asked to attend a 3-hour workshop that the author holds once a month in order to:

- give the athletes a better understanding of the changes and problems seen in association with the malalignment syndrome in order to make it easier to recognize whether or not they are in or out of alignment
- review the contents of the handout
- do a 'hands-on' demonstration of the self-assessment and self-treatment techniques for the various presentations
- stress the avoidance of inappropriate activities, especially those which are asymmetrical or have a torsional component
- discuss the alternate treatment options (e.g. orthotics, or SI belt or ligament injections).

> Athletes are reminded that self-help techniques are no substitute for a formal treatment programme but are intended to supplement it.

The athlete's efforts should be regarded as helping to maintain day-by-day correction, whereas the therapist does the 'fine-tuning'.

In addition, it is emphasized that the self-help manoeuvres should not provoke pain, for fear that pain may trigger reflex spasm, result in a loss of any correction that has been achieved or discourage the athlete from continuing with this approach. It is always wise to have the athlete demonstrate on a subsequent visit how he or she carries out the self-assessment and self-treatment manoeuvres in order to ensure that these are being done correctly.

POST-REDUCTION SYNDROME

Following a successful correction of vertebral malrotation or pelvic malalignment, some athletes experience discomfort from areas that were previously asymptomatic. A typical example is that of the athlete with one of the 'alternate' presentations who has been complaining of discomfort from a tense and tender left TFL/iliotibial band (ITB) complex. Following realignment, he or she is suddenly bothered with symptoms from the same complex on the right side. This phenomenon can be easily explained on the basis of:

1. the shortening of soft tissues put in a relaxed position during the time that malalignment was present. In the example, the tendency to right medial weight-bearing decreased tension in the right TFL/ITB complex and eventually caused it to shorten. In contrast, the tendency to left lateral weight-bearing, facilitation and other factors increased tension in the left TFL/ITB and caused it to lengthen (see Figs 3.33, 3.37, 3.39, 3.40, 4.1 and 4.4).

2. the redistribution of stresses that occurs with realignment. In the example, tension in the shortened right TFL/ITB complex will increase as weight-bearing on the right side shifts from being medial to becoming more neutral or even lateral on realignment (see Fig. 3.29).

Symptoms may occur in the form of localized discomfort and/or referred pain or paraesthesias originating from the affected structure(s). These symptoms usually disappear within 2–4 weeks with natural tissue adaptation supplemented by appropriate stretching.

EXERCISE

During the initial stage of treatment, emphasis should be on symmetrical routines and on strengthening the thoracic and pelvic core muscles in order to increase stability and decrease the chance of recurrence of malalignment. Graduated increases are advised to allow for progressive improvement and to minimize the chance of precipitating pain and reflex muscle spasm.

CONTRA-INDICATED ACTIVITIES

Malalignment presents primarily as a musculoskeletal problem, but the definitive treatment is realignment. Standard treatment approaches to musculoskeletal problems emphasize specific stretching, strengthening and flexibility routines. In the face of malalignment, some of these standard approaches and certain sports activities are contraindicated because they are more likely to cause recurrence of malalignment and/or put the athlete at increased risk of injury.

Contraindicated stretches

As indicated in Chapter 3, malalignment results in an increase in tension in certain muscles. This increase may be the result of a mechanical separation of origin and insertion, a response to pain or instability, or a facilitation, with a change in the setting of the muscle spindle effected at a spinal segmental or possibly even cortical level. A chronic increase in tension eventually results in tenderness to palpation of these muscles, their tendons and points of attachment. Discomfort from these sites perpetuates the increase in tension and initiates a vicious cycle.

It is important to note that some of the standard treatment approaches to muscles that are tight and tender are unlikely to be helpful and may in fact cause further harm.

Stretching a tight muscle may fail if the increase in tension is occurring on the basis of malalignment and/or in reaction to a chronic source of pain. Stretching attempted under these conditions in fact increases the chance of perpetuating the problem by temporarily causing a further restriction of the inflow and exit of blood, increasing tension on the points of attachment and precipitating more pain.

This is not to preclude the gentle stretching that is often carried out:

- to relax muscles just prior to attempts at mobilization
- to decrease any residual increase in tension noted after realignment and thereby decrease the chance of the subsequent recurrence of malalignment.

All muscles that show an increase in tone and tenderness should be included in the routine. Graduated stretching should be carried out three or four, if possible even five or six times a day. Stretching a muscle–tendon unit once or twice a day only lets it creep back to its shortened state in the interval and slows the rate of recovery.

The athlete, unless otherwise instructed, is asked to carry out only symmetrical stretches. Unilateral stretches that exert a rotational force on the innominate bone are frequently the cause of a recurrence of malalignment, hence the emphasis on symmetrical stretching, avoiding any twisting of the trunk, pelvis or extremities. If symmetrical stretching is not possible, the athlete should be cautioned to avoid stretching in a way that creates a torquing effect on the pelvis or that turns the thigh into a lever arm on the innominate. Consider, for example, the following stretches carried out by an athlete who suffers from recurrent right anterior, left posterior innominate rotation:

1. A left hamstring stretch while standing with the left leg up on a fence rail or other support (Fig. 7.22A): as the trunk leans progressively forward, the increasing tension in gluteus maximus and the hamstrings, in addition to the lever effect of the femur, come to exert an unwanted posterior rotational force on the left innominate.
2. A right quadriceps muscle stretch in prone-lying or standing (Fig. 7.22B; see Fig. 3.38). As the hip is progressively extended, the increasing tension in rectus femoris and iliacus, and the lever effect of the femur, all come to exert an unwanted anterior rotational force on the right innominate.

Unilateral stretches carried out on the appropriate side can be used effectively to correct a rotation, but initially that should only be attempted under the express guidance of a therapist. Intensive stretching on one side, in an effort to achieve the same range of motion in a given direction as is possible on the other side, may lead to grief. In the presence of malalignment, a muscle may not be able to respond to such a stretch for completely different reasons. Inability to stretch the hamstrings, for example, may result for the following reasons.

Standing hamstring stretch

The athlete with a right anterior, left posterior innominate rotation may find that, in standing with the right leg propped up on a support, there is a limitation when attempting a right hamstring stretch by bending the trunk forward towards the right leg compared with carrying out the same stretch on the left side (Fig. 7.22C). The right limitation comes from the fact that:

- tension has been increased by a separation of right hamstring origin and insertion (see Fig. 3.38) and probably also by an automatic increase in tension (facilitation)
- anterior rotation of the right innominate bone creates a mechanical block to right hip flexion (see Figs 3.64 and 3.65).

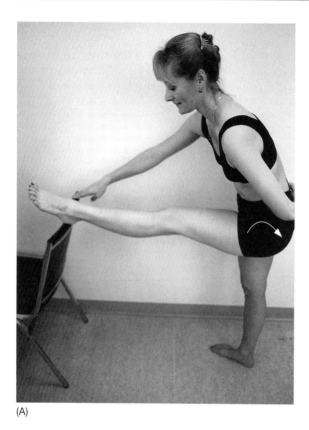

(A)

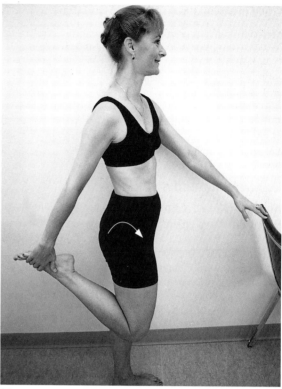

(B)

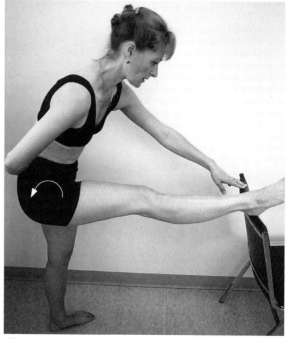

(C)

Figure 7.22 Asymmetrical stretches that result in a unilateral pelvic rotational force. (A) Left hamstring: posterior rotational. (B) Right quadriceps: anterior rotational. (C) Right hamstring: posterior rotational.

Sitting hamstring stretch

When the same athlete attempts a hamstring stretch by sitting on the floor, the legs in front and abducted, the limitation of trunk flexion because of 'hamstring tightness' will be noted on attempts to bend the trunk forwards toward the left leg (see Figs 3.67 and 3.68). The limitation is actually caused mainly by the posterior rotation of the left innominate. Unlike in the standing position, when the innominates are still free to rotate in the sagittal plane, the pelvis is now relatively 'fixed' to the floor in sitting. Forward flexion of the trunk and reaching to the left is literally blocked by the posteriorly rotated left innominate. This limitation is often wrongfully attributed to a tightness of the left hamstrings, but there is usually 'tightness' from the malalignment-related facilitation of the left calf muscles, often with a noticeable restriction of dorsiflexion as well. In contrast, the fact that the right innominate is already in an anteriorly rotated position allows for increased trunk flexion on that side.

On attempts at stretching in these various positions, this athlete may feel increased 'tightness' of the hamstrings and calf muscles on one side as compared with the other. He or she may increase efforts to 'stretch out' the tight groups at all costs, unaware of the true reason for the tightness and of the fact that stretching may not only be futile, but also *dangerous* as the muscle–tendon units involved are put at risk of suffering a sprain or even strain.

Contraindicated strengthening exercises

The bulk of a weak muscle can usually be improved by increasing the size of the individual muscle fibres through a selective strengthening of that muscle. The atrophy in some muscles seen in association with malalignment is, however, the result of reorientation and inhibition and may not respond fully, or as quickly as expected, to this approach. The wasting of vastus medialis on the side of the externally rotated lower extremity is, for example, more likely to respond to first re-establishing the symmetry of lower limb biomechanics by a correction of the malalignment, followed by appropriate strengthening routines (see Figs 3.53B and 3.54).

> The asymmetrical pattern of functional weakness seen so consistently in the lower extremities is determined primarily by factors other than lack of muscle bulk and usually disappears immediately on correction of the malalignment (see Figs 3.49–3.51).

Selective strengthening is unlikely to have an effect on this functional weakness, other than possibly to help prevent or slow down the development of any component of disuse wasting while malalignment is present. Once realignment has been achieved, strengthening efforts should also speed up the reversal of any disuse wasting.

Contraindicated flexibility exercises

There comes a point at which a further limitation of range of motion is not a matter of lack of flexibility but one of a mechanical limitation imposed by the malalignment, a limitation that is unlikely to respond to flexibility exercises other than to achieve basic 'maintenance'. Reference is made to the asymmetrical limitation of both axial and appendicular joint ranges of motion associated with malalignment (see Figs 3.3, 3.9, 3.15, 3.69–3.73). Of interest is the fact that, following realignment, there is often an immediate 5–10 degree increase in the range of motion evident on what was previously the 'good' side, which is matched by the total range on the former 'bad' side (see Fig. 3.45C).

Specific contraindicated activities

The following activities are contraindicated on the basis that they carry a particularly high risk of causing malalignment to recur. These are in general actions that have a rotational component or that create asymmetrical stresses on isolated body segments.

First are those causing torquing of the trunk, such as golf and court sports (e.g. tennis; see Fig. 5.3). Next are those which cause rotation of the trunk relative to a fixed pelvis:

- twisting the trunk from one side to the other while standing and supporting a weight on the shoulders (see Fig. 5.28)
- trunk rotation to reach alternatively towards the right and left leg while seated on the floor with the legs apart (see Fig. 3.67); gymnastic routines with an asymmetrical and/or torquing component (see Fig. 5.9); canoeing in the sitting or half-kneeling position (see Fig. 5.2); and wrestling moves forcing rotation of the trunk when the pelvis is pinned to the floor (see Fig. 5.29).

Also to be avoided are activities leading to rotation of the pelvis relative to a fixed trunk, for example, wrestling moves that force rotation of the pelvis when the trunk is pinned to the floor (see Fig. 5.30). Lying supine, hips and knees flexed to 90 degrees and alternately allowing both knees to drop outwards and down to the right and left side, may be a good way to strengthen the external and internal obliques but not without caution and through a limited range until the pelvis and spine are starting to stabilize (Fig. 7.23).

Activities that can turn a lower extremity into a lever arm capable of causing anterior or posterior rotation of an innominate are also contraindicated:

1. pulling a thigh on to the chest on the side of a recurrent posterior rotation (see Figs 2.32A, 2.76 and 7.16); similarly, lunges that can act like levers when carried out on the wrong side (see Figs 5.8 and 7.18)
2. hip extension (intended for stretching) carried out on the side of the anterior, and hip flexion on the side of the posterior, rotation; both may, however, be flexed or extended together in order to stretch the soft tissues symmetrically and decrease risk of malalignment

Jumping alternately from one leg to the other increases the forces being transmitted through one and then the other SI joint, as in running, high-impact aerobics and some gymnastic and 'aquacise' routines.

Repeated medial and lateral translation with sudden stopping and pushing off occurs in court sports and sports requiring a cutting or crossing action (e.g. football, soccer and hockey) so these are not recommended.

Low-impact aerobics may be a problem, especially if it includes a lot of asymmetrical stretches; sometimes even aerobic classes carried out in water may be too much, particularly if the athlete gets carried away by the gyrations of a fit (and often younger) instructor and the natural, albeit needless, instinct to keep up with the rest of the group, all of which results in temporarily forgetting the risk of recurrence of malalignment.

Repetitive actions with or without twisting, such as occur on the golf course and driving range, during a curling sweep or when bowling, are contraindicated.

All these activities should be avoided until alignment is being maintained. Persistence with asymmetrical exercises and activities of the type listed above frequently results in a recurrence of malalignment following correction and accounts for a large number of so-called 'failures of treatment'.

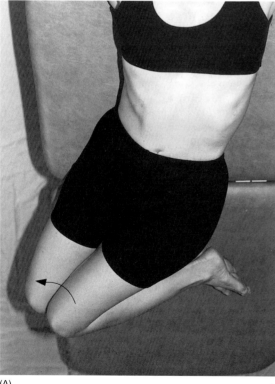

(A)

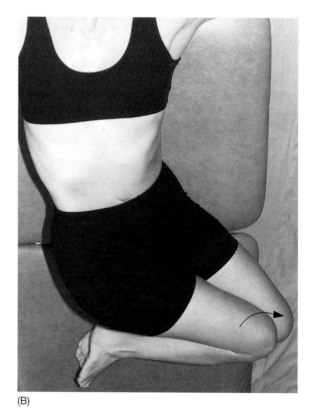

(B)

Figure 7.23 Pelvis torquing on the trunk: supine, alternately letting the flexed hips and knees drop down to the right (A) and left (B).

RECOMMENDED EXERCISES AND SPORTS

Unless otherwise indicated, the emphasis is again on symmetry during the early period of realignment, especially for those in whom malalignment keeps recurring. Training should include the types of exercise outlined below.

Cardiovascular (endurance) training

The following are appropriate in that they are fairly symmetrical types of aerobic activity.

Swimming

Swimming is one of the best exercises for improving and maintaining cardiovascular fitness because weight-bearing is avoided and the buoyancy and warmth of the water has a relaxing effect on the muscles while the water itself offers some resistance to effort.

Rowing

Rowing machines and rowing sports requiring a symmetrical action (e.g. sculling singles and doubles) are suitable as long as the athlete takes care not to twist the trunk and pelvis when getting in and out of the boat and is excused from helping to lift the boat in and out of the water, or off and on a transport vehicle (see Figs 5.13 and 5.14). River and ocean kayaking may also be tolerated, with the same precautions.

Cycling

Leaning forwards to hold on to the handle bars may provoke pain by increasing tension in tight and tender muscles and posterior pelvic ligaments. A mountain bike is therefore preferable to one with dropped handle bars. Better still is to start on a reclining bicycle or, if that is not available, a stationary bicycle, sitting upright initially with the arms relaxed at the side and the legs doing all the work.

Direct pressure on a tender structure (e.g. the sacrotuberous ligament insertion, hamstring origin or coccyx) may necessitate additional padding (e.g. a pillow or visco-elastic gel seat cover). Also now available are seats that have elevations to increase the weight-bearing on the ischial tuberosities, while the groove in between decreases the pressure exerted on the coccyx (see Fig. 5.5B).

Stairmaster and stairs

The emphasis on the stairmaster should be on frequent repetitions initially at low resistance, using a step differential of no more than 10–15 cm to minimize the amount of pelvic torquing and any tilting to alternate sides. For the same reason, the athlete should be warned to go up a flight of stairs only one step at a time and to limit the height of the increasingly popular step-up stations used in circuit training.

It should also be stressed that the stairmaster is intended for a workout of the legs; the arms should be used mainly for balance. Some athletes hang on to the frame so fiercely that they not only do a large part of the work with the arms, but also introduce a major component of twisting of the trunk and pelvis with every step, thereby increasing the risk of recurrence of malalignment.

Strength training

Unless otherwise specified, strengthening exercises (Box 7.4) should be carried out symmetrically.

Any weight training is preferably done lifting balanced weights simultaneously with both arms and legs. If for some reason strengthening is to be limited to a muscle or muscles on just one lower limb, avoid moving that limb to the point at which it turns into a

---

Box 7.4 Strengthening exercises

- *Back extensor and abdominal muscles*, to improve back mechanics and strength (see Figs 7.4 and 7.6)
- *Pelvic 'core' muscles* (Figs 7.24–7.28), exercises for strengthening in particular the elements of the 'inner' (see Figs 2.22 and 2.23) and 'outer' units – the posterior and anterior oblique, deep longitudinal and lateral systems (see Figs 2.24–2.27)
- *The quadriceps, hamstrings* and other muscles that attach to the pelvic bones, particularly those which can affect the SI joint, the emphasis nowadays being on:
  - strengthening the muscles in such a way as simultaneously to re-establish normal sequences of contraction (e.g. posterior oblique system: latissimus dorsi, through the thoracodorsal fascia to the gluteus maximus and finally the hamstrings – see Fig. 2.25A)
  - strengthening the core muscles initially to re-establish stability of the trunk and pelvis (e.g. in strengthening of the pelvic core muscles: the outer ones, such as iliopsoas, piriformis and gluteus maximus, the inner ones, such as obturators, gemelli and pectineus, and those of the pelvic floor; see Fig. 2.36)
- *Alternating isometric contractions of the hip adductors and abductors* to effect realignment of the pubic bones and, at the same, a symmetrical strengthening of these muscles (see Figs 7.15, 7.28 and 'Self-help techniques', above)

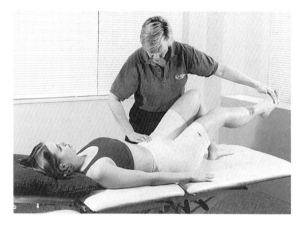

Figure 7.24 Exercises: one leg extension with co-contraction of the inner pelvic muscle unit. (From Lee 1999, with permission.)

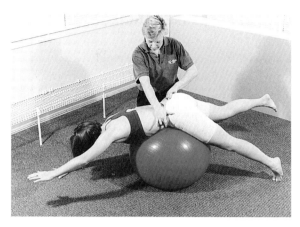

Figure 7.26 Exercises: prone over a ball; one leg, one arm extension with co-contraction of the inner pelvic muscle unit (for the posterior obliques). (From Lee 1999, with permission.)

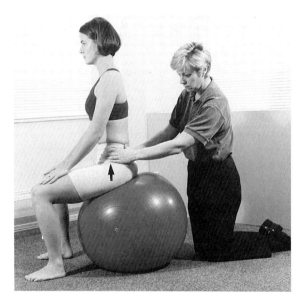

Figure 7.25 Rise and sit with co-contraction of the inner pelvic muscle unit. (From Lee 1999, with permission.)

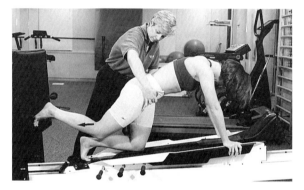

Figure 7.27 Strengthening of one leg extensor in four-point kneeling with a balance challenge on a shuttle MVP. (From Lee 1999, with permission.)

lever arm capable of causing the rotation of an innominate or vertebra.

A typical example is hip abductor strengthening carried out in side-lying. The tendency is to bring the uppermost leg towards the ceiling as far as possible, at the risk of torquing that side of the pelvis through the hip and SI joint (Fig. 7.29A). This risk can be avoided by limiting abduction to the horizontal (Fig. 7.29B). Attention must also be paid to avoiding:

1. excessive forward bending of the trunk, by bending at the hips and knees at the same time

2. actions requiring reaching or incorporating simultaneous lifting and twisting.

Pilates exercise

Joseph H. Pilates developed a dynamic form of exercise that has been very effective for those trying to regain 'form and function' and maintaining realignment. Suffering from asthma, rickets and rheumatic fever during most of his childhood in Germany, Pilates was greatly influenced by holistic medicine and learned to use it to heal himself. While interned in England during World War I and training to become a nurse, he developed Pilates mat work and also a form of resistance training that used springs attached to the hospital bed, in order to facilitate the rehabilitation of the immobilized patients. After moving to New York

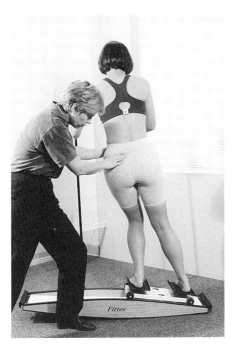

Figure 7.28 Strengthening of the lateral system with co-contraction of the inner unit on a FITTER. (From Lee 1999, with permission.)

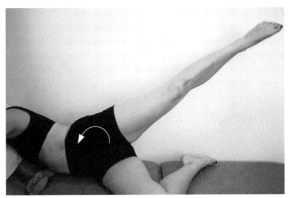

(A)

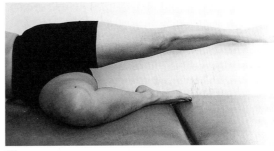

(B)

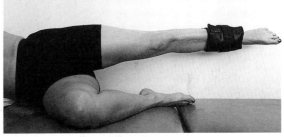

(C)

Figure 7.29 Hip abductor strengthening. (A) Excessive abduction, creating a torsional stress on the left innominate through the left sacroiliac joint and symphysis pubis. (B) Abduction limited to the horizontal to decrease torsional strain. (C) Initial progression with the addition of 0.5–1kg ankle weight.

in 1926, he refined his method by developing over 500 exercises on 10 different pieces of apparatus over the next 60 years.

The Pilates technique relies on working out with springs, which can elongate and contract, to resemble muscles. This method is in contrast to weight training, which relies on a resistance to gravity. Pilates is based on the 'six principles':

1. *Concentration* – you move your limbs while stabilizing your torso and coordinating your breathing, to bring an awareness to all parts of the body
2. *Control* – you are in control of your body and of the equipment: you move the equipment, it does not move you
3. *Centring* – the exercise helps you to focus on your 'power centre' in the lower abdominal region
4. *Flowing movement* – you move with grace, ease, coordination, control, efficiency and enjoyment
5. *Precision* – you perform a few repetitions in an exacting manner to develop awareness, efficient form and posture
6. *Breathing* – your breathing flows with the movements, your consciousness expands, and you feel revitalized.

The method probably has proved so successful in helping athletes recover from malalignment because it:

- Uses muscles synergistically rather than in isolation
- Stretches muscles and increases joint range of motion, as well as strengthening the muscles
- Improves postural alignment and increases coordination, getting the muscles to work efficiently in an effortless and graceful movement

- Takes care to work on the deeper, smaller muscle groups intrinsic to joint stability, thereby strengthening the core of the body
- Looks at the function and strength of the whole body and tries to improve on this in a graduated manner.

RETURN TO REGULAR SPORTS

Unless otherwise instructed by their therapist, athletes should restrict themselves to symmetrical types of exercise until they have maintained alignment for at least 2 or 3 months. If malalignment recurs on reintroduction to regular sports, the programme needs to be re-evaluated to see whether any one component is responsible for the recurrence. All that may be needed is to modify or eliminate the particular exercise(s) for a while.

If the athlete absolutely insists on running early on, while malalignment is still recurring, he or she might try running in water: initially suspended with a life jacket or belt to avoid complete weight-bearing, progressing to the toes just touching the pool floor, and eventually running in more shallow water in preparation for a return to dry land.

SHOES

Weight-bearing problems related to malalignment can be compounded by wearing shoes built to accommodate a specific weight-bearing pattern: pronation or supination. Shoes built for a pronator are usually constructed with medial reinforcement of the midsole and upper. In addition, some have a wedge of higher-density material tapering from medial to lateral (see Fig. 3.31). These so-called 'double-density' shoes typically also have a straight last to decrease the tendency towards longitudinal arch collapse.

A pair of 'pronator' shoes, when worn by an athlete who presents with one of the 'alternate' patterns of malalignment, and the not uncommon picture of right pronation and left supination, will:

- decrease the tendency towards right pronation
- increase the tendency towards left supination, because of the straight last and medial reinforcement of the midsole
- result in even less ability to dissipate shock at the level of the left foot because of the high-density wedge and the fact that the foot is now even more rigid by having been forced into further supination (see Fig. 3.26B).

This type of shoe has been identified as one cause of new or ongoing problems in athletes presenting with malalignment, for example complaints of lateral hip, thigh and knee pain related to excessive tension on the TFL/ITB complex on the side of the lateral shift of weight-bearing and increased tendency to supinate. It is interesting to speculate whether this type of shoe might not also increase the chance of suffering ankle inversion sprains and stress fractures on that side.

As mentioned above, there has been a preoccupation with pronation over the past two decades.

> As a result, those dealing with athletes are generally more adept at recognizing pronation than supination.

An athlete presenting with malalignment is therefore much more likely to be labelled a 'pronator' even though pronation is occurring only on one side, usually the right, whereas the tendency is towards a neutral position or even supination on the other side, usually the left. This athlete stands a good chance of being prescribed shoes intended for a pronator, and risking the consequences noted above.

In a few cases, the supination on one side may be so blatantly obvious that athletes are labelled 'supinators' and are prescribed single-density shoes with a curved last to allow for collapse of the longitudinal arch. This has the effect of accentuating any tendency towards pronation on the opposite side.

FOOT ORTHOTICS

A trial of longitudinal arch supports should be considered when malalignment keeps recurring, in the hope that the orthotics will increase the chances of maintaining alignment. The athlete may actually report a feeling of increased pelvic stability when wearing orthotics. In addition, a previously weak and 'sloppy' foot and ankle may feel stronger and more stable on weight-bearing, at push-off and when executing turns.

ORTHOTICS: WHEN, WHAT AND WHAT NOT
Off-the-shelf arch supports

These may be adequate but tend to be wider than custom-made orthotics. There may thus be difficulty trying to fit them into day shoes, which are usually narrower than running shoes. These supports may, however, be helpful in terms of:

- being readily available 'off the shelf'
- allowing for a quick assessment of whether or not orthotics would really make a difference in the first place, at a price most athletes can afford (approximately a tenth of the price of custom-made ones)
- allowing for a trial of modifications to see whether any of these modifications would be worthwhile incorporating into a subsequent custom-made orthotic; for example:
  - a lateral raise of the heel/forefoot section to counteract excessive lateral traction forces
  - right lateral and left medial forefoot raise to create a counterclockwise torquing force in an externally and internally rotated right and left leg, in order to counter malalignment (see 'Risks associated with orthotics' below).

Custom-made orthotics

If the decision is to use custom orthotics, casting should be carried out at a time when the athlete is in alignment. The malalignment-related asymmetry affects the static and dynamic attitude of the feet, the passive ranges of motion possible at the foot and ankle, and hence the eventual shape and fit of the orthotics (see Figs 3.21, 3.23 and 3.77).

> Asymmetrical orthotics worn by an athlete who is now in alignment can result in asymmetrical proprioceptive signals from the sole and exert an asymmetrical torquing effect through the lower extremities all the way up to the pelvis. In other words, these orthotics can cause a recurrence of the malalignment.

To prevent this complication, the athlete's alignment should be checked just prior to the fitting, and a correction carried out if necessary.

In the same light, all old custom orthotics should be suspect, especially if there is difficulty maintaining realignment when they are being worn. They were probably cast at a time when the athlete was out of alignment and could now be setting up unwanted asymmetrical forces at foot level.

RISKS ASSOCIATED WITH ORTHOTICS

The athlete presenting with malalignment is at risk of further insult with the provision of orthotics that are posted or incorporate a medial or lateral raise. The tendency is, for example, to provide an increasing amount of medial posting in an attempt to counteract the pronation that is sometimes so blatantly obvious on the side of the externally rotated lower extremity. Aggressive medial posting (e.g. of 4 degrees or more, which equates to about 4 mm) actually results in further torquing of the lower extremity by augmenting, at foot level, the forces already tending towards external rotation of that extremity.

Torquing forces are more likely to occur if the medial posting is limited to the forefoot section. By increasing the amount of external rotation, the medial posting may fail to counteract the excessive pronation or may actually worsen it. Similarly, aggressive lateral posting increases the forces promoting internal rotation and may augment the tendency to supination, especially if posting is limited to the forefoot section.

The problem amounts to more than just augmenting or perpetuating an abnormal weight-bearing pattern. Increasing the forces responsible for the pathological internal and external rotation of the lower extremities augments the rotational forces acting on the hip and SI joint region. In other words, injudicious posting will help to perpetuate the malalignment. The corollary is that malalignment can sometimes be corrected with judicious posting that sets up a torquing force to counteract the tendency towards internal or external rotation (Fig. 7.30). Malalignment can be corrected from the ground up, so to speak. A combination of appropriate

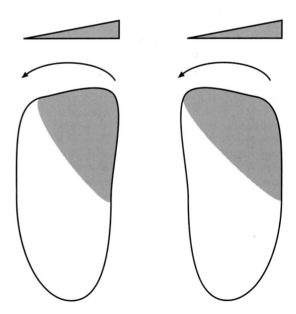

Figure 7.30 An example of a simple approach using a forefoot posting of orthotics for the correction of malalignment: right lateral posting to counteract external rotation; left medial posting to counteract internal rotation.

postings, for example, may result in the correction of a rotational malalignment:

1. A lateral posting of the forefoot on the side of the externally rotated lower extremity would set up torquing force towards internal rotation.
2. A medial posting of the forefoot on the side of the internally rotated extremity would have the opposite effect.

If the athlete presenting with an upslip or rotational malalignment has been mistakenly labelled a 'pronator' because pronation or the inward collapse of a heel cup is so blatantly obvious on one side, the subsequent pro-vision of orthotics having a medial raise bilaterally in the forefoot section will serve only to increase the forces promoting supination that in fact exist on the other side (see Fig. 5.33). On the pronating side, they may improve medial support to counteract pronation, but they could also result in a further, unwanted, external rotation of that lower extremity. The athlete may present with an aggravation of previous symptoms, for example:

- *on the supinating side*: increased pain from the lateral structures (e.g. TFL/ITB complex), which are now put under even greater stress
- *on the pronating side*: problems relating to increased external rotation, knee valgus and stress on the medial aspect of the knee.

> It must also be remembered that the weight-bearing pattern may change once the malalignment has been corrected.

This change is most dramatically evident in children, who are usually referred for assessment because they have been noted to pronate excessively and/or display marked in-toeing or out-toeing. Again, the pronation, in-toeing or out-toeing is often actually unilateral, or worse on one side than the other, in keeping with the presence of a malalignment. On realignment, the tendency towards pronation will usually be markedly decreased or may no longer be discernible: the pattern has become one of neutral weight-bearing or may have completely reversed to become one of symmetrical supination. In fact, a surprising 5–10% of athletes who were seemingly pronating on one or both sides when out of alignment end up with a neutral to slight supin-ation pattern following correction (see Fig. 3.29). Reorientation of the lower extremities may also reduce any in-toeing or out-toeing.

It is therefore very important to reassess the gait, along with a new pair of shoes worn regularly for 2–3 months after the correction, and to recommend appro-priate changes to the orthotics and footwear if the weight-bearing pattern has changed. Should the athlete now have a neutral to supination pattern, for example:

- remove any medial posting if there are ongoing signs or symptoms consistent with lateral traction forces
- consider the addition of a lateral raise if lateral traction signs or symptoms have failed to settle
- replace rigid or semi-rigid orthotics with a soft-shell type and recommend shoes with a curved last and 15–20 mm single-density midsole cushion to improve shock absorption at foot level.

WHEN MALALIGNMENT CANNOT BE CORRECTED

Orthotics may still play a role when the correction of malalignment just cannot be achieved or maintained. They may provide an unexplained sensation of increased pelvic stability, felt sometimes even when the athlete is still out of alignment. More easily explained is the ability of the orthotics to decrease some of the bio-mechanical stresses attributable to the malalignment.

Minimizing stresses caused by apparent leg length difference

When malalignment cannot be corrected, it would seem appropriate to provide a lift on the side of the apparent or functional 'short' leg when standing. This will decrease stress, particularly on the lumbosacral region and the spine, by decreasing the pelvic obliquity and the compensatory curvatures of the spine. It should, however, be remembered that sacral rotation can com-pensate for up to 5 mm of LLD. It is therefore more important that a lift correct any residual obliquity of the sacral base rather than obliquity of the pelvis *per se*.

The lie of the sacrum is preferably assessed on a standing anteroposterior X-ray view of the pelvis. If the sacral base is level, no lift is indicated, even though there may be persistent obliquity of the pelvis (see Fig. 3.83). If no X-ray is available, a trial with a lift may be worthwhile. The functional LLD should be measured while standing, from the iliac crest, anterior superior iliac spine (ASIS) or other pelvic landmark down to the floor. A safe rule is initially to limit cor-rection to 5 mm, using a simple heel lift (Fig. 7.31A). There are two possible outcomes to consider.

The 5 mm lift is well tolerated. In this case, consider increasing the lift by another 5 mm every 2–3 months until the pelvis is level, or as tolerated. It usually takes that long for soft tissue adaptations to occur. If the total difference is 1 cm, a heel lift or a simple partial or

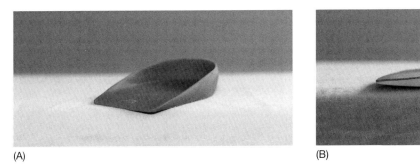

(A)   (B)

Figure 7.31 Progressive heel lifts. (A) A simple 5 mm heel lift, used for the initial correction of a difference of 5 mm or more. (B) A 10 mm heel lift, tapering to 5 mm in the forefoot.

full-length insole, 10 mm high at the heel and tapering down to 5 mm at the forefoot, may suffice (Fig. 7.31B). Any additional correction required usually has to be added to the heel and sole of the shoe.

The lift is not tolerated. The soft tissues may have changed so much over the years as a result of the functional LLD that they can no longer adapt to the biomechanical changes imposed by the lift. Alternately, levelling of the sacral base may already be compensating, and the addition of the lift now creates unwanted stresses by unlevelling the base, something that could be confirmed radiologically.

Medial or lateral posting of an orthotic or shoe

Posting should be guided by ongoing signs or symptoms that can be related to the altered pattern of movement and weight-bearing. The intent is to decrease the tension on structures that are tender as a result of being put under increased stress from persistent malalignment. This may call for medial posting on one side to counteract stress from pronation, lateral posting on the other to counteract traction attributable to a neutral or supination pattern. It is best to start with a posting of no more than 2 degrees – approximately 2–3 mm – and evaluate its effectiveness in 3–4 weeks. Further increases should be guided by the response to temporary posting with moleskin or adhesive felt, added one layer at a time at 2–3 day intervals.

> Always be aware that the posting may cause increased torquing of a lower extremity.

As an alternative, or in addition to posting, consider reinforcing the heel cup of the shoe medially or laterally to counteract excessive pronation or supination forces respectively (Schamberger 1983).

WHY DO ORTHOTICS HELP TO MAINTAIN ALIGNMENT?

Some of the possible mechanisms to consider include the following.

First, an orthotic increases the stability at foot level by providing contact for weight-bearing across a larger part of the sole. Pressure is therefore distributed more evenly across the entire area provided by the orthotics (Fig. 7.32A). Contrast this with the kidney-shaped imprint of a bare foot in sand: weight-bearing is primarily at the heel, lateral sole and ball of the foot (Fig. 7.32B).

Second, orthotics can be used to decrease any persistent tendency of the feet to roll inwards into pronation, or outwards into supination, once the athlete is in alignment. They may thereby decrease any torquing forces on the legs that could cause a recurrence of rotational malalignment, especially if these forces are in any way asymmetrical.

Third, by providing support over the major part of the sole of the foot, the orthotics increase both the amount and the symmetry of the sensory input from the surface of the sole. Stimulation of the cutaneous proprioceptive receptors has been postulated to result in pain control. There are three neurophysiological mechanisms currently in vogue (Box 7.5).

There are several end results of these mechanisms, as affected by the increased cutaneous input from the larger weight-bearing area and more uniform pressure distribution on the orthotic, including the following:

1. A decreased perception of pain results in a reflex relaxation of the muscles. This could decrease the recurrence of malalignment by decreasing or actually eliminating any asymmetry in muscle tension.

2. The barrage of proprioceptive signals could also decrease excitatory input to the muscle spindle, again resulting in a reflex relaxation of the muscles in the immediate area.

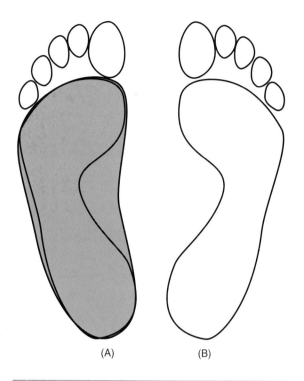

(A)   (B)

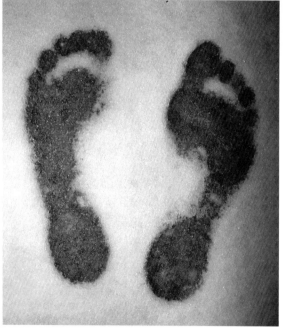

(C)

Figure 7.32 Foot contact surface. (A) On an orthotic versus (B) barefoot on sand. (C) Barefoot weight-bearing pattern, reflecting the malalignment-related shift: medially on the right – increasing foot surface contact; laterally on the left – decreasing surface contact (see also Fig. 3.21A, B).

Box 7.5 Theories of pain modulation

- *The gate theory of Melzack & Wall* (1965)
  Pain signals travel along the small-diameter, unmyelinated and slow-conducting C-fibres. Proprioceptive signals, in contrast, travel along large-diameter, myelinated and fast-conducting A-fibres. Signals from both pass through the substantia gelatinosa in the dorsal horn of the spinal cord before ascending to the brain. A barrage of proprioceptive signals arriving by way of the A-fibres may cause the substantia gelatinosa to block the signals arriving through the C-fibres. This effectively 'closes the gate', preventing pain signals from ascending further in the spinal cord and reaching the brain.
- *The central biasing mechanism* (Mayer & Liebeskind 1974, Melzak 1981)
  Pain signals ascending in the spinal cord can be prevented from reaching the brain if their transmission is subjected to the powerful inhibitory influence of the raphe nucleus in the brain stem. Cutaneous stimulation is one mechanism known to trigger activity in this nucleus, which in turn 'closes the gate' to further ascent of pain signals.
- *Release of endorphins* (Pomeranz 1975)
  The stimulation of cutaneous touch and pressure receptors results in the release of endorphins from the anterior pituitary gland.

---

3. The proprioceptive signals are ultimately transmitted to the sensory cortex where they may:

- effectively decrease excitatory signals to the muscles, signals that would otherwise facilitate these muscles and cause them to tense up
- result in a more symmetrical output from the motor cortex, which would in turn decrease any tendency to torquing attributable to an asymmetry of motor output.

SACROILIAC BELTS AND COMPRESSION SHORTS

The application of a compressive force across the SI joints and symphysis pubis can afford relief from pain in these areas by decreasing the likelihood of displacement of these joints and recurrence of malalignment.

THE SACROILIAC BELT

The sacroiliac belt, also known as an intertrochanteric belt, fits into the space just below the anterior superior iliac spine and above the symphysis pubis anteriorly and the greater trochanter laterally (Fig. 7.33A). It runs

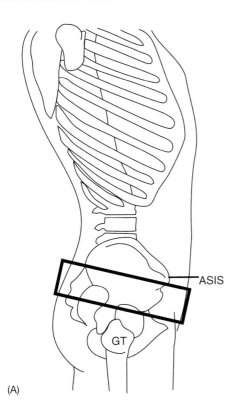
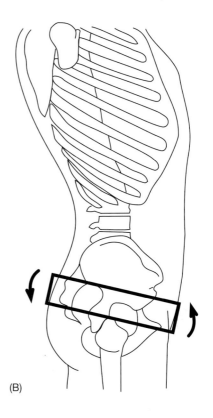

(A)

(B)

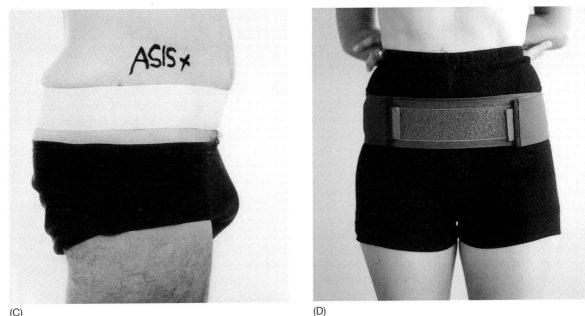

(C)

(D)

Figure 7.33 Placement of a sacroiliac belt. (A) Correct: anteriorly below the anterior superior iliac spine (ASIS) and overlying or just above the symphysis pubis, laterally above the greater trochanter (GT) and posteriorly across the lower one-third of the sacroiliac joint; see also (C). (B) Incorrect: too low over sacrum, creating a rotational force into counternutation. (C) Sacroiliac belt: correct location. (D) Sacroiliac belt worn over clothing (Serola model – see Fig. 7.34A).

across the lower third of the sacrum posteriorly; if applied too low over the sacrum, it will exert a rotational force into counternutation (Fig. 7.33B).

The belt was developed to enhance the stability of the SI joints and symphysis pubis and has proved effective in reducing pain from these sites (Walheim 1984). Athletes wearing the belt have spontaneously reported a decrease in pelvic pain, increased comfort sitting, a tendency for the back to be straighter when sitting, and a feeling of increased pelvic girdle strength and stability. The belt also appears to be effective in decreasing the frequency of recurrence of malalignment, if not preventing it altogether, once correction has been achieved.

How the belt works

Possible mechanisms by which the belt exerts its effects include:

1. It brings the adjoining sacral and iliac surfaces of the SI joint closer together. As confirmed by cadaver studies, the result is an increase in the friction coefficient of the joint, decreasing the ease with which one surface can slide over the other (Vleeming et al 1990b).

2. It enhances the 'self-bracing' mechanism (Snijders et al 1992a; see Ch. 2) that normally ensures stability of the SI joint and allows for a transfer of the lumbosacral load to the legs while minimizing the shear between the iliac and sacral surfaces (see Figs 2.20 and 2.21).

3. It decreases the amount of anterior rotation of the innominates and posterior tilting of the lower part of the sacrum by exerting a direct pressure against these structures (Fig. 7.33A).

Cadaver studies suggest that the belt can increase the friction coefficient, and hence the stability of the SI joint, by bringing the apparently matching valleys and elevations on the sacral and iliac surfaces closer together (Vleeming et al 1990b). It is, however, hard to conceive of a belt that is applied just snugly enough to prevent it from slipping up or down actually being capable of mechanically decreasing or stopping any movement of the pelvic bones. In addition, in some athletes a corset or tube-top has had equally dramatic results in helping to maintain pelvic alignment, even though these would exert only minimal pressure on the skin.

In the cadaver studies mentioned above (Vleeming et al 1990b), doubling the tension on a belt from 50 N to 100 N decreased the amount of rotation possible at the SI joint only from 18.8% to 18.5%. Conway & Herzog (1991) hypothesized that if the SI belt did indeed stabilize the SI joint by restricting joint mobility, ground reaction forces measured in patients with SI joint problems should differ depending on whether or not they were wearing the belt. The authors were, however, unable to detect any statistically significant differences.

Other mechanisms can also be considered when trying to explain the effectiveness of the belt.

First, does it favourably influence the orthokinetic reflex? Abnormal tension in the ligaments that stabilize a joint results in a change of strength in the muscles acting on that joint. By helping to maintain the SI joint surfaces in normal apposition, the belt may equalize the tension in the ligaments and thereby the strength in the surrounding muscles.

Second, could some of the belt's effects be exerted by way of the proprioceptive system? The belt applies pressure symmetrically to a large surface area. By stimulating cutaneous pressure receptors, it could flood the system with input along the fast conducting A-alpha proprioceptive fibres. In other words, the belt may be able to decrease pain by closing the 'pain gate' (Melzack & Wall 1965). Decreasing the pain allows for a relaxation of these muscles in which tone has increased, either in a reflex response to pain or as a result of facilitation. If relaxation evened out tension in muscles on the right and left sides, it would decrease any tendency towards SI joint torquing.

Third, the belt applies even pressure against the hip abductor and buttock muscles. Some of these muscles are consistently tense and tender, in particular the left hip abductors and right piriformis. Applying gentle pressure may have the same effect as applying a forearm band for a tennis elbow to dimple the wrist extensor muscles: the band decreases the strength of the maximum contraction possible in these muscles, thereby decreasing the torsion and traction forces they can exert on the inflamed and tender muscle origins and insertions.

Finally, the belt may favourably influence posture. One athlete, for example, felt that perhaps the belt, by serving as a reminder, 'trained her to take more care' to avoid the movements and activities that would put her at risk of going out of alignment. Another felt that a pad over the sacrum caused her back to straighten when sitting, increasing the lumbar lordosis to the point at which she no longer needed to use a back support with a lumbar roll.

Indications and contraindications

The belt is used primarily for a problem of hypermobility of either SI joint or of the symphysis pubis, pain originating from any of these joints, a feeling of pelvic instability and recurrent malalignment.

The belt is particularly likely to be helpful if:

- stressing the joint(s) in the anterior-posterior or craniocaudal directions provokes the athlete's pain
- The passive straight leg raising test is positive; that is, passive compression of the SI joints allows the athlete to extend or flex the leg on one or both sides further and/or more easily (see Figs 2.91B and 2.92B). The belt is likely to provide similar passive reinforcement to a symphysis pubis or SI joint(s) rendered unstable by ligament laxity or osteoarthritic degeneration (see Figs 2.70 and 4.30).

The belt is unlikely to be helpful if manoeuvres that compress the SI joints or the symphysis pubis provoke pain. The belt itself has the effect of bringing the anterior SI joint lines and superior pubic rami closer together and may therefore aggravate pain from these sites. If that is the case, Lee (1993b) advises resting the joint(s) by using a cane or crutches. One should not try an SI belt until the compression of these joints no longer proves painful.

Problems

Problems encountered with the SI belt include the following.

The belt is too wide and moves up and down too easily. This becomes a nuisance particularly when sitting down. A 5 cm belt is probably adequate for most athletes whose height is 180 cm or less, whereas those who are taller do well with a belt 7.5 cm in width.

The belt is applied too tightly. Excessive pressure from the belt, buckles or stitching can result in actual maceration of the skin. The belt should be applied snugly and is best worn over the top of clothing, inside or out, especially if wearing it against the skin proves too uncomfortable (see Figs 7.33C, D and 7.34A).

The belt is not worn in the proper position. The belt should lie between the ASIS and the greater trochanter. Snijders et al (1992b) have postulated that, in this position, the belt is able to exert its maximum effect to counteract any tendency of the ilium to rotate on the sacrum, as well as to enhance the 'self-bracing' of the SI joint referred to above.

Of interest here is their hypothesis that the belt worn by weight-lifters, rather than acting to give extra support to the back by increasing intra-abdominal pressure, actually works by enhancing this self-bracing of the SI joint in the stooped position and squat. Snijders et al were able to show on magnetic resonance imaging (MRI) studies that the weight-lifter's belt, which is applied using exactly the same landmarks, was level with the cranial part of the SI joints.

The belt was therefore in an optimal position to stabilize the joint by narrowing the joint space. These authors felt that if the belt lay too high, it could be useless or even detrimental, in that it would open up the caudal (lower) aspect of the joint and decrease its overall stability.

The belt increases pain from the SI joint. It may do so by compressing the inflamed anterior joint surfaces and/or gapping the joint posteriorly and stressing tender interosseous and posterior SI joint ligaments.

The belt material evokes an allergic reaction. This is easily solved by wearing the belt over clothing, a habit already adopted by many athletes for the sake of comfort.

The belt presses on a painful structure. The belt may not be tolerated because it exerts direct pressure on one of the structures that has become tender with the malalignment. The problem usually turns out to lie with the left gluteus medius/minimus and/or the piriformis (usually the right). Always rule out, however, that the pain is not resulting from pressure on some unrelated problem, such as a lipoma or neurofibroma.

Instructions for use

> The belt should be worn when the athlete is up and about, and preferably when in alignment.

It may still, however, provide some comfort even when the athlete is not in alignment, possibly by increasing the general stability of the SI joints and symphysis pubis. The occasional athlete derives benefit from wearing the belt at night as well, perhaps by decreasing any tendency to lose alignment when lying or turning in bed, or by easing tension on some tender structure. In some athletes, malalignment is noted to recur readily on standing, in which case the belt is best applied while still lying supine. For the pregnant athlete, there are belts that can be let out to accommodate the progressive increase in girth. Some belts incorporate a triangular posterior support to lie over the sacrum.

COMPRESSION SHORTS

These shorts, commonly used in football and other sports for 'groin injuries', are now also being advocated for pain originating from the SI joints or symphysis pubis as a result of instability or inflammation. They are usually made with neoprene and non-elastic materials in a way that minimizes any restriction of range of motion (see Fig. 7.34A, B). They have several benefits (Box 7.6).

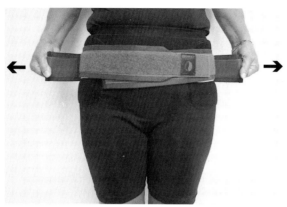

(A)

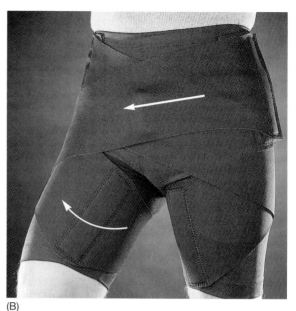

(B)

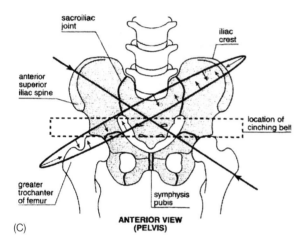

(C)

Figure 7.34 Compression pants. (A) Incorporating a sacroiliac belt (Serola model – note the elastic side-straps stretched out sideways to be secured with Velcro anteriorly to reinforce the support). (B) With cross-straps secured to leggings and wrapped upwards around the trunk (figure-of-eight). (C) Diagonal stabilizing forces created across the sacroiliac joints by the cross-straps. (From Active Orthopaedics Inc.1999, with permission.)

Box 7.6 Beneficial effects of compression shorts

- *Heat retention:* this may be particularly helpful when there is injured groin tissue but will also help to relax muscles that are tense and tender as a result of malalignment
- *Compressive forces:*
  - These forces are spread over a larger surface area and may therefore be more easily tolerated by the athlete
  - Some shorts incorporate an SI belt for an additional compressive force to help to immobilize these joints; the belt also helps to keep the shorts in place (Fig. 7.34A)
  - The addition of 'figure-of-eight' hip and thigh straps provide adjustable compressive forces (Fig. 7.34B). One strap, for example, may be anchored to the inside of the groin, wrapped anteriorly around the thigh and then across the buttocks, before being anchored anteriorly to a strap originating from the opposite thigh. The result is a diagonal compression force across both SI joints (Fig. 7.34C)

These shorts, in combination with the belt, have helped many patients finally to achieve some stability and comfort when the belt alone has failed.

ALTERNATE FORMS OF TREATMENT

The aim of treatment is to achieve and maintain alignment, re-establish normal muscle tension, strength and activation, create stability of pelvis and spine and decrease or abolish pain.

> In the process of trying to achieve realignment, other methods of treatment may be helpful, particularly those which can temporarily reduce or eliminate muscle spasm and pain.

To this end, treatment with massage, acupuncture or biofeedback may assist the therapist in making realignment easier to achieve and subsequently more likely to be maintained between mobilization or manipulation sessions. None of these methods is, however, likely to bring any more than temporary relief if simultaneous attempts at achieving and maintaining realignment are neglected. Analgesics, anti-inflammatory medication and muscle relaxants may initially be more effective for pain control when taken on a preventative basis regularly around the clock; they are less likely to have an effect when taken on an 'as needed' basis to counteract an established pain pattern or aggravation.

Transcutaneous electrical nerve stimulation may also be worth a trial to help to decrease pain and relax the muscles, but this modality is again more likely to be helpful when used by the athlete on a regular basis several times a day (e.g. 20–30 minutes 3 or 4 times a day), in the hope of preventing the pain from worsening or manifesting itself in the first place.

Magnetic devices in the form or insoles or pads applied to the skin may bring relief by improving the circulation to localized sites of tender muscle or connective tissue (e.g. ligaments and fascia); more generalized, and less clearly defined, effects may result with the use of pillows and mattresses.

Methods such as extracorporeal shock wave therapy and pulsed signal therapy may be worthwhile trying in an attempt to resolve residual painful areas localizing to deep musculoskeletal tissue, in particular sites that have become a chronic source of pain as a result of the insults to which they have been subjected by the malalignment and which now fail to respond to other treatment measures, even though realignment is being maintained.

INJECTIONS

Injection is a treatment option for those presenting with:

- Recurrent malalignment caused by ligament laxity
- Ongoing pain despite correction of the malalignment, this arising from:
  - inflamed and/or weakened ligaments and tendons
  - trigger points within ligaments, tendons and muscles
  - inflamed facet and/or SI joints.

The stability of any joint depends on the fit of the joint surfaces and the proper function of the supporting structures, the strength and tension in the muscles acting on that joint, and the strength and tightness of its ligaments and capsule. Malalignment, whether it involves vertebral malrotation or a shift of the sacral–

innominate complex, increases tension in some soft tissue structures while relaxing others.

> The connective tissue structures put under tension by persistent or recurring malalignment will eventually lengthen, and with time, the joint may become hypermobile because of a failure of these supportive structures.

Even the SI joint that shows the movement restriction or 'locking' may actually turn out to be hypermobile on correction, a reflection of the lengthening that has occurred in the supporting ligaments and joint capsule. There is often also weakening of the muscles that act across the joint.

Hypermobility of a joint can also develop because its supporting structures are being put under increased stress by the restriction of movement in another joint. Locking of the right SI joint, for example, increases the stress on the left SI joint, the decreased movement of a hip joint increases stress on the ipsilateral SI joint and the lumbosacral junction, and the decreased movement of a vertebral complex increases the stress on the level above and below, all of these restrictions possibly also affecting more distant joints. Realignment may put the joint surfaces back into proper position, but malalignment or malrotation may now keep recurring because of a failure of the supporting structures.

Strengthening the muscles acting on the joint may prove inadequate to maintain realignment; worse still, the instability may have advanced to the point at which any realignment achieved is quickly lost by these attempts at strengthening or even simple exercise routines. In these cases, an injection technique known as prolotherapy may be helpful to increase the tightness and strength of the ligaments and capsule.

Cortisone temporarily weakens connective tissue structures and is therefore more appropriate for the injection of persistently tender and inflamed ligaments in those cases in which alignment is being maintained, as well as for injection directly into an inflamed facet or SI joint space in the hope of calming any inflammation.

PROLOTHERAPY INJECTIONS

Prolotherapy is based on the premises that:

- Following injury, the inadequate repair of fibrous tissue can result in chronic pain from musculoskeletal tissue (e.g. the fibro-osseous junction or enthesis)
- The complete healing of injured ligaments and tendons is compromised by their limited blood supply

- A lack of cells, in particular fibroblasts, may be another factor to account for the slow healing, or even failure of healing, of injured ligaments and tendons
- Irritant solutions can be injected to stimulate fibroblasts to produce collagen and promote healing.

Prolotherapy injections have proved helpful in treating the problems of persistent ligament/tendon (enthetic) pain, and of the laxity of the supporting tissues that now results in joint hypermobility and a recurrence of malalignment. The technique aims to strengthen the connective tissue, when the natural healing process:

1. has been too slow or has proven inadequate
2. has failed altogether to repair an insufficient collagen matrix that has resulted from:
   - a single major traumatic disruption of these tissues (e.g. a shear injury to the SI joint or joint dislocation)
   - a repeated and/or chronic stretching and lengthening (e.g. recurrent malalignment, and joint hyperextension or subluxation).

Prolotherapy stimulates healing by initiating a localized inflammatory reaction, which in turn triggers the natural connective tissue 'healing cascade'. Following a sprain, strain or other injury to a ligament, capsule or tendon, the release of mediators (e.g. cytokines) from damaged tissues normally results in blood vessel dilatation and increased permeability, with an increase in blood flow to the injured area, increased warmth and the development of oedema (Fig. 7.35). An initial infiltration of granulocytes is followed by one of monocytes, macrophages and other scavenger cells intent on the removal of necrotic tissue.

Next comes the inflammatory phase, during which the release of growth factors (e.g. growth hormone) and other derivatives from platelets, macrophages, lymphocytes and similar cells stimulates fibroblasts to migrate to this area. By the second or third day after the injury, these activated fibroblasts are already synthesizing an immature collagen.

Over the next 2 weeks, the inflammatory phase gradually gives way to the early reparative phase, also called the 'proliferative' phase because of ongoing fibroblast proliferation (Fig. 7.36A). The process of new collagen formation continues for another 3–4 weeks and then gradually decreases as the number of activated fibroblasts declines. During the weeks that follow, known as the 'remodelling' or maturation phase, collagen fibrils mature by becoming longer, thicker and 'close-packed' through cross-linkage and orientation along the lines of stress (Fig. 7.36B). The process of maturation continues for some time: it may take up to 12–18 months before the tissue reaches its maximum post-injury tensile strength.

When this natural process fails to take place during the initial 6 months post-injury, one is usually left with a weakened, and often painful, ligament no longer capable of healing spontaneously. With an injury to the SI joint ligaments, for example,

1. failure to heal may occur because:
- the initial trauma resulted in a partial or complete disruption of ligaments (see Fig 2.34B)
- poor blood supply has delayed the onset of healing
- any new collagen fibres that form are elongated by being subjected to increased stress, either constantly with persistent malalignment and the separation of the surfaces, or repeatedly with recurrence of malalignment because of a lack of adequate stabilizing support from the ligaments (and often also muscles) and recurrent muscle spasm
2. the pain can arise from:
- excessive tension on the nerve fibres, which: cannot elongate as much as the elastic tissue; may get entrapped in scar tissue; are particularly abundant in the fibro-osseous junction, which is often weakened and under increased tension as a result of malalignment

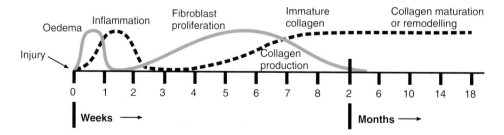

Figure 7.35 Phases of natural connective tissue repair following sprain or strain (immature collagen = thin, short, randomly oriented fibres; mature collagen = thick, long, cross-linked fibres, oriented along lines of stress).

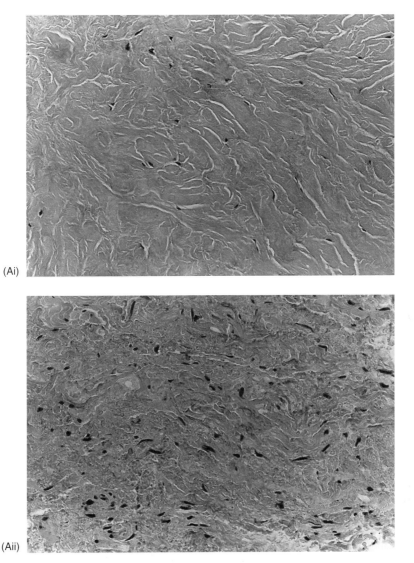

(Ai)

(Aii)

Figure 7.36 Biopsy of the posterior pelvic ligaments before and then 3 months after a course of 6 weekly prolotherapy injections; note the fibroblastic hyperplasia, with a 60% increase in average fibre diameter. (A) Black and white haematoxylin and eosin representative slides of ligament histology (Ai) before and (Aii) after prolotherapy. Note the increased waviness representing collagen and the increased number of fibroblast nuclei. Of significance is the *absence* of inflammation or disease. (B) Electron microscopy longitudinal cuts of ligament tissue (Bi) before and (Bii) after prolotherapy. Note the increase in size of the collagen fibres as well as the increase in variation of the size of these fibres. (From Dorman 1997, with permission.)

Figure 7.36 (B), see overleaf

– the development of trigger points in ligaments and muscles.

> Prolotherapy may become the treatment of choice in that it can decrease the pain at the same time as it increases the tensile strength of the tissue by promoting collagen formation.

The technique relies on the injection of an irritant that causes an inflammatory response in the connective tissue. The subsequent course of developments exactly follows the natural cascade: the migration of fibroblasts to the area, with the initial production of immature collagen fibres that subsequently mature over the next 12–18 months (Fig. 7.35). In other words, one artificially induces the sequence that would normally follow these

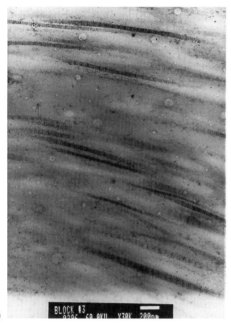

(Bi)

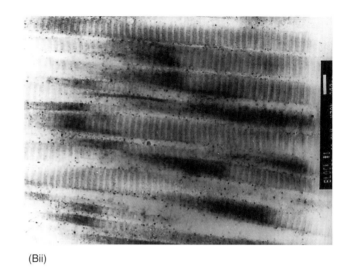

(Bii)

Figure 7.36 *Continued.*

injuries, while continuing attempts to maintain alignment so that the new collagen is not subjected to abnormal tensile stresses and can therefore mature to reach maximum strength.

There are a number of irritants being used to induce inflammation, but a hyperosmolar sugar solution is gradually becoming the most commonly used 'proliferant' and probably remains one of the safest. Dextrose solution 15–20% draws fluid out of the surrounding connective tissue to such a degree that it causes tissue breakdown and incites inflammation, the 'injury response' described above eventually being set in motion. The inflammatory response subsides as soon as the dextrose becomes diluted again by cell fluid (Banks 1991).

Hackett pioneered research in this area and published the first monograph on prolotherapy in 1956. Based on his clinical experience and the results of animal studies, Hackett (1958) proposed the theoretical model outlined in Box 7.7.

Hackett felt that the ideal treatment would be to strengthen the fibro-osseous junction by stimulating the proliferation of fibrous tissue in this region. Solutions to induce such proliferation were readily available as they already enjoyed popularity in the treatment of venous and oesophageal varices, hernias and haemorrhoids, a treatment method commonly referred to as 'sclerotherapy'.

Hackett (1958) thought the term 'prolotherapy', or 'proliferant therapy', was more appropriate given that there was indeed a proliferation of normal tissue. This usage would get away from the concept of scarring, which was commonly held to be the basis of the beneficial effect of these so-called 'sclerosing' injections. He indicated that the confusion in terminology arose from the fact that:

> In the early days the name 'sclerosing solution' was given to any solution which produced abundant fibrous tissue because it resembled scar tissue formation [whereas] the action of the stimulating solution has always been that of a proliferant, which Webster's Dictionary defines biologically as the production of new cells [in this case fibroblasts] in rapid succession. (p. 100)

Experimental evidence

Early studies into the effects of proliferant solutions by Rice & Mattson (1936), Maniol (1938) and Harris et al (1938) had already confirmed that the injection of a chemial irritant into tissue such as muscle, tendon or ligament caused an initial inflammatory response, then a proliferant phase and subsequently a maturation of the collagen produced. Rice (1937) reported how the conversion to adult fibrous tissue was essentially complete in approximately 7 weeks.

Hackett & Henderson (1955), reporting on the effect of injecting a proliferant solution into the Achilles

---

Box 7.7 Hackett's model of prolotherapy
• The 'relaxation' or lengthening of the ligaments that span the joints of the spine and pelvis is a major cause of chronic low back pain.
• The relaxation of a ligament or tendon can result from:
– inadequate healing following trauma (e.g. major trauma such as a sprain or strain or repetitive microtrauma, resulting from chronic or recurrent activity, or related to malalignment)
– congenital laxity
– ligament laxity associated with pregnancy
• Such relaxation of the ligaments and tendons can be the cause of pain from the 'fibro-osseous' junction, the site where the ligaments and tendons insert on to the bone.
• Because of this increased laxity, these structures must now be considered incompetent in terms of providing adequate support to the bones and joints.
• Pain arises as a result of:
– irritation of the relatively inelastic sensory nerves that lie within the ligaments and tendons Even relatively normal tension forces will cause stretching of the now incompetent elastic components, whereas the relatively inelastic sensory fibres fail to stretch to an equal extent. This results in irritation of the sensory fibres, with localized and/or referred pain.
– increased wear and tear of the now excessively mobile joints
• Pain, ligament laxity and 'loose joints' lead to a vicious cycle of further ligament relaxation and decalcification of bone in the region of the fibro-osseous junction. Either one can induce the other: bone strength is dependent on stress imparted to the bone by the attaching ligaments or tendons, just as ligament strength is favourably affected by the stress imparted to the ligament through its connections to the bone and myofascia.

tendon of rabbits, documented a progressive increase in both fibrous tissue and bone in the region of the fibro-osseous junction at 3 months. By 9 months, the diameter of the injected tendons had increased 40% and tensile strength 100% compared with control tendons. The authors remarked particularly on the increase of continuous fibrous tissue that extended from the tendon, through the periosteum and into the bone in order to increase the strength of the 'weld' at the fibro-osseous junction. They also felt that:

the increase of bone is significant because it results in a strong fibro-osseous union where sprains, tears and relaxation of the ligament chiefly take place and where sensory nerves are abundant. (p. 972)

Several studies have now clearly validated the theories put forth by Hackett and proved the effectiveness

of prolotherapy injections into the ligaments of the human pelvis and spine. Naeim et al (1982) carried out a single-blind study that indicated that a combination of lidocaine and dextrose was more effective in treating chronic iliolumbar syndrome than was the use of lidocaine alone. Ongley et al (1987) published the first double-blind controlled study on human beings that proved the effectiveness of prolotherapy in the treatment of chronic low back pain.

Klein et al (1989) presented the first histological documentation of ligament proliferation in three human subjects involved in a double-blind study into the effectiveness of prolotherapy for the treatment of chronic low back pain of at least 2 years' duration (Fig. 7.36 above). Biopsies of the posterior sacroiliac ligaments carried out 3 months after the completion of a course of 6 weekly injections of a proliferant solution showed fibroblastic hyperplasia and a 60% increase in average fibre diameter. The three patients also demonstrated a statistically significant improvement in the range of motion in the three major axes of lumbar movement, and improved visual analogue pain and disability scores, compared with 20 controls.

Proulx (1990), injecting with a solution of lidocaine mixed with either hypertonic dextrose (12.5%) or the corticosteroid triamcinolone (10 mg), commented that, on follow-up at 8 months, the results suggest that:

1. compared with steroid therapy, prolotherapy was more beneficial the more chronic the fibrous tissue ailments
2. symptoms of prolonged immobility (theatre cocktail party syndrome, night pain and morning stiffness) were good predictors of a favourable response only for the prolotherapy group
3. the SI joint dysfunction tests and ligament stress tests were of no value as predictors of outcome in either group
4. the study proves that dextrose is an 'active medication'.

Klein et al (1993) reported on a randomized, double-blind clinical trial of xylocaine/hypertonic glucose (prolotherapy) versus xylocaine/saline injections into the posterior pelvic ligaments, fascia and joint capsules of 79 patients with chronic low back pain resistant to previous conservative treatment. The prolotherapy group showed greater improvement on visual analogue, disability and pain grid scores. Of interest was the finding that MRI and computed tomography (CT) scans 'showed significant abnormalities in both groups but these did not correlate with subjective complaints and were not predictive of response to treatment' (p. 23), a finding that has been echoed in a number of other reports (e.g. Jensen et al 1994, Kieffer et al 1984, Magora & Schwartz 1976, Weishaupt et al 1998).

Proliferent solutions

Dorman & Ravin (1991) have reported that the most frequently used proliferant in contemporary practice is 'Ongley's solution', known also as P25G: a solution of phenol 2.5%, glucose 25%, glycerine 25% and pyrogen-free water to 100%. There are, however, a number of advocates for the use of dextrose alone. Hirschberg (1985, p. 682) writes that 'Neither phenol nor glycerine are required. A sclerosant solution containing only 25% dextrose gives excellent results'. Pomeroy (1983, p. 1) emphasizes that:

the incidence of serious complication from the dextrose solution itself is negligible... The skill of the physician, the cooperation of the patient and anatomical variations within the patients seem to be the only significant factors that lead to complications.

Concentrations of dextrose ranging between 12.5% and 25% have now been shown to be adequate; concentrations in excess of 25% should be avoided for fear of causing tissue necrosis.

Barring allergic reactions, xylocaine is probably the ideal local anaesthetic in that it is less likely to produce pain on intradermal and subcutaneous injection (Morris et al 1987) and has a rapid onset of action (5–10 minutes). These advantages may, however, be offset by its short duration of action (1–2 hours). If the ligament pain does indeed stem from the irritation of hypersensitive nerve fibres at the fibro-osseous junction, longer-acting anaesthetics, such as marcaine 0.25% and procaine 2%, may be more effective for actually 'desensitizing' these nerve endings at the same time.

Indications for injection

Prolotherapy may be the treatment of choice in the following situations:

• if the malalignment has been corrected, but the ligaments continue to be an ongoing source of pain. This may relate to the severity of the initial injury, the length of time the malalignment has been present or the development of a hypersensitivity of the sensory endings that has failed to respond to the normalization of tension

• if the malalignment keeps recurring, and laxity of the supporting tissues is evident or suspected. Remember that muscles, in particular iliopsoas, coccygeus and piriformis, may be chronically con-

tracted and stabilizing what would otherwise prove to be an unstable SI joint.

Scheduling of injections

There is no consensus in the literature on how often one should inject and at what interval. Suggestions range anywhere from one injection a week for 6 weeks, to one injection every 4 weeks for a total of three or four injections. Fibroblastic activity subsides within 6–8 weeks following an injection (see Fig. 7.35). Common practice is to give repeat injections within 1–2 weeks in order to stimulate an ongoing inflammatory response and thereby boost the changes initiated by the preceding injection(s). In addition, given that the response rate for partial or complete relief is about 60–70% following 3–6 injections (Klein et al 1989, Ongley et al 1987), it seems wise to try an initial course of six injections, 2 weeks apart, in order to spare the majority either inadequate or unnecessary injections. Those who respond only partially, or not at all, to this initial course will then proceed to a set of further 'booster' injections.

The author's preference is to see the athlete 2 months after the last of the initial course of six injections, when the fibroblast count can be expected to have returned to the pre-injection level. The response to this first set of injections is assessed in terms of pain relief and improved stability. If this response appears to be inadequate, a course of booster injections is initiated. These boosters are spaced further apart, starting with three boosters at 1-month intervals. There follows a further reassessment 2 months later and, if necessary, further boosters, usually spaced 2 months apart, until stability has been achieved.

The treatment protocol obviously needs to be tailored to each athlete. He or she (and those involved in their care) must be made aware that:

1. improvement occurring during the course of initial injections to some extent reflects the effect of local anaesthetic on painful structures
2. the actual process of connective tissue tightening and strengthening depends on the maturation of the newly formed collagen, a process that continues over several months; that is, treatment effects may not become evident for several months
3. 60–70% of cases will show some improvement at the time of the initial reassessment, which usually takes place approximately 4–5 months after the first injection
4. if at all possible, efforts to achieve and maintain alignment should continue during the course of injections and while waiting for the completion of the matur-

ation process, in order to minimize excessive tension on the immature collagen fibres that have been formed.

Injection technique

For information, the reader is referred to Dorman & Ravin (1991), the two more recent adaptations and expansions of Hackett's original 1956 monograph, by Mirman (1989) and Hackett et al (1991), and the very informative book *Prolo Your Pain Away* by Hauser (1998). Workshops with hands-on teaching for prolotherapy injection techniques are offered on a regular basis by both the American and Canadian Associations of Orthopaedic Medicine.

The choice of which connective tissues to inject is determined by the problem at hand (Fig. 7.37). If alignment is being maintained, injections may be limited to those ligaments and tendons which are persistently tender. When the SI joint is involved, injection may be localized to several ligaments (Box 7.8; see Figs 2.2, 2.3, and 3.56–3.63).

To stabilize any segment of the spine (see Fig 3.63), injection must include the supra- and interspinous lig-

---

Box 7.8 Ligaments injected for sacroiliac joint involvement

- For a *recurrent right inflare* in isolation, the right iliolumbar, posterior SI joint, sacrotuberous, sacrospinous and long dorsal sacroiliac ligaments
- For *right anteroposterior instability*, the above ligaments; the interosseous, and ideally the anterior SI joint ligaments and capsule, may be added by injection directly into the right SI joint
- For a *current right SI joint upslip*, the right posterior sacroiliac, sacrospinous, sacrotuberous and long dorsal sacroiliac ligaments
- For *right craniocaudal instability*, as for a recurrent right inflare, with the exception of the iliolumbar ligament
- For *recurrent rotational malalignment and/or upslip*, injection can be limited to one side if there is evident unilateral SI joint laxity. If laxity is found bilaterally, however, or if the anterior/posterior rotation or upslip keeps switching from one side to the other or if there is usually a compensatory rotation in the opposite direction, one should include the posterior pelvic ligaments bilaterally.

---

aments and facet joint ligaments and capsules one or two levels above and below the affected vertebra(e). In the thoracic segment, injection should include the costovertebral, costotransverse and costochondral ligaments at the affected levels (see Figs 2.63, 3.13 and 3.14). Remember that instability, particularly of the atlanto-axial-occipital region and L4 and/or L5 vertebra(e), is common and must be considered as a possible trigger of recurrent pelvic malalignment.

If the injection of tender superficial iliolumbar ligament insertions fails to bring relief, the pain may be arising from an involvement of the deep insertions. These, like the SI joints, are best injected under fluoroscopic visualization using a needle of 7.5 cm or longer.

The coccyx tends to be the most tender site to inject. With recurrent coccygeal malalignment or instability, the ligaments inserting along the lateral borders, those running from the tip to the rectum and those crossing the posterior aspect of the sacrococcygeal joint should all be included.

The injections are usually well tolerated and can be carried out in a clinic setting. Some therapists like to carry out the procedure under intravenous sedation. The author prefers local anaesthetic and has those with a lower pain threshold or excessive pain take Demerol 50 mg and Gravol 50 mg 1 hour beforehand. The needle entry sites are anaesthetized with xylocaine 1% using a 'pop' gun, for the skin surface (Figs 7.37 and 7.38), followed by a deeper injection using a 25 mm 30

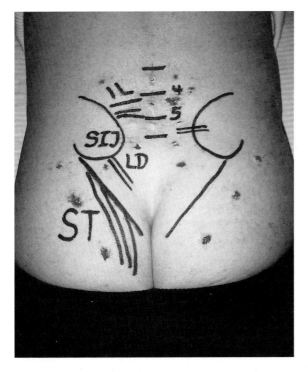

Figure 7.37 Typical ligaments injected: IL, iliolumbar; SIJ, posterior sacroiliac joint; LD, long dorsal sacroiliac; ST, sacrotuberous; L4/L5/S1, lumbosacral ligaments (inter- and supraspinous, and facet joints).

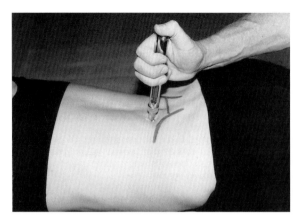

Figure 7.38 'Pop' gun dermal anaesthetization of the needle entry sites, supplemented with the injection of local anaesthetic into the subcutaneous tissue using a 2.5 cm 30 gauge needle, in order to minimize discomfort from the actual prolotherapy injection.

gauge needle, before proceeding with the injection of the proliferate solution itself. The athlete is advised:

- to apply ice repeatedly, for 10–20 minutes at a time during the first day following each injection in order to alleviate any pain and swelling
- to keep active by walking about in order to speed up the absorption and dispersion of the injected fluids, and to counteract development of stiffness
- not to plan any strenuous activity for the rest of the day
- to avoid public swimming pools until the wheals from the 'pop' gun and the needle sites have healed over (usually within 2 or 3 days)
- to avoid further irritation of the injected ligaments during the course of the injections; this includes strenuous or jarring activities and activities that put an excessive or prolonged stretch on the injected ligaments (e.g. deep squats, weight-lifting and gardening)
- to avoid all anti-inflammatory medications during the initial course of injections, and for at least 2–3 weeks following the more widely spaced booster injections, given the timing of the inflammatory phase (see above)
- to continue with exercises that 'work' the ligaments being injected in a reasonable manner, for example, repeated sets of trunk flexion and extension following injection of the lumbosacral and posterior pelvic ligaments.

Gentle, short exercise periods with frequent rests seem to work best for most athletes. Problems are often related to overdoing things and then suffering the consequences. This is frequently the result of being misled by the temporary feeling of improvement that may follow an injection and which is probably attributable to the temporary effect of the analgesic in decreasing the chronic discomfort arising from the deep ligamentous structures.

> Common sense and moderation are the key!

Reassessment for the effectiveness of injections

Reassessment is carried out about 2 months after the last injection, at which time the reaction in the tissues will largely have subsided. In 20–30% of cases, the ligament tenderness will have disappeared by this time. In another 30–40%, there are now only localized areas of tenderness rather than the generalized tenderness seen on initial examination. As indicated, 60–70% will already show improved stability by this time. Booster injections may be appropriate in an effort to eliminate any residual tenderness, instability or recurrence of malalignment, should these still be a problem.

In 20–30% of athletes, there will be a persistence of the previously noted generalized tenderness, 30–40% showing no, or only a partial, improvement of the recurrent malalignment and previously noted instability. The athlete may report some temporary beneficial effect. Such improvement often does not occur until several days after the injection, some time after the local anaesthetic has worn off. In these cases, it may be worthwhile initiating a second course of six injections spaced 2 weeks apart, or proceeding to the 3 monthly boosters, possibly with addition of a chemical irritant such as phenol or sodium morrhuate (cod liver oil concentrate), followed by another reassessment 2 months after the last injection. By this time, feedback from the therapists may indicate that they have noticed increasing stability of a previously unstable SI joint or vertebral complex. This feedback is helpful in deciding whether the athlete may derive benefit from further boosters, in combination with ongoing attempts to maintain alignment.

Some athletes return for a 'booster' injection some months or a year or more after the initial injections. They have seemingly had a good result that lasted some time but now appears to be 'wearing off'. This is sometimes attributable to a recurrence of the malalignment, but the athlete may be in alignment with just a tenderness of the posterior pelvic ligaments. 'Repeaters' usually respond well to another short course of three injections, only to return again some time in the future for yet another 'booster'. Others do best with a single booster spaced 4 to 12 months apart. It seems as if the healing response of their ligaments is either inadequate or has been interfered with by repeatedly excessive demands.

Side-effects and complications

The most common side-effect is the increased pain associated with the injection. This usually lasts no more than 1 or 2 days but can go on for a week, in which case one might consider increasing the time between the injections to 3 or 4 weeks. Other less frequently encountered problems include:

1. fainting, usually because of transient hypotension and bradycardia triggered by the stimulation of a vasovagal attack
2. allergy to the local anaesthetic, glucose, cod liver oil or other component
3. bleeding and bruising from the puncture of a subcutaneous vessel
4. referred pain from the transiently damaged and distended tissue
5. infection of the injection site
6. pneumothorax following injection in the thoracic region.

In a survey carried out by Dorman (1992), a total of 66 'minor' and 14 'major' complications were reported by 95 practitioners on a patient pool of 494 845 treated with prolotherapy. 'Major' was defined either as requiring hospitalization or having transient or permanent nerve damage. The conclusion was that the risk-to-benefit analysis for prolotherapy indicated a low complication rate.

Other applications for prolotherapy

Prolotherapy injections are appropriate for the treatment of any accessible ligament that is a problem on account of laxity, pain or both. Prolotherapy has, for example, proved effective in:

1. increasing the stability of:
   - subluxing or repeatedly dislocating shoulders, especially when surgery is no longer an option
   - ankles prone to recurrent sprains when ligament laxity is evident
   - wrists (e.g. the ligaments of specific carpal bones)
2. strengthening lax cruciate or collateral knee ligaments in patients who are not candidates for surgery (Ongley et al 1988)
3. the treatment of enthesopathies such as chronic 'tennis elbow'.

Case history

A lady 7 months postpartum suffered a shear injury of her left sacroiliac joint in a motor vehicle accident in which her car was rear-ended and subsequently pushed into the car ahead. Her feet were braced on the floor in anticipation of both impacts. A failure to respond to ongoing attempts at realignment and strengthening of the inner and outer pelvic units was eventually attributed to persistent ligament laxity, maximal in the craniocaudal (vertical) plane.

Active left straight leg raising was restricted to 50 degrees compared to 70 on the right (see Figs 2.90 and 2.91). Form closure augmented by compression of the SI joints with pressure on the sides of the innominates increased her ability to transfer forces through the hip girdle so that left straight leg raising came to match the 70 degrees on the right. An attempt to increase force closure by recruiting the right anterior oblique system (right external and internal abdominal obliques connected to the left adductors by way of the anterior abdominal fascia) was effected with pressure against her right shoulder to resist her attempt to do an oblique sit-up. This manoeuvre decreased her left straight leg raising to 40 degrees, possibly by decreasing or shutting off contraction in the inner unit

The findings were consistent with a lack of form closure caused by ligament disruption; this could not be overcome by an attempt at augmenting force closure. Recommendations were for:

- having her use a cane in the right hand to decrease weight-bearing through the left SI joint
- prolotherapy injections to strengthen the ligaments that controlled vertical joint displacement
- a decreased emphasis on exercises aimed at augmenting force closure until form closure had been improved with prolotherapy.

INJECTION OF CONNECTIVE TISSUE: CORTISONE VERSUS PROLOTHERAPY

Ligaments, in particular the posterior pelvic ligaments, may continue to be acutely tender even though realignment is being successfully maintained. This ongoing tenderness relates in part to:

- *the severity of the initial injury to the ligaments*: typical of these is a ligament sprain or strain seen in association with a shear injury of the SI joint (see Fig 2.34)
- *the length of time the malalignment has been present*: in those athletes who present with malalignment and a history of pain having come on within the past 2–3 months, the ligament tenderness almost always disappears spontaneously within a matter of days or weeks following realignment. When malalignment has been present for years, it may

take up to 1 or 2 years for the ligaments to heal and the pain finally to settle down.

It is sometimes a low-grade inflammatory response that is the main cause of the ongoing ligament pain, in which case a course of anti-inflammatory medication may be helpful. As long as the athlete is maintaining alignment, a trial with cortisone injections may be warranted. In these cases:

1. if there is no improvement after one or two injections of cortisone spaced 2 weeks apart, the author prefers to proceed with a course of prolotherapy injections, which can both decrease the pain and strengthen these structures

2. if there is some improvement with the initial cortisone injection, repeat injections carried out every 2 weeks can be tried. These injections are restricted to any remaining sites of tenderness noted at the time of each visit until the area involved has been reduced to about 10–20% – any residual tenderness will usually resolve on its own. In most athletes, this goal is achieved after four or five visits.

3. if alignment is still being maintained on reassessment 3 months after the last cortisone injection, and there has overall been a further improvement but the athlete is still symptomatic and there are still areas of localized tenderness, it should be safe to initiate another short course of 1–3 cortisone injections, limited to the persistently tender sites. The sacrotuberous origins and coccygeal ligaments are the most likely to be involved.

OTHER TYPES OF INJECTION

Pain arising from any structure can predispose to a recurrence of asymmetry if it creates asymmetrical torquing forces by altering movement patterns, or precipitates an asymmetrical voluntary or reflex contraction of muscles in the immediate vicinity in an attempt to splint the site of the pain. Therefore, the painful site should if at all possible be treated. Treatment may include the following:

Injection of trigger points.

Injection of tender tendons, capsules and fascia. Cortisone may quickly settle inflammation. The fact that it also weakens connective tissue structures by disrupting the cross-linking of collagen fibres precludes injection directly into a tendon for fear of rupture. This same feature, however, makes it useful for injection into tight and tender fascia and scar tissue, to help loosen up the tissue in conjunction with deep massage and stretching.

If pain persists or recurs after one or two cortisone injections around a tendon or into a capsule, consider a course of prolotherapy injections instead.

Injection of tense or tender muscle. Temporarily decreasing muscle tension or breaking up muscle spasm with an injection of a short-acting local anaesthetic into multiple points in the muscle itself, the motor point(s) or the nerve supplying that muscle may interrupt the vicious cycle of an increase in tension or spasm causing more pain and perpetuating the abnormal increase in tone. The injections should be followed by deep massage and stretching while the anaesthetic is active.

Injection of the sacroiliac joint(s). If injection of the posterior pelvic ligaments brings only partial or no relief, if SI joint stress tests are positive, and especially if there is a history of a shear injury, consider injecting the SI joint(s) proper. One may not be able to pinpoint the painful structure because it is hard to stress the joint surfaces without simultaneously stressing the ligaments and capsule. A bone scan will help to narrow the differential as it may be abnormal for some time following a shear injury.

If the first injection dramatically reduces or eliminates the pain, but only temporarily, the block may have to be repeated two or three times for an adequate trial of therapy. Two common approaches to SI joint injection are currently being used (Aprill 1992, Bernard & Cassidy 1991, Derby 1986, Haldeman & Soto-Hall 1983):

- *direct joint injection* (Fig. 7.39A): this should decrease or eliminate pain from all joint structures because it will also anaesthetize the branches of the lumbosacral plexus from L3 to S2 that innervate the anterior joint capsule
- *blocking of the posterior primary rami* (Fig. 7.39B): these supply the posterior ligamentous portion of the joint. The block will not anaesthetize the anterior joint capsule.

Neural therapy. This technique is aimed at the chronic pain from nerve irritation that is often a component of the malalignment syndrome, especially when the problems related to the malalignment and/or additional insults (e.g. previous trauma or surgery) have been present for some time. Pain is reduced by injecting local anaesthetic into autonomic ganglia, peripheral nerves, scars, glands, acupuncture points and trigger points, as well as directly into tender tissues. With the decrease in pain, there is often an immediate improvement in the range of motion and ability to use and strengthen muscles, something that may increase the chance of achieving and maintaining realignment.

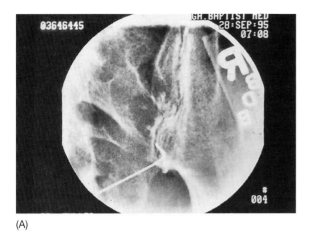

(A)

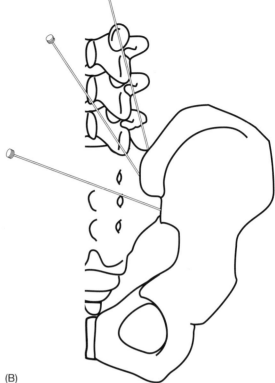

(B)

Figure 7.39 Injection of the sacroiliac joint. (A) Direct joint injection: the position of a needle in the nexus of the ilium and sacrum is verified on fluoroscopy in preparation for sacroiliac joint arthrogram or arthrodesis. (B) Needle placement for blocking the posterior primary rami that innervate the sacroiliac joint. (From Keating et al 1997, with permission.)

TREATMENT OF INTERNAL STRUCTURES

Recurrent malalignment and ongoing pain can be the result of malalignment of the sacrococcygeal joint and/or pelvic floor dysfunction, with chronic tension and at times trigger point development in the pelvic floor musculature and internal ligaments. Particularly likely to be involved are the levator ani muscle complex and the sacrospinous and sacrococcygeal ligaments (see Figs 2.16, 2.36, 3.59, 3.60, 4.15 and 4.34). Tenderness is easily confirmed by a palpation of these structures per rectum or per vagina. Treatment consists of:

1. realignment of the sacrococcygeal joint
2. external massage and stretching of the tender soft tissue structures immediately alongside the coccyx
3. internal massage of the coccygeal structures and gentle stretching of the tense and tender pelvic floor musculature and ligaments (using either a rectal or a vaginal approach) for persistent tenderness in these structures

4. biofeedback, using sensors in the rectum, vagina or both, to teach pelvic floor strengthening and relaxation routines
5. ongoing efforts at correcting pelvic and spine malalignment
6. the possible addition of visceral manipulation.

> The treatment of pelvic floor dysfunction often reveals that there is a coexisting problem involving the internal viscera.

Typical of these is a tightness, adhesion or scarring of visceral ligaments that interferes with the proper function of the bowel and can precipitate visceroso-matic reflexes (see Ch. 4 and Fig. 4.33). In addition to tackling the malalignment and pelvic floor dysfunction, visceral manipulation may be required in order finally to resolve the problems typically related to these internal structures: episodic diarrhoea, urinary frequency, urgency, nocturia, coccydynia, vaginal wall pain, dyspareunia and stress incontinence.

The discussion that follows focuses on the diagnosis and treatment of pelvic floor dysfunction, reference being made to Barral (1989) and Barral & Mercier (1988) regarding visceral manipulation, as well as to the discussion in Chapter 4.

DIAGNOSTIC AND TREATMENT AIDS FOR PELVIC FLOOR DYSFUNCTION

Kegel (1948) advocated a 'physiological' treatment for poor tone and function of the genital muscles and for urinary stress incontinence. He developed a set of exercises aimed at improving the tone of the pelvic floor muscles, in particular pubococcygeus.

In an attempt to obtain an objective measure of pelvic floor tension, Kegel invented the 'perineometer', which is basically a rectal/vaginal probe linked to a manometer. It proved helpful for giving patients feedback on how to contract these muscles appropriately and for allowing them to document an improvement in strength. Perry modified this with the addition of an electromyography monitor to give simultaneous objective pressure measurements and an electromyograph read-out. This unit, the PerryMeter, has been used successfully for biofeedback (Craig 1992; Perry et al 1988; Selby 1990).

Using this device, patients are trained to appreciate when the pelvic floor muscles are overactive or underactive and what they need to do to relax or strengthen them respectively. Perry & Hullett (1990) have also reported a high success rate in the treatment of stress incontinence using the PerryMeter in conjunction with Kegel's pelvic exercises.

Wallace (1993) has presented a combined approach to pelvic floor dysfunction in athletes that includes simultaneous correction of any SI joint malalignment and pelvic floor strengthening exercises using Femina cones of gradually increasing weight. The tendency of a vaginal cone to slip out with the pull of gravity provides the athlete with immediate feedback on which muscles to contract in order to retain the cone and helps to strengthen the appropriate pelvic floor muscles.

Treatment: non-invasive techniques

Non-invasive approaches include the frictioning and deep pressure release advocated by Selby (1990), the correction of pelvic and spine malalignment, acupressure, myofascial release of the soft tissues inserting into the lateral aspect of the sacrum and coccyx, deep psoas and piriformis release, and the use of electrical modalities (e.g. transcutaneous electrical nerve stimulation, laser and ultrasound) over the coccyx and adjacent soft tissue structures. Kegel exercises and biofeedback approaches help to ensure that the athlete is actually contracting the pelvic floor muscles, rather than intraabdominal muscles by mistake. Acupuncture and deep needling in the area of piriformis and the greater sciatic foramen, while 'invasive', are best mentioned in this connection.

Non-invasive techniques must also include the following.

Instruction regarding proper sitting postures

The emphasis is on shifting weight-bearing onto the ischia by restoring the lumbar lordosis (sitting upright with use of a lumbar roll, Obus form or other supportive seating). Weight-bearing on the sacrum or coccyx must be minimized by not slouching and not sitting for prolonged periods on hard or soft furniture or in bucket seats.

Coccygeal relief cushion

Doughnut cushions should be avoided. The coccyx often ends up directly bearing weight by chaffing against the inside of the cushion posteriorly. Letting the coccyx sag down into a hole will increase tension on the soft tissue attachments to the coccyx, which are often already tender.

An appropriate coccygeal pillow is usually made out of firm foam about 5–10 cm thick. It has a cut-out in its central posterior aspect, either square (approximately 10 cm along each edge) or triangular in shape (Fig. 7.40). The cut-out is the soft part that accommodates the coccyx; it can be filled simply with a piece of soft foam or by re-using the foam that was cut out and then shredded. The firm part of the pillow to either side provides support for the ischial tuberosities, where weight-bearing should occur.

A home exercise programme

- In those presenting with pelvic floor laxity, traditional Kegel exercises to strengthen the pelvic floor muscles, supplemented with biofeedback and other methods (e.g. intravaginal cones), can be used.
- In those presenting with pelvic floor hypertonicity, the emphasis is on relaxation exercises, including deep rhythmic abdominal breathing and visualization; muscle tightening is used only to 'get in touch' with how it feels to hold tension and to learn how to let this tension go.
- In those with pelvic instability, pelvic core strengthening exercises are prescribed.

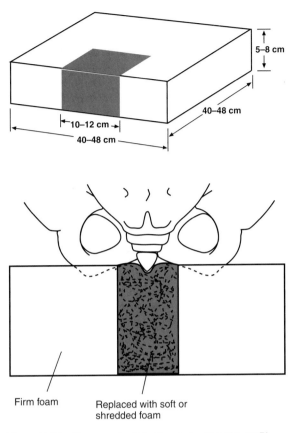

Figure 7.40 Coccygeal relief pillow (see also Fig. 5.5B).

Treatment: invasive technique

> The results using the non-invasive techniques may unfortunately be only temporary; it is sometimes not until one uses an invasive technique that the sacrococcygeal articulation is actually mobilized or the pelvic floor dystonia reversed and one finally notes improvement.

Any subsequent reintroduction of the non-invasive techniques may then help to ensure that the gains established with the invasive techniques will be maintained and that the malalignment will not keep on recurring.

Invasive techniques approach the sacrococcygeal articulation and pelvic floor structures by way of either the rectum or the vagina. The rectal approach is sometimes not feasible because of personal preference, marked and/or painful spasm of the anal sphincter, anal fissures or other pathology. The vaginal approach is felt by some (Barral & Mercier 1988; Craig 1992; Selby 1990) to be superior; it is usually more comfort-

able and allows the therapist to reach more of the pelvic floor musculature than would be possible using the rectal approach. Unfortunately, issues relating to professional ethics and medicolegal considerations may prohibit using this form of treatment.

SURGERY

Surgery plays an important role in the treatment of problems related to malalignment. The diagnosis of malalignment may unfortunately have been missed, unwarranted surgery being undertaken in an attempt to rid the athlete of symptoms that might well have responded simply to a correction of the malalignment.

SURGICAL FUSION

Athletes who fail to respond to the conservative course of treatment outlined above may be candidates for immobilization in a final attempt to gain relief from chronic pain attributable to an unstable vertebral complex or recurrent malalignment involving the SI joints and/or symphysis pubis. They are often those with generalized joint hypermobility. Before considering surgical immobilization, one must be absolutely certain of several factors (Box 7.9).

The very nature of the surgery may mean that the athlete cannot return to the previous sport.

Immobilization of a vertebral complex

Immobilization of a vertebral complex puts increased stress on the disc and facet joints immediately above and below the level(s) of fusion and predisposes to an earlier development of degenerative change at these levels. This may preclude a return to sports that repeatedly load the spine, especially if loading is accompanied by torsional stresses (e.g. in gymnastics, ballet or wrestling).

Immobilization of the sacroiliac joints

The immobilization of one or both SI joints impairs the normal reciprocal movement that occurs in these joints during the gait cycle, with a loss of the normal shearing motion that facilitates weight transfer and helps to dissipate any residual shock from the ground forces transmitted up through the legs. The hip joint, lumbosacral junction and lower lumbar spine in particular are subjected to increased stress because they now have to accommodate the loss of movement at the SI joint(s).

Box 7.9 Factors to assess before contemplating surgery

- *The pain is arising from the structure considered for fusion*: in the case of the sacroiliac joint, for example, there should be a dramatic temporary decrease or abolition of the pain following the injection of local anaesthetic into the joint. Some surgeons may also have the athlete undergo a 2-week trial with an external 'fixator' device (Fig 7.41) in an attempt to establish whether or not fusion would really be helpful (Sturesson 1999).
- *The athlete has complied fully with all recommendations and the conservative approach has definitely failed*: the author has unfortunately repeatedly been made aware of the fact that athletes who have 'failed' the conservative course of treatment are frequently also those who have compromised the results of that approach. Their inability to comply with the treatment programme to date only increases the chance that they are likely to compromise the results of a surgical procedure as well. These are typically the athletes who:
  - prematurely attempt a return to running or some other activity that repeatedly loads the SI joints asymmetrically and result in a torsional stress
  - repeatedly exceed the amount of exercise that they are able to tolerate without precipitating pain, a reflex tightening of the muscles and a recurrence of the malalignment.

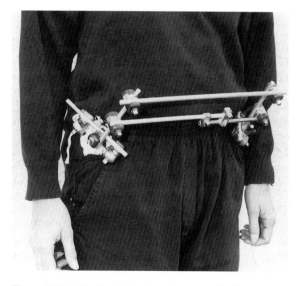

Figure 7.41 'Fixator device' used preoperatively to determine whether subsequent sacroiliac joint fusion is likely to relieve the pain, and postoperatively to ensure the fusion.

For these reasons, immobilization may preclude a return to sports in which an impairment of stride length, shock absorption and the ability to deal with torsional stresses is particularly detrimental (e.g. running, high-impact aerobics and gymnastics).

Immobilization of the symphysis pubis

Immobilization of the symphysis pubis will also impair the normal reciprocal movement of the SI joints. Bone grafting with the introduction of a bone plug is particularly likely to lead to new problems. By separating the pubic bones at the symphysis, the plug causes an outflare of both innominates, this outflare resulting in an anterior opening of the SI joints, a stretching of the anterior capsule and a posterior closing with compression of the posterior joint margins. The overall effect is to increase stress on the SI joints and to impair their movement and weight-transfer function. These stresses may eventually aggravate pre-existing pain or cause pain in SI joints that were previously asymptomatic.

SI joint arthrodesis rather than fusion is currently being advocated for patients who have failed conservative treatment. The majority have SI joint dysfunction attributed to postpartum instability, previous trauma or transitional SI joint instability following solid lumbosacral fusion (Kurica 1995). Percutaneous posterior screw fixation is carried out as an outpatient procedure in some clinics. Lippitt (1995) advocates:

1. fixation with two screws because using only one screw often results in a recurrence of the pain after a year (Fig. 7.42A)
2. bilateral fixation for patients who have previously undergone a lumbosacral fusion (Fig. 7.42B).

UNWARRANTED SURGICAL INTERVENTIONS

Below are examples of some problems that may be treated surgically because of a failure to realize that malalignment, rather than the entity listed, is the primary cause of the symptoms and signs.

Disc problem: bulging, protrusion and herniation

Disc bulging, protrusion and even herniation are not infrequently noted on imaging of symptomatic and

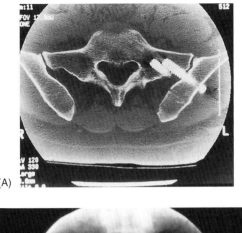

(A)

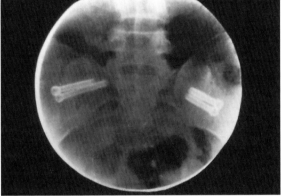

(B)

Figure 7.42   Surgical fixation of the sacroiliac joint.
(A) Unilateral single screw arthrodesis: postoperative
computed tomography scan checking screw placement.
(B) Bilateral screw fixation (with two screws bilaterally).
(From Keating et al 1997, with permission.)

asymptomatic populations alike (Kieffer et al 1984,
Klein et al 1993, Jensen et al 1994, Magora & Schwarz
1976, Weishaupt et al 1998). This finding is more likely
to be exaggerated if there are also:

- referred sensory symptoms that appear to fall
  within the dermatome pattern of the suspected
  compressed root (see Figs 3.10, 3.42, 3.56, 3.58, 3.62,
  4.10 and 5.32)
- weak muscles within the anterior myotome of that
  particular root (see Figs 3.49–3.51).

A right lateral disc bulge or protrusion at L4–L5 is,
for example, going to take on much more significance
when there is:

- a report of paraesthesia on the lateral aspect of the
  right calf or dorsum of the foot or toes, or possibly

even a report of a decreased pinprick or touch
appreciation on testing these areas
- weakness in the right extensor hallucis longus,
  extensor digitorum brevis and tibialis anterior and
  posterior
- a 'positive' test for root irritation: a limitation of
  straight leg raising; a report of back pain on straight
  leg raising, bowstring and/or Lasegue's test; acute
  back pain on the slump test; or the precipitation or
  aggravation of paraesthesia.

All the above symptoms and signs are, however,
also frequently noted in association with malalignment alone. In the presence of malalignment with
anterior rotation of the right innominate, for example,
the following may be seen.

There will usually be weakness ranging from 3+ to
4+/5 in right extensor hallucis longus, extensor digitorum brevis and tibialis anterior and posterior muscles,
whereas their left counterparts remain strong (see
Ch. 3). The fact that the strength is full in the L5- and
S1-innervated right medial hamstrings and peroneus
longus/brevis can easily be rationalized as being due
to the 'intact' S1 nerve root contribution to these
muscles.

Paraesthesias lying with this 'L5 dermatome'
pattern are not unusual. Hackett (1958) and others
have documented how paraesthesia associated with
lumbosacral and/or SI joint instability can be referred
into the typical L5 distribution: from the upper half of
the posterior sacroiliac ligaments to the lateral calf
region (see Fig. 3.58B), and from the ligaments around
the hip joint to the anterolateral calf and the dorsum of
the foot (see Fig. 3.62).

> Root stretch tests put tension on not only nerve roots,
> but also other soft tissue structures.

These include the sacrotuberous ligament, which is
tender in over 50% of those presenting with malalignment. This ligament will be put under increased
stretch by straight leg raising and, if it happens to be
continuous with biceps femoris, also by the bowstring,
Lasegue's and slump tests, and any other manoeuvres
that further increase tension in the hamstrings.

Irritation of the ligament can precipitate or augment
the referral of pain and paraesthesias to the lower
extremity, something that can easily be misinterpreted
as an indication of increased irritability of a nerve root
or the sciatic nerve. Malalignment-related piriformis
facilitation or spasm may irritate the sciatic nerve,
especially the peroneal component (see Fig. 4.17).

The following should trigger a suspicion that the problem is likely to be caused by something other than root irritation or compression:

Patchiness of the paraesthesias

Paraesthesias may, for example, involve the lateral calf region or the dorsum of the foot, not necessarily both at once (as would be more likely to be the case with an L5 root lesion). In addition, these sites are often clearly separated from one another; in the example cited above, the athlete may distinguish a patch overlying the lateral calf region and another, distinctly separate, patch overlying the dorsum of the foot at times when both sites are symptomatic.

Variability of the paraesthesias

The location and intensity of the paraesthesias may vary. There may, for example, be paraesthesias in the lateral calf region on one day, the dorsum of the foot on another and both sites or neither one at other times.

Asymmetry of muscle strength

The asymmetry involves muscles from more than one myotome on the 'affected' right side, whereas other muscles in these same myotomes have retained full strength. A typical finding is weakness of the right iliopsoas (L2 and L3) but a strong quadriceps (L2, L3 and L4), and weakness in right hip extensors but strong ankle evertors and hip abductors (all L5 and S1).

Asymmetrical weakness of muscles in the opposite limb

On the 'good' left side, there is weakness in different muscles but involving the same myotome(s) as on the 'affected' side. The right ankle evertors (L5 and S1) are, for example, strong, whereas their counterparts on the left will be weak, yet the right hip extensors (also L5 and S1) may be weak, whereas those on the left are strong.

Ligamentous discomfort

Discomfort arises from specific ligaments, usually lateralizing to the ipsilateral right or left lumbosacral region or buttock area (rather than being central, as in a disc or root problem). Of particular concern are the ligaments that are put under stretch by straight leg raising: the sacrotuberous, posterior SI joint, sacrococcygeal and sacrospinous. Discomfort precipitated by increasing the tension in these ligaments is usually reported as being off-centre.

> With a disc protrusion, the pain is more likely to localize to the centre or just to the side of the spine as the cord and roots are subjected to increased tension or compression.

Sometimes pain from the central low back region can also arise from tender interspinous, supraspinous and coccygeal ligaments put under stretch. Low back pain in association with malalignment is, however, more likely to be to the right or left lumbosacral region. If it is in the midline, check for a malrotation of L4 or L5, pain from the high-stress lumbosacral area, and tenderness localizing to the inter- and supraspinous ligaments in particular.

In the presence of malalignment, the failure to find a well-defined neurological deficit on clinical examination takes on even more significance if imaging fails to show any diminution or loss of fat around the root and there is no evidence of contact between the disc and root, or of root displacement. If there is any doubt about the diagnosis, the first step should not be disc surgery but a correction of the malalignment in conjunction with an appropriate exercise programme to see whether that will resolve some or all of the symptoms.

If, after realignment of the athlete described above, one were to find residual weakness limited to the right L5 myotome and a persistence of sensory changes and paraesthesias confined to the L5 dermatome region, that would certainly strengthen the argument that the problem stemmed from L5 root irritation or compression (see also the case history in Ch. 3). Further investigations, including electromyography and nerve conduction studies, a root block and possibly a discogram, should then be considered if they have not already been carried out.

These steps are, however, often not taken, and a discectomy is carried out on the basis of an unfortunate coincidence of symptoms and signs suggesting the irritation or compression of a nerve root, with a disc bulge or even protrusion at the level at which it is the most likely to catch that root. In this regard, the following observations by Kieffer et al (1984) should be kept in mind:

- the incidence of disc bulging increases with age after the third decade
- a bulging disc is usually not associated with nerve root compression.

MRI and CT scanning has in the past led to an overdiagnosis of a disc protrusion being the cause of a patient's back pain. More recent studies using these imaging techniques indicate that anywhere from 10% to 30% of asymptomatic subjects may show evidence of disc protrusion. As observed by Klein et al (1993, p. 23), MRI and CT scans:

showed significant abnormalities … but these did not correlate with subjective complaints and were not predictive of response to treatment.

Jensen et al (1994) found a disc bulge on MRI at least one level in 52%, a protrusion in 27% and an extrusion in 1% of 98 asymptomatic subjects. The findings suggested that 'the discovery by MRI of bulges or protrusions in people with low back pain may frequently be coincidental' (p. 69).

The author has repeatedly had to deal with patients who have undergone futile disc resection only to have the pain finally disappear with a subsequent correction of the real cause, the malalignment. The pain typically decreases or even disappears for a few days, sometimes weeks, following the resection. In retrospect, patients often volunteer that this 'interlude' was probably the result of a combination of post-operative inactivity and an increased intake of analgesic medication, or the use of stronger analgesics, to counteract the pain caused by the surgery.

The recurrence of their previous pain often coincides with their first attempts at becoming more active. The pain is frequently even worse than before; this may relate to a loss of muscle and ligament strength with the imposed rest. Extensive investigations are repeated but are usually negative or inconclusive. In the absence of definite pathology relating to the disc, there is now the risk that one of the following scenarios will evolve:

1. Ongoing symptoms are attributed to scar tissue formation and/or adhesions around the nerve root that are probably the result of chronic irritation and inflammation from the previous disc protrusion and/or the surgical intervention. The patient is told to 'live with it', often without the benefit of instruction on how to do so. Nerve blocks or epidurals may provide temporary relief. Ongoing symptoms may actually, however, be stirred up by an underlying, and so-far neglected, malalignment syndrome.

2. Symptoms are attributed to 'segmental instability' caused by the previous disc resection. The recommendation of a one- or two-level fusion of the 'unstable' segment or segments usually follows, even though flexion and extension views of the spine either fail to show a movement of 3 mm or more, or fail to do so conclusively.

The decision may be mistakenly 'strengthened' by coincident evidence of degenerative disc changes at the level(s) in question, although such degenerative changes are not uncommon on routine imaging and, in a large number, are unlikely to be the cause of their symptoms (Jensen 1994, Magora & Schwarz 1976, Weishaupt et al 1998).

Assuming that a fusion of L5–S1 or L4–L5–S1 is carried out, it is unlikely to relieve the pain stemming from pelvic malalignment. Fusion at these levels may be helpful when the underlying problem is a recurrent malrotation of L4 or L5 that has precipitated the malalignment of the pelvis. Following such a fusion, realignment of the pelvis may still result in a resolution of symptoms, provided that secondary changes related to the chronicity of the pain and the two surgeries have not progressed to the point of having become irreversible.

Either way, the hypomobility of the fused segment(s) results in stresses that increase mobility and accelerate degeneration at the disc spaces immediately above and below, as well as increasing the stress on the SI joints and hips. The end result is superimposed mechanical back pain, sometimes leading to the fusion of yet another level for advancing disc and/or facet joint degeneration.

This is a sad scenario indeed, but one unfortunately all too familiar to those working with problems relating to malalignment. It is therefore this author's heartfelt conviction that patients in whom there is any question of whether their symptoms are caused by disc protrusion should be seen in consultation by someone familiar with the diagnosis and treatment of malalignment-related problems. Hackett (1958, p. 49) said as much over 40 years ago when he advised that:

Every surgeon who operates on the spine should have a conferee that is competent to diagnose the case for him unless he fully understands ligament disability.

He was referring here to the importance of recognizing that 'sciatica' can result from causes other than disc protrusion, such as a 'relaxation' of the ligaments that support the lower portion of the sacrum (see Figs 3.58B, 4.10 and 5.32).

It is encouraging to note that a large number of articles on malalignment and secondary back problems has now been published in reputable medical journals such as *Spine* and the *Journal of Bone and Joint Surgery*, as attested to by the reference lists in this book.

Surgical 'derotation' of the tibia

The author was recently dismayed to hear a surgeon present at an international sports medicine meeting the case of a female athlete who came to the office with obvious outward rotation of the right 'foot'. This was attributed to right 'tibia varum', the solution being to cut through the tibia and fibula in order to rotate the distal part of these bones, and with it the ankle and foot, counterclockwise until the toes were more or less pointing straight ahead like the ones on the left side. There was no mention of any preoperative attempt to look for evidence of malalignment. On being questioned, it became obvious that the surgeon was unaware that malalignment even existed.

As indicated throughout this text, 'alternate' presentations and upslips are associated with external rotation of the right and internal rotation of the left lower extremity, and that was exactly what was evident on a preoperative standing view of this athlete. An outward rotation of 45 degrees from the midline, the other foot pointing straight ahead or even across midline, is not an unusual finding prior to realignment (see Figs 3.3, 3.16, 3.71 and 3.72).

'Trochanteric bursitis' and/or iliotibial band 'tendonitis'

Several athletes who have failed to respond to repeated injections of cortisone for left 'trochanteric bursitis' and/or attempts at decreasing pain arising from the tense and tender ITB have undergone resection of the left greater trochanter, the ITB or both, the other possible causes of pain in this area, such as malalignment, trigger points and referral from other structures, having been neither considered nor explored (see Figs 3.37, 3.42, 3.58 and 4.21). Typical of the latter is referral from the iliolumbar ligament to a sclerotome involving the greater trochanter region (see Figs 3.42 and 3.58); in the case of the thoracolumbar syndrome, there may be a hypersensitivity of the overlying skin from irritation of the lateral perforating cutaneous branch from T12 and L1 (see Fig. 4.21A3, B3).

Needless to say, these resections have failed to bring relief. The long scar subsequently increases tension in the skin overlying the lateral thigh and the underlying muscles, causing them to become tender with time. Correction of the malalignment, combined with stretching and strengthening, may resolve the pain, but the unsightly scar remains, and the biomechanical advantages attributable to the trochanter and the TFL/ITB complex are lost forever.

MALALIGNMENT THAT FAILS TO RESPOND TO TREATMENT

In the athlete who may or may not derive temporary relief from correction but fails to maintain that correc-

tion, the vertebral or pelvic malalignment may itself be one manifestation of an underlying problem that has so far escaped detection (see Appendix 13). In addition, it should also be borne in mind that malalignment can mimic a number of other conditions. It is therefore extremely important to avoid falling into the trap of attributing all symptoms to the malalignment and failing to rule out underlying pathology by a thorough clinical examination and investigations, especially if there is any suspicion of abnormality that cannot be explained simply on the basis of the malalignment.

The following are examples of conditions that can result in possible overlap of symptoms and signs, and may be responsible for the recurrence of malalignment.

Unilateral vertebral lumbarization or sacralization

The fact that the vertebral complex is fixed on one side and free to move on the other introduces a torquing effect every time the athlete bends forwards or backwards (see Figs 4.23 and 4.24). This torquing results in direct asymmetrical forces on the spine and the sacrum. It also exerts indirect asymmetrical forces on the innominates by way of the iliolumbar ligament attachments to the posterior iliac crests (see Fig. 2.35).

Unilateral pseudo-arthrosis or pseudo-joint

This usually involves a large L5 transverse process abutting the sacral ala, with definite or suggestive evidence of a joint space and sclerotic margins (see Fig. 4.22). An impingement of the transverse process on only one side can result in a torquing effect with any flexion, extension or rotation forces through the lumbosacral region. The pseudo-arthrosis can also become a source of pain, although the pain may manifest itself only when malalignment is present.

Disc protrusion or herniation

Pain from the disc itself or from irritation of the dura and/or nerve roots can result in asymmetrical muscle tension that predisposes to recurrent malalignment.

> Central disc protrusions are more likely to be missed because of a lack of findings on clinical examination. They should be suspected if there is a report of acute central low or mid-back pain, or even neck pain, attributable to stretching and irritation of the dura on Maitland's (slump) test.

Symptoms commonly occur when the head is brought down on the flexed trunk and/or the ankle is dorsiflexed (see Fig. 3.68).

Central protrusion must be excluded by an MRI or CT scan in those athletes whose examination otherwise reveals no obvious cause for their failure to maintain alignment (see the case history in Ch. 3).

Facet joint pathology

Facet joints can be a source of both localized and referred pain, as well as of secondary asymmetrical muscle splinting, often as the result of osteoarthritic changes.

Abdominal and pelvic masses

Masses, including uterine fibroids and ovarian cysts, can exert direct pressure on the iliopsoas and piriformis, and trigger spasm in these muscles. Iliopsoas of course crosses both the hip and the SI joint, and can exert rotational effects by way of its attachments to the spine, ilium, sacrum and femur (see Figs 2.31, 2.40, 3.38, 4.2 and 4.13). Piriformis can exert a rotational effect on the sacrum and femur (see Figs 2.31 and 7.20). Masses can also cause pain and asymmetrical muscle tension by exerting direct pressure on the pelvic floor and anterior lumbosacral plexus (see Figs 2.36 and 4.15).

Visceral pathology

Pathology can occur in the form of:

- adhesions, scar tissue or the tightness of structures such as suspending ligaments, all of which can cause restriction of the mobility of organs and viscera
- a malpositioning of the organs and viscera (e.g. upward or downward displacement, or excessive rotation).

These have all been implicated as either causative or perpetuating factors for malalignment (Barral 1989, Barral & Mercier 1988). Visceral manipulation has not infrequently finally allowed for a correction of malalignment and brought relief where other attempts of treatment aimed primarily at realignment have failed.

Lipomas

Tender lipomas, especially those which lie directly over the posterior SI joint margins and posterior pelvic ligaments, can mimic pain arising from the SI joint region and give one the mistaken impression that it is the joint or a ligament that is tender. When subjected to pressure, such as from seat backs, belts or objects carried in a back pocket (e.g. a wallet), they may trigger a reflex spasm of muscles in the vicinity, which can in turn cause a recurrence of malalignment. Sacroiliac belts sometimes cannot be tolerated for the same reason.

Some of the manoeuvres carried out as part of the back examination can cause pain by entrapping a lipoma in this region, for example as the back is extended, or by simultaneous extension, side flexion and rotation to one side. This pain may be confused with a facet or SI joint problem.

Scar tissue

Nerve fibres entrapped in scar tissue can become a source of chronic localized or referred pain that in turn triggers a reflex, asymmetrical increase in muscle tension. Those who practise neural therapy preach that all scars should be suspect until proven otherwise, something that can easily be done by injection of the scar with a short-acting local anaesthetic.

Referred pain

Pain referred to the lower extremities can result from a number of causes other than malalignment. These include trigger points, a degenerating or protruding disc, sciatic nerve irritation, facet joint degeneration or compression, and increased tension or inflammation affecting the pelvic ligaments. Intrapelvic lesions (e.g. adhesions, post-surgical scars, endometriosis, fibroids and cysts) can also be a source of referred pain.

Investigations have in such cases to be guided by the clinical presentation and availability of diagnostic equipment. In most centres, this will include:

1. a blood screen (e.g. anti-nuclear antibody, complement factor C4 level and erythrocyte sedimentation rate for underlying connective tissue disease, and HLA-B27 typing for possible ankylosing spondylitis)
2. a bone scan for inflammatory arthropathy
3. X-rays of the lumbosacral spine and SI joints
4. a CT or MRI scan to rule out disc protrusion, scar tissue or other pathology affecting the spinal cord and nerve roots
5. ultrasound of the abdomen and pelvis to rule out organomegaly and masses.

A local anaesthetic block of a facet joint, pseudo-arthrosis, nerve root, scar tissue or lipoma can quickly establish whether or not that structure is the cause of some or all of the athlete's pain. If the block provides temporary partial or complete relief, it should be repeated with the addition of cortisone, in the hope of obtaining long-term relief. Lipomas sometimes fail to respond to anything other than excision, and the fusion of a facet joint or pseudo-arthrosis may be necessary for a permanent cure. There is unfortunately still a rotational element following a unilateral fusion, just as there is with unilateral sacralization or lumbarization, and fusion of the opposite side may be necessary to prevent the recurrence of malalignment in these situations. Sensitive scar tissue may respond to attempts at desensitization with repeated injections of local anaesthetic; an initial course of 10 weekly injections usually suffices, but repeat courses may become necessary.

X-ray correlation with the presence or absence of malalignment has been in large part ignored. Malalignment is usually evident on films on a side-to-side comparison of major pelvic landmarks or joints (see Figs 2.45, 2.70, 3.75, 4.6, 4.22, 4.25, 4.26 and 4.28). An upslip and a rotational malalignment of the innominates both, for example, create a step deformity at the superior aspect of the symphysis pubis. A rotation of the lower extremities in opposite directions results in an apparent difference in the size of the lesser trochanters, which may look larger by having rotated into view on one side, and come to look smaller because of increased overlap with the shaft of the femur on the other (see Figs 2.44, 2.45 and 4.25). Different aspects of the SI joint space will be prominent on the right compared with the left side because the joints are angulated differently to the beam; often one part of the joint will be more clearly defined on one side, another on the other side (see Figs 4.22, 4.25–4.27). Aitken (1986) has clearly shown how sacral torsion around one of the oblique axes becomes evident on an X-ray, in terms of the changes in sacral alignment relative to the vertical axis, before and after correction of the malalignment (see Fig. 4.29). This is not, however, to advocate the use of X-rays to establish or confirm whether malalignment is present or whether realignment has been achieved. In addition, one must caution against trying to rely on the use of X-rays taken with the athlete lying supine when looking at pelvic obliquity and curvatures of the spine. A standing view allows for a more accurate assessment of the changes attributable to malalignment, as well as providing information on LLD and sacral base tilt (see Fig. 3.83).

UNNECESSARY INVESTIGATIONS AND TREATMENT

It is unethical and financially unjustifiable to embark on, or persist with, standard physiotherapy treatment if the underlying problem of malalignment is not being addressed at the same time. A typical example is that of the athlete with one of the 'alternate' presentations of rotational malalignment who suffers recurrent left ankle sprains.

> Limiting care to the treatment of symptoms and signs – pain, oedema, inflammation, weakness and tightness – while failing to treat the underlying predisposing condition, the malalignment, may in fact be responsible for the recurrences.

Similarly, it is unjustifiable to persist with manipulation or a specific mobilization technique indefinitely. If a trial of one technique over a 3–6 month period fails to achieve lasting realignment, a trial of another technique, or a combination of techniques, should be considered. Failure to get the athlete involved in the effort to regain or maintain realignment, by using self-assessment and self-treatment techniques, will also prolong recovery time or even prevent full recovery altogether.

The diagnosis of problems attributable to malalignment starts with an index of suspicion. Particular attention has to be paid to the possible mechanism of injury and the presenting complaint(s) that implicate structures typically put under increased stress by malalignment. It is the conglomeration of symptoms and signs, rather than any one specific test, that establishes the diagnosis of a 'malalignment syndrome'.

Malalignment can obviously coexist with other conditions involving the spine, viscera or soft tissues. If there is any doubt over whether it is the malalignment or another condition that is the cause of the problems, the first step is usually to correct the malalignment to see whether that makes any difference. To write the problems off as being caused by one of these other conditions, or worse still to proceed with surgery when the diagnosis is still suspect, is to do these athletes a great disservice and invite medicolegal repercussions.

Injured athletes are usually driven by an intense desire to get back to their sport as quickly as possible. As a result, they are probably more aware of, and more willing to try out, alternate treatment approaches. They are swift to register that a given treatment has failed and another one succeeded. If their problems do indeed arise from malalignment, they will have no difficulty eventually realizing that they underwent needless investigation and received improper, futile or aggravating treatment because the correct diagnosis had been missed.

TREATMENT IS A LONG-TERM COMMITMENT

Failure of treatment is more likely to arise from the athlete's failure to participate in the realignment process rather than from a failure to diagnose and treat one of the 'underlying problems' listed above. The athlete will sometimes give up on the manual therapy and exercise programme after 1 or 2 months because there have been no obvious dramatic results. The length of treatment may in some countries be governed by the number of therapy sessions covered by an insurance plan. Unfortunately, not everyone can be expected to respond fully in the time span of 12 therapy sessions or whatever limit is set by a regional plan.

Whereas most athletes respond to realignment procedures within 3–4 months, this is not always the case. The athlete must therefore be advised that treatment may be a long-term proposition, which requires a full commitment on his or her part: 1 or 2 years may be required to undo the effects of malalignment that has been present for several years or even decades.

Malalignment results in long-term problems primarily related to connective tissue structures. Tendons, ligaments, capsules and myofascial structures that have either contracted or become lax over the years take time to regain their normal length as they adapt to the realignment. The healing response may be compromised by the poor blood supply of connective tissues. Any recurrence of the malalignment serves only to slow down the recovery process, and any interruption of the treatment programme, for whatever reason, can only have the same detrimental effect.

Some athletes are happy to settle for short-term results and are not willing to participate in long-term treatment and a regular home exercise programme, preferring instead to return for treatment whenever their symptoms flare up. It is for this reason that athletes should be taught right at the start how malalignment puts them at risk of recurrent injury, and how they play a major part in the recovery process.

> Treatment should not be a sporadic event, limited to time spent with the therapist at weekly or biweekly intervals but should become a process that requires their involvement.

Athletes must be told firmly that they have to be willing to forego some activities for a time in order to increase the chance of regaining and maintaining alignment, and to allow the injured tissues to heal. The aim is to allow them eventually to return to all their activities, regular self-assessment and self-treatment thereafter becoming the key to the prevention of recurrent symptoms and injury. If athletes fail to heed this advice, and fail to play an active part in their recovery process, they are merely compromising their chances of ever making a complete recovery and reaching their full athletic potential.

8

Treatment: manual therapy modes

There are many therapies and professions that offer potential solutions to body malalignment problems. This chapter will outline some effective choices of therapeutic technique and consider the health-care professionals who address musculoskeletal malalignment. The resolution or persistence of a malalignment syndrome depends to large extent on the level of training, skill and experience of the health-care professionals from whom an athlete seeks help. From the chapter, the reader will observe the author's strong bias towards hands-on, manual therapy approaches.

MANUAL THERAPY

Manual therapy consists of a wide variety of hands-on techniques applied to the body's tissues. The disruption of any body tissue structure will disturb the functioning of those tissues, that is, it will result in a somatic dysfunction. Manual therapy techniques are particularly effective in helping to correct somatic dysfunctions because of the ability of the therapist's trained hands to sense subtle changes occurring in the treated tissues. The approach chosen by a therapist is influenced by the therapeutic model that the therapist uses to understand and influence the body's tissues. What follows is an outline of the therapeutic models that can be considered when addressing the malalignment syndrome (Box 8.1).

CONNECTIVE TISSUE BIOMECHANICAL AND NEUROPHYSIOLOGICAL CHARACTERISTICS

Manual techniques that change the tissue characteristics of the body require an understanding of the biomechanical and neurophysiological properties of these tissues, which include muscle, bone and pervasive connective tissues. A common denominator

---

Box 8.1 Therapeutic models used to treat
malalignment syndrome

Biomechanical approach
Direct techniques
- Thrust technique, i.e. chiropractic-type high-velocity, low-amplitude joint manipulation
- Non-thrust techniques
  - joint oscillation, joint mobilization and articulations, e.g. range of motion exercises
  - muscle energy technique
  - functional and neuroreceptive techniques
  - soft tissue procedures such as Swedish massage and stretching

Indirect techniques
- Counterstrain and other functional techniques
- Myofascial release

Neuroreceptive approach
Disruption of body rhythms
- Craniosacral therapy
- Functional technique
- Myofascial technique

Total body reintegration
- Structural integration (Rolfing)
- Upper cervical 'Grostic' (NUCCA) chiropractic method
- Alexander technique
- Feldenkrais method

Disruption of sensory and motor points
- Counterstrain
- Travell trigger point therapy
- Touch for health and applied kinesiology
- Intramuscular stimulation (Gunn dry-needling technique)
- Acupuncture

Combined techniques with elements from all of the above techniques
- Craniosacral therapy
- Myofascial release
- Functional techniques

---

not return to its original condition when the mechanical load is removed.
3. Tissue failure will occur at some point when the collagen tissue can no longer continue to deform. The end result is usually an acute injury with an accompanying inflammatory response.

The author hypothesizes that those techniques which reduce tissue stress patterns are particularly successful in re-establishing good body alignment and the neuromuscular tone necessary to maintain it. Connective tissue fibres align along lines of stress. Malalignment creates abnormal stress patterns in connective tissues strong enough to deform it beyond its original elastic characteristics. The gel-like matrix between and around the collagen fibres has lost some of its fluid-retaining abilities and reduced the distance between collagen molecular chains. This allows a more random cross-linking of collagen strands that resist standard therapeutic stretching. In addition, DeVries (1986) writes that:

the importance of the fascial tissues [connective tissues] has been shown by a recent experiment in which a small slit in the epimysium of the fascia resulted in 15% loss in muscle strength.

The changed characteristics of organized connective tissue that is biomechanically dysfunctional as a result of abnormal stress patterns or direct trauma affect the function of the enclosed tissues and organs. The release of biomechanically induced stress patterns in connective tissues reduces the afferent barrage of proprioceptive signals into the central nervous system.

It is the author's contention that, in living beings, biomechanical dysfunctions are ultimately the result of reactions and responses to gravitational and neural stresses. Correcting physical tissue dysfunctions lays the groundwork for removing many of the stimuli that keep the nervous system in a state of alarm.

---

between all of these is the presence of a large amount of collagen. Collagen has several physical properties when subjected to mechanical loading:

1. Collagen fibres can initially stretch because of their visco-elastic properties (see below), and recover from the deformation soon after the mechanical loading is removed.
2. With increased loading, the collagen tissues enter a 'plastic' phase of tissue deformation in which, it is thought, some of the intermolecular cross-links between the collagen strands separate. At this point, the affected tissue will 'yield' to the load and will

PROPRIOCEPTIVE AND CONNECTIVE TISSUE CONCEPTS IN TREATMENT

Connective tissue surrounds every body tissue. A form of organized connective tissue – myofascia – envelops muscles. A considerable afferent innervation of connective tissue surrounding the joints influences the tone of muscles around these joints. Sensory input into the central nervous system by passive joint movements may temporarily override the brain's output of the inhibitory signals that increase local muscle tension and restrict a joint's range of movement.

In addition, the sensory input from nerve endings in the muscles and joints from adjacent spinal segments will eventually overcome local inhibitory sensory input through the proprioceptive influence of larger musculoskeletal postural patterns in the body. Engles (1989) writes that type III proprioceptor endings:

being similar to Golgi tendon organs, can totally inhibit the excitability of the alpha motoneuron in nearby muscles when they are strongly stimulated.

Freeman & Wyke (Engles 1989) have demonstrated that muscle resists passive stretching when muscle tone is increased through a reflex action involving the intense stimulation of alpha motorneurons (see below). The mechanical characteristics of the connective tissue change after a deforming force has been present for a long time. The sensory stimulation of joint mechanoreceptors through joint mobilization or manipulation may fail to counteract physical tissue changes. Examples in this chapter demonstrate that the biomechanical treatment of connective tissue elements restricting joint range of motion is also important to the successful resolution of musculoskeletal malalignment.

Joint proprioceptors

Wyke (1973) has classified the proprioceptors around joints into four categories (Box 8.2).

Mechanoreceptive nerve endings in the joint capsule and tendons stimulated with mobilization techniques provide various feedback nerve loops. These nerve

---

Box 8.2   Joint proprioceptors

- **Type I endings:** an encapsulated ending supplied by myelinated nerves that are physiologically slow-adapting and provide a conscious awareness of joint position and joint movement. These endings are important for postural control
- **Type II endings:** an encapsulated ending supplied by myelinated afferent nerve fibres that are rapidly adapting and highly sensitive to movement and pressure changes around joint capsules
- **Type III endings:** endings that are identical to Golgi tendon organs in structure and function, and are located in the pericapsular ligaments. They are slow-adapting and serve to protect joints from excess stress through a reflex inhibition of the surrounding muscles
- **Type IV endings:** these endings are free and unencapsulated, also supplied by myelinated nerve fibres and thought to sense excessive joint movement primarily by signalling pain

---

endings reflexly reduce or eliminate limitations of the joint's range of motion by creating conditions for releasing muscle tension.

MECHANICAL LOADING OF CONNECTIVE TISSUE

Clinically, the author has observed that the symmetry of muscle tone often improves immediately upon the re-establishment of good body alignment. Muscle tone may change because both biomechanical and proprioceptive factors are beneficially altered in the surrounding myofascia. Connective tissue mobilization inevitably involves the proprioceptive facilitation of associated muscles; the therapeutic forces need not be intense in order to counteract this state of deformation.

Engles (1989, p. 27) aptly expresses the therapeutic limitations of some rehabilitation approaches that can apply to the malalignment syndrome when she states the following:

When procedures are more specific, forces can be continually controlled and modified according to the response of the tissue and the patient. Without knowledge of the normal structure of the tissues we are dealing with, of the changes in these tissues with injury, immobilization, healing, and remobilization, and the response of these tissues to the mechanical forces placed on them during physical therapy procedures, treatment is at best only minimally therapeutic.

A surprising number of the athletes treated by these manual therapy methods do, however, respond even though the exact nature of the changes that their neuromusculoskeletal tissues have undergone with the malalignment is not readily apparent.

Muscle energy techniques

Sawtell (1982) describes muscle energy techniques (METs) as an area of manual therapy that addresses the treatment of musculoskeletal (somatic) dysfunction. Muscle energy principles were developed by the osteopaths F. L. Mitchell Sr and F. L. Mitchell Jr, who organized and promoted the treatment concepts in their book *An Evaluation and Treatment Manual of Osteopathic Muscle Energy Procedures* (Mitchell & Mitchell 1979). METs have proved valuable in addressing some of the major musculoskeletal imbalances that occur in athletes with malalignment problems. These techniques are not only ones that the therapist can apply, but also include some that the athlete can use for self-treatment and the prevention of malalignment problems (see below).

Somatic dysfunctions

On the subject of somatic dysfunctions and MET, Sawtell (1982) writes:

The term *'somatic dysfunction'* can be defined as 'impaired or altered function of related components of the somatic (body framework) system: skeletal, arthrodial, and myofascial structures, and related vascular, lymphatic and neural elements'. In other words, it is a malfunction of a segment or segments of the spinal column, pelvis or extremities that may produce limited motion in an area, muscle spasm, pain, tenderness, and even remote symptoms. In our practices, we commonly see terms such as 'myositis', 'neuralgia', 'limited range of motion', 'spasm', etc.; which are synonymous with and amplifications of the above concept. As musculoskeletal dysfunctions and syndromes often defy easy classification under conventional medical diagnostic conventions, many models of somatic function have been used to provide a basis for therapeutic intervention. These include Neurologic Models, Postural-Structural Models, Respiratory-Circulatory Models and Bio-Energy Models. The many 'schools of thought' within the area of manual therapy base their principles and philosophies on one or more of these models in their approach to the biomechanical treatment of somatic dysfunction.

Muscle Energy Technique

The Muscle Energy Technique utilizes all of the above-mentioned models in its approach to somatic dysfunction. The principle modality for determining appropriate treatment using muscle energy techniques is that of palpation. With educated hands one is able to detect and discriminate qualities such as softness and hardness, shape, texture, size–depth–thickness, position, temperature and moisture. These qualities are perceived by the examiner and integrated with other information such as motion, pulses and reactions of tissues. Interpretation of this information is necessary to establish possibilities, relationships, and techniques applicable to our findings. Most of us repeat this process several times every day. However, what determines their treatment (to stretch, to strengthen, to facilitate, to inhibit …) is how we interpret and what significance we put on what our proprioceptive touch is telling us.

In addition to palpation, direct inspection is an important part of evaluating the athlete with somatic dysfunction. While touch gave us a wealth of information within the Respiratory-Circulatory Model (edema, autonomic dysfunction such as skin texture, temperature and moisture) and the Neurologic Model (muscle tone, excitability, etc.), direct inspection will give the examiner valuable information within the Postural-Structural Model (gravitational adaptations, gross motion, anomalies and observable injury).

Basic to the use of Muscle Energy Technique as a treatment approach is the understanding of the various systems within the body and the relationships that these systems form in both a state of health and a pathological state. [If a hypomobile segment is the cause of a hypermobility elsewhere] it makes no sense to treat a pain producing hypermobility symptomatically while leaving the non-pain-producing hypomobility untreated. [If a scoliosis is an adaptation to an unlevel sacral base] it makes no sense to treat an adaptive scoliotic curve without first treating an unlevel sacral base. Stress in many forms can influence the sympathetic nervous system and manifest itself in somatic disorders and dysfunction. Recognition and treatment of both go hand in hand if one expects a good result. The somatic component of disease, the neurophysiological and the biomechanical/biochemical relationships of the body must be considered.

Also basic to the Muscle Energy Technique is the concept of soft tissue restrictions. Primary or secondary to the underlying pathology there may be edema, histological changes, muscle spasm, and/or biomechanical/biochemical restriction to normal somatic function. These restrictions are referred to as 'Pathological Motion Barriers'. Muscle Energy Technique is aimed at 'disengaging' these barriers. In normal tissue no resistance to movement is encountered until approaching the (normal) anatomical barrier….

The quality of the restrictive barrier is determined by the examiner, i.e., muscle shortening, spasm, joint restriction, edema, etc., and the appropriate Muscle Energy Technique is employed to disengage this barrier. This differs from many of the mobilization techniques in where the restrictive barrier (usually presumed joint restriction) is engaged and some force is directed into the barrier only in the technique used…

Performing a Muscle Energy Technique requires that both the therapist and the athlete are relaxed and balanced and that care is taken by the therapist to localize his or her efforts so that least energy and force will accomplish the desired result. With the above criteria, the Muscle Energy Technique involves: (1) active contraction by the athlete, (2) controlled joint positioning, (3) specific direction, (4) distinct counterforce and (5) controlled contraction intensity. The specific types of muscle contractions utilized vary with the desired result. Isometric contraction would be used to lengthen a shortened muscle. Neurophysiological phenomena including relaxation and reciprocal inhibition are used. Structural relationships and posture can be directly influenced via the reverse action of a particular muscle using isometric exercises. Isotonic exercises are used to increase muscle strength and an 'isolytic contraction' involves a mobilization technique superimposed on an isometric contraction. A specific stimulus is directed to achieve a specific response. These stimuli are mediated via the somatic system to influence the sympathetic nervous system, the gamma-alpha loop, direct structural and postural relationships, and the function and mobility of joints. The responses desired include stretching of muscles and fascia, toning muscles, mobilizing restricted joints and relieving passive congestion.

No one approach to the treatment of somatic dysfunction can be used exclusive of all others. However the Muscle Energy Technique, as a concept and as a skill, is a valuable treatment modality which has good neurophysiological basis, is easily learned by most manual therapists if they so desire and, most importantly, yields good results in the clinic with those athletes whose main problem is somatic dysfunction. (Sawtell 1982; adapted by permission from the Ursa Foundation)

Functional technique

The 'functional technique' is an osteopathic indirect technique. It aims to correct body movement dysfunctions by re-establishing a balanced neural function that indirectly leads to balanced structures, that is, alignment. There are in general three types of functional technique (Greenman 1989).

The balance and hold method

The aim of this method is to achieve a dynamic balance of relaxed tissues surrounding a dysfunctional spinal segment. A segment of the spine may, for example, have limited rotation. A segment is said to be therapeutically 'stacked' when it is put through a series of separate and precise physiological movements. The surrounding soft tissue structures are relaxed in the primary biomechanical ranges of motion of that segment:

- The therapist assesses and assists the athlete to relax and rotate his or her spine into the mid-range of that segment's range of rotation.
- Next, the therapist assesses and positions the same area in its mid-range of flexion and extension, then
  - its mid-range of side flexion, and perhaps
  - its axial compression/distraction.

Once the body segment is appropriately 'stacked', the athlete is asked to breathe in and out fully. The therapist determines whether the athlete is most at ease in breathing in or out. The athlete is asked to hold the breath in that phase of respiration for as long as is comfortably possible, usually between 5 and 30 seconds. The result is the re-establishment of a symmetrical and comfortable functional movement at that segment.

The functional technique relaxes the muscles in the stacked 'facilitated segment' of the spine. This relaxation normalizes the actions of the joints of that segment and leads to a rebalancing of the body posture. The concept (Bowles 1981) behind the use of functional movements is that of achieving a positive segmental response rather than an idealized segmental position of the joints.

The 'facilitated segment' is a concept developed by Korr (1986); it suggests that a neurological segment of the spine, when injured, results in dysfunction in the associated dermatome, myotome, sclerotome and visceral distribution. These act like an amplifier to increase the awareness of body dysfunction. In other words, there are effects distant from the affected spinal segment. Treatment that helps to restore the neuromuscular function of a segment with an approach such as the functional technique described also helps to resolve these distant effects.

Dynamic functional method

This method involves having the therapist hold one hand (the monitoring hand) over a dysfunctional body segment and having the athlete move either actively or passively around the affected segment in such a way that a normal movement pattern is 'dynamically' recaptured. The involved segment contributing to an overall malalignment is often the lumbosacral segment. By placing the monitoring hand over the lumbosacral junction, the therapist can assist the athlete through a series of localized movements. A significant correction of alignment can be observed when the movements succeed in temporarily shutting off the spasms in resting muscles that to this point have resisted the re-establishment of normal movement patterns in a body segment.

Counterstrain (release by positioning)

Jones (1981), an osteopath, developed the use of a positional release therapy that he named *counterstrain*. This involves placing body segment(s) into their most relaxed and comfortable position for 30–90 seconds. A point of localized tenderness to palpation within the soft tissue that may correspond to a trigger point, or so-called 'Jones point', is monitored through palpation. The surrounding body parts and tissues are positioned to normalize inappropriate proprioceptive activity and nociceptive sensory input until the pain at this site completely disappears.

For example, if the left quadratus lumborum muscle became tense and hypertonic in comparison to the right muscle, the effect of its tension will be to pull the lumbar spine into left side-bending and relative right rotation – a condition that contributes to malalignment. Using counterstrain principles, the therapist will palpate for a tender point(s) in the hypertonic quadratus lumborum muscle. Monitoring the tension around that point and with constant feedback from the athlete, the therapist then assists the athlete into a position in which the painful stimulus of the palpated trigger point completely subsides. The therapist then maintains this position for 30–90 seconds while continuing to maintain pressure over the trigger point area. On returning the body part to the original position, the point is no longer painful to palpation, and the tissues involved demonstrate a greater range of motion.

Myofascial release

Myofascial release is a combined technique that manipulates the connective tissue of the body, especially the fascia, in such a way until it achieves, as Greenman (1989, p. 106) states:

the common goal of all manual medicine procedures of attempting to achieve symmetrical function of the entire musculo-skeletal system in postural balance.

Myofascial release, as an approach, encompasses elements from many other techniques. In myofascial release, the therapist has the choice of manually moving the myofascia either away from the joint or tissue of perceived restriction or towards the restriction. The primary motive of myofascial release is to achieve a biomechanical release of the myofascia. Greenman (1989) describes this with the mnemonic P.O.E. $(T)^2$. The approach requires:

- a *point of entry* into the musculoskeletal system, in which the therapist's hands are placed in a comfortable position on the athlete to allow stretching forces to be introduced
- T^2 equals the application of a *traction* force through the longitudinal alignment of the underlying body fascia followed by a *twisting* force through the body that allows the ensuing stretch to equalize the tensions in the fascia along the spiral-form arrangement of most organized body connective tissue.

TREATMENT METHODS USING DISRUPTION OF BODY RHYTHMS

The qualities of three physiological rhythms are palpable almost anywhere in the human body: the cardiovascular, the respiratory and the craniosacral. The cardiovascular and respiratory rhythms are used both diagnostically and therapeutically. A very valuable method for treating musculoskeletal malalignment involves affecting the quality of a particular body rhythm such as the respiratory or craniosacral rhythm.

With the functional technique, the established breathing pattern is therapeutically altered. During treatment, an athlete may be asked to hold his or her breath during the inspiration or expiration phase of breathing. The therapeutic aim is based on a neurological model of body functioning. A musculoskeletal dysfunction transmits an abnormal flow of afferent impulses into the central nervous system. This flow may be altered when the body is positioned in a pain-free position and the breathing pattern, which may be shallow or rapid, is interrupted.

> For an optimal result, the functional technique and counterstrain aim to disrupt the facilitating effect of the muscle spindles on muscle tone for 30–90 seconds. The change of afferent flow into the central nervous system helps to normalize the control of the dysfunctional segment.

Craniosacral therapy uses the craniosacral rhythm to assess the body's functioning and therapeutic changes. Palpation of the more subtle craniosacral rhythm is easily learned. Musculoskeletal malalignment can be treated manually by disrupting the rhythm while assisting the athlete to move into various postures. When the craniosacral rhythm subsides and the individual's body stops moving at an internally significant position, profound tissue changes tend to occur. An analysis of the craniosacral therapy approach follows.

Craniosacral system

The craniosacral system (Upledger Institute 1991) is a physiological system that exists in humans as well as those animals possessing a brain and spinal cord. Its formation begins in the womb, and its function continues until death. Its name is derived from the most cephalic and caudal bones to which the dural membranes enclosing the system are connected. A biomechanical imbalance in the craniosacral membrane system surrounding the central nervous system can adversely affect the development and function of the brain and spinal cord. Sensory, motor and intellectual dysfunctions can result.

Craniosacral therapy and the 'still point'

Craniosacral therapy involves the treatment of the body's organized connective tissues. The tissues may be myofascial, dural-meningeal, tenoligamentous or visceral.

> Craniosacral therapy involves a gentle proprioceptive facilitation of the afferent nervous system to promote an 'unwinding' of tortions in the connective tissues.

The process is 'dynamic' and involves the palpation of continual tissue movement and changes in tissue tension.

The function and alignment of the pelvis are inextricably connected with the functioning of the craniosacral system and its dural connections from the cranium to the sacrum. The rhythmic fluctuation in the volume and pressure of the cerebrospinal fluid produced in the cranial ventricles affects the intracranial dural membranes as well as the spinal dura. This fluctuation of the craniosacral rhythm is a natural physiological rhythm of between 8 and 14 cycles per minute that is transmitted throughout the body via the connective tissue, such as the myofascia.

Many parts of the body, including the cranial bones and sacrum, can be used as points of contact to palpate and influence the rhythm. The rhythm is palpable as an alternating increase in the tension of the muscles or fascia affecting the internal and then the external rotators of the hips, forearms and shoulders, for example. Retzlaff (1987) and Upledger (1977) confirm that fluctuations in the cardiac and respiratory rhythms do not affect this rhythm.

Facilitating a 'still point' or temporarily arresting the craniosacral rhythm produces a valuable therapeutic response. A still point is gently achieved by temporarily restricting the physiological motion of the bones that are influenced by the craniosacral rhythm. This can be done using an occipital hand-hold called the 'CV4 technique' or via a similar constraining hold on the sacrum, the feet and so on.

During a still point, the athlete usually experiences a profound relaxation effect. Musculoskeletal dysfunctions often spontaneously self-correct and the breathing becomes very relaxed. The craniosacral rhythm resumes within a few seconds or a few minutes. The motion of the body tissues usually exhibits a better symmetry and a larger amplitude throughout the craniosacral system.

Craniosacral therapy analogy

The author has found that a combination of the direct and indirect biomechanical approaches inherent to craniosacral therapy often works best in helping correct malalignment. The following analogy can be used as an introduction to this therapy.

A tangled telephone cord can not be untangled simply by stretching it: the tangles recur and often are magnified when the tension on the cord is released. They can, however, easily be eliminated by suspending the handset by its attached cord and unwinding the cord. The handset goes through a series of spins and turns within the gravitational field until the cord reaches its optimal length.

What is the meaning behind this analogy? First, the telephone cord and handset represent a system, one which can transmit, absorb or disperse the forces imposed on it. When the system is the human body, the absorption or dispersion of forces has the most negative impact on the athlete. The dispersion of a physical force through the body often arises from an acute injury such as a haematoma, strain, sprain or fracture. When the body absorbs the impact of a force or a 'stressor', the telephone cord analogy applies.

Forces imposed upon the system create a dysfunctional system, as the tangles demonstrate. Stretching the cord will not reduce its tendency to tangle when the tension is removed, but, suspending the handset by its cord allows the system to unwind on its own. The handset spins in one direction and then the other as the cord releases its kinks and tangles. Afterwards, the cord responds 'normally' to stretching, by recovering from a stretch without increasing the amount of tangling or kinking in the cord.

Using the analogy above, the telephone cord can be equated to the human body. After absorbing a serious blow, the body begins a process of adaptation. An athlete who 'suddenly' develops a physical dysfunction without a blatant injury may find it difficult to explain, especially when such a dysfunction persists. His or her body may have absorbed the forces either from instantaneously introduced trauma or cumulative repetitive forces. The dysfunction may be the result of the inability of the body tissues to adapt to any further 'quantums' of absorbed energy common to the type of, and intensity of, athletic activities. Appropriate therapy to the connective tissue elements that make up the local and distal connections with the pelvis aims to help to 'disperse' the energy manually.

The telephone cord analogy illustrated a spiral-form system, the system by which the human body functions mechanically. Gracovetsky & Farfan (1986) describe important spiral-form elements in human gait in their discussion of electromyographic pattern of activity of the trunk musculature in walking. This arthrokinematic description of human gait serves to underline the essentially spiral-form function of body movement.

In this process, the pelvis functions as a torque converter, transferring the energy of leg movements during the gait cycle into a spinal torque that conserves energy in the ligaments and fascia of the trunk. This makes the smooth functioning at the sacroiliac joints and pubic symphysis pivotal to efficient body mobility.

Any injury or stress disturbs the normal pattern of tissue mobility. Tissue unwinding re-establishes a more biomechanically efficient gait and movement pattern. Given that movement is inherently a function of the nervous system, efficient biomechanics lead to efficient nerve function.

Energy cyst model for body dysfunctions

Upledger & Karni (1990) developed an 'energy cyst' hypothesis relating to the impact of forces on the body (Box 8.3).

Craniosacral therapy: a 10-step protocol

This protocol is a hands-on approach developed by Upledger and addresses pivotal areas of the body that affects the craniosacral system. The malalignment

---

Box 8.3 Upledger & Karni's 'energy cyst' theory

An 'energy cyst' is created when body tissues absorb a physical force, this energy cyst disrupting the normal molecular and energetic order of these tissues and raising their state of disorder or entropy. The authors hypothesize that the body system's protective-adaptive response is to wall off the energy cyst area in order to allow the rest of the body to function as effectively as possible. Upledger's opinion is that '[the] major determinant for the formation of these energy cysts ... is the emotional state of the individual at the time of the accident or injury' (Manheim & Lavett 1989, p. 12). Extra physiological and biochemical energy is needed to maintain the malalignment of body tissues perpetuated by an energy cyst. The adaptive stresses on the body system reach a maximum limit and the athlete experiences the result as a myriad of complaints.

---

syndrome can usually be treated effectively by using the protocol as a therapeutic basis.

Myofascial diaphragms. The organized connective tissue of the body permeates the whole body, the body's fascial sheets being predominantly longitudinally aligned. In several areas in the body, however, there are transverse structural or functional orientations of the body's connective tissues, the respiratory diaphragm being the most obvious example. Upledger also describes the plantar fascia, the pelvic floor, the thoracic outlet, the suboccipital region and the submandibular region as functional, horizontally aligned myofascial diaphragms. Any hypertonicity of these diaphragms can significantly restrict the fascial mobility of the longitudinally oriented fascial planes.

In healthy people, fascial tissue, influenced by the craniosacral rhythm, moves in a balanced and symmetrical manner. Trauma will distort this balance, causing asymmetrical motion and a contracture of the connective tissues around the muscles, bones and organs. Within the 10-step protocol, the therapist uses hands-on placement over the areas of the diaphragms to achieve a release and relaxation of the underlying tissues. A discussion of the treatment rational of some of the body's diaphragms follows.

Respiratory diaphragm. The respiratory diaphragm may develop hypertonus or contracture under the influence of its efferent nerves, such as the branches of the ventral primary divisions of thoracic nerves 9–12, and the phrenic nerve, which has its origins primarily from the IVth cervical nerve with contributing branches from C3 and C5 (Upledger & Vredevoogd 1983). In addition, visceral problems such as those affecting the liver and gall bladder, or inflammation of the pleura, can create diaphragmatic hypertonus

(see Fig. 4.33). Even when some of the initial pathologies or injuries that may have contributed to diaphragmatic hypertonus resolve, the hypertonus may itself become self-perpetuating. As part of the treatment protocol used with craniosacral therapy, the respiratory diaphragm is 'unwound' to achieve a new balance of myofascial elements.

Pelvic and urogenital diaphragms. The pelvic and urogenital diaphragms function as one unit. Given the anatomy of the area, the tone of the myofascial tissue of this diaphragm has a significant effect on the mobility of the coccyx and sacrum, and its function of anchoring the dural tube to the sacrum and coccyx.

Coccygeal release methods

The internal pelvic floor treatment of abnormalities of the sacrococcygeal joint and the pelvic floor lives outside the 10-step protocol of Upledger-based craniosacral therapy, but Upledger refers three times to the direct treatment of the coccyx in his book *Craniosacral Therapy* (Upledger & Vredevoogd 1983).

The functioning of the pelvic floor is integral to the functioning of many structures. In many sports, such as figure-skating, falls onto the coccyx frequently occur, whereas in other sports, for example the luge, the coccyx is at risk of being subjected to the repeated impact of contusive forces. The example of a broad- or long-jumper propelled by an asymmetrical push off the take-off board followed by a jarring stop when landing on the buttocks and inevitably on the coccyx provides a common scenario that leads to and perpetuates the malalignment syndrome.

Recognizing the structural interconnections of the fascia and muscles on the pelvic floor to the sacrum, pelvis and internal organs, there is a broad range of possible body symptoms, especially in the low back and pelvis, that may have their origins in structural dysfunctions and will therefore benefit from manual therapy. The pelvic floor release included in the 10-step protocol involves unwinding the pelvic floor diaphragm by a hand placement on the lower abdominal wall and sacrum. This is not, however, always enough to resolve a pelvic floor dysfunction: it may be necessary to assess and treat the sacrococcygeal joint directly via gentle internal manipulation of the coccyx and its surrounding tissues, like the sacrotuberous ligament, through the anus and sometimes intravaginally.

Prior to attempting an invasive technique on a physically and psychologically sensitive body area such as the anus, Selby (1990) proposes a trial of a treatment technique that will be summarised here as it has already been alluded to in more detail in Chapter 4:

1. Evaluate the gross range of motion of the whole spine, including the neck. Evaluate sacroiliac mobility using the techniques mentioned in Chapter 2.
2. Evaluate the spinal dural system for irritability using such tests as Maitland's slump test (see Fig. 3.68), carefully noting the ranges of motion in the lower extremity and spine as the dural barrier is engaged.
3. Palpate the coccyx through the clothing, noting its anterior–posterior angulation, any deviation to one side, any tenderness around its tip and any thickening or hypertrophy of the soft tissue inserting into it.
4. Briefly massage around the edges of the coccyx deeply through the clothing. Note its flexibility and end-feel while attempting to release tension in the soft tissues. Gently mobilize the joint. Alternatively, with the athlete either in sitting, prone or side-lying, apply sustained pressure deeply onto the lateral margins of the coccyx.
5. Immediately re-evaluate the range of motion in the spine and neck and re-examine the slump test if it was positive.

In Selby's experience, blatant coccyodynia is associated with a loss of lumbosacral extension, unilateral or bilateral side-bending and sometimes flexion. In his experience, it is not uncommon, after rubbing the coccygeal margins deeply for only 30 seconds, to observe a doubling or tripling of spinal motion in patients with post-traumatic hypertonicity of the pubococcygeal muscle.

Connective tissues have a good afferent proprioceptive innervation, and the stimulation of some proprioceptors in the ligaments can have a positive reflex effect on the tone of the surrounding muscles (Heinrich 1990, Midttun & Bojsen-Moller 1986). A relaxation of the muscles in the pelvic floor through some form of myofascial release can facilitate a removal of myofascial tissue stress imposed by various traumatic forces.

BODY REINTEGRATION METHODS

Other forms of manual therapy or exercise can also address the complaints accompanying a malalignment syndrome. Below are examples of body reintegration approaches that can counteract the body imbalances resulting from not only trauma and injury, but also habitual movement and postural patterns.

The neuromuscular influences on motion include, in addition to frank neurological diseases, alterations in neuromuscular organization and coordination. Neuromuscular shock following significant tissue trauma may produce unequal tone, muscle weakness,

fibrosis and a loss of coordination. A joint may become inflamed and undergo physical or chemical changes in its various collagen elements, including the synovial fluid, with resultant pain. Pain may itself become an additional neurogenic factor in the limitation of motion.

A common situation involves an ankle sprain. With injury to the ankle ligaments, there is usually a reduction in the proprioceptive signalling from the ankle. Pain and muscle splinting result in a reduction of the movement that would normally activate the many proprioceptive receptors in the ankle ligaments. The reduction of proprioceptive information can then result in an alteration of movement patterns at the ankle and eventual postural maladaptation affecting proximal parts of the lower extremity and finally the pelvis and trunk.

In speaking of the process of postural adaptation, Steindler (1955) calls attention to the principle of 'the path of least resistance'. This means in essence that the body will rearrange its posture in adapting to a deformity or functional deficit in order to allow for the least amount of muscular effort expenditure. Such postural accommodation requires changes in neuromuscular coordination.

Structural integration: Rolfing

The direct hands-on work of Rolfing practitioners is aimed at 'structural integration'. Rolf, a doctor of biochemistry and physiology, originally developed this treatment approach in the 1930s. Its aim is to bring the body into a better alignment with gravity through a system of deep and often painful stretching of the body fascia. The work consists of a series of 10 60–90 minute treatment sessions, summarised in Box 8.4 (Faldiman & Frager 1976, p. 139).

The emphasis in Rolf's approach is on pelvic biomechanics. In the author's experience, this is one area which, when treated, leads to a significant impact on the functioning of other areas of the body.

Upper cervical 'Grostic' chiropractic technique

A unique approach to the treatment of the malalignment syndrome comes from within the chiropractic profession. The 'Grostic' technique (Portman 1992) was developed by chiropractors J. Grostic and R. Gregory in the 1940's in the USA. Their technique has evolved into the National Upper Cervical Chiropractic Association (NUCCA). The NUCCA acronym has become synonymous with the technique.

Given the wide repercussions of the malalignment syndrome, it appears remarkably simple to suscribe

---

Box 8.4 Structure of Rolfing treatment sessions

1: Includes much of the body, with special focus on those muscles of the chest and abdomen that govern breathing, and the hip joint, which controls pelvic mobility.

2: Concentrates on the feet, reforming the foot and ankle hinges and aligning the legs with the torso.

3: Devoted primarily to lengthening the sides, especially the large muscles between the pelvis and rib cage.

4–6: Devoted primarily to freeing the pelvis: Rolf has stressed that most people hold their pelvis rotated toward the rear [with anterior innominate rotation, lumbar hyperlordosis and accompanying changes like shortened hamstring muscles that restrict full pelvic mobility (Rolf 1977).] Because of the tremendous importance of the pelvis in posture and in movement, one of the major emphases of rolfing is to make the pelvis more flexible, and better aligned with the rest of the body.

7: Concentrates on the neck and head and also on the muscles of the face.

8–10: Deal mainly with organizing and integrating the entire body.

---

most of these problems to a condition that NUCCA calls the 'atlas subluxation complex' (A.S.C.). Foran (1999) describes this as:

Verifiable elements such as spastic contracture, pelvic distortions, contractured leg, center of gravity displacement, and deviations of the spinal vertebrae from the vertical axis are objective signs that can be measured, tested, and reciprocally related to the A.S.C. A misaligned atlas causes unilateral shortening of the leg length and causes compensatory postures often affecting the spine. As the head shifts off center, the pelvis must also shift.

Many manual therapy methods described in this book are aimed at re-establishing normal biomechanical functioning, with an emphasis on reducing the stress on the nerves and musculoskeletal structures of the body. With the possible exception of craniosacral therapy, to which we will return, the NUCCA technique places a primary emphasis on restoring normal central nervous system functioning by removing physical stresses on the brainstem and spinal cord at the level of C1 and C2.

At the level of the foramen magnum and occipital base, there are many vital neural structures that are particularly vulnerable to pressure and to being stretched as a result of upper cervical vertebral displacement and cranial base distortions. Pressure on and stretching of the neural structures can lead to the creation of a facilitated segment (see above).

A brief examination of neuroanatomy will indicate that, at the level of the cranial base and the atlas, the central nervous system contains the nuclei for the glossopharyngeal, vagus, accessory and hypoglossal cranial nerves. The pyramidal decussation of the spinal cord tracts also occurs at this level. In addition, the reticular activating system of the brainstem reaches down through the foramen magnum and is vulnerable to stresses imposed on the spinal cord either directly by a subluxed atlas or by its surrounding dural membranes. A thorough neuroanatomical discussion of this area is available in Upledger (1987).

NUCCA treatment technique

The NUCCA treatment technique relies on a direct and precise manual treatment protocol for the C1 and C2 levels based on an X-ray analysis of the cranium in weight-bearing on the atlas and axis vertebrae. To be treated, the athlete lies on one side with the cranium supported on the mastoid process. With the offending C1/C2 transverse process exposed superiorly and the head side-flexed and rotated to expose the transverse process, the chiropractor applies a very gentle, controlled pressure on the transverse process with his pisiform bone. The treatment direction or vector of pressure is determined by the X-ray analysis. The treatment method is best classified as a direct, non-thrust, proprioceptive technique.

Complementary treatment approach to craniovertebral dysfunctions

Using craniosacral and osteopathic principles, the author offers an alternate approach to NUCCA techniques that can, in many cases, achieve an equal therapeutic goal while using equally gentle techniques. In other cases, this method may serve as an initial treatment measure to help to relieve central nervous system pressure around the cranial base. The response to this approach can aid the decision of whether a standard NUCCA treatment system is needed and whether pelvic malalignment can be significantly influenced by cervico-occipital techniques.

First, the therapist carries out a postural assessment of the athlete. The relative position in the coronal and horizontal planes of the mastoid processes, the shoulder girdles and pelvic crests are noted.

Next, the athlete actively lifts first each leg straight up in the air, then carrying out an active double straight leg raise. The relative active elevation of each leg is noted. Any lag in the ease of movement between the legs is noted during the double straight leg raise. After the legs are again at rest, any leg length discrepancy is noted. The relative symmetry of the pelvis is noted at the anatomical landmarks overlying the anterior superior iliac spine.

The C1 transverse processes are then palpated in the supine position to determine the ease of lateral passive intervertebral movement and the relative distance from the associated mastoid process. A common dysfunctional pattern is one in which the C1 transverse process that is most tender on palpation is also the transverse process that is held in spasm in occipitoatlantal side-flexion on the corresponding side. The same transverse process is also more prominent in that the biomechanics of the subluxation laterally displace the atlas while rotating C1 on the occipital facets into a jammed position.

The athlete receives appropriate explanations about the principles behind the treatment, especially if their presenting problem(s) is situated much lower in the body. Hands-on treatment starts with:

- a thoracic outlet myofascial release
- an anterior cervical myofascial release of the subhyoid and infrahyoid myofascia.

The occipitomastoid sutures are then individually mobilized while the athlete lies supine. The release of bony restrictions between the occiput and the temporal bones is crucial. The jugular foramen can be considered to be similar to a 'wide spot on the road' created along the occipitomastoid suture. A restriction of sutural mobility or a jamming of these two cranial bones affects the passage of a wide variety of cranial nerves passing through the foramen. This may have an equally profound effect on postural alignment, similar to the effect that upper cervical subluxation is proposed to have on body alignment.

This author considers the use of techniques to mobilize the occipitomastoid suture to be complementary to the NUCCA method (Gehin 1985).

Some of the facilitation of the reticular activating system proposed as the cause for postural malalignment is created by physical traction on the brainstem and its dural membranes.

There may also, however, be an autonomic nervous system dysfunction in the efferent flow of cranial nerve signals passing through the jugular and hypoglossal foramina in the cranial base.

Next, the mouth is assessed and treated for maxillary tortions or shears, zygomal suture restrictions and sublingual myofascial restrictions. Combining a stabilizing hold on the occiput with one hand and an application of unilateral intraoral counterstresses to the maxilla with the other can have a significant impact on the release of suboccipital tensions most

probably affecting the patency of the particular jugular foramen and its enclosed structures.

The relative position of the transverse processes of C1 is then reassessed. If there continues to be increased discomfort on palpation of the C1 transverse process and restricted C1/occiput passive side-flexion, the athlete is positioned in side-lying in order to expose that C1 transverse process superiorly. The athlete's neck is supported in neutral (the sagittal plane) on a firm pillow. Using functional technique principles, the head is positioned so as to reduce the amount of fascial tension on the elevated C1 transverse process.

The therapist stands in front of the side-lying athlete and manually supports the inferior mastoid and occiput on the finger-tips of his or her lower hand. The therapist's free hand gently applies a steady pressure on the superior C1 transverse process for approximately 10–20 seconds. As the vector of the force is not predefined using X-ray analysis, the therapist determines the direction of applied pressure by palpation. The therapist gently follows the subtle movements of the upper cervical transverse process on the restricted side as local tissue tension softens in response to the proprioceptive input from the therapist's hand.

Finally, leg length and pelvic and mastoid symmetry are re-examined. The author has found that this approach frequently balances leg length and pelvic symmetry. If the therapeutic results from the complementary approach or NUCCA approach are short-lasting, the author applies an integrated full-body myofascial and intraosseous release approach with the athlete. This requires an intricate knowledge of anatomy, and essentially goes through a systematic release of energy cysts throughout the body.

It is important to continue to monitor closely the athlete's condition on a regular basis to allow time for the sensitive central nervous system structures to heal. The occipitoatlantal area needs to be symmetrical for at least 1 month to keep pressure off these structures to allow adequate time for this healing to occur. As hypertonicity subsides, the athlete can gradually increase the level of activity, and the body musculature will respond much better to strengthening and toning routines. To achieve this, it is advised to keep the athlete on a weekly schedule of appointments so that the therapist can assess and, if necessary, treat the upper cervical area or the rest of the body malalignments.

Alexander technique

The Alexander technique had its origins outside the medical community. At the turn of the 20th century, Australian actor F.M. Alexander developed a set of exercises aimed at reorganizing the posture for more efficient body movement, choosing the term 'disorganization' rather than 'malalignment' to describe the disintegration of human posture.

> The Alexander method revolves around a gradual training programme to develop a subconscious and efficient maintenance of posture. This often starts with a student proprioceptively and kinaesthetically learning how to stand up from a seated position.

Feldenkrais functional integration method

Moshe Feldenkrais, a Russian-born Israeli physicist, developed a system for teaching clients kinaesthetic movement awareness during the 1940s. Feldenkrais developed his methods after having initially studied the Alexander technique with Alexander, as well as neurology and other bodies of relevant knowledge.

The Feldenkrais method integrates biomechanics with functional movements and learning theories. The method is designed to inhibit patterns of habitual neuromuscular rigidity that maintain patterns of pain and dysfunction. The method also expands motor options and provides strategies for new ways of moving. An increased awareness of movement patterns, reduced muscular stress and expanded motor possibilities result in improved motor learning, efficiency and ease of movement.

The method involves two parallel modalities:

- exercises (verbally guided movement lessons), called 'awareness through movement'
- a system of manual facilitation called functional integration.

The exercises and lessons consist of a large array of precisely structured movement explorations based on developmental movements and ordinary functional activities.

DISRUPTION OF SENSORY AND MOTOR POINTS

This section deals with some therapeutic approaches that disrupt the afferent–efferent reflex loops to the musculoskeletal system. As with a large number of the techniques highlighted in this chapter, the principles underlying many of the approaches fit into several of the categories outlined. Thus, the functional technique of counterstrain, besides therapeutically employing a disruption of body rhythms, also utilizes a disruption of sensory points.

Anatomical acupuncture: dry-needling and trigger point therapy

The puncture of trigger points is effective whether carried out by dry-needling, by injec-tion with saline or with a short-acting local anaesthetic. Dry-needling requires the greatest precision, or most repetitions. Long-acting anaesthetics and cortisone require the least precise placement of the injection, but their use for this purpose is discouraged because they can cause muscle necrosis, impaired healing, weakened tissue elements, a local atrophy of fatty tissue and inflammation as a result of crystal deposition (Gunn 1989, Travell & Simons 1983).

The principle behind the use of this form of acupuncture in the treatment of malalignment problems is to disrupt trigger points that produce pain and muscle spasm. The trigger points are selected for their neurologically based pain distribution. If one invokes the gate theory of pain (Melzack 1973; see Ch. 7), the effect of the stimulation is to relax any hypertonic muscles. In addition, the resulting central nervous system output of endorphins causes an overall pain reduction and an opportunity for improved active exercise or more passive tissue mobilization.

Intramuscular stimulation

Botek (1990) summarizes the principles of Intramuscular Stimulation, a modified system of dry-needle therapy developed by Canadian physician, C.C. Gunn (1989) as follows:

Needle therapy, as in classical acupuncture and trigger-point therapy, can be effective in the treatment of chronic pain. But, as all experienced therapists know, their results are often temporarily palliative, rather than definitively and totally curative. Where they seem to fail is that they generally regard painful peripheral muscle areas as isolated, free-standing entities. According to the Gunn model, most musculoskeletal pain conditions of neuropathic origin are related to radiculopathy (i.e. pathology at the root). Consequently, peripheral muscle-piercing should nearly always be accompanied by the additional needling of associated paraspinal muscles. (Palpation quickly reveals that both areas are tender.)

Gunn's model for chronic pain explains 'entropathic' pain as supersensitivity in neuropathic or partially denervated structures. Various types of treatment modalities, such as heat or massage, are energy sources that desensitize pain by re-establishing the homeostatic equilibrium. However, these modalities are passive and limited in scope. The energies introduced end when treatment is terminated. In contrast, needle therapies are more effective and long-lasting because the tissue injury that they produce can unleash the body's own healing source of bio-energy through the continuing stimulation the needle-induced injury produces. The tissue injury at the needling site creates a change in tissue electrical potentials that are of several microamperes in intensity. This 'current of injury' [Gunn, 1978] can persist for days until healing in the area is complete. The local tissue injury also releases the platelet-derived growth factor which promotes healing.

Gunn and his colleagues have aptly labelled this dry-needling technique as 'IntraMuscular Stimulation'. Although it resembles acupuncture or trigger point injection in that a needle is employed, it is the antithesis of earlier needling techniques. IMS promotes a total hands-on approach and involvement with the patient's musculature unlike orthodox acupuncture where, too often, the therapist inserts needles and then leaves the patient unattended for a time. In IMS, a single needle is inserted into muscle. Manual or electrical stimulation is then applied to the needle. When spasm has eased, the needle is removed and another painful area treated. (pp. 4–5)

MANUAL THERAPY AND THERAPISTS

> Manual therapy involves the use of a hands-on manipulation of the tissues aimed at restoring function or reducing pain.

Historically, several separate professions have practised manual therapy. These include physical therapists, chiropractors, osteopathic physicians, massage therapists, some naturopaths and some medical physicians such as physiatrists, orthopaedic surgeons, sports medicine specialists and those practising orthopaedic medicine. Although all of the professionals listed possess skills and training that can have a positive influence on the biomechanical functioning of athletes experiencing the symptoms associated with the malalignment syndrome, the athlete as well as the coaching staff should be aware of the variations in therapeutic approach that these professions provide.

ACQUIRING MANUAL THERAPY SKILLS

The successful treatment of musculoskeletal dysfunctions associated with the malalignment syndrome significantly depends on skillfully applied manual therapy techniques. Some health-care professionals acquire their manual therapy skills as a result of their initial professional training. The techniques discussed in this chapter are, however, generally available for postgraduate training to a broad cross-section of such professionals through workshops offered by various organizations.

As described above, Craniosacral Therapy™ is a therapeutic approach developed by John Upledger of the Upledger Institute, Florida. The level of skill required to utilise craniosacral approaches can be gained through a series of 3–5 practical hands-on workshops, each lasting 3 or 4 days. These workshops are accessible to health-care professionals. Other professionals may be permitted to attend these workshops if, by the nature of their work, they encounter clients whom they could then refer to an appropriate therapist. After the initial workshop, the therapist has learned enough skills to address and help to temporarily relieve many easily discerned pelvic malalignments and their consequences.

On the athletic field, this skill level can relieve athletes of significant discomfort and in some cases allow them to return immediately to their activity. However, the impact of accumulated forces on the body leaves a neuromuscular adaptive postural pattern that requires time and facilitation to relearn and re-establish a more lasting, balanced and stable musculoskeletal alignment. This occurs through a combined process consisting of a series of craniosacral therapy sessions, corrective exercises, increased body awareness and appliances (e.g. foot orthotics) when necessary.

Other techniques, when successfully applied, can help athletes with a malalignment syndrome on the road to recovery. Sacro-occipital technique addresses problems in the craniosacral system from a certain chiropractic perspective. Cranial osteopathy techniques, which remain the basis of the historical evolution of craniosacral therapy, are taught to non-osteopaths by several organizations. MET workshops are widely available in North America to physical and massage therapists.

A relatively recent organization – the Physical Medicine Research Foundation – has undertaken also to be a facilitator of manual medicine therapy workshops in both North America and Europe. These are aimed at attracting and training a broad range of health-care professionals in physical medicine approaches to chronic pain including counterstrain techniques and sensorimotor integration.

Athletes themselves may be interested in taking training in 'Touch for Health' approaches. Such workshops are specifically directed at training the general public in self-help techniques that can positively influence malalignment syndromes.

SUMMARY

The author has attempted to provide here an overview of the more successful methods used in manual therapy and manual medicine approaches for the treatment of symptoms associated with musculoskeletal malalignment, emphasizing the value of the craniosacral therapy biodynamic concept of treatment as being, in his experience, the most comprehensive form of manual therapy that can be used to address malalignment problems.

9

Conclusion

The biomechanical changes associated with the malalignment syndrome turn the athlete into a split personality, most noticably from the waist down. With the asymmetry of weight-bearing, the athlete may now pronate on one side and supinate on the other. Lower extremity joint ranges of motion, muscle strength and tone are typically asymmetrical. There are associated asymmetries of trunk, shoulder and neck ranges of motion. Some of these asymmetries are predictable from the pattern of malalignment present.

Also predictable are the restrictions that these asymmetries impose on athletic activities and the most likely injuries that can occur as a result. We have seen how anterior rotation of the right innominate relative to the sacrum automatically limits left pelvic rotation in the transverse (horizontal) plane, making it harder for a skier to make a turn to the left than to the right. A skater with this presentation will probably find it easier to execute a circle counterclockwise because the tendency to pronate on the right and supinate on the left makes it easier to get onto the right inside and left outside edge respectively. An increased tendency to supinate predisposes to recurrent ankle inversion sprains.

It is easy to fall into the trap of attributing these restrictions and recurrent injuries to habit, laterality (handedness or footedness) or problems related to previous injury such as 'ligament laxity'. If, however, we carry on taking this approach, we will continue to miss the real cause of these phenomena in a large number of athletes: malalignment. Failure of treatment then often reflects the fact that the malalignment has not been addressed.

One factor that has interfered with the recognition of malalignment as a cause of symptoms and signs is the tenacity with which certain influential health providers have clung to misconceptions regarding the biomechanics of the pelvis. As a result, athletes and the general public alike have often undergone needless investigations, been deprived of appropriate therapy or been subjected to totally inappropriate treatment, including surgery.

> One point that relates specifically to malalignment is the mistaken notion, despite numerous studies to the contrary, that the sacroiliac joint does not move and cannot therefore be a cause of pain other than when afflicted by an inflammatory process (sacroiliitis) or when subjected to an acute disruptive force such as a shear stress, fracture or dislocation.

This viewpoint is particularly puzzling when one realizes that the sacroiliac (SI) joint was the object of considerable study and research as a cause of back pain during the late 19th and early 20th centuries. Interest in the SI joint started to wane following the 1934 publication by Mixter & Barr that correctly identified disc protrusion or herniation as a cause of back pain. Unfortunately, the disc soon seemed to become the only cause of back pain, to the exclusion of all previously espoused causes and mechanisms.

How did this come about? It can largely be attributed to the fact that there are fashions in medicine, and fashions have both a good and a bad side. The good side is that they can channel energy in order to rapidly advance knowledge in a particular area. The discovery that the disc could cause back pain, for example, quickly led to the development of new investigative and treatment approaches. The bad side is that fashions can sometimes suppress the understanding of another area and make it suspect. When the SI joint ceased to be a fashionable cause of back pain, research in this area withered, and those who spoke of it just a decade later were felt to be out of touch with 'current thinking'.

In 1944, *Gray's Anatomy* (Johnson & Whillis) classified the SI joint as an 'amphi-arthrosis', which means that it would allow for hardly any movement. This classification was based on the dissection of three cadavers aged over 70 years of age. Interestingly, Diemerbroeck correctly stated in 1689 that the SI joint has some form of mobility in subjects other than those who are pregnant, and in 1864, Von Luschka correctly classified the joint as a diarthrosis. Nevertheless, the misclassification in the eminent anatomy text, based as it was on a limited sampling of cadavers of advanced age, nailed the lid on the coffin of the SI joint. The idea that this joint could be a cause of back pain was unceremoniously buried, and the writing and research into this area prior to 1934 were basically ignored.

But medical fashions, unlike designer fashions, tend to die hard. It should therefore come as no surprise that the misconceptions surrounding the SI joint per-

sisted for five decades. These misconceptions were initially instilled into a whole generation of doctors, who in turn used their authority and vested interests to promote the errors and foist them onto the next generation, no questions asked. So it has come to be that the SI joint has the honour of being the only joint in the body that for some reason cannot move and therefore cannot cause pain.

Luckily, even medical fashions are eventually displaced, or at least put into a proper perspective. This is what is now happening after disc surgery has failed to bring the expected results in many patients. Chymopapain injections were in favour for a short while but often bought only short-term relief at the cost of some dire long-term consequences. These consequences were predictable on purely biomechanical grounds, given the contracture of the disc material, the settling phenomenon and the resulting increase in pressure on the now-approximated facet joint surfaces.

Computed tomography and now magnetic resonance imaging have given us an appreciation not only that disc protrusions can decrease in size or even be absorbed completely with time, but also that protrusions are present in 10–30% of subjects who are asymptomatic in terms of back pain. After five decades, the role of the disc as 'the cause' of back pain is starting to be put in perspective, and the search for other possible explanations is gathering momentum. The SI joint and surrounding soft tissues are being rediscovered.

Publications of clinical findings and research results relating to malalignment are timely as this condition remains a poorly understood cause of problems in medicine and sports. The next breakthrough will come with the recognition of malalignment as a diagnostic entity and cause for an array of dysfunctions. In the light of current pressure on medical insurance budgets, recognition will hopefully give cause to reconsider expensive, and possibly incorrect, investigations and treatment options.

The literature available in this area in medical publications is unfortunately lagging behind the subject's rediscovery. Articles are published primarily in the chiropractic, osteopathic and physiotherapy literature; they are either not readily available to the medical profession or are just not being sought out. Only in the past decade have relevant articles started to appear in reputable medical journals. In addition, the literature continues to concentrate primarily on the manifestations of malalignment in the pelvic and spinal regions, to the almost complete exclusion of its effects on the rest of the body. Publications on force plate studies by researchers with a medical background may comment on side-to-side differences, which they invariably attribute to a leg length difference, usually in retrospect and often with no indication of how this difference was actually determined. The results of any research that has ignored the issue of malalignment should be suspect, especially if the results could be influenced by the asymmetries that are part of the malalignment syndrome.

I have tried to emphasize the importance of recognizing the pattern of change that results with malalignment, the so-called 'malalignment syndrome', so that the reader does not fall into the trap of investigating or treating the athlete for a condition that either does not exist or is not responsible for the pain. Some of the referred pain patterns from the posterior pelvic ligaments can, for example, mimic a dermatome distribution, and this, combined with the weakness typically associated with malalignment, can launch unnecessary investigations for a possible root compression.

More serious is the risk of the athlete being subjected to needless back surgery because the back pain and/or referred pain caused by the malalignment has mimicked a root problem. The following scenario is not unfamiliar to those working in this area. Pain is wrongly attributed to a coincidental bulging or protruding disc discovered with imaging techniques. When the pain fails to respond to a partial or complete discectomy, it is then wrongly attributed to segmental 'instability' and a fusion is carried out. Persistence of the symptoms eventually leads to the discovery and treatment of the malalignment, at which point the pain does finally settle. The athlete is now unfortunately left with a restriction of back ranges of motion and the prospect of accelerated degeneration of the disc and facet joints above and below the level of the fusion.

A mistake more specific to sports medicine is that of providing the athlete with medially posted orthotics 'to counteract pronation' bilaterally, when in reality pronation is only occurring on one side while the other stays in neutral or actually supinates. The consequences are all too readily apparent: the medial raise augments lateral weight-bearing on the neutral or supinating side, which has the effect of increasing:

- the risk of ankle inversion sprain
- the stress (tension) on lateral structures such as the lateral ankle ligaments and the tensor fascia lata/iliotibial band
- the possibility of developing stress fractures as the ability of the foot to absorb shock is further decreased.

Misdiagnosis leads to mistreatment. Needless to say, a failure to recognize the presentations of malalignment and the malalignment syndrome can also have major medicolegal implications.

The days of looking at an injury in isolation are over. The athlete presenting with left lateral knee pain may well, for example, have pain localizing to the distal iliotibial band. Treating that area with standard physiotherapy, anti-inflammatory medication, ice and rest may get the athlete back on the road, but if one ignores the fact that the athlete is a supinator and that the presence of malalignment has shifted weight-bearing even more to the outside on the left, the athlete is set up for a recurrence of the same injury. Inattention to these factors may also prolong the recovery from the initial injury; worse yet, it may result in a failure to recover at all. The constant increase in tension exerted on the inflamed iliotibial band by the malalignment may interfere with the healing process.

A recognition of the malalignment syndrome will hopefully lead to a greater awareness of these various kinetic chains, their interactions and the appropriate treatment process, not least of which is the involvement of the athlete on a day-by-day basis to ensure its success.

Appendices

APPENDIX 1. SACROILIAC JOINT ROTATIONAL MALALIGNMENT

Examination findings with the most common presentation:

- Anterior rotation of the right innominate, posterior rotation of the left
- Dysfunction of movement: usually 'locking' of the right sacroiliac (SI) joint
- Weight-bearing: right foot pronating, left supinating
- Gait: right leg turned outwards, left inwards

Standing:

- Compensatory, contrasting lumbar and thoracic curves
- Pelvic obliquity: most often right side high
- Bony landmarks: the right anterior superior iliac spine (ASIS) has rotated downwards, the right posterior superior iliac spine (PSIS) upwards; the reverse has occurred on the left side
- Pelvic rotation (transverse plane): decreased to the left (into the side of posterior innominate rotation)

Sitting on a hard surface:

- Pelvic obliquity: present (most often right side high)

Supine-lying:

- Right ASIS and pubic ramus caudad (down) to those on left
- Right leg turned outwards relative to the left; right inner thigh appears to face more anterior compared to the left

Prone-lying:

- The right PSIS lies cephalad (up) compared with that on the left

Changing position from long-sitting to supine-lying:

- The apparent leg length difference changes, the most frequent presentation being: right leg shorter in long-sitting, longer in supine-lying

Squatting:

- Right thigh usually higher and longer compared to left one.

APPENDIX 2. SACROILIAC JOINT UPSLIP (RIGHT SIDE)

Standing:

- Pelvic obliquity: right side high
- Bony landmarks: all elevated on right side
- Compensatory, contrasting lumbar and thoracic curves
- Pelvic rotation (transverse plane): right = left

Sitting on a hard surface:

- Pelvic obliquity persists: right side high

Supine and prone-lying:

- Right leg shorter than left in both positions
- Bony landmarks: right anterior superior iliac spine, posterior superior iliac spine, pubic ramus all cephalad (up)

Changing position from long-sitting to supine-lying:

- Right medial malleolus cephalad in both positions (right leg appears short)
- The actual difference between the two legs does not change with position change

Tests for sacroiliac joint locking:

- Negative

Other observations:

1. Suspect an upslip when hip extension/flexion symmetrical but other ROMs still asymmetrical, all landmarks on one side elevated, pelvic obliquity persists on sitting, and an LLD does not change on going from long-sitting to supine-lying
2. A downward force on the right leg may correct the upslip
3. Squat: thighs level, right shorter than left
4. Findings are similar for 'downslip' of the left innominate, but would fail to correct with traction on right leg.

APPENDIX 3. ASYMMETRY OF LOWER EXTREMITY RANGES OF MOTION

Pattern of ranges of motion associated with the 'alternate' presentations having right anterior innominate rotation.

	Right (degrees)		Left (degrees)	
Hip joints				
Abduction	Increased	e.g. 45	Decreased	e.g. 35
Adduction	Increased	e.g. 45	Decreased	e.g. 35
Rotation:				
external	Increased	e.g. 50	Decreased	e.g. 40
internal	Decreased	e.g. 20	Increased	e.g. 30
total		e.g. 70		e.g. 70
Flexion*	Decreased	e.g. 45	Increased	e.g. 60
Extension*	Increased	e.g. 20	Decreased	e.g. 5
total:		e.g. 65		e.g. 65

* i.e. right anterior innominate rotation restricts hip flexion, left posterior rotation restricts hip extension.

Tibio-Talar joints

Flexion – angle compared with neutral plantigrade foot; knee straight:

Dorsal	Increased	e.g. 25	Decreased	e.g. 20
Plantar	Decreased	e.g. 25	Increased	e.g. 30
Total		e.g. 50		e.g. 50

Subtalar joints

Inversion	Increased	e.g. 25	Decreased	e.g. 15
Eversion	Decreased	e.g. 5	Increased	e.g. 15
Total		e.g. 30		e.g. 30

APPENDIX 4. ASYMMETRY OF LOWER EXTREMITY MUSCLE STRENGTH

Manual assessment with sacroiliac joint rotation or upslip

	Right	Left
Hip		
Flexors	Weak	Strong
Extensors	Weak	Strong
Abductors	Strong	Weak
Adductors	Weak	Strong
Rotators:		
internal	See text	See text
external	See text	See text

Knee
Flexors:

hamstrings	Strong	Weak
extensors:		
quadriceps	*	*

Ankle
Invertors:

tibialis anterior	Weak	Strong
tibialis posterior	Weak	Strong
Evertors:		
peroneus longus	Strong	Weak
gastrocnemius soleus	*	*

* Minimal weakness hard to detect in these muscles manually.

APPENDIX 5. CLINICAL CORRELATIONS SPECIFIC TO RUNNING

Athlete with one of the 'alternate' presentations of SI joint rotational malalignment or right SI joint upslip

- *Problems related to a tendency towards pronation on the right*:
- Increased right hallux valgus and first metatarsophalangeal bunion
- Right 'pump bump', or right one larger than left
- Right plantar fasciitis, Achilles tendonitis
- Increased tension on right medial structures: medial knee (collateral) and ankle ligaments, medial plica, tendon origins and insertions (hip adductors, pes anserinus and tibialis posterior) and periosteum (medial 'shin splints')
- Increased right knee Q-angle and knee flexion: patellofemoral syndrome, patellar off-tracking/subluxation, patellar tendonitis and Osgood–Schlatter's traction epiphysitis

Problems related to a tendency towards supination on the left:

- Painful left 4th and 5th metatarsal shafts and toes
- Increased tension on left lateral structures: lateral knee and ankle ligaments, hip abductor muscles, iliotibial band, lateral compartment muscles/tendons, and peroneal and sural nerve
- Recurrent left ankle inversion sprains

Problems related towards lower extremity contrary rotation:

- Right external rotation: the right heel hitting the left foot or calf on swing-through; left internal rotation: the left toes clipping the right foot or calf on swing-through
- Ankle muscle 'functional weakness': a fish-tailing of either foot or heel or both, especially when weight-bearing on the toes

APPENDIX 6. CLINICAL FINDINGS WITH ANATOMICAL LONG RIGHT LEG

Standing position:

- Pelvic obliquity: right side high
- Bony landmarks all elevated on right: anterior superior iliac spine, posterior superior iliac spine (PSIS), iliac crest and greater trochanter
- Compensatory curvatures of lumbar and thoracic spine: lumbar convexity may be to the left or right, usually with the thoracic convexity in the opposite direction and a further reversal in the upper thoracic spine or cervicothoracic junction
- Right shoulder/scapula depressed if the thoracic convexity is to the left
- Pelvic rotation (transverse plane): right = left

Sitting on a hard surface:

- Pelvis level: the effect of the lower extremities is eliminated as the weight is now borne on the ischial tuberosities
- Compensatory curvatures: decreased or eliminated

Supine and prone-lying:

- Bony landmarks (pelvis and greater trochanter) all level
- Right medial malleolus lies caudad compared with the left

Changing position from supine-lying to long-sitting:

- Right medial malleolus caudad in both positions
- Actual difference between the malleoli does not change

Tests for sacroiliac joint locking:

- Negative; on the standing sacral flexion test, the right PSIS higher by the difference in leg length – this difference does not change on forward flexion and extension of the trunk

Squatting:

- thighs equal height, right longer than left

APPENDIX 7. COMBINATION OF ASYMMETRIES IN ATHLETE 1

Presentation: an athlete with a right anterior innominate rotation, 'locked' right sacroiliac (SI) joint, upslip of the right SI joint and an anatomically longer right leg.

Presentation on initial examination:

- Stand and sit: pelvic obliquity – right iliac crest high
- Right anterior superior iliac spine (ASIS) caudad (down) and posterior superior iliac spine (PSIS) cephalad (up) compared with left
- Sacral flexion, kinetic rotational test: positive on right
- Asymmetrical leg ranges of motion as for 'alternate' presentations (1)
- Asymmetry of leg muscle strength in keeping with the malalignment
- Long-sitting to supine-lying: right leg lengthens, left shortens

Following successful correction of the anterior rotation:

- Sacral flexion, kinetic rotational test: now negative
- Standing: persistence of pelvic obliquity; landmarks now *all* higher on the right (ASIS, PSIS, iliac crest and greater trochanter)
- Long-sitting, supine-lying: no change; right leg may be shorter, longer or equal to left depending on the amount of leg length difference (LLD)

Persistence of following indicates right SI joint upslip:

- The pelvic obliquity persists in sitting and lying
- Persistent asymmetrical muscle strength and hip adduction

After correction of the upslip, findings consistent with a residual anatomical LLD include:

- Symmetrical strength, ranges of motion and sitting/lying landmarks
- Long-sitting to supine-lying: right leg consistently longer to equal extent

APPENDIX 8. COMBINATION OF ASYMMETRIES IN ATHLETE 2

Presentation: athlete with left anterior rotation, 'locked' right SI joint, right upslip and an anatomically longer right leg.

Findings on initial examination:

- Stand and sit: pelvic obliquity, left or right crest high
- Left anterior superior iliac spine (ASIS) caudad (down), left posterior superior iliac spine (PSIS) cephalad (up) compared with right
- Sacral flexion, kinetic rotational test: positive on right
- Asymmetry of lower extremity muscle strength and joint ranges of motion
- On supine-lying: left leg lengthens relative to right

Following correction of left anterior rotation:

- Sacral flexion, kinetic rotational test: now negative
- Standing and sitting: right iliac crest high in both positions; bony landmarks all higher on the right side
- Long-sitting to supine-lying: no change in length; leg length may or may not be different depending on how anatomical leg length difference (LLD) affects the right 'shortening' caused by the right upslip
- Persistence of asymmetrical strength

NB. Right upslip is indicated by: all right landmarks elevated, obliquity sitting, asymmetrical strength

After correction of the upslip, the only findings remaining were consistent with an LLD, right leg long:

- Standing: bony landmarks all high on right side
- Site and lie (prone/supine): level crests, ASIS and PSIS
- Long-sitting to supine-lying: right leg longer to an equal extent

APPENDIX 9. THORACOLUMBAR SYNDROME

Diagnostic signs

- The 'iliac crest point' sign: pain and deep tenderness localizing to the site on the iliac crest where the posterior sensory branches become cutaneous
- Skin-rolling test: the skin and subcutaneous tissue in an area supplied by the specific cutaneous branch feels thickened, and hypersensitive when rolled.
  - anterior branch: lower lateral abdomen and groin
  - lateral perforating branch: lateral hip (crest to greater trochanter)
  - posterior branch: iliac crest and buttock area
- Pain localizing to the thoracolumbar region with pressure: creating a rotatory force on each vertebra by applying pressure to the spinous processes from the right and left elicits a pain response from involved segment(s), usually unilaterally.
- Facet joint pain: deep, vertical pressure applied 1 cm lateral to each spinous process elicits pain at the level of involved facet joint(s)
- Diagnostic block with local anaesthetic: 2 ml local anaesthetic solution (xylocaine or procaine) is infiltrated around the painful facet joint(s). A positive block temporarily decreases or abolishes the above signs

Treatment

- Correct any minimal vertebral displacement (e.g. manipulate)
- Infiltrate corticosteroids around the facet joint(s)
- If the pain persists: consider surgical denervation of the facet joint(s) or percutaneous posterior rhizotomy

APPENDIX 10. NON-SPECIFIC CLINICAL CORRELATIONS

Sports that can be affected by:

- Limitation of trunk rotation (transverse plane): golf, baseball, cricket, rowing, hockey, kayaking, court sports, baseball, gymnastics, wrestling and ice/field hockey
- Limitation of pelvic rotation (transverse plane): skiing, golf, gymnastics, wrestling, baseball and canoeing
- Limitation of limb ranges of motion:
  - anterior innominate rotation predisposing to hamstring tears: jumping competitions – long, triple, high; running – leaving the blocks, hurdles, steeplechase, cross-country; martial arts; soccer, football, rugby
  - asymmetrical arm extension: swimming (e.g. butterfly)
  - restriction of right leg internal rotation, left adduction and external rotation: ice- and ski-skating, horseback riding
- Combinations of limitations – trunk, pelvis, and limbs: fencing, court sports, balance beam, martial arts, gymnastics, wrestling, soccer, windsurfing, snow-boarding, high jump, throwing events (hammer, discus, shot and javelin)

Sports in which symmetry and/or style is rewarded: synchronized swimming, gymnastics, ice-skating (figures competition), ballet and other dances, diving and weight-lifting

Sports in which symmetry of leg strength is important: cycling, running, swimming, skiing, skating, gymnastics, weight-lifting, body-building and power-lifting

APPENDIX 11. CLINICAL CORRELATIONS TO SPECIFIC SPORTS

An athlete with sacroiliac (SI) joint upslip or one of 'alternate' SI joint rotational malalignment presentations, right anterior.

Skiing:

- Problem initiating or carrying out turns to the left
- Problem 'getting a good inner edge' with the right ski (a weak or 'sloppy' right pronating foot and ankle)

Skating:

- Problem turning to the right – tendency towards pronation on the right interferes with getting on to the outer edge of the right skate; tendency towards supination on the left facilitates left turns
- Right ankle feels 'weak', 'sloppy' and 'collapses inward'

Golf:

- Restrictions of trunk or pelvic rotation to the right or left; gradually increasing back pain as the game progresses

Cycling:

- Awareness of asymmetry of form (e.g. right knee moves further away from the crossbar when the knee is flexed = external rotation; inwards when extended = pronation; knee valgus stress)
- Awareness of asymmetry of strength (e.g. feeling that the right leg cannot generate as much power as the left)
- Right pronation: right foot feels 'weak' and 'falls inwards'

Swimming:

- Detrimental effects on the execution of strokes from asymmetries (e.g. head/neck rotation, shoulder extension and rotation); compensatory torquing requires more energy
- Contrary effect of leg internal/external rotation

APPENDIX 12. FACTORS CONTRIBUTING TO RECURRENCE OF INJURIES

Athlete with an 'alternate' rotational malalignment or upslip.

Left hip abductor and tensor fascia lata/iliotibial band (TFL/ITB) complex sprain/strain:

- Tendency towards supination on the left side
- Increased muscle tension in the left hip abductors
- Increased tension in the left TFL and ITB

Left ankle inversion sprains/strains:

- Tendency towards supination on the left side
- 'Functional weakness' of peroneus longus and brevis
- Fitting with orthotics intended for a pronator (medial raise)
- Wearing double-density shoes intended for a pronator

Right patellofemoral compartment syndrome:

- Tendency towards pronation on the right side, knee valgus strain
- Increased right Q-angle and outward tracking of the patella
- Tendency towards flexion of the relatively 'longer' right leg when standing to lower the high right iliac crest: increases tension in the quadriceps muscle and across the patellofemoral compartment

Back 'strains':

- Stresses from compensatory movements required because of limitations of trunk, pelvic and limb ranges of motion in certain directions; for example, increased left trunk rotation to compensate for the limitation of left pelvic rotation when the left innominate is rotated posteriorly
- Minor insults (e.g. repetitive lifting, bending and squatting) superimposed on tissue already tender from chronic compression, distraction and/or torsional forces

APPENDIX 13. CAUSES OF RECURRENT MALALIGNMENT

- Unilateral lumbarization, sacralization and pseudo-joint formation
  - creates rotational moment on trunk flexion and extension
- Degeneration affecting structures capable of producing 'deep', poorly defined, or referred pain*
  - hip joints, facet joints and discs
- Disc protrusion or herniation
  - central disc protrusion may irritate the dura and spare the nerve roots or sleeves; secondary reflex muscle spasm
- Unsuspected underlying arthritic condition*
  - ankylosing spondylitis, Reiter's syndrome, gout, ulcerative colitis and Crohn's disease (regional ileitis)
- Spinal stenosis, arachnoiditis, root sleeve fibrosis, intra- or extradural tumours
- Abdominal or pelvic masses: uterine fibroids, ovarian cysts, tumours; capable of irritating muscles (e.g. the iliopsoas), which can in turn exert rotational forces on the vertebrae, the pelvic bones and the lower extremities
- Pre-menstrual relaxin hormone release – causing a transient increase in ligament laxity; stress associated with menses

* NB. Bone scans may show an increased uptake in the sacroiliac joint(s) and/or symphysis pubis, leading to a diagnosis of 'sacroiliitis' and 'osteitis pubis'. Laboratory tests for inflammatory arthropathy are usually negative, and symptoms often settle with realignment of the sacroiliac joints and pubic bones

Glossary

abduction moving a part of the body away from the midline or, in the case of the hands/fingers and feet/toes, away from the axial line of the limbs

adduction moving a part of the body toward the median plane or, in the case of the hands/fingers and feet/toes, toward the axial line of the limb

Adson's manoeuvre a test for compression of the nerves and blood vessels to the arms at the site where they run through the thoracic outlet (the space between the collar bone and the underlying 1st rib) – Fig. 3.11

afferent carrying toward a center (e.g. a nerve fibre sending signals toward the spinal cord or brain)

'aids' the signals by which the rider communicates with the horse

AIIS Anterior Inferior Iliac Spine, a landmark on the lower part at the front of each pelvic bone; serves as attachment point for the origin of the rectus femoris part of the quadriceps muscle – Fig. 2.31C

'alternate' presentation one of the presentations of 'rotational malalignment' other than the 'left anterior and locked' presentation

amphiarthrodial joint a joint that allows for little motion, the apposed bony surfaces being connected by fibrocartilage (e.g. symphysis pubis)

ankylosis immobilization and consolidation of a joint as a result of disease, injury, or surgical procedure

anterior on the front or forward part; referring to the front (chest and stomach) surface of the body

aponeurosis a white, flattened or ribbon-like tendinous expansion, serving mainly to connect a muscle with the parts that it moves (e.g. the conjoint tendons of the extenal oblique and transverse muscles on the abdomen that connects them to the superior pubic bone – Figs 2.24a, b)

appendicular skeleton referring to the bones in the arms and legs (the parts that are suspended from the axial skeleton)

apprehension test a test to check for evidence of increased irritability/tenderness at the back surfaces of the knee cap or the underlying groove that it tracks up and down on as the knee straightens and bends, respectively

arthrodesis a surgical fixation of the joint that promotes proliferation of bone cells to achieve eventual fusion of the joint surfaces

arthrodial referring to a joint with flat opposing surfaces (e.g. SI joint)

ASIS Anterior Superior Iliac Spine, a landmark on the upper part of the front of the pelvic bone that serves as origin for the TFL muscle and the inguinal ligament – Figs 2.2, 2.37

autonomic nervous system the part of the nervous system that regulates the activity of cardiac muscle, smooth muscle and glands; composed of the sympathetic (thoracolumbar) and parasympathetic (craniosacral) nervous system

axial skeleton referring to the bones of the head, spine, ribs and sternum (breast bone)

axial rotation rotation of the axial bones relative to an axis drawn through the axial skeleton

axon in the peripheral nervous system, the nerve fibre that carries impulses from the neuron (nerve cell body) to its terminal branches, at which point the impulses are transmitted to another nerve cell or to cells of the organ that it acts on

bowstring test test for irritability of the nerve roots and spinal cord; to stretch these structures, the knee is straightened (extended) when the hip is maximally flexed

brachialgia pain in the arm(s)

bursa a sac filled with a viscous fluid, situated at places where friction between structures would otherwise develop; e.g. iliopectineal bursa between the iliopsoas tendon and the iliopectineal eminence (a diffuse enlargement on the anterior aspect of the acetabulum or hip socket – Fig. 4.2); trochanteric bursa between the greater trochanter and the overlying hip abductor–ITB complex – Fig. 3.37

calcaneus heel bone

caudad directed down, toward the coccyx (tail bone)

cephalad directed up, toward the head

cellulalgia pain arising from cells

chymopapaine 'discectomy' a treatment method for disc protrusion popular in the 1980s consisting of the injection of chymopapaine (an enzyme capable of breaking down the mucopolysaccharide–protein complexes in the protruded disc); unfortunately, the long-term effect was to accelerate development of osteoarthritis at the level injected, with complicating mechanical back pain

cervicogenic originating from the neck region

coccydynia pain originating from the tailbone

coccyx the tailbone

contralateral located on, pertaining to, or influencing the opposite side (vs. ipsilateral)

'core' muscles muscles that act to stabilize the SI joints, consisting of an 'inner' (Fig 2.22) and 'outer' (Figs 2.24–2.27) unit

counternutation backward movement of the sacral base relative to the adjacent iliac bone(s) (Fig. 2.8B)

conjoint muscle a muscle that has several components, each of which is capable of a specific action but all of which can also act together (e.g. iliopsoas made up of psoas major and minor and the iliacus – Fig. 2.40)

CNS central nervous system

crepitus the sensation of dry surfaces of muscle when rubbed between the fingers, indicative of chronic spasm and replacement with fibrotic tissue (increased connective tissue content)

curved last referring to the sole of the foot (last) which has an indentation on the inner border to promote inward collapse (pronation) of the foot – Fig. 3.31

cranio-caudal running from head to tail

craniosacral rhythm an alternating increase in tension of muscle and fascia, produced by the rhythmic fluctuation in the flow of the cerebrospinal fluid (CSF) from the brain down to the tailbone (see Ch. 8)

dermatome the area of the skin supplied by one nerve root

dorsiflexion bending the foot upward (decreasing the angle at the ankle)

dextroscoliosis vertebrae turning to the right along the length of a curved segment of the spine (e.g. lumbar vertebrae will turn to the right, into a curve that is convex to the right – Fig. 2.65A, 4.22)

double blind study a research study in which neither the subject nor the person administering the treatment knows which treatment any particular participant is receiving

double-density midsole a midsole that is reinforced with more dense material on the inside underneath the arch of the foot, to counter any tendency to pronation – Fig. 3.31

downslip downward displacement of a pelvic bone relative to the sacrum, with lengthening of the leg on that side

dura the outermost covering of the brain and spinal cord

dysmenorrhoea painful menstruation

dyspareunia painful intercourse

dyseasthesias impaired sensation, or abnormal unpleasant sensations provoked by normal stimuli

edema accumulation of excessive amounts of fluid in the spaces between cells of tissues, most easily evident within the subcutaneous tissue lying immediately below the skin

efferent carrying away from a center (e.g. a nerve transmitting signals from the brain or spinal cord)

enthesis the site where a ligament, tendon, or muscle attaches to bone

enthetic pain pain arising from an enthesis

epiphysis the expanded articular end of a long bone (e.g. humerus at the elbow, articulating with the radius and ulna), developed from a secondary ossification centre, which during its period of growth is either entirely cartilagenous or is separated from the shaft by the epiphyseal cartilage

eversion a turning or tipping outward (e.g. as of the ankle in an 'eversion sprain')

evertors muscles that act to evert a body part (e.g. peroneus longus everts the foot – Fig. 3.33)

facilitation   the increase in tension in a muscle resulting from an increased efficiency of transmission of nerve impulses and/or an increased number of impulses traveling in the nerve supplying that muscle

fascia   a sheet or band of fibrous connective tissue (e.g. thoracodorsal fascia lying deep to the skin and surrounding the muscles of this complex – Fig. 2.25; anterior abdominal fascia surrounding the rectus abdominis muscles and serving as an anchor point for transversus abdominis – Figs 2.24A,B,C)

femur   thigh bone

fibrosis   replacement with excessive amounts of fibrous connective tissue

fibro-osseous junction   where ligament, muscle, tendon, or capsule inserts into bone

fins   the spinous processes of a horse

foramen   a natural opening, in particular one into or through bone (e.g. at the base of the skull: foramen magnum for exit of the brainstem/spinal cord; hypoglossal foramen for exit of the 12th cranial nerve to the tongue; the foramina for the exit of nerve roots from either side of each vertebra and the sacrum)

'forehand'   the front legs of a horse

frontal (coronal) plane   any plane which passes longitudinally through the body (from side to side, at right angles to the median plane), dividing the body into front and back parts; one of these planes roughly parallels the frontal suture, another the coronal suture of the skull (Fig. 2.6)

Gaenslen's test   a test to stress the hip–SI joint–lumbosacral region by having the athlete flex one thigh onto the chest while achieving hyperextension on the opposite side by applying downward pressure on that thigh as it hangs over the edge of the table; pain that occurs does not define the specific site(s) affected (hip, SI joint and/or lumbosacral) – Fig. 2.75B

genu valgum   inward collapse of the knee joint

genu varum   outward collapse of the knee joint

Gillet test   kinetic rotational test – see below (Figs 2.88–90)

Golgi tendon organs   a mechanoreceptor found in tendons, arranged in series with the muscle and therefore sensitive to the mechanical distortion that results with passive stretch of the tendon or isometric muscle contraction and capable of signalling changes in muscle tension; it is the receptor responsible for the 'lengthening' or 'clasp-knife' reflex, whereby stimulation of the tendon (= Golgi receptor) result in relaxation of the muscle–tendon complex which may prevent tearing but results in giving-way of the joint (e.g. knee joint giving way on sudden relaxation of the quadriceps muscle induced by activation of the tendon organs with excessive stretching of the tendon)

greater trochanter   a bony process protruding outward below the neck of the femur (Fig. 3.37)

Grostic   a chiropractic technique that limits adjustments to C1 and C2 vertebrae (see Ch. 8)

hallux rigidus   painful limitation of movement of the joints of the first toe, which may be associated with flexion deformity

hallux valgus   angulation of the big toe away from the midline, possibly to the point of riding over or under the 2nd and even 3rd toes

hypertonia   abnormal increase in tension in a muscle–tendon complex

hypotonia   abnormal decrease in tension in a muscle–tendon complex

inhibition   a decrease in muscle tension resulting from a decreased efficiency in the transmission of nerve impulses and/or a decreased number of impulses in the nerve supplying that muscle

innominate   the pelvic bone on either side of the sacrum, each made up of an iliac, ischial and pubic bone (Figs 2.2, 2.3)

inversion   a turning or tipping inward (e.g. as of the calcaneal bone with an inversion sprain of the ankle)

invertor   a muscle that acts to invert a body part (e.g. tibialis anterior and posterior invert the foot – Fig. 3.33)

ipsilateral   located on, pertaining to, or influencing the same side (vs contralateral)

ischial tuberosities   the bones on the lower aspect of each pelvic bone which become the weight-bearing part on sitting (Figs 2.3, 2.4)

isometric contraction   muscle contraction maintained without any movement of the joint that the muscle acts on

isotonic contraction   movement of a joint carried out while maintaining uniform tension in the muscle acting on the joint

kinetic rotation test (Gillet test)   test for intra-pelvic torsion (ability for the pelvis to twist) and the ability to transfer weight through the pelvis when standing on one leg (Fig. 2.88–90)

lateral   on the outside, away from the median plane or midline

Lasegue's test   pain elicited on flexing the hip when the knee is extended but abolished with the knee flexed is likely to result from irritation of the sciatic nerve, a nerve root, or the spinal cord rather than originating from a hip joint

LCL   lateral collateral ligament, running across the outside of the knee from attachments to the femur above and the head of the fibula below (Fig. 3.33)

lesser trochanter   a bony process that protrudes inward below the neck of the femur and serves as the insertion for the iliopsoas muscle (Figs 2.40, 3.46)

lumbarization   partial or complete separation of the first segment of the sacrum (S1) from the second; when complete, the new vertebral segment is usually designated 'L6' (see 'sacralization' and Figs 4.22–4.24)

levator ani syndrome   pelvic floor muscle hypo or hypertonia/reactive spasm, with resulting pelvic floor dysfunction syndrome and recurrent malalignment (Fig. 2.36)

levoscoliosis   vertebrae turning to the left along the length of a curved segment of the spine (e.g. lumbar vertebrae will turn to the left, into a curve that is convex to the left – Figs 2.29, 4.24)

linea alba on the anterior abdomen, a white line in the midline between the rectus abdominus muscles, formed by the fascia/connective tissue that surrounds and binds these muscles together (Fig. 2.24)

Maitland's slump test a test for nerve root/spinal cord irritability such as occurs with disc protrusion; the test involves putting the roots and cord under progressively more stretch by first sitting with the hip flexed and knee extended and then, in succession, flexing the trunk, then the head, and finally dorsiflexing the foot

malrotation in this text, referring to abnormal and/or excessive rotation of one or more vertebrae, with or without the simultaneous presence of malalignment of the pelvis (Fig. 2.65B)

MCL Medial Collateral Ligament, running from its attachment to the inside of the femur above and tibia below (Fig. 3.33)

medial on the inside, or towards the median plane or midline

meniscus a 'spacer' or pad of fibrocartilage or dense connective tissue found in a number of joints (e.g. the crescent shaped medial and lateral menisci in the knee joint)

micturition referring to the act of voiding

Morton's neuroma a benign thickening of a nerve in the foot that results from repeated irritation of a natural nerve enlargement formed by the junction of branches contributed by the medial and lateral plantar nerves, usually located between the 3rd and 4th metatarsal heads (Fig. 4.16)

Morton's toe for various reasons the 2nd and sometimes also 3rd toe end up longer than the 1st (e.g. developmental, hallux valgus); this results in a shift of weight-bearing from the 1st to the 2nd/3rd metatarsal heads and may result in pain on weight-bearing and excessive callus formation

myelinated nerve fibre an insulated nerve fibre, which can conduct signals more quickly than an unmyelinated fibre

myofascial referring to tissue consisting of muscle and its fascia

myositis inflammation of muscle

myotome all the muscles supplied by one nerve root

neuralgia paroxysmal pain that spreads out in the course of one or more nerves

neurovascular bundle a bundle of nerves and blood vessels that supplies a specific part of the body (e.g. femoral bundle to the leg – Fig. 4.14; cervicobrachial to the arm – Fig. 3.11)

nutation forward movement of the sacral base relative to the adjacent iliac bone(s) – Fig. 2.8A

Ober's test a test of the hip abductor–ITB complex for an increase in tension or evidence of contracture – Fig. 3.40

olecranon the tip of the elbow

Osgood–Schlatter's disease affects the tuberosity of the tibia (the bump or ephysisis that serves as an attachment point for the tendon of the knee cap); initially there is inflammation and degeneration (osteochondrosis) of the

growth centre of the epiphysis, followed by regeneration and recalcification – by the time growth has been completed, the tuberosity often ends up enlarged and protruberant to the point that it may get in the way (e.g. when attempting to kneel)

osteoarthritis noninflammatory degenerative disease of joints, characterized by degeneration of the joint cartilage, protruding bone growths along the margins (osteophytes), and thickening of the synovial lining on the inside of the capsule which may or may not cause pain; joints are likely to be painful with activity and to stiffen with rest

osteoarthrosis chronic noninflammatory arthritis

parasympathetic nervous system that part of the autonomic nervous system consisting of a cranial (ocular, bulbar part of the brainstem) and sacral division; in general, stimulation of this system has a calming effect (e.g. lowering of the heart rate and blood pressure)

paravertebral running alongside the spine (e.g. the paravertebral muscles lying on either side of the vertebral spinous processes)

patella kneecap

patellar facets the medial (inside) and lateral (outside) surface on the back of the knee cap

patellofemoral compartment syndrome tender inflamed joint surfaces, involving the back of the kneecap (facet surfaces) and the underlying groove that the knee cap tracks up and down in on knee extension and flexion, respectively; pain is most likely to be felt with activities that load the knee joint in flexion, increasing the pressure exerted by the kneecap against the femur – going up and down stairs, rowing, cycling, jumping, squatting

pathognomonic distinctive or characteristic of a disease or pathological condition, or a sign (finding on examination) or symptom (complaint) on which a diagnosis can be made (e.g. jaundice is pathognomonic of a probable disease process involving the liver or gallbladder)

periosteal referring to the periosteum, a specialized connective tissue that covers the bones of the body and has the potential to form bone

PIIS Posterior Inferior Iliac Spine, a landmark on the inferior aspect of the back of the ilium just below the PSIS; serves as iliac attachment point for the lower 'short' and the long 'dorsal' sacroiliac ligaments (Figs. 2.3, 2.4, 2.16)

Pilates a dynamic form of symmetrical exercises that aims at a graduated recovery of strength and mobility/movement patterns, particularly suited for those presenting with problems relating to malalignment (see Ch. 7, p. 354–356)

planar joint a joint with flat adjoining surfaces (e.g. symphysis pubis; SI joint early in life)

plantarflexion pointing the foot downward (increasing the angle at the ankle)

pleura the membrane that lines the thoracic cavity (chest cage) and surrounds the lung on each side, enclosing a potential space known as the pleural cavity

plica a ridge or fold of connective tissue that may be noted as a thickening (e.g. the medial plica of the knee that results from an 'infolding' of the inner knee capsule; it may become tender and painful, particularly when put under increased tension by being strung across the underlying enlarged end of the thigh bone, such as occurs with increased inward collapse of the knee joint as a result of pronation – Fig. 3.33)

posting a raise added to build up the inside or outside of an orthotic – Fig. 7.30

pneumothorax an accumulation of air or gas in the pleural space; a needle that accidentally pierces the pleura can result in formation of a 'tension pneumothorax' when tissues surrounding the opening into the pleural cavity act like a one-way valve that allows air to enter, but not escape, the cavity – the patient experiences shortness of breath that worsens as the increasing positive pressure pushes the lung to the opposite side

posterior referring to the back or 'dorsal' surface of the body, or to a part 'located in the back of' or 'the back part of' a structure

prolotherapy a treatment method that involves injection of an irritant to promote proliferation of collagen, with the aim of strengthening a ligament, tendon, or capsule (see Ch.7, p. 365–374)

pronation a rolling-inward of the weight-bearing foot, with simultaneous fore-foot abduction, calcaneal (heel bone) eversion and ankle dorsiflexion – Figs 3.18, 3.33, 5.33

prone lying on the stomach

proprioception the part of the nervous system concerned with providing information regarding movements and the position of the body, information that is provided by sensory nerve terminals located primarily in the muscles, tendons and the labyrinth of the ear

PSIS Posterior Superior Iliac Spine, a landmark on the back of each pelvic bone (ilium) that serves as origin for both the long 'dorsal' sacroiliac and long dorsal sacrotuberous ligaments – Figs 2.3, 2.4, 2.10, 2.16

pudendal nerve the nerve that comes off the sacral plexus (S2–S4) and supplies the muscles, ligaments, skin and erectile tissue of the pelvic floor

raphe a 'seam' formed by the joining of tissues, usually in the midline (e.g. linea alba of the abdomen)

relaxin hormone a hormone secreted in increasing amounts toward the later part of a pregnancy, to help relax the connective tissue (ligaments, joint capsules etc.) in the pelvis to facilitate delivery at term; some increase in blood levels is also noted with breast feeding and at the time of ovulation and menstruation

reticular activating system – RAS the 'net' of cells of the reticular formation of the medulla oblongata, which is part of the brainstem – with the brain above and the spinal cord below – and contains ascending and descending tracts as well as important collections of nerve cells that deal with vital functions, such as respiration, circulation, and special senses; the RAS receives collaterals from the sensory ascending pathways and projects to higher centres of the brainstem and brain to control the overall degree of central nervous system activity (including attentiveness, wakefulness and sleep)

sacralization incorporation of the 5th lumbar vertebra into the sacral base by the formation of bone that partially or fully joins the transverse process of L5 to the sacrum – Figs 4.22–4.24

sacro-coccygeal joint the joint between the tailbone (coccyx) and the sacrum – Figs 2.1, 2.11, 2.15, 4.34

sagittal plane any vertical plane that runs through the body parallel to the median plane/sagittal suture and therefore divides the body into a right and left portion – Fig. 2.6

sagittal split in synchronized swimming, this refers to separating the legs by full extension of one and flexion of the other leg; that is, separation in the sagittal plane

scapula shoulder blade

scapulothoracic (joint) referring to the shoulder blade and the underlying rib cage (= the joint between the two)

Scheuermann's disease osteochondrosis of the vertebrae, which can result in premature (juvenile) kyphosis or excessive forward angulation of the thoracic spine with collapse of the anterior part of one or more vertebral epiphyses

sclerotherapy injection of an irritant into connective tissue or vessels, with the intent of producing scarring (e.g. injection for the treatment of varicose veins)

sclerotome all the parts of bone supplied by one nerve root

serratus anterior muscle originates from the outer surface of ribs 1–8 and inserts primarily into the inner border and lower angle of the shoulder blade; it rotates the blade and will draw it forward while keeping it applied to the chest cage when reaching or pushing against a resistance (e.g. an object, wall) with the arm straight out in front

sesamoid small bone of the foot, located underneath the big toe within the tendon that bends that toe downward (flexor hallucis longus)

single blind study a study in which the researcher is aware of the treatment being administered, but the participant is not

single-density midsole midsole of uniform density to improve cushioning, useful for supinators

somatovisceral reflexes inhibition or stimulation of visceral (intestinal) functions initiated by signals from the musculoskeletal system

somatic referring to the musculoskeletal system (as opposed to the viscera)

spondylolisthesis forward or backward displacement of one vertebra relative to another or to the sacrum; L4 or L5 are frequently involved because developmental separation of the pars interarticularis (see 'spondylolysis') allows L4 to move forward relative to L5, or L5 relative to the sacral base

spondylolysis developmental or traumatic dissolution of the vertebral complex, which includes separation of the pars interarticularis (connects the vertebral body to the bony part that surrounds the spinal cord), such as can occur as a result of stress fractures through the pars with repeated back extension (e.g. gymnastics)

sprain injury to muscle, tendon, ligament, or capsule that has resulted in rupture of some of the fibres, but the continuity of the structure(s) affected remains intact

straight last   the pattern of the sole of the shoe (last) that has the area under the inner arch of the foot filled in to provide more support – Fig. 3.31

strain   injury to muscle, tendon, ligament or capsule that results in complete disruption (tearing) of the structure(s) involved

subtalar joint   the joint between the talus (that the tibia or shin bone sits on at the ankle) and the calcaneus (the heel bone that sits underneath)

sulcus   a groove or trench

supination   a rolling outward of the weight-bearing foot, with simultaneous fore-foot adduction, calcaneal (heel bone) inversion and ankle plantarflexion – Figs 3.18, 3.33, 5.33

supine   lying on the back

sympathetic nervous system   the part of the autonomic nervous system originating from the thoracolumbar region; in general, stimulation has an excitatory effect (increased heart rate and blood pressure, spasm of blood vessels, formation of goose flesh)

synostosis   a fusion between bones that are usually distinct, as a result of calcification of connecting cartilage or fibrous tissue

thoracic outlet syndrome   irritation or actual compression of the cervicobrachial neurovascular bundle (Fig. 3.11) from narrowing of the thoracic outlet (the space between the 1st rib and collar bone) as seen in association with drooping of the shoulder girdle or continual hyperabduction, abnormal 1st rib, cervical rib or large transverse process, fibrous band, tight anterior scalene muscle edge; presents with arm pain, arm/finger paraesthesia, vasomotor changes (e.g. oedema, cyanosis, pallor), weakness and wasting (with C8 and T1 fibres most vulnerable)

tibia   shin bone

upslip   upward displacement of one or other pelvic bone relative to the sacrum, with shortening of the leg on that side (Fig. 2.40A, B)

urethra   the outlet from the bladder (Fig. 2.36)

uterine fibroid   a fibrous mass (fibroma) within or attached to the wall of the uterus

valgus   leaning or bent/twisted outward, angulating away from midline (right leg in Figs 3.27B, 3.32)

varus   leaning or bent/twisted inward, angulating toward midline (left leg in Figs 3.27B, 3.32)

viscera   referring to the contents in the three great cavities of the body (e.g. lungs, bowels and organs)

visceral manipulation   a form of manual therapy that concerns itself with the viscera (e.g. freeing up adhesions, repositioning organs)

viscero-somatic reflex   a reflex effect on the musculoskeletal system triggered by stimulation of some part of the visceral system

whiplash   excessive movement of the head and neck, typically hyperextension followed by hyperflexion in the case of a rear-end collision

vaso-vagal attack   a reaction that can be triggered by emotional stress, fear, or pain; the response involves the circulatory and neurological systems and is characterized by nausea, pallor, slowing of the heart rate and a fall in blood pressure which can lead to loss of consciousness

Yeoman's test   a test to stress the hip–SI joint–lumbosacral region by passively hyperextending the thigh on one side while the athlete is lying prone; pain occurs on the affected side(s) but, as with Gaenslen's test, it fails to define the specific site(s) of the problem (hip, SI joint and/or lumbosacral?) – Fig. 2.75A

References

Adrian MJ, Cooper JM. Biomechanics of human movement. Indianapolis, IN: Benchmark Press; 1986.

Aitken GS. Syndromes of lumbo-pelvic dysfunction. In: Grieve GP, ed. Modern manual therapy of the vertebral column. Edinburgh: Churchill Livingstone; 1986:473–478.

Andrish JT. Knee injuries in gymnasts. Clin Sports Med 4:111–121.

Aprill CN. The role of anatomically specific injections into the sacroiliac joint. In: Vleeming A, Mooney V, Snijders C, Dorman T, eds. Low back pain and its relation to the sacroiliac joint. Rotterdam: European Conference Organizers; 1992:373–380.

Armour PC, Scott JH. Equalization of limb length. J Bone Joint Surg 1981; 63B:587–592.

Ashmore E. Osteopathic mechanics. Kirksville, MO: Journal Printing; 1915.

Aspden R Intra-abdominal pressure and its role in spinal mechanics. Clin Biomech 1987; 2:168–174.

Baker PK. Musculoskeletal problems. In: Steege JF, Metzger DA, Levy BS, eds. Chronic pelvic pain: an integrated approach. Philadelphia: WB Saunders; 1998:215–240.

Balduini FC. Abdominal and groin injuries in tennis. Clin Sports Med 1988; 7:349–357.

Banks AR. A rationale for prolotherapy. J Orthop Med 1991; 13:54–59.

Barral J-P, Mercier P. Manipulations viscerales. Paris: Maloine; 1983.

Barral J-P, Mercier P. Visceral manipulation. Seattle, WA: Eastland Press; 1988.

Barrel J-P. Visceral Manipulation II. Seattle, WA: Eastland Press; 1989.

Basmajian JV. Primary anatomy. Baltimore: Williams & Wilkins; 1964.

Beal MC. The sacroiliac problem: review of anatomy, mechanics and diagnosis. J Am Osteopath Assoc 1982; 81:667–679.

Beighton PH, Grahame R, Bird H. Hypermobility of joints. 3rd edn. London: Springer-Verlag; 1999.

Bellamy N, Park W, Rooney PJ. What do we know about the sacroiliac joint? Semin Arthr Rheum 1983; 12:282–312.

Bernard TN Jr, Cassidy JD. The sacroiliac joint syndrome: pathophysiology, diagnosis and management. In: Frymoyer JW, ed. The adult spine: principles and practice. New York: Raven Press; 1991:2107–2131.

Bernard TM, Kirkaldy-Willis WH. Recognizing specific characteristics of nonspecific low back pain. Clinical Orthopedics and Related Research 1987; 217:266–280.

Botek ST. Book critique: Treating myofascial pain: intramuscular stimulation (IMS) for myofascial pain syndromes of neuropathic origin, by C. Chan Gun, MD. Phys Med Rev (Fall):4–5.

Bowen V, Cassidy JD. Macroscopic and microscopic anatomy of the sacroiliac joint from embryonic life until the eighth decade. Spine 1981; 6:620–628.

Cassidy JD. The pathoanatomy and clinical significance of the sacroiliac joints. J Manip Physiol Ther 1992; 15:41–42.

Cibulka MT, Rose SJ, Delitto A, Sinacore DR. Hamstring muscle strain treated by mobilizing the sacroiliac joint. Phys Ther 1986; 66:1220–1223.

Ciullo JV, Jackson DW. Pars interarticularis stress reaction, spondylolysis, and spondylolisthesis in gymnasts. Clin Sports Med 1985; 4:95–110.

Colachis SC, Worden RE, Bechtal CO, Strohm BR. Movement of the sacroiliac joint in the adult male: a preliminary report. Arch Phys Med Rehabil 1963; 44:490–498.

Conway PJW, Herzog W. Changes in walking mechanics associated with wearing an intertrochanteric support belt. Journal of Manipulative and Physiological Therapeutics 1991; 14(3):185–188.

Costello K. Myofascial syndromes. In: Steege JF, Metzger DA, Levy BS, eds. Chronic pelvic pain: an integrated approach. Philadelphia: WB Saunders; 1998:251–266.

Craig C. Notes for a workshop on pelvic floor dysfunction: examination techniques and treatment. West Vancouver, Canada, 1992.

Dal Monte A, Komor A. Rowing and sculling mechanics. In: Vaughan CL, ed. Biomechanics of sport. Boca Raton, FL: CRC Press; 1989:53–119.

Derby R. Diagnostic block procedures: use in pain location. Spine: State of the Art Reviews 1986; 1:47–65.

d'Hemecourt P, Micheli L. Acute and chronic adolescent thoracolumbar spine injuries. Sports Med Arthrosc Rev 1997; 5:164–171.

Dihlmann W. Roentgendiagnostik der Iliosakralgelenke und Ihrer Nahen Umgebung. Stuttgart: George Thieme; 1967.

Dijkstra PF. Basic problems in the visualization of the sacroiliac joint. In: Vleeming A, Mooney V, Dorman T, Snijders C, Stoechart R, eds. Movement, stability and low back pain. The essential role of the pelvis. Edinburgh: Churchill Livingstone; 1997:333.

DonTigny RL Function and pathomechanics of the sacroiliac joint. A review. Phys Ther 1985; 65:35–44.

DonTigny RL Anterior dysfunction of the sacroiliac joint as a major factor in the etiology of idiopathic low back pain syndrome. Phys Ther 1990; 70:250–265.

DonTigny RL. Sacroiliac dysfunction: recognition and treatment. In: Vleeming A, Mooney V, Snijders C, Dorman T, eds. Low back pain and its relation to the sacroiliac joint. Rotterdam: European Conference Organizers; 1992:481–499.

DonTigny RL. Mechanics and treatment of the sacroiliac joint. In: Vleeming A, Mooney V, Dorman T, Snijders C, Stoechart R, eds. Movement, stability and low back pain. The essential role of the pelvis. Edinburgh: Churchill Livingstone; 1997:461–476.

Dorman TA. Prolotherapy: a survey. Journal of Orthopaedic Medicine 1993; 15:2–3.

Dorman TA. Failure of self-bracing at the sacroiliac joint: the slipping clutch syndrome. J Orthop Med 1994; 16:49–51.

Dorman T. Failure of self-bracing at the sacroiliac joints: the slipping clutch syndrome. In: Vleeming A, Mooney V, Dorman T, Snijders CJ, eds. Second interdisciplinary world congress on back pain. San Diego, CA, 9–11 November 1995; 653–656.

Dorman TA. Pelvic mechanics and prolotherapy. In: Vleeming A, Mooney V, Dorman T, Snijders C, Stoeckart R, eds. Movement, stability, low back pain: the essential role of the pelvis. New York: Churchill Livingstone; 1997:501–522.

Dorman TA, Ravin TH. Diagnosis and injection techniques in orthopedic medicine. Baltimore: Williams & Wilkins; 1991.

Dorman T, Brierly S, Fray J, Pappani K. Muscles and pelvic gears: hip abductor inhibition in anterior rotation of the ilium. J Orthop Med 1995; 17:96–100.

Dorman TA, Brierly S, Fray J, Pappani K. Muscles and pelvic clutch; hip abductor inhibition in anterior rotation of the ilium. In: Vleeming A, Mooney V, Tischler H, Dorman TA, Snijders C, eds. Proceedings of the third interdisciplinary world congress on low back and pelvic pain, Vienna, 19–21 November 1998:140–148.

Dunn J, Glymph ID. Investigating the effect of upper cervical adjustment on cycling performance. Vector 1999; 2(4).

Egund N, Olsson TH, Schmid H, Selvik G. Movement of the sacroiliac joint demonstrated with roentgen stereophotogrammetry. Acta Radiolog Diagn 1978; 19:833–846.

Fadiman J, Frayer R. Personality and personal growth. New York: Harper and Row; 1976.

Fitt SS. Corrective exercises for two muscular imbalances: tight hip flexors and pectoralis minor syndrome. J Health Phys Educ Recreation 1987; 58(5):45–48.

Foran P. Upper cervical adjustment's impact on athletic performance. Can Chiropract 1999:10–12.

Foran P. NUCCA technique. Can Chiropract 1999; 4:6–8.

Fowler C. Muscle energy techniques for pelvic dysfunction. In: Grieve GP, ed. Modern manual therapy of the vertebral column. Edinburgh: Churchill Livingstone; 1986:805–814.

Fraser DM. T-3 revisited. J Orthop Med 1993; 13:5–6.

Freeman MAR, Dean MRE, Hanham IWF. The etiology and prevention of functional instability of the foot. J Bone Joint Surg 1965; 47B:678–685.

Frigerio NA, Stowe RR, Howe JW. Movement of the sacro-iliac joint. Clini Orthop Related Res 1974; 100:370–377.

Fryette HH. Principles of osteopathic technique. Carmel, CA: Academy of Applied Osteopathy; 1954.

Garn SN, Newton RA. Kinesthetic awareness in subjects with multiple ankle sprains. Phys Ther 1988; 68:1667–1671.

Gilmore KL. Biomechanics of the lumbar motion segment. In: Grieve GP, ed. Modern manual therapy of the vertebral column. Edinburgh: Churchill Livingstone; 1986:103–111.

Glencross D, Thornton E. Position sense following joint injury. J Sports Med Phys Fitness 1981; 21:23–27.

Gracovetsky SA. Linking the spinal engine with the legs: a theory of human gait. In: Vleeming A, Mooney V, Dorman T, Snijders C, Stoeckart R, eds. Movement, stability and low back pain. New York: Churchill Livingstone; 1997:243–251.

Gracovetsky S, Farfan HF. The optimum spine. Spine 1986; 11:543–573.

Greenman PE. Clinical aspects of sacroiliac function in walking. In: Paterson JK, Burn L, eds. Back pain – an international review. Kluwer, 1990:125–130.

Greenman PE. Clinical aspects of sacroiliac joint in walking. In: Vleeming A, Mooney V, Dorman T, Snijdere CJ, Stoeckart R, eds. Movements, stability and low back pain. Edinburgh: Churchill Livingstone, 1997: 235–242.

Grieve GP. The sacro-iliac joint. Physiotherapy 1976; 62:384–400.

Grieve GP. Treating backache – a topical comment. Physiotherapy 1983; 69:316.

Grieve GP. Movements of the thoracic spine. In: Grieve GP, ed. Modern manual therapy of the vertebral column. Edinburgh: Churchill Livingstone; 1986a:86–102.

Grieve GP. Thoracic joint problems and simulated visceral disease. In: Grieve GP, ed. Modern manual therapy of the vertebral column. Edinburgh: Churchill Livingstone; 1986b:377.

Grieve GP. Common vertebral joint problems. Edinburgh: Churchill Livingstone; 1988.

Gunn C. Transcutaneous neural stimulation, acupuncture and the current of injury. American Journal of Acupuncture 1978; 6(3):191–196.

Guymer AJ. Proprioceptive neuromuscular facilitation for vertebral joint conditions. In: Grieve GP, ed. Modern manual therapy of the vertebral column. Edinburgh: Churchill Livingstone; 1986:622–639.

Hackett GS. Ligament and tendon relaxation (skeletal disability) treated by prolotherapy (fibro-osseous proliferation), 3rd edn. Springfield, IL: Charles C Thomas; 1958.

Hackett GS, Henderson DG. Joint stabilization. An experimental, histological study with comments on the clinical application in ligament proliferation. Am J Surg 1955; 89:968–973.

Hackett GS, Hemwall GA, Montgomery GA. Ligament and tendon relaxation treated by prolotherapy, 5th edn. Oak Park, IL: Gustav A Hemwall; 1991.

Haldeman KO, Soto-Hall R. The diagnosis and treatment of sacro-iliac conditions by the injection of procaine (novocain). J Bone Joint Surg 1983; 20(3):675–685.

Harris FI, White AS, Biskind GR. Observations on solutions used for injection treatment of hernia. Am J Surg 1938; 39:112–119.

Hauser RA. Prolo your pain away! Curing chronic pain with prolotherapy. Oak Park, IL: Beulah Land Press, 1998.

Hayes HM. Veterinary notes for horse owners. London: Random House; 1987 (revd edn PD Rossdale).

Heardman H. Physiotherapy in obstetrics and gynecology. Edinburgh: E & S Livingstone; 1951.

Herman H. Urogenital dysfunction. In: Wilder E, ed. Obstetric and gynecologic physical therapy. New York: Churchill Livingstone; 1988:83–111.

Herzog W, Nigg BM, Read LJ. Quantifying the effects of spinal manipulation on gait using patients with low back pain. J Manip Physiolog Ther 1988; 11:151–157.

Hesch J, Aisenbrey JA, Guarino J. Manual therapy evaluation of the pelvic joints using palpatory and articular spring tests. In: Vleeming A, Mooney V, Snijders C, Dorman T, eds. Low back pain and its relation to the sacroiliac joint. Rotterdam: European Conference Organizers; 1992:435–459.

Hill C. Making, not breaking: the first year under saddle. Ossining, NY: Breakthrough Publications; 1993.

Hirschberg GG. Sclerosant solution in low back pain. West J Med 1985; 143:682–683.

Hobusch FL, McClellan T. Sports performance series: The karate roundhouse kick. J Strength Cond Res 1990; 12:6–9.

Hodges PW, Richardson PA Inefficient muscular stabilization of the lumbar spine associated with low back pain. A motor control evaluation of transversus abdominis. Spine 1996; 21(22):2640–2650.

Hollingshead WH. Textbook of anatomy. New York: Harper and Row, 1962.

Howse J. Disorders of the great toe in dancers. Clinics in Sports Medicine 1983; 2:499–505.

Jacob HAC, Kissling RO. The mobility of the sacroiliac joints in healthy volunteers between 20 and 50 years of age. Clin Biomech 1995; 10(7):352–361.

Janda V. Muscles, central nervous motor regulation and back problems. In: Korr I, ed. The neurobiological mechanisms in manipulative therapy. London: Plenum Press; 1978:27.

Janda V. Muscle weakness and inhibition (pseudoparesis) in back pain syndromes. In: Grieve GP, ed. Modern manual therapy of the vertebral column. Edinburgh: Churchill Livingstone; 1986:197–201.

Jensen MC, Brant-Zawadski MN, Obuchowski N, Modic MT, Malkasian D, Ross RS. Magnetic resonance imaging of the lumbar spine in people without back pain. New Engl J Med 1994; 331:69–73.

Johnson TB, Whillis J, eds. Gray's Anatomy: descriptive and applied. London: Longmans & Green; 1944.

Jones LH. Strain and counterstrain. Colorado Springs, CO: American Academy of Osteopathy, 1981.

Jull G, Richardson C, Toppenberg R, Comerford M, Bui B. Towards a measurement of active muscle control for lumbar stabilization. Austral J Physiother 1993; 39:187–193.

Jurriaans E, Friedman L. CT and MRI of the sacroiliac joints. In: Vleeming A, Mooney V, Dorman T, Snijders C, Stoeckart R, eds. Movement, stability and low back pain. New York: Churchill Livingstone; 1997:347.

Kapandji IA. The physiology of the joints. III. The trunk and vertebral column, 2nd edn. Edinburgh: Churchill Livingstone; 1974.

Kegel AH. Progressive resistance exercise in the functional restoration of the perineal muscles. American Journal of Obstetrics and Gynaecology 1948; 56(2):238–248.

Kesson M, Atkins E. The thoracic spine and sport. J Orthop Med 1999; 21(3):80–86.

Kieffer SA, Cacayorin E, Sherry RG. The radiological diagnosis of herniated lumbar intervertebral disc. A current controversy. J Am Med Assoc 1984; 251:1192.

Kirkaldy-Willis WH, Cassidy JD. Spinal manipulation in the treatment of low back pain. Can Fam Phys 1985; 31:535–540.

Kissling RO, Jacob HAC. The mobility of sacroiliac joints in healthy subjects. In: Vleeming A, Mooney V, Dorman T, Snijders C, Stoeckart R, eds. Movement, stability and low back pain. New York: Churchill Livingstone; 1997:177–185.

Klein KK. Progression of pelvic tilt in adolescent boys from elementary through high school. Arch Phys Med Rehabil 1973; 54:57–59.

Klein KK, Buckley JC. Asymmetries of growth in the pelvis and legs of growing children. Am Correct Ther J 1968; 22:53–55.

Klein RG, Dorman TA, Johnson CE. Proliferant injections for low back pain: histologic changes of injected ligaments and objective measurements of lumbar spine mobility before and after treatment. J Neurolog Orthop Med Surg 1989; 10:123–126.

Klein RG, Eek BC, DeLong WB, Mooney V. A randomized double-blind trial of dextrose-glycerine-phenol injections for chronic, low back pain. J Spinal Disord 1993; 6:23–33.

Korr IM. Neurobiological mechanisms of manipulative therapy. New York: Plenum Press; 1978.

Kurica KB. A prospective study of sacroiliac joint arthrodesis with one to six year patient follow-up. In: Vleeming A, Mooney V, Dorman T, Snijders CJ, eds. The integrated function of the lumbar spine and sacroiliac joint. Rotterdam: European Conference Organizers; 1995:367–368.

Lee DG. The relationship between the lumbar spine, pelvic girdle and hip. In: Vleeming A, Mooney V, Snijders C, Dorman T, eds. Low back pain and its relation to the sacroiliac joint. Rotterdam: European Conference Organizers; 1992:464–478.

Lee DG. Biomechanics of the thorax: a clinical model of in vivo function. J Man Manipulative Ther 1993a; 1:13–21.

Lee DG. Biomechanics of the thorax. In: Grant R, ed. Physical therapy of the cervical and thoracic spine. New York: Churchill Livingstone; 1994a: ch 3.

Lee DG. Manual therapy for the thorax: a biomechanical approach. Delta, BC: Delta Orthopedic Physiotherapy Clinic; 1994b.

Lee DG. Instability of the sacroiliac joint and the consequences for gait. In: Vleeming A, Mooney V, Dorman T, Snijders C, Stoeckart R, eds. Movement, stability and low back pain. Edinburgh: Churchill Livingstone; 1997a:231–233.

Lee DG. Video teaching tapes. 1: Assessment – articular function of the sacroiliac joint. 2: Manual therapy techniques for the sacroiliac joint. 3: Exercises for the unstable pelvis. Delta, BC: Delta Orthopedic Physiotherapy Clinic; 1998.

Lee DG. The pelvic girdle: an approach to the examination and treatment of the lumbo–pelvic–hip region. Edinburgh: Churchill Livingstone; 1999.

Lee DG, Walsh MC. Workbook of manual therapy techniques for the vertebral column and pelvic girdle. 2nd edn. Altona, Manitoba: Friesen Printers; 1996.

Lehmann RC. Thoracoabdominal musculoskeletal injuries in racquet sports. Clin Sports Med 1988; 7:267–276.

Lentell GL, Katzman LL, Walters MR. The relationship between muscle function and ankle stability. J Orthop Med 1992; 14:85–90.

Lippitt AB. Percutaneous fixation of the sacroiliac joint. In: Vleeming A, Mooney V, Dorman T, Snijders CJ, eds. The integrated function of the lumbar spine and sacroiliac joint. Rotterdam: European Conference Organizers; 1995:369–390.

Lovett RW. A contribution to the study of the mechanics of the spine. Am J Anat 1903; 2:457–462.

Luttgens K, Deutsch H, Hamilton N. Kinesiology: scientific basis of human locomotion. 8th edn. Dubuque, IA: Brown & Benchmark; 1992.

McArdle WD, Katch FI, Katch VL. Exercise physiology: energy, nutrition and human performance. Philadelphia: Lea & Febiger; 1986.

McCall IW, Park WM, O'Brien JP. Induced pain referral from posterior lumbar elements in normal subjects. Spine 1979; 4:441–446.

McGivney JQ, Cleveland BR. The levator syndrome and its treatment. South Med J 1965; 58:505–509.

McGuckin N. The T4 syndrome. In: Grieve GP, ed. Modern manual therapy of the vertebral column. Edinburgh: Churchill Livingstone; 1986:370–376.

Maffetone P. Complementary sports medicine. Champaign, IL: Human Kinetics; 1999.

Magora A, Schwartz A. Relation between the low back pain syndrome and x-ray findings. 1. Degenerative osteoarthritis. Scand J Rehabil Med 1976; 8:115–125.

Maigne R. Low back pain of thoracolumbar origin. Arch Phys Med Rehabil 1980; 60:389–395.

Maigne R. Thoraco-lumbar junction syndrome: a source of diagnostic error. J Orthop Med 1995; 17(3):84–89.

Maigne J-Y. Lateral dynamic X-rays in the sitting position and coccygeal discography in common coccydynia. In: Vleeming A, Mooney V, Dorman T, Snijders C, Stoeckart R, eds. Movement, stability and low back pain. New York: Churchill Livingstone; 1997:385–391.

Maigne J-Y, Lazareth JP, Guerin-Surville H, Maigne R. The lateral cutaneous branches of the dorsal rami of the thoracolumbar junction: an anatomical study of 37 dissections. J Surg Radiol Anat 1986; 8:251–256.

Maigne J-Y, Aivaliklis A, Pfefer S. Results of sacroiliac joint double block and value of sacroiliac pain provocation tests in 54 patients with low back pain. Spine 1996; 21:1889–1892.

Maitland GD. Vertebral manipulation. London: Butterworth; 1977.

Maniol L. Histologic effects of various sclerosing solutions used in the injection treatment of hernia. Arch Surg 1938; 36:171–189.

Mann R. Biomechanics of running. In: Mack RP, ed. American Academy of Orthopedic Surgeons symposium on the foot and leg in running sports. St Louis: CV Mosby; 1982:1–29.

Mayer D, Liebeskind J. Pain reduction by focal electrical stimulation of the brain: an anatomical and behavioral analysis. Brain Res 1974; 68:73–93.

Melzack R. Myofascial trigger points: relation to acupuncture and mechanisms of pain. Arch Phys Med Rehabil 1981; 62:114–117.

Melzack R, Wall P. Pain mechanisms: a new theory. Science 1965; 150:971–979.

Mens JMA, Stam HJ, Stoeckart A, Vleeming A, Snijders CJ. Peripartum pelvic pain: a report of the analysis of an inquiry among patients of a Dutch patients' society. In: Vleeming A, Mooney V, Snijders C, Dorman T, eds. Low back pain and its relation to the sacroiliac joint. Rotterdam: European Conference Organizers; 1992:519–533.

Mens JMA, Vleeming A, Snijders CJ, Stam HJ. Active straight leg raising test: a clinical approach to the load transfer function of the pelvic girdle. In: Vleeming A, Mooney V, Dorman T, Snijders C, Stoeckart R, eds. Movement, stability and low back pain. Edinburgh: Churchill Livingstone; 1997:425–431.

Micheli LJ. Low back pain in the adolescent: differential diagnosis. Am J Sports Med 1979; 7:362–364.

Micheli LJ. Back injuries in dancers. Clin Sports Med 1983; 2:473–484.

Micheli LJ. Back injuries in gymnastics. Clin Sports Med 1985; 4:85–93.

Midttun A, Bojsen-Moller F. The sacrotuberous ligament pain syndrome. In: Grieve GP, ed. Modern manual therapy of the vertebral column. Edinburgh: Churchill Livingstone; 1986:815–818.

Miller JAA, Schultz AB, Andersson GBJ. Load-displacement behaviour of sacroiliac joints. J Orthop Res 1987; 5:92–101.

Mirman MJ. Sclerotherapy. 4th edn. Springfield, PA: 652 E. Springfield Road; 1989.

Mitchell FL Sr, Mitchell FL Jr. An evaluation and treatment manual of osteopathic muscle energy procedures. Valley Park, MO: Moran and Pruzzo Associates; 1979.

Mixter WJ, Barr JS. Rupture of the intervertebral disc with involvement of the spinal canal. New Engl J Med 1934; 211:210–215.

Money V, Robertson J. The facet syndrome. Clin Orthop 1976; 115:149–156.

Mooney V, Pozos R, Vleeming A, Gulick J, Swenski D. In: Vleeming A, Mooney V, Dorman T, Snijders C, Stoeckart R, eds. Movement, stability and low back pain. The essential role of the pelvis. New York: Churchill Livingstone; 1997:ch. 7, 115–122.

Morris R, McKay W, Mushlin P. Comparison of pain associated with intradermal and subcutaneous infiltration with various local anaesthetic solutions. Anaesth Analges 1987; 66:1180–1182.

Mueller MJ, Minor SD, Schaaf JA, Strube MJ, Sahrmann SA. Relationship of plantar–flexor peak torque and dorsiflexion range of motion to kinetic variables during walking. Phys Ther 1995; 75(8):684–693.

Nacim F, Froetscher L, Hirschberg GG. Treatment of the chronic iliolumbar syndrome by infiltration of the iliolumbar ligament. West J Med 1982; 136:372–374.

Nixon JE. Injuries to the neck and upper extremities of dancers. In Clin Sports Med 1983; 2:459–472.

Norman GF. Sacroiliac disease and its relationship to lower abdominal pain. Am J Surg 1968; 116:54–56.

O'Brien CP. Case history: footballer's ankle (anterior impingement of the ankle). J Orthop Med 1992; 14:91.

Oestgaard HC. Assessment and treatment of low back pain in working pregnant women. In: Vleeming A, Mooney V, Tischler H, Dorman T, Snijders C, eds. Third interdisciplinary world congress on low back and pelvic pain. Rotterdam: European Conference Organizers; 1998:161–171.

Ongley MJ, Klein RG, Dorman TA, Eek BC, Hubert LJ. A new approach to the treatment of chronic low back pain. Lancet 1987; 2:143–146.

Ongley MJ, Dorman TA, Eek BC, Lundgren D, Klein RG. Ligament instability of knees. A new approach to treatment. Man Ded 1988; 3:152–154.

Pace JB, Nagle D. Piriformis syndrome. West J Med 1976; 124:435–439.

Paish W. Track and field athletics. London: Lupus Books; 1976.

Panjabi MM. The stabilizing system of the spine. I. Function, dysfunction, adaptation, and enhancement. J Spinal Disord 1992; 5(4):383–389.

Pansky B, House EL. Review of gross anatomy. New York: Macmillan; 1975.

Paris SV. Foundations of clinical orthopaedics. St Augustine, FL: Institute Press; 1990.

Parker P. Free heel skiing: the secrets of telemark and parallel techniques – in all conditions. Chelsea, VT: Chelsea Green Publishing; 1988.

Pearson WM. A progressive structural study of school children. J Am Osteopath Assoc 1951; 51:155–167.

Pearson WM. Early and high incidence of mechanical faults. J Osteopath 1954; 61:18–23.

Perry JD, Hullett LT, Bollinger JR. Biofeedback treatment of incontinence: California Biofeedback 1988; Summer: 7–9, 18–19.1

Pitkin HC, Pheasant HC. Sacrathrogenetic telalgia. A study of sacral mobility. J Bone Joint Surg 1936;18A;365–374.

Pitman B. Fencing: techniques of foil, epée and saber. Swindon: Crowood Press; 1988.

Pomeranz B. Brain's opiates at work in acupuncture. New Scient 1975; 73:12–13.

Pomeroy KL. Position statement of the American Association of Orthopedic Medicine on prolotherapy. Phoenix Physical Medicine Centre, Phoenix, Arizona.

Prechtl JC, Powley TL. B-afferents: a fundamental division of the nervous system mediating homeostasis? Behav Brain Sci 1990; 13:289–331.

Proulx WR. Comparison of efficacy of prolotherapy versus steroid injection in the treatment of low back pain. Presented at the annual meeting of the American Association of Orthopedic Medicine, Denver, CO; 1990.

Resnick D, Niwayama G, Georgen TG. Degenerative disease of the sacroiliac joint. Invest Radiol 1975; 10:608–621.

Rice CO. Injection treatment of hernia. Philadelphia: FA Davis; 1937.

Rice CO, Matson H. Histologic changes in the tissues of man and animals following the injection of irritating solutions intended for the cure of hernia. Ill Med J 1936; 70:271–278.

Richard R. Osteopathic lesions of the sacrum. Physio-pathology and corrective techniques (trans. D Louch). Wellingborough: Thorsons Publishing; 1986 (original work published in 1978).

Richardson AR. The biomechanics of swimming: the shoulder and knee. Clin Sports Med 1986; 5:103–113.

Richardson CA, Jull GA. Muscle control – pain control. What exercises would you prescribe? Man Ther 1995; 1:2–10.

Richardson C, Jull G, Hodges P, Hides J. Therapeutic exercise for stabilization in low back pain: scientific basis and clinical approach. Churchill Livingstone: Edinburgh; 1999.

Sammarco GJ. The dancer's hip. Clin Sports Med 1983; 2:485–498.

Sapsford RR, Hodges PW, Richardson CA. Activation of the abdominal muscles is a normal response to contraction of the pelvic floor muscles. Abstract, International Continence Society Conference, Japan; 1997.

Sapsford RR, Hodges PW, Richardson CA, Cooper DA, Jull GA, Markwell SJ. Activation of pubococcygeus during a variety of isometric abdominal exercises. Abstract, International Continence Society Conference, Japan; 1997.

Sashin D. A critical analysis of the anatomy and the pathologic changes of the sacro-iliac joints. J Bone Joint Surg 1930; 12A:891–910.

Schamberger W. Orthotics for athletes: attacking the biomechanical roots of injury. Can Fam Physician 1983; 29:1670–1680.

Schamberger W. Nerve injuries around the foot and ankle. In: Shephard RJ, Taunton JE, eds. The foot and ankle in sport and exercise. Med Sport Sci 1987; 23:105–120.

Schwarzer AC, Aprill CN, Bogduk N. The sacroiliac joint in chronic low back pain. Spine 1995; 20:31–37.

Shaw JL. The role of the sacroiliac joint as a cause of low back pain and dysfunction. In: Vleeming A, Mooney V, Snijders C, Dorman T, eds. Low back pain and its relation to the sacroiliac joint. Rotterdam: European Conference Organizers; 1992:67–80.

Snijders CJ, Vleeming A, Stoeckart R. Transfer of lumbosacral load to iliac bones and legs. I. Biomechanics of self-bracing of the sacroiliac joints and its significance for treatment and exercise. Clin Biomech 1992a; 8:285–294.

Snijders CJ, Vleeming A, Stoeckart R. Transfer of lumbosacral load to iliac bones and legs. II. The loading of the sacroiliac joints when lifting in a stooped posture. In: Vleeming A, Mooney V, Snijders C, Dorman T, eds. Low back pain and its relation to the sacroiliac joint. Rotterdam: European Conference Organizers; 1992b:255–271.

Snijders CJ, Vleeming A, Stoeckart R, Kleinrensink GJ, Mens JMA. Biomechanics of sacroiliac joint stability: validation experiments on the concept of self-locking. In: Vleeming A, Mooney V, Snijders C, Dorman T, eds. The integrated function of the lumbar spine and the sacroiliac joint. Rotterdam, European Conference Organizers; 1995a:75–91.

Snijders CJ, Vleeming A, Stoeckert R, Mens JMA, Kleinrensink GJ. Biomechanical modelling of sacroiliac stability in different postures. Spine: State of the Art Reviews. Philadelphia: Hanley & Belfus; 1995b:23.

Solonen KA. The sacroiliac joint in the light of anatomical, roentgenological and clinical studies. Acta Orthop Scand Suppl. 1957; 27:1–127.

Steege JF, Metzger DA, Levy BS, eds. Chronic pelvic pain: an integrated approach. Philadelphia: WB Saunders; 1998.

Stevens A. Side-bending and axial rotation of the sacrum inside the pelvic girdle. In: Vleeming A, Mooney V, Snijders C, Dorman T, eds. Low back pain and its relation to the sacroiliac joint. Rotterdam: European Conference Organizers; 1992:209–230.

Stinson JT. Spondylolysis and spondylolisthesis in the athlete. Clin Sports Med 1993; 12:517–528.

Strachan WF. Applied anatomy of the pelvis and perineum. J Am Osteopath Assoc 1939; 38:359–360.

Strasser HA. Lifetime of soundness 1998.

Sturesson B. External fixator. Acta Orthop Scand 1999.

Sturesson B, Selvik G, Uden A. Movements of the sacroiliac joints. A roentgen stereophotogrammetric analysis. Spine 1989; 14:162–165.

Sweeting RC, Fowler C, Crocker B. Anterior knee pain and spinal dysfunction in adolescents. J Man Med 1989; 4:65–68.

Thiele GH. Coccydynia: cause and treatment. Paper presented at the meeting of the American Proctology Society, May 1963.

Travell JG, Simons DG. Myofascial pain and dysfunction. The trigger point manual. Baltimore: Williams & Wilkins; 1983.

Travell JG, Simons DG. Myofascial pain and dysfunction: the trigger point manual. The lower extremities. Baltimore, MD: Williams & Wilkins; 1992.

Tsai L, Wredmark T. Spinal posture, sagittal mobility, and subjective rating of back problems in former female elite gymnasts. Spine 1993; 18(7):872–875.

Upledger JE. Craniosacral therapy II: beyond the dura. Seattle, WA: Eastland Press; 1987.

Upledger JE, Larni Z. Somato-emotional release and beyond. Palm Beach Gardens, FZ: U1 Publishing; 1990.

Upledger J. Vrredevoogd JD. Craniosacral therapy. Chicago: Eastland Press; 1983.

Valojerdy MR, Salsabili N, Hogg DA. Age changes in the human sacroiliac joint: joint fusion. Clin Anat 1989; 2:253–261.

Van Ingen Schenau GJ. The influence of air friction in speed skating. J Biomech 1982; 15:449–458.

Van Ingen Schenau GJ, De Boer RW, De Groot G. Biomechanics of speed skating. In: Vaughan CL, ed. Biomechanics of sport. Boca Raton, FL: CRC Press; 1989:121–167.

Vleeming A, Stoeckart R, Snijders DJ. The sacrotuberous ligament: a conceptual approach to its dynamic role in stabilizing the sacro-iliac joint. Clin Biomech 1989a; 4:201–203.

Vleeming A, Van Wingerden JP, Snijders CJ, Stoeckart R, Stijnen T. Load application to the sacrotuberous ligament; influences on sacro-iliac joint mechanics. Clin Biomech 1989b; 4:204–209.

Vleeming A, Stoeckart R, Volkers ACW, Snijders CJ. Relation between form and function in the sacroiliac joint. 1. Clinical anatomical aspects. Spine 1990a; 15(2):130–132.

Vleeming A, Van Wingerden JP, Dijkstra PF, Stoeckart R, Snijders CJ, Stijnen T. Mobility in the sacroiliac joints in the elderly: a kinematic and radiological study. Clin Biomech 1992a; 7:170–176.

Vleeming A, Stoeckart R, Snijders CJ. A short history of sacroiliac research. Developmental biology of the sacroiliac joint. Regional anatomy of the sacroiliac joint. Investigating sacroiliac mobility: In Vleeming A, Mooney V, Snijders C, Dorman T, eds. Course proceedings of the first interdisciplinary world congress on low back pain and its relation to the sacroiliac joint, San Diego, 5–6 November. Rotterdam: European Conference Organizers; 1992b:1–64.

Vleeming A, Volkers ACW, Snijders CJ, Stoeckart R. Relation between form and function in the sacroiliac joint. II. Biomechanical aspects. Spine 1990b; 15(2):133–136.

Vleeming A, Pool-Goudzwaard AI, Stoeckart R, van Wingerden JP, Snijders CJ. The posterior layer of the thoracolumbar fascia; its function in load transfer from spine to legs. Spine 1995; 20:753–758.

Vleeming A, Snijders CJ, Stoeckart R, Mens JMA. The role of the sacroiliac joint in coupling between spine, pelvis, legs and arms. In: Vleeming A, Mooney V, Dorman T, Snijders C, Stoeckart R, eds. Movement, stability and low back pain. New York: Churchill Livingstone; 1997:53–71.

Wagner-Chazalon A. Back in the saddle. Chiropractor and vet find link between horses, riders and backs. Canadian Horseman 2000; Mar/Apr:18–21.

Walheim GG. Stabilization of the pelvis with the Hoffman frame. Acta Orthop Scand 1984; 55:319–324.

Walker JM. The sacroiliac joint: a critical review. Phys Ther 1992; 72:903–916.

Wallace KA. Pelvic floor muscle dysfunction and its behavioral treatment. In: Agostini R, ed. Medical and orthopedic issues of active and athletic women. Philadelphia: Hanley & Belfus; 1994:200–212.

Wanless M. Ride with your mind: a right brain approach to riding. London: Reed; 1995.

Watanabe K. Ski-jumping, alpine-, cross-country- and nordic-combination skiing. In: Vaughan CL, ed. Biomechanics of sport. Boca Raton, FL: CRC Press; 1989:239–261.

Weinberg SK. Medical aspects of synchronized swimming. Clin Sports Med 1986; 5:159–167.

Weishaupt D, Zanetti M, Hadler J, Boos N. MRI imaging of the lumbar spine: prevalence of intervertebral disk extrusion and sequestration, nerve root compression, end plate abnormalities, and osteoarthritis of the facet joints in asymptomatic volunteers. Radiology 1998; 209:661–666.

Weisl H. Movements of the sacro-iliac joint. Acta Anat 1955; 23:80–91.

Wells PE. Movement of the pelvic joints. In: Grieve GP, ed. Modern manual therapy of the vertebral column. Edinburgh: Churchill Livingstone; 1986:176–181.

Whatmore, Kohli. The pathophysiology and treatment of functional disorders. New York: Grune & Stratton; 1974.

Willard FH. The lumbosacral connection: the ligamentous structure of the low back and its relation to pain. In: Vleeming A, Mooney V, Dorman T, Snijders CJ, eds. The integrated function of the lumbar spine and sacroiliac joint. Rotterdam: European Conference Organizers; 1995:29–58.

Williams PL, Warwick R, eds. Gray's Anatomy. 36th edn. The joints of the lower limb: the sacro-iliac joint. Edinburgh: Churchill Livingstone; 1980:473–477.

Wingerden JP van, Vleeming A, Snijders CJ, Stoeckart R. A functional anatomical approach to the spine–pelvis mechanism interaction between the biceps femoris muscle and the sacrotuberous ligament. Eur Spine J 1993; 2:140–144.

Woo C-C. World class female windsurfing championships: a pilot study of physical characteristics and injuries. Sports Chiropractic Rehab 1997; 11(1):11–17.

Worth DR. Movements of the cervical spine. In: Grieve GP, ed. Modern manual therapy of the vertebral column. Edinburgh: Churchill Livingstone; 1986:77–85.

Worth S, ed. The rules of the game. New York: St. Martin's Press; 1990.

Wyke BD. Articular neurology and manipulative therapy. In: Glasgow EF, Twomey LT, Scull ER, Kleynhans AM, eds. Aspects of manipulative therapy. 2nd edn. New York: Churchill Livingstone; 1985:72–77.

Yeomans W. The relation of arthritis of the sacro-ilic joint to sciatica. Lancet 1928; 2:1119–1122.

Further reading

Adams C, Logue V. Studies in cervical spondylotic myelopathy. Brain 1971; 94:557–568.

Beighton PH, Solomon L, Soskolne CL. Articular mobility in an African population. Ann Rheum Dis 1973; 32:413–418.

Bourdeau Y. Five-year follow-up on sclerotherapy/prolotherapy for low back pain. Man Med 1988; 3:155–157.

Bourdillon J. Spinal manipulation. 2nd edn. London: Heinemann; 1973.

Breig A. Biomechanics of the central nervous system. Stockholm: Almquist & Wiksell; 1960.

Breig A. Adverse mechanical tension in the central nervous system. Stockholm: Almquist & Wiksell; 1978.

Brennan LJ. A comparative analysis of the golf drive and seven iron with emphasis on pelvic and spinal rotation. Thesis, University of Wisconsin; 1968.

Bromley M. Equine manipulation and therapy. New York: Howell Book House; 1987.

Campbell-Smith S. Long leg arthropathy. Ann Rheum Dis 1964; 28:359–365.

Chamberlain E. The symphysis pubis in the roentgen examination of the sacroiliac joint. Am J Roentgenol, Radium Ther Nucl Med 1930; 24:621–625.

Cyriax J. Textbook of orthopedic medicine. Vol. 1. Diagnosis of soft tissue lesions. 5th edn. London: Baillière, Tindall & Cassell; 1970.

Denslow JS. An analysis of the variability of spinal reflex thresholds. J Neurophysiol 1944; 7:207–216.

Denslow JS, Korr IM, Krems AD. Quantitative studies of chronic facilitation in human motoneuron pools. Am J Physiol 1947; 150:229–238.

Diemerbroech I. The anatomy of human bodies (trans. W. Salmon). London: Brewster, 1689.

Epstein JB. Temporomandibular disorders, facial pain and headache following motor vehicle accidents. J Can Dental Assoc 1992; 58:488–495.

Fraser DM. The forgotten joint: superior tibiofibular joint. J Orthop Med 1989; 2:52–53.

German National Equestrian Education. The principles of riding. The complete riding and driving system. Book 1. Addington, Buckingham: Kenilworth Press; 1992.

Greenman PE. Clinical aspects of the sacroiliac joint in walking. In: Vleeming A, Mooney V, Dorman T, Snijders C, Stoeckart R, eds. Movement, stability and low back pain. New York: Churchill Livingstone, 1997:235.

Greenman PE. Clinical aspects of sacroiliac function in walking. J Man Med 1990; 5:125–130.

Hackett GS. Joint ligament relaxation treated by fibro-osseous proliferation. Springfield, IL: Charles C Thomas; 1957.

425

Hackett GS, Huang TC. Prolotherapy for sciatica from weak pelvic ligaments and bone dystrophy. Clin Med 1961; 8:2301–2316.

Heinrich S. Treatment of sacro-coccygeal dysfunction: dealing with a delicate issue in therapy. Available from W. Schamberger, 5450 Moreland Drive, Burnaby, B.C., Canada, V5G 1Z7; 1990.

Henriques P. Balanced riding: a way to find the correct seat. Middleton, MD: Half Halt Press; 1990.

Hirschberg GG, Froetscher L, Naeim F. Iliolumbar syndrome as a common cause of low back pain. Arch Phys Med Rehabil 1979; 60:415–419.

Hruby RJ. The total body approach to the osteopathic management of temporomandibular joint dysfunction. J Am Osteopathic Assoc 1984; 8:502–510.

Hussar CJ, Curtis JD. TMJ syndrome: an integrative approach. In Retzlaff EW, Mitchell FL Jr, eds. The cranium and its sutures: anatomy, physiology, clinical applications and annotated bibliography of research in the cranial field. New York: Springer-Verlag; 1987:48–58.

Kegel AH. Progressive resistive exercise in the functional restoration of the perineal muscles. Am J Obstet Gynecol 1948; 56:238–248.

Korr IM. Somatic dysfunction, osteopathic manipulative treatment, and the nervous system: a few facts, some theories, many questions. J Am Osteopath Assoc 1986; 86:109–114.

LaBan MM. Collagen tissue: implications of its response to stress in vitro. Arch Phys Med Rehabil 1962; 43:461–466.

Lee DG. A workbook of manual therapy technique for the upper extremity. Delta, BC: DOPC; 1989.

Lee DG. The pelvic girdle: an approach to the examination and treatment of the lumbo-pelvic-hip region. Edinburgh: Churchill Livingstone; 1989.

Lee DG. When to use a sacroiliac belt. Can Physiother Assoc Orthop Div Rev 1993; 19.

Lee DG. Treatment of pelvic instability. In: Vleeming A, Mooney V, Dorman T, Snijders C, Stoeckart R, eds. Movement, stability and low back pain. Edinburgh: Churchill Livingstone; 1997:445.

Lee DG, Walsh M. A workbook of manual therapy techniques for the vertebral column and pelvic girdle. Delta, BC: Nascent Publishing; 1985.

Louis R. Vertebroradicular and vertebromedullary dynamics. Anatom Clin 1981; 3:1–11.

McCaw ST, Bates RT. Biomechanical implications of mild leg length inequality. Br J Sports Med 1991; 25(1):10–13.

Maigne R. Orthopaedic medicine. Springfield, IL: Charles C Thomas; 1972.

Massey AE. Movement of pain sensitive structures in the neural canal. In: Grieve GP, ed. Modern manual therapy of the vertebral column. Edinburgh: Churchill Livingstone; 1986:182–193.

Meagher J. Beating muscle injuries for horses. Hamilton, MA: Hamilton Horse Associates; 1992.

Moran M. Evaluation and treatment of the sacrum: direct and indirect technique. Edmonds, WA: Ursa Foundation; 1992.

Morgan D. Understanding your horse's lameness. Middletown, MD: Half Halt Press; 1992.

O'Connell JEA. Clinical signs of meningeal irritation. Brain 1946; 69:9–21.

Panjabi MM, Brand RA, White AA. Mechanical properties of the thoracic spine. J Joint Bone Surg 1976; 58A:642–652.

Perry JD, Hullett LT. The role of home trainers in Kegel's exercise program for treatment of incontinence. Ost Wound Manage 1990; 30:46–57.

Perry J, Hullett LT, Bollinger JR. EMG biofeedback treatment of incontinence. Calif Biofeed 1988; 7–9:18–19.

Pine J. Your guide to coping with back pain. Toronto: McClelland & Stewart; 1985.

Polsdorfer R. Coccydynia and the orthopaedic rectal examination. J Orthop Med 1992; 14:13–17.

Porac C, Coren S. Lateral preferences and human behaviour. New York: Springer-Verlag; 1981.

Rees L. The fundamentals of riding. London: Roxby Paintbox; 1991.

Reid J. Effects of flexion–extension movements of the head and spine upon the spinal cord and nerve roots. J Neurol Neurosurg Psychiatr 1960; 23:214–220.

Rigby BJ. The effect of mechanical extension upon thermal stability of collagen. Biochim Biophys Acta 1964; 79:634–636.

Rigby BJ, Hirai N, Spikes J, Eyring H. The mechanical properties of rat tail tendon. J Gen Physiol 1959; 43:265–283.

Roy S, Irvin R. Sports medicine: prevention, evaluation, management and rehabilitation. Englewood Cliffs, NJ: Prentice-Hill; 1983.

Schamberger W. Low back pain treatment: let's get our act together. Mod Med Can 1986; 41:999–1014.

Schamberger W. Malalignment: implications for cardiac rehabilitation. Can Assoc Cardiac Rehabil Newsletter 1998; 7(3):5–8.

Smith CG. Changes in length and position of the segments of the spinal cord with changes in posture in the monkey. Radiology 1956; 66:259–266.

Snijders CJ, Vleeming A, Stoeckart R. Transfer of lumbosacral load to iliac bones and legs. I. Biomechanics of self-bracing of the sacroiliac joints and its significance for treatment and exercise. In: Vleeming A, Mooney V, Snijders C, Dorman T, eds. Low back pain and its relation to the sacroiliac joint. Rotterdam: European Conference Organizers; 1992:233–254.

Snijders CJ, Vleeming A, Stoeckart R. Transfer of lumbosacral load to iliac bones and legs. II. The loading of the sacroiliac joints when lifting in a stooped posture. In: Vleeming A, Mooney V, Snijders C, Dorman T, eds. Low back pain and its relation to the sacroiliac joint. Rotterdam: European Conference Organizers; 1992:255–271.

Spinder SI, Schamberger W. Malalignment of the pelvis as a cause of chronic pain complaints in athletes. Med Sci Sports Exer 1993; 25(5 suppl.):S203.

Thie JF. Touch for health: a practical guide to natural health using acupressure touch and massage to improve postural balance and reduce physical and mental pain and tension. Pasadena, CA: TH Enterprises; 1987.

Thiele GH. Tonic spasm of the levator ani, coccygeus and piriformis muscles. Trans Am Practit Soc 1936; 37:145–155.

Thiele GH. Coccydynia and pain of the superior gluteal muscle. J Am Med Assoc 1937; 109:1271.

Thiele GH. Tonic spasm of the levator ani, coccygeus and piriformis muscles. Trans Am Proctol Soc 1937; 37:145–155.

Upledger JE. SomatoEmotional release and beyond. Palm Beach Gardens, FL: UI Publishing; 1990.

Upledger JE. SomatoEmotional release study guide. West Palm Beach, FL: UI Publishing; 1992.

Ursa Foundation. Manual therapy: the language. Ursa Foundation Course Materials. Edmons, WA: Ursa Foundation.

Vale MM, Wagner DM. The illustrated veterinary encyclopedia for horsemen. Tyler, TX: Equine Research; 1977.

Van de Graaf KM, Fox SI. Concepts of human anatomy and physiology. Dubuque, IA: WC Brown; 1992.

Vleeming A, Mooney V, Snijders C, Dorman T, eds. Course proceedings of first interdisciplinary world congress on low back pain and its relation to the sacroiliac joint. San Diego, CA, 5–6 November. Rotterdam: European Conference Organizers, 1–64.

Vleeming A, Buyruk HM, Stoeckart R, Karamursel S, Snijders CJ. Towards an integrated therapy for peripartum pelvic instability: a study of the biomechanical effects of pelvic belts. Am J Obstet Gynecol 1992; 166:1243–1247.

Vleeming A, Mooney V, Dorman T, Snijders CJ, Stoeckart R, eds. Movement, stability and back pain. Edinburgh: Churchill Livingstone, 1997.

Vleeming A, Snijders CJ, Stoeckart R, Mens JMA. A new light on low back pain: the selflocking mechanism of the sacroiliac joint and its implications for sitting, standing, and walking. In: Vleeming A, Mooney V, Dorman T, Snijders CJ, eds. The integrated function of the lumbar spine and sacroiliac joint. Rotterdam: European Conference Organizers; 1995:147–168.

Wallace KA. Why Jane stopped running: pelvic floor dysfunction. Clinical lecture presented at the 40th Annual American College of Sports Medicine meeting, Seattle, WA; 1993.

Wallace KA. Female pelvic floor functions, dysfunctions, and behavioral approaches to treatment. Clinics in Sports Medicine 1994; 13(2): 459–481.

White AA, Panjabi MM. Clinical biomechanics of the spine. Philadelphia, PA: JB Lippincott; 1978.

Wildman F. A motor learning approach to orthopaedic dysfunction: the Feldenkreis method. In: Canadian Physiotherapy Association Orthopaedic Division Review 1992; Nov/Dec.

USEFUL ADDRESSES

Upledger Institute, 11211 Prosperity Farms Road, Palm Beach Gardens, Florida, 33410, USA.

Myofascial Release Treatment Centers & Seminars. John Barnes, P.T., Rts. 30 & 252, Suite 1, 10 S. Leopard Rd. Paolo, PA, USA.

Rolf Institute, P.O. Box 1868, Boulder, CO 80306, USA.

New Mexico School of Natural Therapeutics, 117 Richmond N.E. (Ste. E), Albuquerque, NM 87106, USA.

Ursa Foundation, 2329 Robinhood Drive, Edmonds, WA 98020, USA. Attn: Executive Director.

International Directory of Chiropractors Trained in Sacro Occipital Technic: c/o Dr Major B. DeJarnette, 722.5 Central Avenue, Nebraska City, NE 86410, USA.

National Upper Cervical Chiropractic Association, Inc., 217 West Second Street, Monroe, MI 48161, USA.

American Academy of Osteopathy, PO Box 750, Newark, OH 43055, USA.

Physical Medicine Research Foundation, 510–207 West Hastings Street, Vancouver, BC, Canada.

North America Touch for Health Association, PO Box 430009, Maplewood, MO 93143, USA.

International Kinesiology College, PO Box 3347, CH-8031, Zurich, Switzerland

Index

Note: Page numbers in *italics* refer to pages on which figures/tables or boxed material appears.